Bone Formation and Repair

American Academy of Orthopaedic Surgeons

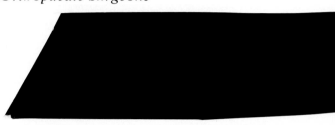

The cover picture is a photograph of the preserved skeleton of a 39-year-old man who had fibrodysplasia ossificans progressiva. It shows extensive synostoses between the clavicle, scapula, sternum, humerus, and ribs through bridges of flat and tubular heterotopic bone. Note also the extensive enveloping sheets of heterotopic bone about the left humerus and elbow. (Reproduced with permission from Kaplan FS, Strear CM, Zasloff MA: Radiographic and scintigraphic features of modeling and remodeling in the heterotopic skeleton of patients who have fibrodysplasia ossificans progressiva. *Clin Orthop* 1994;304:238–247. Grateful acknowledgments to the Mutter Museum of The College of Physicians of Philadelphia and to Joanne Diethorn, photographer.)

Bone Formation and Repair

Edited by
Carl T. Brighton, MD, PhD
Paul B. Magnuson Professor of Bone and Joint Surgery
Department of Orthopaedic Surgery
University of Pennsylvania School of Medicine
Philadelphia, Pennsylvania

Gary E. Friedlaender, MD
Professor and Chairman
Department of Orthopaedics and Rehabilitation
Yale University School of Medicine
New Haven, Connecticut

Joseph M. Lane, MD
Professor/Chairman Orthopaedic Surgery
UCLA Medical School
Los Angeles, California

With 159 illustrations

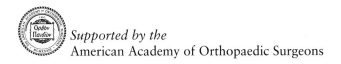
Supported by the
American Academy of Orthopaedic Surgeons

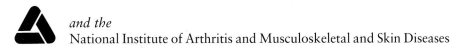
and the
National Institute of Arthritis and Musculoskeletal and Skin Diseases

American Academy of Orthopaedic Surgeons
6300 North River Road
Rosemont, IL 60018

Bone Formation and Repair
American Academy of Orthopaedic Surgeons

First Edition
Copyright © 1994 by the
American Academy of Orthopaedic Surgeons

ISBN 0–89203–116–6

Library of Congress Cataloging-in-Publication Data
Bone formation and repair / edited by Carl T. Brighton, Gary E.
  Friedlaender, Joseph M. Lane. — 1st ed.
  543 p. cm.
    International workshop sponsored by the American Academy of
  Orthopaedic Surgeons and the National Institute of Arthritis and
  Musculoskeletal and Skin Diseases.
    Includes bibliographical references and index.
    ISBN 0-89203-116-6
    1. Bones—Growth—Congresses. 2. Bone remodeling—Congresses.
  I. Brighton, Carl T. II. Friedlaender, Gary E. III. Lane, Joseph
  M., 1939–   . IV. American Academy of Orthopaedic Surgeons.
    [DNLM: 1. Bone Development—congresses. 2. Bone Remodeling—
  congresses. WE 200 B7115 1994]
  RD684.B66 1994
  612.7′5—dc20
  DNLM/DLC
  for Library of Congress   94-24323
                                                                  CIP

American Academy of Orthopaedic Surgeons

Contributors and Participants

James Aronson, MD*†
  Associate Professor, Orthopaedics
    and Pediatrics
  University of Arkansas for Medical
    Sciences
  Chief of Pediatric Orthopaedics
  Arkansas Children's Hospital
  Little Rock, Arkansas

Roland Baron, DDS, PhD*†
  Professor
  Yale University School of
    Medicine
  New Haven, Connecticut

Mark E. Bolander, MD*†
  Senior Associate Consultant
  Department of Orthopaedics
  Mayo Clinic
  Rochester, Minnesota

Jeff Bonadio, MD*
  Assistant Professor of Pathology
  University of Michigan Medical
    School
  Ann Arbor, Michigan

Adele Boskey, PhD*†
  Director of Research
  The Hospital for Special Surgery
  New York, New York

Harold Brem, MD*†
  Ohio State University Hospital
  Columbus, Ohio

Carl T. Brighton, MD, PhD*†
  Paul B. Magnuson Professor of
    Bone and Joint Surgery
  Department of Orthopaedic
    Surgery
  University of Pennsylvania School
    of Medicine
  Philadelphia, Pennsylvania

James T. Bronk†
  Associate in Orthopaedic Research
  Orthopaedic Research
  Mayo Clinic
  Rochester, Minnesota

Susan V. Brooks, PhD†
  Postdoctoral Research Fellow
  University of Michigan
  Ann Arbor, Michigan

Arnold I. Caplan, PhD*†
  Professor of Biology
  Director, Skeletal Research Center
  Case Western Reserve University
  Cleveland, Ohio

Charles N. Cornell, MD†
  Associate Attending Orthopaedic
    Surgeon
  The Hospital for Special Surgery
  New York, New York

Dwight T. Davy, PhD†
  Professor
  Department of Mechanical and
    Aerospace Engineering
  Case Western Reserve University
  Cleveland, Ohio

Henry Donahue, PhD†
Assistant Professor
Musculo-Skeletal Research
Laboratory
Department of Orthopaedics
Health Sciences Center
State University of New York
Stony Brook, New York

Thomas A. Einhorn, MD*†
Professor of Orthopaedics
Mount Sinai School of Medicine
New York, New York

John L. Esterhai, Jr, MD*†
Associate Professor of
Orthopaedic Surgery
Hospital of the University of
Pennsylvania
University of Pennsylvania School
of Medicine
Philadelphia, Pennsylvania

David R. Eyre, PhD*†
Burgess Professor of Orthopaedics
Department of Orthopaedics
School of Medicine
University of Washington
Seattle, Washington

John A. Faulkner, PhD*†
Professor of Physiology
Associate Director for Biological
Research
Institute of Gerontology
University of Michigan
Ann Arbor, Michigan

Judah Folkman, MD†
Julia Dyckman Andrus Professor
of Pediatric Surgery
Professor of Cell Biology
Harvard Medical School
Boston, Massachusetts

Gary E. Friedlaender, MD*†
Professor and Chairman
Department of Orthopaedics and
Rehabilitation
Yale University School of
Medicine
New Haven, Connecticut

André Gächter, MD†
Department for Orthopedics and
Traumatology
University Hospital
Basel, Switzerland

Julie Glowacki, PhD*†
Associate Professor of
Orthopaedic Surgery
Brigham and Women's Hospital
Boston, Massachusetts

Victor M. Goldberg, MD†
Professor and Chairman
Department of Orthopaedics
Case Western Reserve University
Cleveland, Ohio

Steven A. Goldstein, PhD*†
Professor of Surgery
Director of Orthopaedic Research
University of Michigan Medical
School
Ann Arbor, Michigan

Stephen L. Gordon, PhD*
Chief, Musculoskeletal Diseases
Branch
National Institute of Arthritis and
Musculoskeletal and Skin
Diseases
National Institutes of Health
Bethesda, Maryland

James A. Goulet, MD†
Assistant Professor of Surgery
(Section of Orthopaedic Surgery)
University of Michigan Medical
School
Ann Arbor, Michigan

Ted Gross, PhD†
Post-Doctoral Fellow
Musculo-Skeletal Research
Laboratory
Department of Orthopaedics
Health Sciences Center
State University of New York
Stony Brook, New York

Farshid Guilak, PhD†
Assistant Professor
Musculo-Skeletal Research
Laboratory
Department of Orthopaedics
Health Sciences Center
State University of New York
Stony Brook, New York

Robert Guldberg, MS†
Graduate Student Research
Assistant
University of Michigan Medical
School
Ann Arbor, Michigan

Gregory V. Hahn, MD*†
Fellow, Molecular Orthopaedics
Department of Orthopaedic
Surgery
University of Pennsylvania School
of Medicine
Philadelphia, Pennsylvania

Wilson C. Hayes, PhD*†
Maurice E. Mueller Professor of
Biomechanics
Harvard Medical School
Boston, Massachusetts

David G. Hicks, MD†
Assistant Professor
Department of Pathology
University of Rochester
Rochester, New York

Jeffrey O. Hollinger, DDS, PhD*†
Professor of Surgery, Anatomy,
and Cell Biology
Oregon Health Sciences University
School of Medicine,
Department of Surgery
Portland, Oregon

Ralph E. Holmes, MD*†
Associate Professor of Surgery
(Plastic)
University of California at San
Diego
San Diego, California

Mark C. Horowitz, PhD*†
Associate Professor of
Orthopaedics and Rehabilitation
Yale University School of
Medicine
New Haven, Connecticut

Ernst B. Hunziker, MD†
University of Bern
M.E. Muller Institute for
Biomechanics
Bern, Switzerland

Karl Insogna, MD*
Associate Professor of Medicine
Director, Yale Bone Center
Yale University School of
Medicine
New Haven, Connecticut

Mitsukazu Ishii, MD†
Assistant Professor
Department of Orthopaedic
Surgery
Gifu University School of
Medicine
Gifu, Japan

Peter R. Jay, MD†
Medical Student
Yale University
New Haven, Connecticut

Sudha Kadiyala†
Department of Biomedical
Engineering
School of Medicine
The Johns Hopkins University
Baltimore, Maryland

Frederick S. Kaplan, MD*†
Chief, Division of Metabolic Bone
Disease and Molecular
Orthopaedics
Departments of Orthopaedic
Surgery and Medicine
University of Pennsylvania School
of Medicine
Philadelphia, Pennsylvania

Patrick J. Kelly, MD*†
  Emeritus Professor of Orthopaedic
    Surgery
  Orthopaedic Research
  Mayo Clinic and Mayo Medical
    School
  Rochester, Minnesota

Joseph M. Lane, MD*†
  Professor/Chairman Orthopaedic
    Surgery
  UCLA Medical School
  Los Angeles, California

Cato T. Laurencin, MD, PhD*†
  Assistant Professor of Orthopaedic
    Surgery
  Medical College of Pennsylvania
    and Hahnemann University
  Research Assistant Professor of
    Chemical Engineering
  Drexel University
  Philadelphia, Pennsylvania

Phoebe S. Leboy, PhD*
  Professor of Biochemistry
  School of Dental Medicine
  University of Pennsylvania
  Philadelphia, Pennsylvania

Kam W. Leong, PhD*†
  Associate Professor
  Department of Biomedical
    Engineering
  School of Medicine
  The Johns Hopkins University
  Baltimore, Maryland

Joan B. Levy, PhD†
  Associate Research Scientist
  Yale University
  New Haven, Connecticut

Meir Liebergall, MD†
  Senior Lecturer in Orthopaedic
    Surgery
  Department of Orthopaedics
  Hebrew University Medical School
  Jerusalem, Israel

Hungnan Lo†
  Graduate Student
  Department of Chemical
    Engineering
  The Johns Hopkins University
  Baltimore, Maryland

Peter C.D. Macpherson, MA†
  University of Michigan
  Ann Arbor, Michigan

Kenneth McLeod, PhD†
  Associate Professor
  Musculo-Skeletal Research
    Laboratory
  Department of Orthopaedics
  Health Sciences Center
  State University of New York
  Stony Brook, New York

Naoto Ozawa, MD†
  Orthopaedic Surgeon
  Yokohama Municipal Citizen's
    Hospital
  Yokohama, Japan

Richard R. Pelker, MD, PhD†
  Professor, Orthopaedics and
    Rehabilitation
  Yale University School of
    Medicine
  New Haven, Connecticut

Ortun Pohler, PhD*
  Head of Research and
    Development in Materials
  Stratec Medical
  Waldenburg, Switzerland

He-Ying Qian, PhD†
  Associate Research Scientist
  Department of Orthopaedics and
    Rehabilitation
  Yale University School of
    Medicine
  New Haven, Connecticut

Lawrence G. Raisz, MD*†
  Professor of Medicine
  Division of Endocrinology and
    Metabolism
  University of Connecticut Health
    Center
  Farmington, Connecticut

A. Hari Reddi, PhD*†
  Percy Professor and Director
  Laboratory of Musculoskeletal
    Cell Biology
  Johns Hopkins University School
    of Medicine
  Baltimore, Maryland

James H. Reese, PhD†
  Assistant Professor, Department of
    Pharmacology
  Center for Applied Pharmacology
  College of Pharmacy
  University of Toledo
  Toledo, Ohio

Pamela Gehron Robey, PhD*†
  Chief, Skeletal Biology Section
  Bone Research Branch
  National Institute of Dental
    Research
  National Institutes of Health
  Bethesda, Maryland

Gideon A. Rodan, MD, PhD*
  Distinguished Senior Scientist
  Merck Research Laboratories
  West Point, Pennsylvania

Vicki Rosen, PhD*†
  Senior Scientist
  Genetics Institute, Inc.
  Cambridge, Massachusetts

Randy Rosier, MD, PhD*†
  Professor of Orthopaedics and
    Oncology
  Department of Orthopaedics
  University of Rochester
  Rochester, New York

Clinton Rubin, PhD*†
  Professor and Director
  Musculo-Skeletal Research
    Laboratory
  Department of Orthopaedics
  Health Sciences Center
  State University of New York
  Stony Brook, New York

Robert K. Schenk, MD*†
  Professor Emeritus of Anatomy
  Institute of Pathophysiology
  University of Bern
  Bern, Switzerland

Laura Senunas, BS†
  Graduate Student Research
    Assistant
  University of Michigan
  Ann Arbor, Michigan

William J. Sharrock, PhD*
  Extramural Program
  Bone Biology and Bone Diseases
    Branch
  National Institute of Arthritis and
    Musculoskeletal and Skin
    Diseases
  National Institutes of Health
  Bethesda, Maryland

Thomas G. Skoulis, MD†
  Instructor, Division of Plastic
    Surgery
  Associate Director International
    Microsurgical Fellowship
    Program
  Eastern Virginia University
  Norfolk, Virginia

Harald Steen, MD, PhD†
  Orthopaedic Research
    Laboratories
  University of Michigan
  Ann Arbor, Michigan

Julia Terzis, MD, PhD*†
  Professor, Department of Plastic
    and Reconstructive Surgery
  Microsurgery Program Director
  Eastern Virginia Medical School
  Microsurgical Research Center
  Norfolk, Virginia

Stephen B. Trippel, MD*†
  Assistant Professor of Orthopaedic
    Surgery
  Harvard Medical School
  Boston, Massachusetts

Nancy Troiano, MS†
  Research Associate II
  Department of Orthopaedics and
    Rehabilitation
  Yale University School of
    Medicine
  New Haven, Connecticut

Rocky S. Tuan, PhD*†
  Director of Orthopaedic Research
  Professor of Orthopaedic Surgery
    and Biochemistry and Molecular
    Biology
  Thomas Jefferson University
  Philadelphia, Pennsylvania

Nicholas Waanders, MS†
  Graduate Student Research
    Assistant
  University of Michigan Medical
    School
  Ann Arbor, Michigan

Paul P. Weitzel, BA†
  University of Pennsylvania School
    of Medicine
  Philadelphia, Pennsylvania

Randell G. Young, DVM†
  Manager, Preclinical Studies
  Osiris Therapeutics, Inc.
  Cleveland, Ohio

* Workshop Participant
† Contributor to Volume

Table of Contents

Preface

Understanding the mechanisms of bone formation as well as the manner by which this extraordinary tissue repairs or regenerates serves as the basis for much of the clinical practice of orthopaedic surgery. We are in the midst of an explosion of knowledge in cellular and molecular biology in general, and much of this new information is focused on cellular control mechanisms of the musculoskeletal system, including growth factors, cytokines, membrane receptor activation, matrix cell interaction, induction, differentiation, and the response of cells to their biologic and physical environment. It is crucial for us as orthopaedic surgeons and basic scientists interested in musculoskeletal research and its clinical applications to revisit the concepts of bone formation and repair utilizing these latest findings and techniques.

To that end, an interdisciplinary workshop, jointly sponsored by the American Academy of Orthopaedic Surgeons and the National Institute of Arthritis and Musculoskeletal and Skin Diseases of the National Institutes of Health, was held in Tampa, Florida, November 13–16, 1993. International experts in cell biology, biochemistry, biophysics, molecular biology, embryology, morphology and ultrastructure, biomechanics, and cell physiology presented the results of their latest research. Many of these talented basic scientists are also practicing orthopaedic surgeons. The participants were challenged to identify

clinically relevant gaps in current knowledge and to point out future research directions. This book is the result of that workshop.

The material in the text is arranged in six sections corresponding to the six sessions held at the workshop. At the end of each section in the book is a summary of recommendations for future research. Section one reviews our current knowledge of normal and abnormal bone formation, including the structure of bone, characteristics of different types of bone, the nature of matrix components and mineralization, available information pertaining to developmental skeletogenesis, and the systemic and local regulation and control of bone formation. Section two focuses on bone regeneration and repair and examines the cascade of cellular events leading to callus formation and maturation, how this process is regulated, and whether or not these activities can be augmented. Section three describes bone remodeling, including local and systemic factors that regulate bone turnover. Abnormal turnover, as in Paget disease and following chemotherapy and irradiation, is discussed. The exciting new emerging technology of bone markers is revealed.

The next section explores biosynthetic approaches to bone grafting and includes information on osteoinduction; osteoconduction; novel delivery systems for bone morphogenetic proteins and growth factors; as well as bone and cartilage stem cells and how they can be isolated, grown, and implanted back into a bony defect. It is evident from the work presented here that the time is rapidly approaching when conventional bone grafting procedures, as they currently exist, will be eclipsed by a variety of less morbid and more reliable approaches. The fifth section documents an enormous amount of work on distraction osteogenesis that has been accomplished in a relatively short period of time. Included are descriptions of cellular and molecular biologic events that occur during distraction osteogenesis, as well as injury and repair to nerve and other soft tissue that can accompany distraction. The last section covers the topic of fracture etiology, including mechanical and intrinsic factors that determine whether or not a fall results in a fracture. The biomechanics of fracture management, the effect of immobilization on healing, characteristics of biomaterials used in internal fixation devices, and fracture outcomes and functional assessment are all covered in this final section. This information is of great interest to the practicing orthopaedic surgeon as well as the orthopaedic basic scientist.

The material discussed at the workshop and presented in this volume, including the latest research findings and techniques as well as future directions and opportunities in musculoskeletal research, will serve as a benchmark in the discipline of bone formation and repair for the next several years. The amount of new knowledge that has accrued in terms of bone formation and repair during the last several years is staggering. However, this new understanding is only a preface to what is coming in the next decade. Truly, orthopaedic surgery is on the threshold of its golden era, a time of accomplishment related to cellular, molecular, and structural biology and biomechanics that will revolutionize the way we practice. If this book is a small beginning to that end, then the workshop and this text will have fulfilled their purposes.

CARL T. BRIGHTON, MD, PHD
GARY E. FRIEDLAENDER, MD
JOSEPH M. LANE, MD

Section 1

Bone Formation: Normal and Abnormal

Section Editors:
Frederick S. Kaplan, MD
Phoebe S. Leboy, PhD

Adele Boskey, PhD
Henry Donahue, PhD
Ted Gross, PhD
Farshid Guilak, PhD
Gregory V. Hahn, MD
David G. Hicks, MD
Frederick S. Kaplan, MD

Kenneth McLeod, PhD
Pamela Gehron Robey, PhD
Randy Rosier, MD, PhD
Clinton Rubin, PhD
Stephen B. Trippel, MD
Rocky S. Tuan, PhD

Chapter 1

Normal Bone Formation: Structure

Pamela Gehron Robey, PhD

Introduction

Bone is a uniquely designed composite of extracellular matrix proteins that mineralize under the tight surveillance of intimately associated cells that maintain the structural integrity of the bone while responding to the metabolic requirements of the organism. This chapter contains a brief description of different types of bone, the cells within bone, and the molecular components of bone matrix itself.

Types of Bone

During development there are two primary processes of bone formation. Intramembranous bone formation occurs independently of a preexisting model; endochondral bone formation occurs via replacement of a cartilaginous structure.[1] During intramembranous bone formation, mesenchymal cells that are producing a loose connective tissue receive a signal, from as yet unidentified sources, that causes them to commit to the osteoblastic lineage. During endochondral bone formation, cartilage proceeds through a stage of hypertrophy and becomes calcified. The mechanism by which this provisional calcified tissue is produced is quite different from that by which true bone is formed as evidenced by the cells that produce the calcified cartilage (chondrocytes) and the composition of the matrix proteins. Removal of calcified cartilage is accomplished by the invasion of osteoclasts and blood vessels.[2] Following eradication of this temporary mineralized matrix, osteogenic precursors, thought to be associated with the invading vasculature, repopulate the area and begin deposition of true bone. However, there is some evidence that a particular subset of chondrocytes has the ability to become osteoblastic, thereby potentially contributing to the pool of cells available for bone formation.[3]

Independent of whether the initial bony matrix is produced by the intramembranous or endochondral pathway, the outcome is the deposition of woven bone, which is composed of a poorly organized matrix scaffolding upon which hydroxyapatite has been deposited.[4] Although woven bone represents a large percentage of the total bone mass during early stages of development, as development continues, it is removed by osteoclasts and replaced by lamellar bone, a highly organized mineralized matrix that is supported by the Haversian canal system.[5] This form of bone is mechanically superior to woven bone and is by far the predominant form in the healthy adult skeleton.

Finally, two spatially and functionally distinct regions within a bone are delineated: (1) cortical bone, lying immediately underneath the periosteum, forms the outer casing; this bone houses (2) trabecular or cancellous bone, lying in the interior.[6] Cortical bone, which is highly dense and relatively acellular, functions primarily to provide strength. Trabecular bone exhibits highly convoluted surfaces that form cavities occupied by red or yellow marrow. Cortical bone is less metabolically active than trabecular bone in which bone turnover occurs with greater frequency as a result of the proportionately larger surface area. Trabecular bone also contributes an element of strength to the bone via formation of struts and crossbridges within the interior spaces.

Bone-Associated Cells

Bone-associated cellular constituents change depending on the type of bone formation and the stage of development. Thus, mesenchyme and cartilage are intimately associated during development, whereas cells of the periosteum and of the marrow are close neighbors at maturity. In all cases, blood vessels are of critical importance, not only for the exchange of nutrients, but also as a source of precursor cells of osteoclastic (and perhaps osteoblastic) destiny. While mineralized matrix deposition is the primary task of cells in the osteoblastic lineage, the factors that influence these osteoblasts are generated by different cellular environments, depending on the pattern of bone formation. Due to the capacity of hydroxyapatite to bind many exogenous and endogenous factors,[7,8] an imprint is maintained within the matrix that may regulate bone formation in subsequent rounds of bone turnover. It is likely that differences in the growth factor complement at a particular site may result in slight differences in how bone is formed and in its structural and functional properties.

Cells in the osteoblastic lineage are descendents of mesoderm, with the exception of those in the mandible, which are derived from neuroectoderm.[9] Cells of this lineage pass through different stages of maturation, each of which has a set of characteristics that is somewhat unique, within the site of bone formation.[10–12] Deposition of extracellular matrix parallels stages of maturity, and the cells in the osteoblastic lineage continuously modify the extracellular environment until it is an appropriate site for nucleation of calcium and phosphate ions and, finally, deposition of hydroxyapatite via fleeting precursors that have yet to be definitively identified.

The major proportion of the secretory product of cells in the osteoblastic lineage is represented by extracellular matrix proteins that are critical for the establishment of an appropriate three-dimensional (3-D) structure.[11,13] Autocrine and paracrine products produced in low abundancy are also essential to normal function.[14] However, it must also be noted that although the primary function of the extracellular matrix proteins is undoubtedly structural in nature, it is quite apparent that they also play critical roles in regulating cellular metabolism.

Mineralized Matrix Proteins

Collagen

The primary structural component of all connective tissues, including bone, is the fibrous protein, collagen.[15] This major building block is composed of three polypeptide chains, termed α chains, that contain a characteristic Gly-X-Y repeating amino acid sequence that allows these chains to coil together to form a stable triple helical molecule. The triple helix can be composed of three identical α chains (homotrimeric) or different ones (heterotrimeric). To date, 20 different α chains have been identified, which, in different combinations, form up to 16 different collagens. Bone collagen is primarily composed of type I collagen, the most abundant form in all connective tissues,[11,13] but it is unique in that it contains different types and amounts of glycosylation and cross-linking than those found in soft connective tissues. Bone matrix proper is virtually devoid of types of collagen that usually are associated with type I collagen in other tissues. However, trace amounts of collagens known to influence fibril diameter, such as types III, V, XII, and XIII, have also been detected, although it is not clear if these collagens are in the mineralized matrix proper or are blood-vessel associated.[11,13] It is possible that the large size of bone collagen fibrils is due to the low abundance of the other types of collagen.

Although the collagen molecule contains sequences that are suggestive of activities such as cell attachment in vitro, it is unlikely that the surface of the collagen fibril is exposed. In addition, the collagen molecule is most likely not a direct nucleator of hydroxyapatite deposition because it does not have the predicted 3-D conformation.[16] However, many extracellular matrix proteins associate with collagen. Thus, the purpose of the collagen may be to orient such proteins, exposing active sites for cell-matrix interactions or matrix-ionic interactions in the nucleation of hydroxyapatite deposition. The fact that without collagen there can be no bone formation is perhaps best exemplified by the Mov-13 mouse,[17] which contains a lethal mutation in one of the type I collagen chains. However, the association of a set of noncollagenous proteins with collagen is critical in establishing the metabolic properties of bone.

Noncollagenous Proteins

Although collagen represents approximately 90% of the organic matrix and the noncollagenous proteins the remaining 10%, the significance of noncollagenous proteins in structural and metabolic functions cannot be underestimated. It was hoped that these noncollagenous proteins would be unique to bone; however, chemical identification made possible by the pioneering work of Termine and associates[18,19] indicates that only two of the abundant bone matrix proteins are bone-specific, although several are bone-enriched. Information on the primary structure is rapidly emerging with the application of molecular biologic techniques for the isolation and purification of messenger RNA (mRNA) to form complementary DNA (cDNA) libraries of osteoblastic cells. The predicted amino acid sequences of virtually all of the major structural noncollagenous proteins of bone are available in a variety of animal species.[11,13,20] Analysis of these sequences has revealed many points of interest that suggest particular functions in tissue metabolism, and in vitro experimentation using this information is in progress. In spite of the explosion of knowledge in this area, definite functions for virtually all of the noncollagenous bone matrix proteins have yet to be determined.

Proteoglycans

This class of macromolecules is characterized by a unique posttranslational modification, whereby long carbohydrate chains composed of repeating sulfated disaccharide subunits of varying compositions (glycosaminoglycans) are covalently attached to genetically distinct core proteins.[21] There are several different proteoglycans associated with different stages of development and bone formation.

In loose, interstitial mesenchyme, a large proteoglycan (CSPG) that has chondroitin sulfate glycosaminoglycan side chains and a molecular weight of approximately 1,000 kd (kilodaltons) (core protein of 390 kd and four to five side chains of 40 kd) has been identified;[22] CSPG may be related to versican, a similar molecule found in loose connective tissues. It has been postulated that the purpose of this proteoglycan is to capture space that will eventually become bone, by virtue of the fact that the sulfated chondroitin sulfate side chains are most likely highly hydrated, thereby occupying a relatively large volume.[23] If, in fact, CSPG is similar to versican, there may be epidermal growth factor (EGF)-like sequences in the core protein, as there are in aggrecan, the major large proteoglycan of cartilage.[24] The significance of these EGF-like repeats in proteoglycan core proteins has not been determined, but upon degradation of the molecules, it is possible that they would be free to bind to the EGF receptors on resident cells.

During the conversion of loose interstitial mesenchyme to mineralizing tissue, the large CSPG is replaced by two small proteoglycans, decorin and biglycan.[25] Decorin, with an apparent molecular weight of ~120 kd (core protein of 38 kd and one glycosaminoglycan side chain of 40 kd), is named for its reported ability to "decorate" collagen fibrils, suggesting a role in the regulation of fibril growth.[26] In accord with this potential function, decorin usually colocalizes with collagen in connective tissues and is somewhat ubiquitous in its distribution. The other small proteoglycan, biglycan, has an apparent molecular weight of ~260 kd (core protein of ~37 kd with two glycosaminoglycan side chains of 40 kd). The distribution of biglycan is somewhat limited in comparison to that of decorin and is localized to areas undergoing morphologic delineation and to pericellular environments.[27] Despite the differences in their tissue localization, the predicted amino acid sequences of the decorin and biglycan core proteins indicate that they are highly homologous and are composed of multiples of a 24-amino acid residue leucine-rich sequence that has a characteristic cysteine residue pattern.[28] This leucine-rich repeat sequence is similar to that found in proteins, such as *Drosophila* chaoptin and toll, that are involved in morphogenesis and cell-surface locations, and also in osteoglycin, formerly termed osteoinductive factor (OIF), which is now known to bind to the multifunctional growth factor, transforming growth factor-beta (TGF-β).[29] In fact, both decorin and biglycan have been reported to bind to this factor, and they may regulate its activity in the matrix and pericellular environment.[30]

In addition to proteoglycans that are secreted by the cells in the osteoblastic lineage, there is also a cell-surface-associated heparan sulfate proteoglycan (HSPG), which may be related to syndecan, that has an apparent molecular weight of 400 kd, (core protein of ~80 kd with several side chains of 60 kd). Although it is usually maintained on the cell surface,[31] small amounts of HSPG can be shed into the extracellular environment.[32] It has been demonstrated that there is a type of TGF-β receptor that is a heparan sulfate proteoglycan (betaglycan),[33] and, more recently, it has been determined that activity of basic fibroblast growth factor (b-FGF) is mediated by binding to its receptor in conjunction with an HSPG.[34] Consequently, this class of proteins very likely plays a role in mediating activity of growth factors known to affect bone.

Hyaluronan, a glycosaminoglycan that is not covalently attached to a core protein, has also been isolated from bone, and its synthesis has been demonstrated in bone cell cultures in vitro.[35] Although there is a method for demonstrating the presence of hyaluronan in tissues,[36] this technique has not been applied to bone. Consequently, little is known about its appearance during development and about the maturational stages at which it is synthesized. In comparison to other tissues, it is likely that hyaluronan plays a role in development of bone.[37]

Glycoproteins

A large percentage of the noncollagenous proteins that are not proteoglycans are glycoproteins. These proteins are often modified by phosphorylation and sulfation in addition to N- and O-linked oligosaccharides. The pattern of the modification may be tissue specific and may ultimately distinguish the tissue of origin of a particular glycoprotein.

The dimeric protein, alkaline phosphatase (subunit molecular weight ~80 kd), is most often localized on the surface of cells in the osteoblastic lineage, but it can be released into the extracellular environment by phospholipase C cleavage of a phosphoinositol linkage.[38] In fact, a glycoprotein with alkaline phosphatase activity has been isolated from bone matrix.[39] Although alkaline phosphatase is often considered to be the hallmark of the osteoblastic lineage, its precise function has been yet to be determined. Alkaline phosphatase is postulated (1) to release phosphate from other constituents, thereby increasing the local concentration of this ion; (2) to destroy inhibitors of hydroxyapatite precipitation such as pyrophosphate; or (3) to act as a calcium-binding protein.[40] Patients with hypophosphatasia synthesize reduced levels of the bone/liver/kidney isozyme, yet in some cases they do not exhibit a primary defect in bone formation or matrix mineralization;[41] however, other evidence still points to a significant role for alkaline phosphatase in the bone-formation process.

Osteonectin, which makes up ~10% of the total noncollagenous protein, has an apparent molecular weight of ~43 kd and has been identified in a phosphorylated form.[42] The primary structure is unique in that it contains at least one and possibly two high-affinity calcium binding sites known as "EF hands," in addition to approximately 12 low-affinity calcium binding sites.[43] It is highly unusual for a secreted glycoprotein to contain these EF hand structures. Osteonectin has also been reported to bind to collagen and mediate deposition of hydroxyapatite,[42] to cause endothelial cell detachment in vitro[44] (although this does not appear to be the case with fibroblasts or osteoblasts), to influence progression of cells through the cell cycle,[45] to bind to platelet-derived growth factor (PDGF),[46] and to influence somite activity during development.[47] Further analysis in vitro and in vivo is clearly required in order to determine the function of this complicated molecule.

Another group of glycoproteins is characterized by the presence of the arginine-glycine-aspartic acid (RGD) cell attachment sequence, which is a ligand for a class of cell-surface receptors, the integrins.[48] There are at least six RGD-containing proteins in mineralized matrix: collagen, fibronectin, thrombospondin, vitronectin, osteopontin, and bone sialoprotein.[11,13] All of these proteins mediate cell attachment of bone cells in vitro,[49] although the predicted molecular structure around the RGD sequence is quite different for each protein. In addition, the point at which they appear during bone development and the maturational stages in a bone cell's life history also differ from one protein to another.

Thrombospondin,[50] a homotrimeric molecule, has the ability to bind to a large number of matrix proteins, and interestingly, to TGF-β as well. Although thrombospondin contains an RGD sequence, its availability may be limited because it is buried within a region with a conformation that depends on the local calcium environment. Cell attachment activity has also been demonstrated in an RGD-independent fashion,[49] although cell adhesion, but not spreading, has been observed in the absence of protein synthesis.[51]

Fibronectin, the prototype of the RGD-containing protein, contains two similar, but nonidentical disulfide-linked subunits. The subunits are formed by three different types of repeating sequences, and the arrangement of these sequences conveys the ability of fibronectin to bind to heparin, collagen, and cell surfaces.[52] Bone-derived cells attach to fibronectin in an RGD-independent fashion, indicating the presence of another region that may be responsible.

Another blood-borne protein that may be synthesized by cells in the osteoblastic lineage is vitronectin. This protein is highly active in mediating cell attachment in vitro, but is of relatively low abundance in bone in vivo, and its precise function is not clear at this time.[49]

Other RGD-containing proteins include the sialoproteins, osteopontin, and bone sialoprotein. Although it has not been determined definitively, yet another sialoprotein, bone acidic glycoprotein-75 (BAG-75), may follow suit.[53] Osteopontin and bone sialoprotein are highly unusual in that they contain long stretches of acidic amino acids (aspartic acid in osteopontin[54] and glutamic acid in bone sialoprotein),[55] a property that most certainly conveys hydroxyapatite-binding capabilities. Osteopontin is highly enriched in bone,[56] but is also found in a number of other locations, including mononuclear cells in the marrow.[57] Osteopontin is sharply upregulated by the process of transformation,[58] which may be related to an increased rate of proliferation, and the protein is differentially phosphorylated.[59] Bone sialoprotein is virtually specific to mineralization tissues[60] and it is found only in a subset of hypertrophic chondrocytes, osteoblasts, and osteoclasts. In placental membranes, syncytial trophoblasts that undergo mineralization at late stages of gestation express bone sialoprotein. Bone sialoprotein is highly induced at the initiation of mineralization[61] and has been found to be sulfated at this point.[62] It is possible that this sulfated form may represent the class of sulfated molecules that has been found to migrate rapidly to the mineralization front.[63] In addition, through use of microprobe analysis, it was found that, in the initial mineralizing nodules, calcium colocalized with sulfate rather than phosphate.[64] Although it was first thought that the sulfate may be borne on proteoglycans, bone sialoprotein must now also be considered.

γ-Carboxyglutamic Acid-Containing Proteins

Proteins of this class contain consensus sequences that cause them to be substrates for vitamin K-dependent enzymes that form γ-carboxy glutamic acid (Gla) residues. Matrix Gla protein (MGP) with a molecular weight of 15 kd is found in many soft connective tissues as well as in cartilage and bone.[65] Cells have been reported to attach to MGP in an RGD-dependent fashion, in spite of the fact that it does not contain RGD in its amino acid sequence.[66] Whereas MGP is broadly distributed, its distant relative, osteocalcin, is very bone specific,[67,68] although osteocalcin has been recently identified in platelets.[69] Current studies suggest that this protein may mediate bone turnover, because it appears to be a chemoattractant for mononuclear cells[70] and influences the activity of osteoclasts and their precursors.[71] More recently, protein S, a Gla protein produced primarily in the liver, has also been identified in bone matrix, although the site of origin has not been described.[72] However, because patients with protein S deficiency exhibit bone defects, protein S is likely to play a role in bone metabolism.

Growth Factors and Other Components

The list of growth factors that are produced endogenously and deposited within bone is long, and it is growing by leaps and bounds.[14] Included in this list are

TGF-βs, bone morphogenetic proteins, and insulin-like growth factors and their binding proteins, all of which have been demonstrated to affect bone cell metabolism. While these factors are produced locally, they are also present in the circulation, and it is not known if there are differences in reactivity depending on the origin. In addition to these major regulators, there are numerous reports of other factors that are present at extremely low levels. These reports have been due in part to increased sensitivity in detection of the mRNA for such factors. However, it should be noted that it often is not clear what the cell of origin is for some of these factors, and it also is apparent that cells can contain low levels of mRNA that are not necessarily translated or present in low copy number.

In addition to autocrine and paracrine growth factors, other cell products, such as enzymes and their inhibitors and proteolipids, which may play a role in matrix mineralization, also become entombed within bone. In addition, serum proteins such as albumin and α2- HS glycoprotein are found in quantities that exceed the levels in serum.[11,13] The combination of both exogenous and endogenous products make bone a unique reservoir that can become active during bone turnover or fracture repair.

Summary

The structural elements of bone matrix are represented by a number of different classes of proteins including collagen (primarily type I), proteoglycans (decorin and biglycan) and hyaluronan, glycoproteins (alkaline phosphatase, osteonectin, and RGD-containing proteins such as fibronectin, thrombospondin, vitronectin, osteopontin, and bone sialoprotein) and Gla-containing proteins (MGP, osteocalcin, and protein S). In addition, many of these proteins can alter cell metabolism by binding to growth factors and modulating their activity, or by direct interaction with receptors, thereby triggering intracellular events. Low abundancy components include products of the osteoblastic lineage such as enzymes and their inhibitors, proteolipids, and growth factors. The molecular composition of bone, together with proteins adsorbed from exogenous sources, makes bone uniquely suited to serve as a structural support as well as a reservoir for factors required for its own regeneration.

References

1. Hall BK (ed): *Bone: Bone Growth-A*. Boca Raton, FL, CRC Press, 1992, vol 6.
2. Baron R, Chakraborty M, Chatterjee D, et al: Biology of the osteoclast, in Mundy GR, Martin TJ (eds): *Physiology and Pharmacology of Bone*. New York, NY, Springer Verlag, 1993.
3. Gentili C, Bianco P, Neri M, et al: Cell proliferation, extracellular matrix mineralization, and ovotransferrin transient expression during in vitro differentiation of chicken hypertrophic chondrocytes into osteoblast-like cells. *J Cell Biol* 1993;122: 703–712.
4. Hancox NM: *The Biology of Bone*. Cambridge, MA, Cambridge University Press, 1972.
5. Marie PJ: Structure, organization, and healing, in Cruess RL (ed): *The Musculoskeletal System: Embryology, Biochemistry and Physiology*. New York, NY, Churchill Livingstone, 1982, p 109.
6. Martin RB: Determinants of the mechanical properties of bone. *J Biomech* 1991; 24:79–88.

7. Delmas PD, Tracy RP, Riggs BL, et al: Identification of the noncollagenous proteins of bovine bone by two-dimensional gel electrophoresis. *Calcif Tissue Int* 1984;36: 308–316.
8. Hauschka PV, Mavrakos AE, Iafrati MD, et al: Growth factors in bone matrix: Isolation of multiple types by affinity chromatography on heparin-sepharose. *J Biol Chem* 1986;261:12665–12674.
9. Balinsky BI: *An Introduction to Embryology*, ed 4. Philadelphia, PA, WB Saunders, 1975.
10. Strauss PG, Closs EI, Schmidt J, et al: Gene expression during osteogenic differentiation in mandibular condyles in vitro. *J Cell Biol* 1990;110:1369–1378.
11. Gehron Robey P, Bianco P, Termine JD: The cellular biology and molecular biochemistry of bone formation, in Favus MJ, Coe FL (eds): *Disorders of Bone and Mineral Metabolism*. New York, NY, Raven Press, 1992, pp 241–263.
12. Stein GS, Lian JB, Owen TA: Relationship of cell growth to the regulation of tissue-specific gene expression during osteoblast differentiation. *FASEB J* 1990;4:3111–3123.
13. Gehron Robey P: The biochemistry of bone. *Endocrinol Metab Clin North Am* 1989;18:858–902.
14. Canalis E, McCarthy TL, Centrella M: Growth factors and cytokines in bone cell metabolism. *Annu Rev Med* 1991;42:17–24.
15. Hulmes DJ: The collagen superfamily: Diverse structures and assemblies. *Essays Biochem* 1992;27:49–67.
16. Addadi L, Weiner S: Interactions between acidic proteins and crystals: Stereochemical requirements in biomineralization. *Proc Natl Acad Sci USA* 1985;82:4110–4114.
17. Harbers K, Kuehn M, Delius H, et al: Insertion of retrovirus into the first intron of alpha1(I) collagen gene leads to embryonic lethal mutation in mice. *Proc Natl Acad Sci USA* 1984;81:1504–1508.
18. Termine JD, Belcourt AB, Christner PJ, et al: Properties of dissociatively extracted fetal tooth matrix proteins: I. Principal molecular species in developing bovine enamel. *J Biol Chem* 1980;255:9760–9772.
19. Termine JD, Belcourt AB, Conn KM, et al: Mineral and collagen-binding proteins of fetal calf bone. *J Biol Chem* 1981;256:10403–10408.
20. Young MF, Ibaraki K, Kerr JM, et al: Molecular and cellular biology of the major non-collagenous proteins in bone, in Noda M (ed): *Cellular and Molecular Biology of Bone*. San Diego, CA, Academic Press, 1993.
21. Fedarko NF: Isolation and purification of proteoglycans. *Experientia* 1993;49:369–383.
22. Fisher LW, Termine JD, Dejter SW Jr, et al: Proteoglycans of developing bone. *J Biol Chem* 1983;258:6588–6594.
23. Fisher LW: The nature of the proteoglycans of bone, in Butler WT (ed): *Chemistry and Biology of Mineralized Tissues*. Birmingham, AL, Ebsco Media, 1985, pp 188–196.
24. Baldwin CT, Reginato AM, Prockop DJ: A new epidermal growth factor-like domain in the human core protein for the large cartilage-specific proteoglycan: Evidence for alternative splicing of the domain. *J Biol Chem* 1989;264:15747–15750.
25. Fisher LW, Termine JD, Young MF: Deduced protein sequence of bone small proteoglycan I (biglycan) shows homology with proteoglycan II (decorin) and several nonconnective tissue proteins in a variety of species. *J Biol Chem* 1989;264:4571–4576.
26. Vogel KG, Trotter JA: The effect of proteoglycans on the morphology of collagen fibrils formed in vitro. *Collagen Rel Res* 1987;7:105–114.
27. Bianco P, Fisher LW, Young MF, et al: Expression and localization of the two small proteoglycans, biglycan and decorin, in developing human skeletal and non-skeletal tissues. *J Histochem Cytochem* 1990;38:1549–1563.
28. Fisher LW: Structure/function studies of the sialoglycoproteins and proteoglycans of bone: It is still the early days, in Slavkin HC, Price P (eds): *Chemistry and Biology of Mineralized Tissues*. Amsterdam, Excerpta Medica, 1992, pp 177–186.

29. Bentz H, Thompson AY, Armstrong R, et al: Transforming growth factor-beta2 enhances the osteoinductive activity of a bovine bone-derived fraction containing bone morphogenetic protein 2 and 3. *Matrix* 1991;11:269–275.
30. Ruoslahti E, Yamaguchi Y: Proteoglycans as modulators of growth factor activities. *Cell* 1991;64:867–869.
31. Beresford JN, Fedarko NS, Fisher LW, et al: Analysis of the proteoglycans synthesized by human bone cells in vitro. *J Biol Chem* 1987;262:17164–17172.
32. Fedarko NS, Termine JD, Gehron Robey P: High-performance liquid chromatographic separation of hyaluronan and four proteoglycans produced by human bone cell cultures. *Anal Biochem* 1990;188:398–407.
33. Lopez-Casillas F, Wrana JL, Massague J: Betaglycan presents ligand to the TGF-beta signaling receptor. *Cell* 1993;73:1435–1444.
34. Klagsbrun M: The affinity of fibroblast growth factors (FGFs) for heparin: FGF-heparan sulfate interactions in cells and extracellular matrix. *Curr Opin Cell Biol* 1990;2:857–863.
35. Fedarko NS, Vetter UK, Weinstein S, et al: Age-related changes in hyaluronan, proteoglycan, collagen, and osteonectin synthesis by human bone cells. *J Cell Physiol* 1992;151:215–227.
36. Salustri A, Yanagishita M, Underhill CB, et al: Localization and synthesis of hyaluronic acid in the cumulus cells and mural granulosa cells of the preovulatory follicle. *Dev Biol* 1992;151:541–551.
37. Toole BP: Hyaluronan and its binding proteins, the hyaladherins. *Curr Opin Cell Biol* 1990;2:839–844.
38. Fedarko NS, Bianco P, Vetter U, et al: Human bone cell enzyme expression and cellular heterogeneity: Correlation of alkaline phosphatase enzyme activity with cell cycle. *J Cell Physiol* 1990;144:115–121.
39. deBernard B, Bianco P, Bonucci E, et al: Biochemical and immunohistochemical evidence that in cartilage an alkaline phosphatase is a Ca + 2-binding glycoprotein. *J Cell Biol* 1986;103:1615–1623.
40. Wuthier RE, Register TC: Role of alkaline phosphatase, a polyfunctional enzyme, in mineralizing tissues, in Butler WT (ed): *Chemistry and Biology of Mineralized Tissues*. Birmingham, AL, Ebsco Media, 1985, pp 113–124.
41. Whyte MP: Alkaline phosphatase: Physiologic role explored in hypophosphatasia, in Peck WA (ed): *Bone and Mineral Research*, ed 6. Amsterdam, Elsevier Science Publishers, 1989, pp 175–218.
42. Termine JD, Kleinman HK, Whitson SW, et al: Osteonectin, a bone-specific protein linking mineral to collagen. *Cell* 1981;26:99–105.
43. Bolander ME, Young MF, Fisher LW, et al: Osteonectin cDNA sequence reveals potential binding regions for calcium and hydroxyapatite and shows homologies with both a basement membrane protein (SPARC) and a serine proteinase inhibitor (ovomucoid). *Proc Natl Acad Sci USA* 1988;85:2919–2923.
44. Sage EH, Vernon RB, Funk SE, et al: SPARC, a secreted protein associated with cellular proliferation, inhibits cell spreading in vitro and exhibits Ca + 2-dependent binding to the extracellular matrix. *J Cell Biol* 1989;109:341–356.
45. Funk SE, Sage EH: Differential effects of SPARC and cationic SPARC peptides on DNA synthesis by endothelial cells and fibroblasts. *J Cell Physiol* 1993;154:53–63.
46. Raines EW, Lane TF, Iruela-Arispe ML, et al: The extracellular glycoprotein SPARC interacts with platelet-derived growth factor (PDGF)-AB and -BB and inhibits the binding of PDGF to its receptors. *Proc Natl Acad Sci USA* 1992;89:1281–1285.
47. Purcell L, Gruia-Gray J, Scanga S, et al: Developmental anomalies of Xenopus embryos following microinjection of SPARC antibodies. *J Exp Zool* 1993;265:153–164.
48. Cheresh DA: Structural and biologic properties of integrin-mediated cell adhesion. *Clin Lab Med* 1992;12:217–236.
49. Grzesik WJ, Gehron Robey P: Bone matrix RGD-glcyoproteins: Immunolocalization and their interaction with human primary osteoblastic bone cells in vitro. *J Bone Miner Res* 1994;9:487–496.

50. Bornstein P: Thrombospondins: Structure and regulation of expression. *FASEB J* 1992;6:3290–3299.
51. Gehron Robey P, Young MF, Fisher LW, et al: Thrombospondin is an osteoblast-derived component of mineralized extracellular matrix. *J Cell Biol* 1989;108:719–727.
52. Ruoslahti E: Fibronectin and its receptors. *Annu Rev Biochem* 1988;57:375–413.
53. Sato M, Grasser W, Harm S, et al: Bone acidic glycoprotein 75 inhibits resorption activity of isolated rat and chicken osteoclasts. *FASEB J* 1992;6:2966–2976.
54. Young MF, Kerr JM, Termine JD, et al: cDNA cloning, mRNA distribution and heterogeneity, chromosomal location, and RFLP analysis of human osteopontin (OPN). *Genomics* 1990;7:491–502.
55. Oldberg A, Franzen A, Heinegard D: The primary structure of a cell-binding bone sialoprotein. *J Biol Chem* 1988;263:19430–19432.
56. Prince CW, Oosawa T, Butler WT, et al: Isolation, characterization, and biosynthesis of a phosphorylated glycoprotein from rat bone. *J Biol Chem* 1987;262:2900–2907.
57. Nomura S, Wills AJ, Edwards DR, et al: Developmental expression of 2ar (osteopontin) and SPARC (osteonectin) RNA as revealed by in situ hybridization. *J Cell Biol* 1988;106:441–450.
58. Craig AM, Nemir M, Mukherjee BB, et al: Identification of the major phosphoprotein secreted by many rodent cell lines as 2ar/osteopontin: Enhanced expression in H-ras-transformed 3T3 cells. *Biochem Biophys Res Commun* 1988;157:166–173.
59. Nemir M, DeVouge MW, Mukherjee BB: Normal rat kidney cells secrete both phosphorylated and nonphosphorylated forms of osteopontin showing different physiological properties. *J Biol Chem* 1989;264:18202–18208.
60. Bianco P, Fisher LW, Young MF, et al: Expression of bone sialoprotein (BSP) in developing human tissues. *Calcif Tissue Int* 1991;49:421–426.
61. Ibaraki K, Termine JD, Whitson SW, et al: Bone matrix mRNA expression in differentiating fetal bovine osteoblasts. *J Bone Miner Res* 1992;7:743–754.
62. Hefferan TE, Gehron Robey P: Biosynthetic response of adult human bone cells to extracellular calcium. *J Bone Miner Res* 1991;6:S267.
63. Prince CW, Rahemtulla F, Butler WT: Incorporation of [35S]- sulphate into glycosaminoglycans by mineralized tissues in vivo. *Biochem J* 1984;224:941–945.
64. Arsenault AL, Ottensmeyer FP: Quantitative spatial distributions of calcium, phosphorus and sulfur in calcifying epiphysis by high resolution electron spectroscopic imaging. *Proc Natl Acad Sci USA* 1983;80:1322–1326.
65. Otawara Y, Price PA: Developmental appearance of matrix Gla protein during calcification in the rat. *J Biol Chem* 1986;261:10828–10832.
66. Loeser RF, Wallin R: Cell adhesion to matrix gla protein and its inhibition by an Arg-Gly-Asp-containing peptide. *J Biol Chem* 1992;267:9459–9462.
67. Price PA: Gla-containing proteins of bone. *Conn Tissue Res* 1989;21;51–60.
68. Hauschka PV, Lian JB, Cole DE, et al: Osteocalcin and matrix gla protein: Vitamin K-dependent proteins in bone. *Physiol Rev* 1989;69:990–1047.
69. Thiede MA, Smock SL, Petersen DN, et al: Production of osteocalcin by platelets. *J Bone Miner Res* 1993;8:S147.
70. Malone JD, Teitelbaum SL, Griffin GL, et al: Recruitment of osteoclast precursors by purified bone matrix constituents. *J Cell Biol* 1982;92:227–230.
71. Lian JB, Tassinari M, Glowacki J: Resorption of implanted bone prepared from normal and warfarin-treated rats. *J Clin Invest* 1984;73:1223–1226.
72. Maillard C, Berruyer M, Serre CM, et al: Protein S, a vitamin K-dependent protein, is a bone matrix component synthesized and secreted by osteoblasts. *Endocrinology* 1992;130:1599–1604.

Chapter 2
Developmental Skeletogenesis

Rocky S. Tuan, PhD

Skeletogenesis in the developing embryo involves the distinct processes of cellular differentiation leading to the formation of cartilage and bone. Because the skeleton represents the scaffolding of the vertebrate animal and provides the general architecture of the body, developmental skeletogenesis must follow a highly programmed pathway and is regulated by multiple cellular and humoral control mechanisms. This chapter will briefly describe the major pathways of ossification, the cellular origin of cartilage and bone, the patterning of the embryonic skeleton, and the in vitro experimental systems currently used to study the mechanisms that regulate skeletal cell differentiation.

Intramembranous Endochondral Ossification

Embryonic skeletal development occurs through two major pathways:[1,2] (1) the endochondral pathway, such as in the long bones of the limbs; and (2) the intramembranous pathway, which takes place predominantly in the bones of the craniofacial structures. In the endochondral ossification sequence, mesenchymal cells, such as those in the embryonic limb bud, condense and differentiate into cartilage, which becomes an anlage of the future skeletal components. The cartilage anlage subsequently matures, undergoes hypertrophy, mineralizes, and is then invaded by blood vessels and osteoprogenitor cells.[3] These cells differentiate into osteoblasts and form spicules of bone by the production and mineralization of an osteoid matrix.[4] In contrast, intramembranous bone formation involves direct differentiation of mesenchymal cells into osteoblasts.[5,6] Centers of ossification and mineralization in cranial bones, such as the calvarium, then fuse to form plates of woven bone. No cartilage intermediate is found in the intramembranous bones. Thus, although the final bony tissue in the intramembranous bone and that in the endochondral bone resemble each other, the pathways leading to their formation are distinctly different.

The mechanistic basis underlying the progression of the embryonic mesenchyme along the endochondral or intramembranous pathway is currently unknown. However, it is noteworthy that, in most cases, the origins of the mesenchymal cells, which give rise to the endochondral long bones and the intramembranous craniofacial bones, are most likely also different. For example, the limb mesenchyme is derived from paraxial mesoderm,[7] whereas the calvarium most likely is derived from cranial neural crest cells.[8,9] Nevertheless, it should be pointed out that neural crest cells will differentiate into cartilage, provided that they interact with the appropriate epithelium during their migration to the rostral part of the developing embryo.[10] For example, differentiation of cranial neural crest mesenchymal cells that have anchorin CII receptors for type II collagen may be influenced by interactions with type II collagen on

13

neuroepithelial tissues encountered during migration.[11,12] Also, premigratory neural crest cells from the mesencephalic region that are cultured in vitro with cranial ectoderm or retinal epithelium undergo chondrogenic differentiation; whereas, when the same cells are combined with maxillary epithelia, they produce both cartilage and membrane bone.[13] Thus, very early neural crest cells have the capability to differentiate in response to epithelia encountered during their migration and/or at their final destination. In a similar manner, the formation of intramembranous bone in the mesenchyme of the palate,[14] maxilla,[15] and mandible[16] requires direct contact with the epithelia. In an analogous manner, the differentiation of paraxial mesenchymal cells into chondrocytes, eg, in the embryonic limb bud, is regulated by interaction with the limb epithelium. For example, the limb epithelium inhibits the expression of chondrogenic phenotype in the underlying mesenchyme both in vitro and in vivo.[17,18] These studies, therefore, clearly indicate that both mesenchymally-derived cells and their interactions with adjacent epithelial cells play important roles in skeletal development.

Under certain conditions, the normally intramembranous calvarium also displays a phenotype resembling that of cartilage. For example, in chick embryos that have been made calcium-deficient via long-term maintenance in culture without their eggshells, the calvarium expresses type II collagen, a cartilage-associated matrix molecule, and cells with a chondrocyte-like phenotype.[19–21] Another example is the formation in the calvarium of a fracture callus, which also undergoes chondrogenesis.[22–24] Thus, the two pathways of ossification, intramembranous and endochondral, may actually share some commonalities, particularly with regard to the cellular differentiation potential of the initial mesenchymal cell population.

Mesenchymal cells appear to have the potential to undergo chondrogenesis; therefore, in developing intramembranous bone, there must exist a set of conditions that would either enhance osteogenesis or inhibit chondrogenesis. Understanding the nature of these conditions should shed light on the underlying mechanisms that lead to birth defects involving intramembranous bones, such as those of the craniofacial skeleton. Such knowledge should also facilitate designing protocols to enhance bone formation in endochondral bones, especially during fracture repair, because diaphyseal bone growth proceeds via the intramembranous pathway.

Cellular Origin of Cartilage and Bone

As described earlier, the cells of cartilage and bone can be of similar or different embryonic origin, depending on the type of ossification pathway. The earliest endochondral structures are the prevertebra and the limb bud. Both are derived from paraxial mesodermal cells. The prevertebrae are derived from somites, which emerge as condensations of the paraxial mesodermal cells located lateral to the neural tube, and undergo segmentation as they emerge from the segmental plate.[25] The nascent somites then undergo a process of epithelialization, such that a polarized epithelial layer engulfs a central core of cells contained in a somitocoel cavity. Upon further maturation towards the rostral end of the embryo, the somites then differentiate into a dorsal dermamyotome and a ventral sclerotome. Further maturation involves the bifurcation of the sclerotome into rostral and caudal halves, involving a process known as resegmentation. This process allows the caudal half of an anterior somite to fuse with the rostral end of the immediately posterior somite upon their migration ventrally towards the notochord to give rise to a perichordal sheath that forms the prevertebra.[26-28] In this manner, the prevertebra is located one half segment out of register with the original somite. This resegmentation process is important for the musculature and neuronal orientation with respect to the vertebrae; it allows anchoring of the newly developing muscle to adjacent vertebrae. The sclerotomal mesenchymal cells at the developing prevertebrae then condense and subsequently form cartilage.[29] Upon maturation, hypertrophy, and mineralization, the cartilage is replaced by bone to yield the final vertebral structures.

A developmentally similar process also takes place in the embryonic limb bud. The paraxial mesoderm that forms the embryonic limb bud first undergoes cellular condensation, ie, the cells begin to aggregate and come into close contact with one another.[30] This process is accompanied by the disappearance of extracellular matrix and the appearance of various cell adhesion molecules (see below). Subsequent to cellular condensation, the mesenchymal cells undergo overt chondrogenic differentiation and begin to express copious amounts of cartilage-specific extracellular matrix, including type II collagen,[31] and high-molecular-weight, chondroitin sulfate-rich proteoglycan (aggrecan).[32] Upon maturation, hypertrophy, and mineralization of the growing cartilage, eg, in the growth plate, bone is formed subsequent to vascularization. It is generally believed that the osteoprogenitor cells are derived from the local mesenchyme, and are recruited as a result of the establishment of the vasculature during cartilage maturation and hypertrophy.[2]

In contrast, the cells responsible for intramembranous bone formation differentiate directly into osteoblasts without the presence of a cartilage intermediate. In bones such as the calvaria and the clavicle, the mesenchymal cells also appear to undergo some type of condensation, although the extent of aggregation is considerably less than that seen in mesenchymal cells destined to become cartilage.[1,33] Most of the cells responsible for intramembranous bone formation are derived from the cranial neural crest population;[9] these cells will differentiate directly into bone, unless specific interaction with appropriate epithelial structures takes place.[10] As noted earlier, fracture repair of intramembranous bone involves, in most cases, the elaboration of a cartilage intermediate, which suggests that the cranial neural crest cells do possess a chondrogenic potential.

Patterning of the Embryonic Skeleton

A singular characteristic feature of the skeleton is that its pattern is invariant and specific for each species. Characteristics such as bilateral symmetry and segmentation clearly pose an important requirement for the developmental processes leading to the formation of the embryonic skeleton. A great deal of information on the molecular regulatory mechanisms governing pattern formation has been generated through pioneering work on the fruit fly, Drosophila.[34] Briefly, pattern formation in the developing Drosophila embryo is regulated by a hierarchy of four classes of zygotic pattern-forming genes: (1) the gap genes, whose mutations are characterized by large gaps of missing segments in the overall pattern; (2) the pair rule segmentation genes, which govern the specific order in the pairing of adjacent segments; (3) the segment polarity genes, which dictate the anterior and posterior polarity within each body segment; and (4) the homeotic genes, which endow each segment with a unique identity. Mutations of the homeotic genes result in the transposition of one body segment identity to another. Members of a specific gene family share common structural features; for example, a conserved DNA sequence, known as the homeobox, is found in all homeotic genes. Thus, although the Drosophila embryo develops as a syncytial structure and, therefore, does not exactly resemble vertebrate structures, which are multicellular and highly complex, the knowledge derived from studying the *Drosophila* embryo has greatly facilitated the elucidation of molecular mechanisms governing skeletal patterning.

The best studied patterning genes in vertebrate animals are the homeobox genes, which are characterized by a highly conserved 180 base pair (encoding 60 amino acids) DNA sequence, the homeobox.[35] These genes are found in four chromosomal clusters, each of which contains a set of genes homologous with other sets in terms of both the order of arrangement and DNA sequence. These genes are therefore considered as "parallelogues" on each chromosome, and correspond to others in an analogous location on another chromosome. During development, these genes are expressed in a specific spatiotemporal manner reflecting their order on the chromosome such that the 5'-most genes are expressed in the most posterior embryonic structures and at the latest stages of development. In this manner, each body part is identified by a unique code of homeobox gene expression; regionalization and spatial specification are thought to be established via these specific gene expression events. A similar replication of this scheme is seen in the developing limb, in which the proximodistal axis is essentially analogous to the anteroposterior axis, and the expression of homeobox genes is sequentially and spatially specified to give rise to the regionalization of the limb structure.[36]

In addition to the homeobox genes, much recent attention has been paid to the pair rule genes.[37] These genes, like the homeobox genes, are characterized by the presence of a highly conserved DNA sequence, which is known as the paired box.[38] Genes of this class were first identified in vertebrate animals in 1988.[39] Currently, there are nine paired box-containing genes in the mouse genome; these genes are designated as *Pax* 1–9. Pair rule genes are thought to give rise to the segmentation pattern, ie, the formation of repeated, similar structures, the most obvious of which are the vertebrae in the spinal column. For example, a mouse mutant, *undulated*, which has a phenotype of a kinky tail and fused and symmetric vertebrae,[40] has been shown to have a point mutation in the paired box sequence of a paired box gene, *Pax* 1.[41] Recent work from my laboratory[42] has further elucidated the functional importance of paired box genes during early embryonic development. Paired box gene expression is found along the borders of segmenting somites during the somitic stage of embryonic development in the chick; this expression also is found at the region of sclerotomal bifurcation prior to and during resegmentation. The cells that express the paired box gene, *Pax* 1, in the resegmenting somite appear to migrate ventromedially towards the notochord, strongly suggesting that the expression of paired box genes may be linked to the actual establishment of borders between the early developing somitic structures that will give rise to the prevertebrae.[39,43] Finally, paired box gene expression is seen in the intervertebral disk area between prevertebrae, again suggesting a role for these genes in establishing borders between structures. At this point, it appears that paired box genes are likely to play a fundamental role in the segmentation and resegmentation process during early somite and vertebral development.

The pattern-forming genes are thought to act as transcription factors by binding to specific DNA sequences and regulating transcription of the adjacent gene.[34] The four classes of genes in *Drosophila* act in a hierarchic manner, ie, gap genes regulate pair rule genes and segment polarity genes, and the homeotic genes are at the end of the hierarchy.[44] There are also instances where members of one class can regulate other members of the same class. Whether a similar hierarchic setup also operates in vertebrates has not been clearly established;

moreover, whether analogous genes can be found in all of the classes is unknown. The experimental question of great interest is: What are the target genes regulated by these pattern-forming genes? In order to establish patterns and set up boundaries, distinct cellular or matrix components must participate in an interactive manner to functionally express this spatiotemporal information. The extensive amount of work done on skeletal cell biology clearly indicates that cell-cell and cell-matrix interactions are crucial to the long-term cellular differentiation and structural architecture of the developing skeletal components. It is thus tempting to speculate that, in vertebrates, these pattern-forming genes act by regulating the expression of genes, in particular, those coding for extracellular components, which are involved in these interactions. In fact, recent studies have implicated homeobox genes as candidate regulators of an extracellular matrix molecule, cytotactin (tenascin), and a neural cell adhesion molecule, N-CAM.[45,46] A great deal of work is still needed to elucidate the molecular regulatory mechanisms in skeletal pattern formation.

In Vitro Differentiation of Embryonic Mesenchyme

Both in vitro experimental systems and in vivo approaches are needed to study the mechanistic aspects of skeletal cellular differentiation. In particular, because embryonic mesenchyme gives rise to both bone and cartilage, the in vitro systems should be able to reproduce such differentiation pathways in a faithful manner. A number of systems are currently being used. The most popular is the limb-bud mesenchyme maintained in high density micromass cultures, which was first used by Ahrens and associates.[47] This system involves the isolation and culturing of embryonic limb mesenchyme cells in a high-density droplet to mimic the high cellular density found in the condensing mesenchyme of the developing limb bud.[48] In this system, chondrogenesis is faithfully produced, particularly if the mesenchyme is isolated from the zone of chondroprogenitor cells located in the distal subridge area of the limb.[49] Chondrogenesis is assessed quantitatively by a number of methods, including the counting of cartilage nodules, the incorporation of radioactive sulfate, and the expression of cartilage-specific markers such as collagen type II[48] and chondroitin sulfate rich proteoglycans (aggrecan).[50] This highly reproducible system has been used to carry out a large number of investigations to analyze the extracellular conditions that can affect chondrogenesis.[51] Embryonic frontonasal mesenchyme has been maintained in micromass cultures in a similar manner and has also yielded a great deal of information concerning craniofacial skeletal development.

In terms of osteogenesis, embryonic or neonatal calvarial cells are the most commonly used primary cell culture system.[52,53] These cells are usually derived from either rodents or avian embryos, and in culture they will form distinct bone nodules and mineralize with the production of bone-specific markers, such as osteocalcin, high alkaline phosphatase activity, osteonectin, and responsiveness to parathyroid hormone.[54] It has been proposed that the calvarial osteoblasts exist in at least six stages of differentiation, with specific molecular markers associated with each stage.[55] The characteristics of the differentiation process and the differentiation potential of such osteogenically committed cell types are currently being examined by many investigators.

Regulation of Skeletal Cell Differentiation

The formation of the skeleton requires a coordinated programmed series of cellular differentiations along both the chondrogenic and the osteogenic pathways. Because it is impossible to address all of the candidate regulatory mechanisms underlying skeletal cell differentiation, this discussion will briefly touch only those aspects that relate to cell-cell, cell-matrix, and ionic interactions that are operational in bringing about the appropriate cellular differentiation events leading to the formation of the skeleton.

Cell-Cell Interactions

Cell adhesion is mediated by a number of pathways, most importantly those that involve cell adhesion molecules (CAM), which are broadly divided into calcium-dependent and calcium-independent components.[56,57] The calcium-dependent components consist largely of a class of transmembrane glycoproteins known as cadherins, whereas the calcium-independent pathway is mediated by an immunoglobulin supergene family of membrane glycoproteins known as CAM. Recent work from my laboratory[58] and those of other investigators[59] has clearly shown that cell-cell interactions are important in limb mesenchymal chondrogenesis, involving both N-cadherin and N-CAM. Antibodies to these molecules disrupt chondrogenesis in vitro and in vivo, and interactions mediated by these adhesion molecules are thought to result in yet to be determined signal transduction events. These findings are consistent with earlier in vitro observations that a high cell density is necessary for the process of condensation, which takes place before chondrogenesis, and the subsequent chondrogenic differentiation event.[47,48]

Cell-Matrix Interactions

A number of cell-matrix interactions have been proposed to be important in limb mesenchymal chondrogenesis. These include the involvement of extracellular matrix molecules such as fibronectin,[60] tenascin (cytotactin),[61] and proteoglycans.[62] It has been proposed that fibronectin[60] serves to activate a matrix translocation mechanism such that the physical and mechanical characteristics of the matrix are changed to allow cellular condensation to take place. Similarly, tenascin- and proteoglycan-mediated interactions are also postulated to serve a functional role in cellular condensation. Precondensation mesenchymal cells possess a hyaluronic acid coat that disappears on cellular condensation, suggesting that hyaluronate may serve as a negative regulator of cellular condensation and subsequent chondrogenesis.[63] Because most of the extracellular matrix molecules, in particular fibronectin, bind to cells via their cognate transmembrane receptors, known as integrins,[64] it is generally believed that such cell matrix interactions will serve to transduce specific signals into the interacting cells. What these signals are and how these signals result in the expression of a specific phenotype in developing skeletal tissues are presently unknown. Because a number of growth factors, including TGF-β,[65] FGF-4,[66] and IGF-I,[67] have been shown to influence mesenchymal differentiation, it is conceivable that the interactions of these growth factors with their respective receptors are also modulated by specific cell-matrix interactions.[36] In this manner, cell-matrix interactions can directly affect the outcome of growth factor-mediated cellular activities.

Ionic Interactions

Limb mesenchymal chondrogenesis depends on extracellular calcium.[48,67] Most likely, this dependence results from the functional requirement of N-cadherin for calcium in mediating cell-cell adhesion.[58] Whether calcium availability and the functional state of calcium-mediated cell adhesion can be regulated during limb development is presently unknown. Another group of molecules that affect limb mesenchymal chondrogenesis are the polyionic polymers. Several years ago, a chemically defined polymer, poly-L-lysine, was found to be able to reproducibly enhance chondrogenesis in limb mesenchymal micromass cultures.[48] The dose-dependent action of poly-L-lysine was found to depend on its molecular size and the time of application during culture, suggesting that there are specific interactions between this polyionic macromolecule and the responding cells.[48] Recent studies have strongly indicated that poly-L-lysine interacts with specific heparan sulfate-containing membrane proteoglycans to effect the promotion of chondrogenesis.[50,68,69] Moreover, the chondrogenesis-promoting action of such a cationic polymer was found to require a minimum number of positive charges per molecule, and it was found that it assumes the conformation of a poly-L-lysine-like structure; ie, polypeptides consisting of mixed amino acids are effective in stimulating chondrogenesis in limb mesenchyme only if the lysine composition exceeds 50% to 70%. It is hypothesized that the polycationic portion of poly-L-lysine most likely mimics a naturally occurring polycationic region of a yet to be identified extracellular matrix macromolecule.[51] In this manner, poly-L-lysine may act as an analog to naturally occurring extracellular matrix molecules to exert a stimulatory effect on chondrogenesis. In a recent study,[70] it was observed that poly-L-lysine injection into chick embryonic muscle grafts produces a cartilage-like phenotype. It is tempting to speculate that the mechanism by which poly-L-lysine stimulates chondrogenesis may also be operative during normal cartilage formation as well as fracture repair. Clearly, more work is needed to elucidate these polyionic interactions important in regulating chondrogenesis.

Summary

This chapter has provided a general overview of developmental skeletogenesis with particular attention paid to the cellular interactions, the molecular genetic influences, and the current experimental systems and approaches available to study problems related to developmental skeletogenesis. Another powerful experimental approach is that of developmental transgenesis, in which genes that are suspected to play a role in specific events in developmental skeletogenesis may be increased in gene dosage, mutated, or knocked out by transgenic manipulation of the embryo. In this manner, the putative role of the gene of interest may be surmised from the phenotypic outcome in the transgenic animal. The power of such a "reverse genetics" approach is obvious. However, because the developing embryo is an internally self-regulating biologic system, the phenotypic outcomes are expectedly complex. In fact, observable phenotypic effects clearly depend on the gene product being "essential" for development and morphogenesis and on the absence of redundant functional compensation by related genes. Therefore, it is crucial to combine the reverse genetics transgenic approach and the more manipulatable and defined in vitro systems in order to arrive at the identification of specific pathways and underlying mechanisms in developmental skeletogenesis.

Acknowledgments

This work is supported in part by NIH grants HD 15822 and HD 29937, the Orthopaedic Research and Education Foundation, the March of Dimes Birth Defects Foundation, and the Arcadia Foundation.

References

1. Hall B: The embryonic development of bone. *Sci Am* 1988;76:174–181.
2. Marks SC Jr, Popoff SN: Bone cell biology: the regulation of development, structure, and function in the skeleton. *Am J Anat* 1988;183:1–44.
3. Owen M: The origin of bone cells in the postnatal organism. *Arthritis Rheum* 1980; 23:1073–1080.
4. Sandberg MM: Matrix in cartilage and bone development: Current views on the function and regulation of major organic components. *Ann Med* 1991;23:207–217.
5. Bernard GW, Pease DC: An electron microscopic study of initial intramembranous osteogenesis. *Am J Anat* 1969;125:271–290.
6. Marvaso V, Bernard GW: Initial intramembraneous osteogenesis *in vitro*. *Am J Anat* 1977;149:453–468.
7. Newman SA: Lineage and pattern in the developing vertebrate limb. *Trends Genet* 1988;4:329–332.
8. Noden DM: Interactions and fates of avian craniofacial mesenchyme. *Development* 1988;103(suppl):121–140.
9. Couly GF, Coltey PM, Le Douarin NM: The triple origin of the skull in higher vertebrates: A study in quail-chick chimeras. *Development* 1993;117:409–429.
10. Hall B: Cellular interactions during cartilage and bone development. *J Craniofac Genet Dev Biol* 1991;11:238–250.
11. Thorogood P, Bee J, von der Mark K: Transient expression of collagen type II at epitheliomesenchymal interfaces during morphogenesis of the cartilaginous neurocranium. *Dev Biol* 1986;116:497–509.
12. Thorogood P: The developmental specification of the vertebrate skull. *Development* 1988;103(suppl):141–153.
13. Bee J, Thorogood P: The role of tissue interactions in the skeletogenic differentiation of avian neural crest cells. *Dev Biol* 1980;78:47–62.
14. Tyler MS, McCobb DP: Tissue interactions promoting osteogenesis in chorioallantoic-grown explants of secondary palatal shelves of the embryonic chick. *Arch Oral Biol* 1981;26:585–590.
15. Tyler MS: Epithelial influences on membrane bone formation in the maxilla of the embryonic chick. *Anat Rec* 1978;192:225–233.
16. Tyler MS, Hall BK: Epithelial influences on skeletogenesis in the mandible of the embryonic chick. *Anat Rec* 1977;188:229–239.
17. Solursh M, Singley CT, Reiter RS: The influence of epithelia on cartilage and loose connective tissue formation by limb mesenchyme cultures. *Dev Biol* 1981;86:471–482.
18. Gregg BC, Rowe A, Brickell PM, et al: Ectodermal inhibition of cartilage differentiation in micromass culture of chick limb bud mesenchyme in relation to gene expression and cell shape. *Development* 1989;105:769–777.
19. Tuan RS, Lynch MH: Effect of experimentally induced calcium deficiency on the developmental expression of collagen types in chick embryonic skeleton. *Dev Biol* 1983;100:374–386.
20. Jacenko O, Tuan RS: Calcium deficiency induces expression of cartilage-like phenotype in chick embryonic calvaria. *Dev Biol* 1986;115:215–232.
21. McDonald SA, Tuan RS: Expression of collagen type transcripts in chick embryonic bone detected by *in situ* cDNA-mRNA hybridization. *Dev Biol* 1989;133:221–234.
22. Girgis FG, Pritchard JJ: Experimental production of cartilage during the repair of fractures of the skull vault in rats. *J Bone Joint Surg* 1958;40B:274–281.
23. Hall BK, Jacobson HN: The repair of fractured membrane bones in the newly hatched chick. *Anat Rec* 1975;181:55–69.
24. Takagi K, Urist MR: The reaction of the dura to bone morphogenetic protein (BMP) in repair of skull defects. *Ann Surg* 1982;196:100–109.
25. Lash JW, Ostrovsky D: On the formation of somites, in Browder L (ed): *Developmental Biology: A Comprehensive Synthesis*. New York, NY, Plenum Press, 1986, vol 2, pp 547–563.

26. Keynes RJ, Stern CD: Segmentation in the vertebrate nervous system. *Nature* 1984; 310:786–789.
27. Keynes RJ, Stern CD: Mechanisms of vertebrate segmentation. *Development* 1988; 103:413–429.
28. Stern CD, Keynes RJ: Interactions between somite cells: The formation and maintenance of segment boundaries in the chick embryo. *Development* 1987;99:261–272.
29. Verbout AJ: A critical review of the "Neugliederung" concept in relation to the development of the vertebral column. *Acta Biotheoret (Leiden)* 1976;25:219–258.
30. Thorogood PV, Hinchliffe JR: An analysis of the condensation process during chondrogenesis in the embryonic chick hind limb. *J Embryol Exptl Morphol* 1975;33: 581–606.
31. Dessau W, von der Mark H, von der Mark K, et al: Changes in the patterns of collagens and fibronectin during limb bud chondrogenesis. *J Embryol Exptl Morphol* 1980;57:51–60.
32. Palmoski MJ, Goetinck PF: Synthesis of proteochondroitin sulfate by normal, nanomelic, and 5-bromodeoxyuridine-treated chondrocytes in cell culture. *Proc Natl Acad Sci USA* 1972;69:3385–3388.
33. Hall BK, Miyake T: The membranous skeleton: The role of cell condensations in vertebrate skeletogenesis. *Anat Embryol* 1992;186:107–124.
34. Akam M: The molecular basis for metameric pattern in the Drosophila embryo. *Development* 1987;101:1–22.
35. Izpisua-Belmonte JC, Duboule D: Homeobox genes and pattern formation in the vertebrate limb. *Dev Biol* 1992;152:26–36.
36. Tabin CJ: Retinoids, homeoboxes, and growth factors: Toward molecular models for limb development. *Cell* 1991;66:199–217.
37. Gruss P, Walther C: Pax in development. *Cell* 1992;69:719–722.
38. Chalepakis G, Fritsch R, Fickenscher H, et al: The molecular basis of the *undulated/Pax1* mutation. *Cell* 1991;66:873–884.
39. Deutsch U, Dressler GR, Gruss P: *Pax 1*, a member of a paired box homologous murine gene family, is expressed in segmented structures during development. *Cell* 1988;53:617–625.
40. Gruneberg H: Genetical studies on the skeleton of the mouse. XII. The development of *undulated*. *J Genet* 1954;52:441–455.
41. Balling R, Deutsch U, Gruss P: *Undulated*, a mutation affecting the development of the mouse skeleton, has a point mutation in the paired box of *Pax 1*. *Cell* 1988; 55:531–535.
42. Love J, Tuan R: Pair-rule gene expression in the developing avian embryo. *Differentiation* 1993;54:73–83.
43. Smith C, Tuan R: Human PAX gene expression and development of the vertebral column. *Clin Orthop* 1994;302:241–250.
44. Levine MS, Harding KW: *Drosophila*: The zygotic contribution, in Glover DM, Hames BD (eds): *Genes and Embryos*. New York, NY, IRL Press, 1989, pp 39–94.
45. Jones FS, Chalepakis G, Gruss P, et al: Activation of the cytotactin promoter by the homeobox-containing gene *Evx-1*. *Proc Natl Acad Sci USA* 1992;89:2091–2095.
46. Jones FS, Prediger EA, Bittner DA, et al: Cell adhesion molecules as targets for *Hox* genes: Neural cell adhesion molecule promoter activity is modulated by cotransfection with *Hox-2.5* and *-2.4*. *Proc Natl Acad Sci USA* 1992;89:2086–2090.
47. Ahrens PB, Solursh M, Reiter R: Stage-related capacity for limb chondrogenesis in cell culture. *Dev Biol* 1977;60:69–82.
48. San Antonio JD, Tuan RS: Chondrogenesis of limb bud mesenchyme *in vitro* stimulation by cations. *Dev Biol* 1986;115:313–324.
49. Kosher RA, Savage MP, Chan SC: *In vitro* studies on the morphogenesis and differentiation of the mesoderm subjacent to the apical ectodermal ridge of the embryonic chick limb bud. *J Embryol Exptl Morphol* 1979;50:75–97.

50. San Antonio JD, Jacenko O, Yagami M, et al: Polyionic regulation of cartilage development: Promotion of chondrogenesis *in vitro* by polylysine is associated with altered glycosaminoglycan biosynthesis and distribution. *Dev Biol* 1992;152:323–335.

51. Tuan R: Ionic regulation of chondrogenesis, in Hall B, Newman S (eds): *Cartilage: Molecular Aspects*. Boca Raton, FL, CRC Press, 1991, pp 153–178.

52. Wong G, Cohn DV: Separation of parathyroid hormone and calcitonin-sensitive cells from non-responsive bone cells. *Nature* 1974;252:713–715.

53. Bellows CG, Aubin JE, Heersche JN, et al: Mineralized bone nodules formed *in vitro* from enzymatically released rat calvaria cell populations. *Calcif Tissue Int* 1986;38:143–154.

54. Stein GS, Lian JB, Owen TA: Relationship of cell growth to the regulation of tissue-specific gene expression during osteoblast differentiation. *FASEB J* 1990;4:3111–3123.

55. Bruder SP, Caplan AI: Osteogenic cell lineage analysis is facilitated by organ cultures of embryonic chick periosteum. *Dev Biol* 1990;141:319–329.

56. Edelman GM, Crossin KL: Cell adhesion molecules: Implications for a molecular histology. *Annu Rev Biochem* 1991;60:155–190.

57. Takeichi M: Cadherin cell adhesion receptors as a morphogenetic regulator. *Science* 1991;251:1451–1455.

58. Oberlender SW, Tuan RS: Expression and functional involvement of N-cadherin in embryonic limb chondrogenesis. *Development* 1994;120:177–187.

59. Widelitz RB, Jiang TX, Murray BA, et al: Adhesion molecules in skeletogenesis: II. Neural cell adhesion molecules mediate precartilaginous mesenchymal condensations and enhance chondrogenesis. *J Cell Physiol* 1993:156:399–411.

60. Newman SA, Frenz DA, Hasegawa E, et al: Matrix-driven translocation: Dependence on interaction of amino-terminal domain of fibronectin with heparin-like surface components of cells or particles. *Proc Natl Acad Sci USA* 1987;84:4791–4795.

61. Mackie EJ, Thesleff I, Chiquet-Ehrismann R: Tenascin is associated with chondrogenic and osteogenic differentiation *in vivo* and promotes chondrogenesis *in vitro*. *J Cell Biol* 1987;105:2569–2579.

62. Gould SE, Upholt WB, Kosher RA, et al: Syndecan 3: A member of the syndecan family of membrane-intercalated proteoglycans that is expressed in high amounts at the onset of chicken limb cartilage differentiation. *Proc Natl Acad Sci USA* 1992;89:3271–3275.

63. Knudson CB, Toole BP: Hyaluronate-cell interactions during differentiation of chick embryo limb mesoderm. *Dev Biol* 1987;124:82–90.

64. Hynes RO: Integrins: Versatility, modulation, and signaling in cell adhesion. *Cell* 1992;69:11–25.

65. Kulyk WM, Rodgers BJ, Greer K, et al: Promotion of embryonic chick limb cartilage differentiation by transforming growth factor-β. *Dev Biol* 1989;135:424–430.

66. Niswander L, Martin GR: FGF-4 and BMP-2 have opposite effects on limb growth. *Nature* 1993;361:68–71.

67. Bee JA, von der Mark K: An analysis of chick limb bud intercellular adhesion underlying the establishment of cartilage aggregates in suspension culture. *J Cell Sci* 1990;96:527–536.

68. San Antonio JD, Winston BM, Tuan RS: Regulation of chondrogenesis by heparan sulfate and structurally related glycosaminoglycans. *Dev Biol* 1987;123:17–24.

69. Tuan RS, Yagami M: Poly-L-lysine stimulation of limb mesenchyme chondrogenesis involves interaction with membrane proteoglycan. *Mol Biol Cell* 1992;3:230A.

70. Tuan RS, Turchi DM, Kreitzer DS: Polylysine stimulation of ectopic cartilage formation. *Cell Mater* 1991;1:157–170.

Chapter 3

Bone and Cartilage Mineralization

Adele Boskey, PhD

Introduction

The application of physical chemical techniques, such as x-ray diffraction,[1,2] infrared (IR) and Raman spectroscopy,[3,4] nuclear magnetic resonance (NMR) spectroscopy,[5,6] other structural techniques,[7,8] ultrastructural techniques ranging from light through high resolution electron microscopy,[9-11] and combinations of the two (eg, Fourier transform (FT) IR spectroscopy),[12] to the mineralized tissues has shown that the predominant mineral phase in bone and cartilage is an analog of the geologic mineral, hydroxyapatite ($Ca_5 (PO_4)_3 OH$). Although there is some debate[13,14] as to whether this is the initial phase that forms, there seems to be no doubt that a poorly crystalline hydroxyapatite is the final product. The questions about the nature of the mineral are related to site variations, arrangement, and most importantly, the mechanism of its formation. Specifically, although the predominant mineral in bone and cartilage is apatitic, there is a question as to how or if the apatite mineral in these tissues differs. Other questions include: What controls the arrangement of the mineral? Where does mineralization start? How do mineral crystals spread throughout the matrix? How is the mineralization process regulated? The answers to these questions are the subject of this chapter.

The Nature and Arrangement of the Mineral in Bone and Cartilage

Historic Perspective

In the 1950s,[15] x-ray diffraction and electron microscopic examinations of bone, teeth, and calcified cartilage yielded structural information on the nature of the mineral in these tissues. Studies over the next 35 to 40 years can be thought of as refining or interpreting the questions posed by those data. To perform the x-ray diffraction analyses, tissues were dried and pulverized into fine powders. The diffraction patterns obtained (Fig. 1, *top*) had maxima at the positions of the geologic mineral hydroxyapatite, but the peaks were broader. Chemical analysis of the powdered tissues gave calcium-to-phosphorus molar ratios ranging from 1.3:1 to 2.0:1, which were very different from the expected 1.67:1 of $Ca_5 (PO_4)_3 OH$. These results, initially explained in terms of impurities from the organic matrix, were then interpreted in terms of impurities in the apatite itself.

IR studies[3,16,17] revealed a distinct inorganic carbonate contribution (Fig. 1, *bottom*) and confirmed the concept that bone mineral was an imperfect apatite. Imperfections in the crystal structure could result in the formation of very small

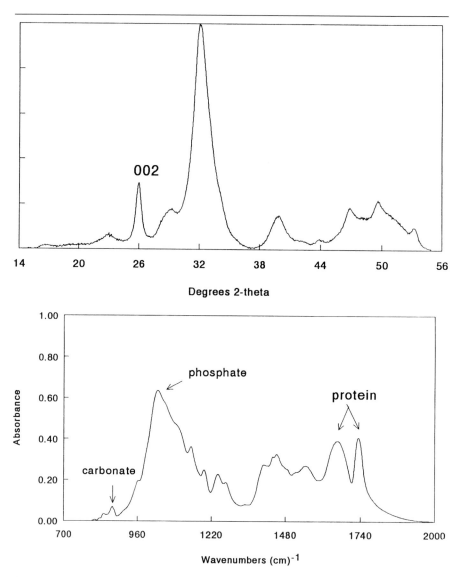

Fig. 1 Top, Wide angle X-ray diffraction patterns of adult rat diaphyseal bone using CuKα radiation. The peak positions correspond to hydroxyapatite. The broadened 002 peak can be used to assess crystallite length as described in the text. **Bottom**, Infrared spectra of bone mineral, a KBr pellet of trabecular bone from a normal dog. The carbonate, phosphate, and protein absorbances are indicated.

crystals, which would produce a poorly defined, broadened x-ray diffraction pattern like that observed. An equation existed from which the particle size (length) of the crystals could be predicted from the extent of broadening of the diffraction bands, using a constant related to the shape of the particles. This equation gave lengths of 200 to 400 Å, assuming the crystals were in the form of a parallelepiped.

Electron micrographs, which showed the presence of crystals 200 to 400 Å long, suggested that the crystals were needle-like (Fig. 2) and, more impor-

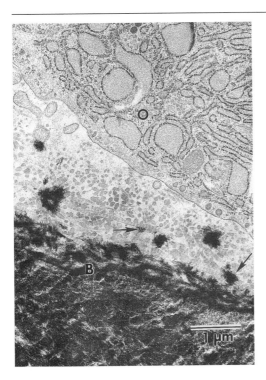

Fig. 2 An electron micrograph of newly mineralizing bone matrix from chick diaphyseal bone. Bone crystallites (arrows) are arranged along type I collagen fibrils. Mineralized bone (B) is seen along the lower portion of the photograph, and the bone forming osteoblast (O) is arranged across the upper portion of the micrograph. (Courtesy of Dr. S.B. Doty.)

tantly, revealed that the needles were aligned along the collagen fibril.[18] Because apatite is soluble and can reprecipitate in solution,[19] the aqueous methods used to prepare the tissues for electron microscopy caused the validity of some of the results to be questioned. This criticism became more significant with the report, based on solution studies,[20] that a noncrystalline basic calcium phosphate phase, more commonly referred to as x-ray amorphous calcium phosphate (ACP), could precipitate from solution and slowly transform into crystalline apatite. The presence of ACP was then used to explain the broadened x-ray diffraction patterns observed for bone and calcified cartilage.[21] As much as 60% ACP was reported in some tissues. The concept that ACP was an obligatory precursor for the formation of bone persisted until physicochemical evidence[5,6] and nonaqueous fixation techniques for electron microscopy (EM)[19] failed to reveal the presence of a noncrystalline phase in bone. Although these techniques might have missed the presence of <5% ACP, the concept of a poorly crystalline, carbonate-enriched apatite as the predominant bone phase was revived.

ACP is not the only calcium phosphate phase suggested to be a precursor of mature apatite in bone. Octacalcium phosphate[22,23] and brushite[24] have also been proposed as precursors. Both of these phases tend to form in acidic environments, such as that around a bone-resorbing cell. Based on radial distribution, NMR,[6] and IR analysis, it appears unlikely that significant (>1%) amounts of these acidic calcium phosphate phases exist in physiologically mineralized tissues.

There have been extensive debates about the shape of the apatite crystals and their distribution within and/or upon the collagen fibrils. The first ultrastructural studies of bone mineral[25] described the crystals as thin platelets 400

Å long and 20 to 30 Å wide. However, as discussed elsewhere,[26] such crystals could not be accommodated within the hole zone of the quarter-staggered array of type I collagen molecules. Thus, the precise arrangement of the mineral within the collagen fibril has remained uncertain.

High resolution transmission EM coupled with three-dimensional (3-D) reconstructions recently has shed light on this question. These tomographic studies show that the poorly crystalline apatite crystals in calcified turkey tendon are irregularly shaped platelets (Fig. 3).[26] These crystals are oriented such that their long (c-axis) dimensions are parallel to one another and lie along the collagen fibrils. They have variable lengths, with widths of 300 to 450 Å and a thickness of about 50 Å. In the turkey tendon, the crystals appear to grow from distinct sites, unhindered by constraints of the hole zone dimension. It is

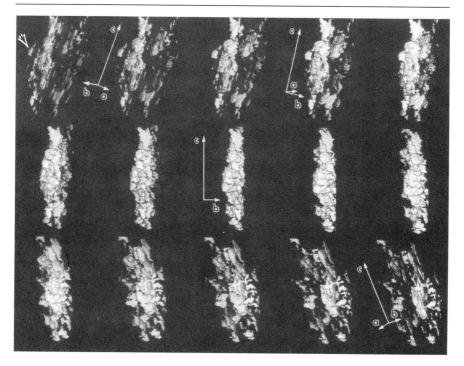

Fig. 3 A series of shaded surface renderings of the mineral component within the region of turkey tendon collagen calcification. Each view has been rotated consecutively 10° and demonstrates that the constituent crystals are platelet-shaped with irregular edges (follow through all views, for example, the individual crystal identified by the arrow in the upper left rendering). The crystallographic c-axes of the platelets, which correspond to the length of the crystals, are directed along and are generally parallel to the collagen long axis. Views in the upper left and lower right, opposed by 140°, show the crystals nearly edge-on and simultaneously parallel. If crystals were to grow along their b,c-axial planes, they would appear to form parallel extended plates or crystals sheets. In views 90° to the edge-on aspects, the crystals fill a 70-nm domain of collagen (middle row of the gallery). The axes marked a and b are operational, not crystallographic, indicators; they are orthogonal to distinguish crystal thickness and width directions, respectively. Crystallographically, a and b are identical for hydroxyapatite. Magnification 105,000 ×. (Reproduced with permission from Landis WJ, Song MJ, Leith A, et al: Mineral and organic matrix interaction in normally calcifying tendon visualized in three dimensions by high-voltage electron: Microscopic tomography and graphic image reconstruction. *J Structural Biol* 1993;110:39–54.)

likely that studies of the mineral in other (less highly oriented) tissues will verify a similar plate-like morphology and similar patterns of growth beyond the hole zones.

With the exception of the microscopic studies, ground, homogenized tissues were used in the above mentioned investigations. Although these studies indicated that age- and disease-dependent changes occurred in the apatite of bone and cartilage[27,28] and that there were differences in the crystalline particle size and carbonate contents of the mineral in these tissues,[28] site-dependent differences between these tissues were described only at the morphologic level.[29]

Coupling a light microscope with an IR spectrometer enabled a map to be made of the site-dependent changes in IR spectra of the mineral in the growth plate and bone.[30] Additional studies, reviewed elsewhere, aided the interpretation of those data.[12] In general, the results of these analyses show that the only detectable mineral is a poorly crystalline apatite. The mineral increases in size and perfection, decreases in carbonate and acid phosphate content, and increases in amount, progressing from the earliest site of mineral deposition in the cartilaginous growth plate to more mature cortical bone. Figure 4 shows selected spectra from a typical FT-IR map. These data, along with results of solubility and chemical composition studies, confirm the current concept that the mineral in bone and cartilage is a single apatite phase, containing adsorbed ions and macromolecules.

Current Concepts of the Distribution of Mineral in Bone and Cartilage

To understand how the first mineral crystals deposit, it is essential to know where this deposition occurs. Although the majority of the mineral in the body is associated closely with type I collagen (the predominant collagen of bone,

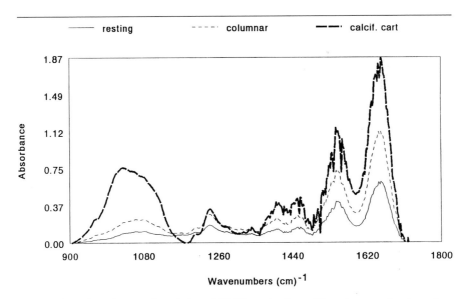

Fig. 4 Selected Fourier transform-infrared (FT-IR) spectra from different zones of an immature mouse growth plate, collected at 4 mm resolution on a BioRad FT-IR microscope. Rest = resting zone, columnar = columnar zone, calcif cart = calcified region below lowermost hypertrophic cell. Note increase in absorbance of the 900 to 1200 cm^{-1} mineral region in the calcified cartilage.

skin, ligament, tendon, dentin, etc), it is not uniformly accepted that type I collagen is the site of the initial mineral deposits.[13,14] For example, in calcified cartilage, the amount of type I collagen expressed is relatively low, and types II, IX, and X collagen are abundant. In cartilage, as well as in newly formed bone, the initial deposition of mineral has been associated with extracellular matrix vesicles (cartilage, bone, dentin), proteoglycan-type X collagen complexes (cartilage only), and chondrocalcin (cartilage only).

Extracellular matrix vesicles released from cell membranes have been reported to be the site of the first mineral crystals in growth plate cartilage[31,32] and chondrocyte cultures,[33] as well as early bone formation[34] and osteoblast cultures.[35] The matrix vesicle-associated mineral deposits are spatially distinct from the collagen-associated deposits, especially in the calcifying tendon where vesicle-associated mineral deposition and type I collagen mineralization appear to occur distinctly albeit simultaneously.[36] Matrix vesicles, as discussed below, may provide a protected site for the accumulation of mineral ions and a mechanism for depositing the earliest mineral crystals. The use of vesicles appears to have been an early system for facilitating mineral deposition in bacteria[37] and may be a vestige of this mechanism in mammalian tissues. To date, it is not known whether cartilage calcification can occur in the absence of matrix vesicles. It is known from cell culture studies that impaired collagen synthesis decreases the extent of calcification.[38]

Based on immunohistochemical and microprobe analyses, other matrix constituents have also been identified at the sites of initial mineral deposition.[39] In elegant light and electron microscopic studies, Poole and associates[39] demonstrated the presence of several macromolecules, distinct from collagen or matrix vesicles, in both tissue sections and tissue culture. Chondrocalcin, the C-propeptide of the predominant cartilage collagen (type II), was reported to be localized alone and/or with two other matrix molecules at the site of initial mineralization.[39] Type X collagen, a unique synthetic product of hypertrophic chondrocytes,[40] and the cartilage aggregatable proteoglycan, aggrecan, were frequently coassociated with mineral. The failure to detect a mineralization abnormality in transgenic animals in which an abnormal, shortened form of type X collagen was expressed,[41] coupled with solution data discussed below, indicates that type X collagen does not have a direct role in mineralization. Because the proteoglycans can serve as calcium reservoirs,[42] their association with mineral in dehydrated fixed sections is not surprising. Detailed arguments for a possible role for chondrocalcin will be presented below.

In order to understand how these matrix components could direct the calcification process, an understanding of the physiology of calcification is required.

The Physicochemistry of Mineralization

The deposition of calcium phosphate crystals on the preformed matrix produced by osteoblasts and chondrocytes is a complex process that can best be understood in terms of the events that occur in better-defined solution systems. The crystal formation process, in general, consists of two steps: the formation of a stable crystal nucleus and the growth and proliferation of the initial crystals.[43] To form a stable nucleus, ions or clusters of ions must come together with the same orientation as in the final crystal. In a supersaturated solution, ie, one in which the ion product of the precipitating ions exceeds the solubility product, interactions occur frequently. The number of such interactions increase with temperature. However, to form a "critical nucleus" that will support proliferation of crystals, the orientation of the interacting ions must match that of those in the crystalline material, and the number of correctly oriented, interacting ions must be sufficient to allow a stable structure to persist in solution long enough for growth to occur. Once a stable nucleus is formed, additional ions can add on, enabling the crystal to get larger. New nuclei may form on the surface of the growing crystals (secondary nucleation) causing an exponential increase in the number of sites for crystal proliferation. These crystal growth and proliferation processes require less energy than the nucleation process. It is rare in nature to form a crystal de novo (homogenous nucleation). Most nuclei form on preexisting particles (a scratch on a glass surface, dust, or another crystal). Heterogenous nucleation from a supersaturated solution is thought to be the mechanism of physiologic mineral deposition. In this situation, the foreign (hetero) nuclei are believed to be the matrix molecules on which the mineral deposits. Mineral deposition is facilitated by cell- and matrix-mediated increases in solution supersaturation ($Ca \times PO_4 \times OH$) product, by the exposure of hetero or epitaxial nucleators, and by the modification or removal of matrix molecules that regulate crystal proliferation.

An epitaxial nucleator has a surface that resembles a surface on the precipitating phase. That surface can then serve as a "homogenous-like" nucleator, or may contain counterions, which bind lattice ions in the correct orientation. For example, it has been suggested that the arrangement of carboxylic acid groups in the matrix protein osteocalcin facilitates the interaction of those groups with calcium on the surface of the apatite crystal.[44] It also has been suggested that the phosphoprotein phosphate groups in the collagen-associated phosphoproteins are distributed in such a way that they resemble the placement of phosphate groups in the apatite structure,[45] thereby providing a partially matched epitaxial surface. Such epitaxial interactions between organic acids and calcium carbonate minerals have been demonstrated based on single crystal structure determinations,[46] and on atomic force microscopic (AFM) investigations.[47] Unfortunately, the quaternary structures of the matrix proteins that interact with hydroxyapatite have not yet been determined, and AFM has not yet been applied to the study of apatitic minerals, in part because of the extremely small size of the crystals.

From a theoretical point of view, these "epitaxial nucleators" as well as anionic and cationic matrix molecules can control mineral deposition in several ways. First, they can increase the local supersaturation by sequestering ions. This has been demonstrated in solution for aggrecan, the large aggregating proteoglycan of cartilage.[42] The highly anionic aggrecan binds calcium, which can be eluted by increasing phosphate concentrations, which, in turn, leads to mineral deposition.[48]

The matrix molecules can act as nucleators per se, or they can stabilize preformed nuclei by binding to one or more faces of the smallest nuclei. As discussed below, there are several matrix molecules that appear to act as nucleators, although their detailed mechanisms of action are not yet delineated. Matrix molecules, by interacting with one or more specific faces on the initial crystals, may regulate the shape of the crystals, the size the crystals can attain, and/or the orientation of the crystals. For example, osteopontin, a phosphorylated bone sialoprotein,[49] retards the elongation of hydroxyapatite crystals in solution, reducing their accumulation in a dose-dependent manner.[50] Further details on the structure and function of specific matrix molecules are presented in chapter 1; the discussion below will deal only with their actions in the mineralization process.

Insights into Cartilage Calcification

During embryonic development and during developmental growth, it is the calcification of cartilage that provides the superstructure for long bone formation. Endochondral ossification, the process occurring in the epiphyseal growth plates of the long bones, has been studied extensively to gain insight into the way the cells (chondrocytes) and the longitudinal extraterritorial matrix regulate the calcification process.

In cell culture[51] and in tissue slices, initial chondrocyte-mediated calcification occurs associated with matrix vesicles.[52] These membrane-bound bodies,[32] whose membranes are enriched in degradative enzymes[53] also contain proteins (annexins)[54] that facilitate calcium transport into the interior of the vesicle. Within the vesicle, as suggested from studies of the synthetic liposomes,[55,56] mineral ions accumulate, increasing the local supersaturation. Nucleation may begin on matrix vesicle membrane-associated calcium-phospholipid phosphate complexes.[52,57] Mineral accumulation within the vesicle occurs in a protected environment, away from the inhibitors present in the matrix that serve to prevent calcification of the other cartilaginous zones. Modification of matrix molecules around the vesicles by the matrix-vesicle degradative enzymes may facilitate the proliferation of mineral crystals, which appear to puncture the vesicle membrane spreading into the matrix (Fig. 5).

The above mechanism is not universally accepted because matrix vesicle and cartilage collagen calcification appear to occur concurrently, vesicle calcification appears to occur at a site distant from collagen calcification, and vesicle-associated calcification has not been observed by all investigators.

Other suggested mechanisms of cartilage calcification are also controversial. Such mechanisms propose that there are specific macromolecules in the cartilaginous matrix that regulate cartilage calcification. To date, only two matrix proteins have been identified as specific products of chondrocytes in the zone preparing for calcification, the hypertrophic zone.[58] One of these proteins, Ch 21, has not been studied in terms of its role in the calcification process or its distribution relative to the mineral.[58] The other, type X collagen,[59] has been morphologically localized to the site of new calcification during limb development. In vitro, type X collagen expression and synthesis occur even when mineral deposition does not,[51] and type X collagen seems to have no effect on de novo hydroxyapatite formation or growth.[60] It has been suggested that type

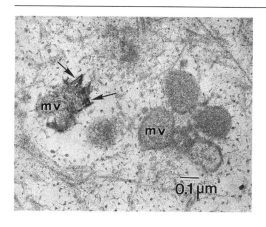

Fig. 5 Electron micrograph illustrating matrix vesicles (mv) in a calcifying cartilage culture. In one instance, the forming mineral (arrows) has penetrated the membrane of the matrix vesicle. (Courtesy of Dr. S.B. Doty.)

X collagen in conjunction with some other macromolecule may be the cartilage "nucleator."[61] This suggestion is refuted by the lack of detectable mineralization abnormality in the type X collagen deficient transgenic mouse.[41]

Chondrocalcin, the C-propeptide of type II collagen, also accumulates in the calcified cartilage zone,[39] and in culture its appearance precedes mineral deposition.[62] The high affinity of chondrocalcin for hydroxyapatite may account for its accumulation within the mineralized zones and for preliminary observations of its concentration-dependent ability to facilitate hydroxyapatite formation in vitro.

The only other cartilage macromolecules that have been linked to the calcification process are the aggregating cartilage proteoglycans. Demonstrated by many to be in vitro inhibitors of hydroxyapatite formation and growth,[63–66] perhaps because of their calcium chelating ability, they also have been proposed[48] as mineralization promoters. This proposal is based on the observation that an increase in phosphate concentration, such as that which occurs in the lower half of the growth plate,[67] elutes bound calcium from glycosaminoglycans, causing mineral deposition to occur.[48] Yet when proteoglycan synthesis is blocked in chondrocyte cultures, mineralization is increased rather than decreased, and in the brachymorphic mouse, a mutant species in which the proteoglycans are undersulfated, there is excessive calcification.[68] These undersulfated proteoglycans, as contrasted to their normal analogs, also facilitate in vitro mineralization,[68] making it unlikely that the sulfated proteoglycans per se are promoting mineral deposition. It is more likely that the sulfated proteoglycans' enzymatic degradation[53] does, in fact, cause an increase in local calcium content, and this increase, along with exposure of other matrix components, may facilitate mineralization. Extracellular cartilage matrix components involved in facilitating mineralization may include the smaller proteoglycans (biglycan and decorin) also found in bone, phosphorylated sialoproteins and perhaps other, as yet uncharacterized, macromolecules.

The chondrocyte is the key player in all these processes. It is the cell that synthesizes the collagens and other matrix molecules, the degradative enzymes, and the enzymes such as alkaline phosphatase, which regulate the flux of ions into the matrix.[69] Further, it is the cell that responds to signals from cytokines[70] and other stimuli. The cell is the origin, be it specific or random, of matrix vesicle generation, and only in the presence of viable cells does cartilage calcification occur.

Insights into Bone Calcification

The osteoblast is to bone what the chondrocyte is to cartilage in the calcification process; the osteoblast synthesizes the type I collagen on which the bone mineral crystals are deposited in an oriented fashion,[26] and produces the matrix components and enzymes that regulate mineralization. Early bone mineralization has been associated with matrix vesicles;[34] however, this association appears to occur only in instances where mineral deposition is impaired.[71] Collagen was long thought to be the "nucleator" of bone mineral;[72] however, when matrix proteins are extracted from collagen, the collagen loses its ability to serve as a "nucleator."[73] Dephosphorylation of collagen-associated phosphoproteins causes the collagen to lose its ability to nucleate hydroxyapatite in vitro.[74] Thus, although collagen in bone appears to act as the template on which the mineral crystals are aligned, other matrix components are responsible for the initial mineral deposition on this matrix.[75] Based on the high-resolution EM studies of calcified turkey tendon, it is apparent that nucleation commences at discrete sites in the hole zones.[26] It is then mandatory that the "nucleating" matrix proteins be located in these areas.

There are several bone matrix molecules that can modulate the calcification process when in solution, and are likely to do the same in vivo. Three of these are phosphorylated sialoproteins:[50] osteopontin, bone sialoprotein, and bone acidic glycoprotein-75 (BAG-75). Osteopontin, on a weight basis, is one of the most effective inhibitors of hydroxyapatite formation and growth that has been studied to date.[50] Bone sialoprotein, on the other hand, is an effective nucleator.[77] BAG-75 has not yet been investigated. In contrast to the phosphoprotein of dentin, which acts as a nucleator at low concentrations and an inhibitor of crystal growth at higher concentrations,[78] the bone phosphoproteins studied to date appear to act as either one or the other. Their mechanisms of action involve binding of specific domains to the apatite crystal, but the nature of the interactions must differ.

Osteonectin, another, albeit nonspecific,[79] bone matrix protein, can both facilitate mineral deposition on denatured collagen[73] and inhibit the growth of apatite crystals.[80] Other highly phosphorylated matrix proteins may similarly be involved in the initiation of bone mineral crystal formation and regulation of crystal growth because of the potential for such molecules to serve as epitaxial nucleators.[76]

The phosphorylation of these bone matrix proteins is modulated by a casein-kinase-like matrix protein kinase.[81,82] A similar enzyme exists in dentin,[83] and there is indirect evidence indicating such an enzyme also exists in cartilage.[84] The factors regulating this enzyme and the enzymes that dephosphorylate bone matrix protein molecules remain to be determined. Because the extent of phosphorylation of these proteins can differ from tissue to tissue and site to site, it is likely that variations in phosphorylation may determine the actions of these proteins in the mineralization cascade.

Most of the mineral in bone is believed to develop by the growth of the initially formed crystals.[72] The size these crystals attain falls in a limited range, increasing with age but not exceeding certain limits. Those matrix proteins that bind to and block the growth of mineral crystals, as well as spatial constraints imposed by the collagen itself, are responsible for the regulation of the crystal sizes. Although structural studies and insight from mutant and transgenic animals will be required to determine which of the matrix proteins are primarily responsible for the regulation of mineral crystal growth, extrapolations from solution and immunohistochemical data offer some suggestions.

In the presence of calcium, osteocalcin,[85] also known as bone Gla protein, has an extremely high affinity for bone mineral.[44] Binding of osteocalcin occurs through its gamma-carboxylated residues.[86] Once the osteocalcin is bound, it is believed from structural predictions[44] that a site chemotactic for bone resorbing osteoclasts is exposed. Thus osteocalcin, which in solution retards hydroxyapatite growth,[80,87] cannot only regulate crystal sizes but also may regulate their turnover. The phosphoproteins mentioned above, as well as many other anionic macromolecules found in bone,[58,75,76] may alone, or via interactions with other matrix molecules, have similar actions.

Studies of bone cell culture and bone organ culture provide insight into the events in the bone/osteoid calcification system.[88–93] Using marrow as a source of osteoprogenitor cells or using osteoblast-like cell lines, investigators have demonstrated the sequence of expression of osteoblast proteins. Histones, type I collagen, fibronectin, osteopontin, and other components involved in matrix development appear before bone sialoprotein, osteonectin, and alkaline phosphatase.[88–93] Osteocalcin appears at an even later stage. This sequence is in accord with the view that the collagen provides a template upon which, via interaction with matrix proteins, mineral deposits. In culture studies, alkaline phosphatase hydrolyzes phosphate esters added to the media, thereby providing an increased concentration of inorganic phosphate and, hence, a higher supersaturation. Whether this enzyme also plays a role in the regulation of matrix protein phosphorylation remains to be determined. Osteocalcin, synthesized coincident with or just after the formation of the first mineral crystals, is apt to be more important in regulating crystal growth and turnover.

Common Themes and Unsolved Questions

The matrix and, therefore, the arrangement and properties of the mineral deposited on that matrix differ in bone and calcified cartilage. Yet there are certain common themes related to their mechanisms of calcification. A viable cell is required in both cases; sulfated and/or phosphorylated proteins function as nucleators and regulators of crystal growth. Noncollagenous matrix proteins rather than collagen act as nucleators, and matrix vesicles may be involved in initial mineral formation. Which of the components are essential and which redundant remain to be defined.

In cartilage, it is likely that calcium binding to proteoglycans increases the local calcium content. How matrix phosphate concentration is increased and how both calcium and phosphate increase in the osteoid are unknown. Other remaining questions include: Does degradation of matrix proteins play a direct role in the regulation of mineralization? How important is the efflux of cell calcium and inorganic phosphate relative to the release of these ions from matrix components?

There probably is a cascade of events that leads to matrix calcification in each tissue. The cells, in response to some as yet undefined signals, secrete and modify a matrix. The components of that matrix essential to proper calcification need to be defined. An increase in $Ca \times P \times OH$ concentration results in nucleation of the initial mineral crystals. Is it the extracellular matrix vesicles that enable this localized cartilage increase in supersaturation to occur or is it specific matrix proteins? Which individual or interacting matrix proteins in bone function as nucleators in situ? The proliferation of the crystals is regulated as the matrix becomes mineralized. Again, the essential players in the regulation of growth require identification.

Verification of the mechanisms suggested in this paper will be forthcoming from detailed structural studies, studies of matrix protein-mineral interaction, and the development of animal and cell-culture models in which these interactions are disrupted or absent.

Acknowledgment

The work described in this review was supported by NIH grants DE04141 and AR037661.

References

1. Posner AS, Eanes ED, Harper RA, et al: X-ray diffraction analysis of the effect of fluoride on human bone apatite. *Arch Oral Biol* 1963;8:549–570.
2. Aspden RM, Hukins DWL: Calcification of the deep zone in pig femoral head cartilage. *Experientia* 1981;37:1333–1334.

3. Legeros RZ, Legeros JP: Phosphate minerals in human tissues, in Nriagu JO, Moore PB (eds): *Phosphate Minerals*. New York, NY, Springer-Verlag, 1984, pp 351–385.

4. Walton AG, Deveney MJ, Koenig JL: Raman spectroscopy of calcified tissues. *Calcif Tissue Res* 1970;6:162–167.

5. Aue WP, Roufosse AH, Glimcher MJ, et al: Solid-state phosphorus-31 nuclear magnetic resonance studies of synthetic solid phases of calcium phosphate: Potential models of bone mineral. *Biochemistry* 1984;23:6110–6114.

6. Casciani FS, Etz ES, Newbury DE, et al: Raman microprobe studies of two mineralizing tissues: Enamel of the rat incisor and the embryonic chick tibia. *Scan Electron Microsc* 1979;II:383–391.

7. Rey C, Shimizu M, Collins B, et al: Resolution-enhanced Fourier transform infrared spectroscopy study of the environment of phosphate ions in the early deposits of a solid phase of calcium-phosphate in bone and enamel, and their evolution with age: I. Investigations in the v_4 domain. *Calcif Tissue Int* 1990;46:384–394.

8. Fratzl P, Fratzl-Zelman N, Klaushofer K, et al: Nucleation and growth of mineral crystals in bone studied by small-angle x-ray scattering. *Calcif Tissue Int* 1991;48: 407–413.

9. Moradian-Oldak J, Weiner S, Addadi L, et al: Electron imaging and diffraction study of individual crystals of bone, mineralized tendon, and synthetic carbonate apatite. *Connect Tissue Res* 1991;25:219–228.

10. Barckhaus RH, Hohling HJ: Electron microscopical microprobe analysis of freeze dried and unstained mineralized epiphyseal cartilage. *Cell Tissue Res* 1978;186: 541–549.

11. Weiner S, Traub W: Crystal size and organization in bone. *Connect Tissue Res* 1989;21:259–265.

12. Boskey AL, Pleshko N, Doty SB, et al: Applications of Fourier transform infrared (FT-IR) microscopy to the study of mineralization in bone and cartilage. *Cells Materials* 1992;2:209–221.

13. Eanes ED: Dynamic aspects of apatite phases of mineralized tissues: Model studies, in Butler WT (ed): *Chemistry and Biology of Mineralized Tissues*. Birmingham, AL, Ebsco Media, 1985, pp 213–220.

14. Boskey AL: Overview of cellular elements and macromolecules implicated in the initiation of mineralization, in Butler WT (ed): *Chemistry and Biology of Mineralized Tissues*. Birmingham, AL, Ebsco Media, 1985, pp 335–343.

15. Posner AS, Betts F, Blumenthal NC: Bone mineral composition and structures, in Simmons DJ, Kunin AS (eds): *Skeletal Research: An Experimental Approach*. New York, NY, Academic Press, 1979, pp 167–192.

16. Baxter JD, Biltz RM, Pellegrino ED: The physical state of bone carbonate: A comparative infra-red study in several mineralized tissues. *Yale J Biol Med* 1966;38: 456–470.

17. Rey C, Renugopalakrishnan V, Collins B, et al: Fourier transform infrared spectroscopic study of the carbonate ions in bone mineral during aging. *Calcif Tissue Int* 1991;49:251–258.

18. Arsenault AL: Crystal-collagen relationships in calcified turkey leg tendons visualized by selected- area dark field electron microscopy. *Calcif Tissue Int* 1988;43: 202–212.

19. Landis WJ, Paine MC, Glimcher MJ: Electron microscopic observations of bone tissue prepared anhydrously in organic solvents. *J Ultrastruct Res* 1977;59:1–30.

20. Boskey AL, Posner AS: Conversion of amorphous calcium phosphate to microcrystalline hydroxyapatite: A pH-dependent, solution-mediated, solid-solid conversion. *J Phys Chem* 1973;77:2313–2317.

21. Termine JD, Posner AS: Infrared analysis of rat bone: Age dependency of amorphous and crystalline mineral fractions. *Science* 1966;153:1523–1525.

22. Brown WE, Chow LC: Chemical properties of bone mineral. *Annu Rev Materials Sci* 1976;6:213–236.

23. Sauer GR, Wuthier RE: Fourier transform infrared characterization of mineral phases formed during induction of mineralization by collagenase-released matrix vesicles in vitro. *J Biol Chem* 1988;263:13718–13724.

24. Roufosse AH, Landis WJ, Sabine WK, et al: Identification of brushite in newly deposited bone mineral from embryonic chicks. *J Ultrastruc Res* 1979;68:235–255.

25. Robinson RA, Watson ML: Crystal-collagen relationships in bone as seen in the electron microscope. *Anat Rec* 1952;114:383–410.

26. Landis WJ, Song MJ, Leith A, et al: Mineral and organic matrix interaction in normally calcifying tendon visualized in three dimensions by high-voltage electron microscopic tomography and graphic image reconstruction. *J Struct Biol* 1993;110:39–54.

27. Grynpas MD, Holmyard D: Changes in quality of bone mineral on aging and in disease. *Scanning Microsc* 1988;2:1045–1054.

28. Burnell JM, Teubner EJ, Miller AG: Normal maturational changes in bone matrix, mineral and crystal size in the rat. *Calcif Tissue Int* 1980;31:13–19.

29. Boyde A, Shapiro IM: Morphological observations concerning the pattern of mineralization of the normal and the rachitic chick growth cartilage. *Anat Embryol* 1987;175:457–466.

30. Mendelsohn R, Hassenkhani A, DiCarlo E, et al: FT-IR Microscopy of endochondral ossification at 20µ spatial resolution. *Calcif Tissue Int* 1989;44:20–24.

31. Anderson HC: Matrix vesicle calcification: Review and update, in Peck WA (ed): *Bone and Mineral Research*. Amsterdam, Elsevier, 1985, pp 109–149.

32. Wuthier RE: Mechanism of de novo mineral formation by matrix vesicles. *Connect Tissue Res* 1989;22:27–33.

33. Wu LN, Sauer GR, Genge BR, et al: Induction of mineral deposition by primary cultures of chicken growth plate chondrocytes in ascorbate-containing media: Evidence of an association between matrix vesicles and collagen. *J Biol Chem* 1989;264:21346–21355.

34. Bernard GW, Peace DC: An electron microscopic study of initial intramembranous osteogenesis. *Am J Anat* 1969;125:271–290.

35. Sudo H, Kodama HA, Amagai Y, et al: In vitro differentiation and calcification in a new clonal osteogenic cell line derived from newborn mouse calvaria. *J Cell Biol* 1983;96:191–198.

36. Landis WJ, Arsenault AL: Vesicle- and collagen-mediated calcification in the turkey leg tendon. *Connect Tissue Res* 1989;22:35–42.

37. Mann S, Hannington JP, Williams RJP: Phospholipid vesicles as a model system for biomineralization. *Nature* 1986;324:565–567.

38. Boskey AL, Stiner D, Doty SB, et al: Requirement of vitamin C for cartilage calcification in a differentiating chick limb-bud mesenchymal cell culture. *Bone* 1991;12:277–282.

39. Poole AR, Matsui Y, Hinek A, et al: Cartilage macromolecules and calcification of cartilage matrix. *Anat Rec* 1989;224:167–179.

40. Poole AR, Pidoux I, Linsenmayer TF, et al: Type X collagen and the calcification of cartilage matrix: An immunoelectron microscopic study. *Trans Orthop Res Soc* 1988;13:155.

41. Jacenko O, LuValle PA, Olsen BR: Spondylometaphyseal dysplasia in mice carrying a dominant negative mutation in a matrix protein specific for cartilage to bone transition. *Nature* 1993;365:56–61.

42. Dunstone JR: Ion-exchange reactions between cartilage and various cations. *Biochem J* 1960;77:164–170.

43. Garside J: Nucleation, in Nancollas GH (ed): *Biological Mineralization and Demineralization*. Berlin, Springer-Verlag, 1981, pp 23–25.

44. Hauschka PV, Wians FH Jr: Osteocalcin-hydroxyapatite interaction in the extracellular organic matrix of bone. *Anat Rec* 1989;224:180–188.

45. Holt C, van Kemenade MJJM: The interaction of phosphoproteins with calcium phosphate, in Hukins DWL (ed): *Calcified Tissue*. Boca Raton, FL, CRC Press, 1989, pp 175–213.

46. Addadi L, Berman A, Oldak JM, et al: Structural and stereochemical relations between acidic macromolecules of organic matrices and crystals. *Connect Tissue Res* 1989;21:127–135

47. Wierzbicki A, Sikes CS, Madura JD, et al: Atomic force microscopy and molecular modeling of protein and peptide binding to calcite. *Calcif Tissue Int* 1994;54:133–141.

48. Hunter GK: Role of proteoglycan in the provisional calcification of cartilage: A review and reinterpretation. *Clin Orthop* 1991;262:256–280

49. Prince CW: Secondary structure predictions for rat osteopontin. *Connect Tissue Res* 1989;21:15–20.

50. Boskey AL, Maresca M, Ullrich W, et al: Osteopontin-hydroxyapatite interactions in vitro: Inhibition of hydroxyapatite formation and growth in a gelatin-gel. *Bone Miner* 1993;22:147–159.

51. Boskey AL, Stiner D, Doty S, et al: Studies of mineralization in tissue culture: Optimal conditions for cartilage calcification. *Bone Miner* 1992;16:11–36.

52. Boyan BD, Schwartz Z, Swain L, et al: Role of lipids in calcification of cartilage. *Anat Rec* 1989;224:211–219.

53. Dean DD, Schwartz Z, Muniz OE, et al: Matrix vesicles are enriched in metalloproteinases that degrade proteoglycans. *Calcif Tissue Int* 1992;50:342–349.

54. Genge BR, Cao X, Wu LN, et al: Establishment of the primary structure of the major lipid-dependent Ca2 + binding proteins of chicken growth plate cartilage matrix vesicles: Identity with anchorin CII (annexin V) and annexin II. *J Bone Miner Res* 1992;7:807–819.

55. Eanes ED: Biophysical aspects of lipid interaction with mineral: Liposome model studies. *Anat Rec* 1989;224:220–225.

56. Eanes ED, Hailer AW: Liposome-mediated calcium phosphate formation in metastable solutions. *Calcif Tissue Int* 1985;37:390–394.

57. Boskey AL: Phospholipids and calcification, in Hukins DWL (ed): *Calcified Tissue.* Boca Raton, FL, CRC Press, 1989, pp 15–243.

58. Heinegard D, Oldberg A: Structure and biology of cartilage and bone matrix noncollagenous macromolecules. *FASEB J* 1989;3:2042–2051.

59. Schmid TM, Linsenmayer TF: Type X collagen, in Mayne R, Burgeson RE (eds): *Structure and Function of Collagen Types.* Orlando, FL, Academic Press, 1987, pp 223–259.

60. Boskey AL, Maresca M, Appel J: The effects of noncollagenous matrix proteins on hydroxyapatite formation and proliferation in a collagen gel system. *Connect Tissue Res* 1989;21:171–178.

61. Poole AR, Pidoux I: Immunoelectron microscopic studies of type X collagen in endochondral ossification. *J Cell Biol* 1989;109:2547–2554

62. Hinek A, Reiner A, Poole AR: The calcification of cartilage matrix in chondrocyte culture: Studies of the C-propeptide of type II collagen (chondrocalcin). *J Cell Biol* 1987;104:1435–1441.

63. Cuervo LA, Pita JC, Howell DS: Inhibition of calcium phosphate mineral growth by proteoglycan aggregate fractions in a synthetic lymph. *Calcif Tissue Res* 1973; 13:1–10.

64. Blumenthal NC, Posner AS, Silverman LD, et al: Effect of proteoglycans on in vitro hydroxyapatite formation. *Calcif Tissue Int* 1979;27:75–82.

65. Chen CC, Boskey AL, Rosenberg LC: The inhibitory effect of cartilage proteoglycans on hydroxyapatite growth. *Calcif Tissue Int* 1984;36:285–290.

66. Chen CC, Boskey AL: The effects of proteoglycans from different cartilage types on in vitro hydroxyapatite proliferation. *Calcif Tissue Int* 1986;39:324–327.

67. Kakuta S, Golub EE, Shapiro IM: Morphochemical analysis of phosphorous pools in calcifying cartilage. *Calcif Tissues Int* 1985;37:293–299.

68. Boskey AL, Maresca M, Wikstrom B, et al: Hydroxyapatite formation in the presence of proteoglycans of reduced sulfate content: Studies in the brachymorphic mouse. *Calcif Tissue Int* 1991;49:389–393.

69. Whyte MP: Alkaline phosphatase: Physiological role explored in hypophosphatasia, in Peck WA (ed): *Bone and Mineral Research*, ed 6. Amsterdam, Elsevier, 1989, pp 175–218.

70. Skjodt H, Russel G: Bone cell biology and the regulation of bone turnover, in Gowen M (ed): *Cytokines and Bone Metabolism.* Boca Raton, FL, CRC Press, 1992, pp 1–70.
71. Anderson HC: Calcium-accumulating vesicles in the intercellular matrix of bone, in *Hard Tissue Growth, Repair and Remineralization.* CIBA Foundation Symposium 11. Amsterdam, Elsevier, 1973, pp 213–246.
72. Glimcher MJ, Krane SM: The organization and structure of bone, and the mechanism of calcification, in Gould BS (ed): *Treatise on Collagen. Vol II. Biology of Collagen, part B.* New York, NY, Academic Press, 1968, pp 68–251.
73. Termine JD, Belcourt AB, Conn KM, et al: Mineral and collagen-binding proteins of fetal calf bone. *J Biol Chem* 1981;256:10403–10408.
74. Endo A, Glimcher MJ: The effect of complexing phosphoproteins to decalcified collagen on in vitro calcification. *Connect Tissue Res* 1989;21:179–190.
75. Glimcher MJ: Mechanism of calcification: Role of collagen fibrils and collagen-phosphoprotein complexes in vitro and in vivo. *Anat Rec* 1989;224:139–153.
76. Boskey AL: Mineral-matrix interactions in bone and cartilage. *Clin Orthop* 1992; 281:244–274.
77. Goldberg HA, Hunter GK: Nucleation of hydroxyapatite by bone sialoprotein. *Proc Natl Acad Sci USA* 1993;90:8562–8565.
78. Boskey AL, Maresca M, Doty SB, et al: Concentration-dependent effects of dentin-phosphophoryn in the regulation of in vitro hydroxyapatite formation and growth. *Bone Miner* 1990;11:55–65.
79. Engel J, Taylor W, Paulsson M, et al: Calcium binding domains and calcium-induced conformational transition of SPARC/BM-40/osteonectin, an extracellular glycoprotein expressed in mineralized and nonmineralized tissues. *Biochemistry* 1987;26:6958–6965.
80. Romberg RW, Werness PG, Riggs BL, et al: Inhibition of hydroxyapatite crystal growth by bone-specific and other calcium binding proteins. *Biochemistry* 1986; 25:1176–1180.
81. Mikuni-Takagaki Y, Glimcher MJ: Post-translational processing of chicken bone phosphoproteins: Identification of bone (phospho)protein kinase. *Biochem J* 1990; 268:593–597.
82. Mikuni-Takagaki Y, Glimcher MJ: Post-translational processing of chicken bone phosphoproteins: Identification of the bone phosphoproteins of embryonic tibia. *Biochem J* 1990;268:585–591.
83. Wu CB, Pelech SL, Veis A: The in vitro phosphorylation of the native rat incisor dentin phosphophoryns. *J Biol Chem* 1992;267:16588–16594.
84. Boskey AL, Doty SB, Binderman I: ATP promotes mineralization in differentiating chick limb-bud mesenchymal cell cultures. *Microsc Res Tech*, in press.
85. Hauschka PV, Lian JB, Cole DE, et al: Osteocalcin and matrix Gla protein: Vitamin K-dependent proteins in bone. *Physiol Rev* 1989;69:990–1047.
86. Poser JW, Price PA: A method for decarboxylation of γ carboxyglutamic acid in protein from calf bone. *J Biol Chem* 1979;254:431–436.
87. Boskey AL, Wians FH Jr, Hauschka PV: The effect of osteocalcin on in vitro lipid-induced hydroxyapatite formation and seeded hydroxyapatite growth. *Calcif Tissue Int* 1985;37:57–62.
88. Aronow MA, Gerstenfeld LC, Owen TA, et al: Factors that promote progressive development of the osteoblast phenotype in cultured fetal rat calvaria cells. *J Cell Physiol* 1990;143:213–221.
89. Gerstenfeld LC, Chipman SD, Kelly CM, et al: Collagen expression, ultrastructural assembly, and mineralization in cultures of chicken embryo osteoblasts. *J Cell Biol* 1988;106:979–989.
90. Pockwinse SM, Wilming LG, Conlon DM, et al: Expression of cell growth and bone specific genes at single cell resolution during development of bone tissue-like organization in primary osteoblast cultures. *J Cell Biochem* 1992;49:310–323.
91. Aubin JE, Bellows CG, Turksen K, et al: Analysis of the osteoblast lineage and regulation of differentiation, in Slavkin HC, Price P (eds): *Chemistry and Biology of Mineralized Tissues.* Amsterdam, Excerpta Medica, 1992, pp 267–276.

92. Rickard DJ, Sullivan TA, Shenker BJ, et al: Induction of rapid osteoblast differentiation in rat bone marrow stromal cell cultures by dexamethasone and BMP-2. *Dev Biol* 1994;161:218–228.

93. Yao KL, Todescan R Jr, Sodek J: Temporal changes in matrix protein synthesis and mRNA expression during mineralized tissue formation by adult rat bone marrow cells in culture. *J Bone Miner Res* 1994;9:231–240.

Chapter 4
Biologic Regulation of Bone Growth

Stephen B. Trippel, MD

Introduction

The normal growth and development of the skeleton reflect the carefully orchestrated actions of a wide variety of cell regulatory factors. Prominent among these are the hormones, growth factors, vitamins, and cytokines that serve as cell-signaling molecules. In any discussion of this subject, a potential source of confusion is the terminology applied to these bioactive agents. To date, no taxonomy for the factors that regulate cells has been developed. The terms used to distinguish categories of factors (eg, hormone, growth factor, cytokine) are principally of historic interest, and the names applied to specific factors (eg, fibroblast growth factor, insulin-like growth factor I, transforming growth factor-beta) are carried over from early descriptions of a factor's action or source.

In light of current knowledge, many of these terms may be misleading. The example of transforming growth factor-beta (TGF-β) is illustrative. This polypeptide was initially characterized on the basis of its ability to promote anchorage-independent growth of nonneoplastic cells whose proliferation is normally anchorage-dependent. The ability to induce neoplastic behavior led to the view that TGF-β may promote the growth of tumors[1] and justified its name. However, further studies demonstrated that TGF-β plays an inhibitory role in a wide variety of cell types, including tumors. In this capacity, which is perhaps its preeminent one, its title is a misnomer. Curiously, the same molecule was independently identified by its ability to induce cartilage formation and was also named cartilage-inducing factor,[2] a description more germane to the skeleton than "TGF-β" but one that was not ultimately adopted. Other cell-signaling factors have experienced similar histories. Thus, the terms used for these substances are best viewed not as descriptors of function, but simply as conventionally used identifiers.

Cell-Signaling Molecules

Growth Hormone

Growth hormone is the classic polypeptide regulator of skeletal growth. Since its identification in 1921,[3] growth hormone has been established as a requisite for normal longitudinal skeletal growth and development. Growth hormone deficiency is associated with profound growth failure and delayed skeletal maturation, resulting clinically in proportionate dwarfism. Conversely, excess growth hormone secretion during skeletal development produces increased linear skeletal growth and, when severe, giantism. For many years, growth hormone derived from pituitary extracts has been used therapeutically to stimulate skeletal growth in children who have growth hormone deficiency. More recently, with the availability of bacterially derived recombinant forms of the molecule, growth hormone has become more widely used in the management of human growth failure from multiple causes.[4] The mechanism of growth hormone action on the skeleton began to be illuminated in 1957 with the observation that its effect on cultured costal cartilage was mediated by a growth hormone-dependent activity in serum.[5] This activity was subsequently found to reflect the actions of a group of peptides called somatomedins or insulin-like growth factors (IGFs).

Insulin-Like Growth Factor-I

Two classes of somatomedins have been demonstrated by amino acid and DNA sequence analysis: IGF-I, or somatomedin-C, and IGF-II. IGF-I is functionally distinct from IGF-II in being more highly human growth hormone-dependent and in possessing greater growth promoting activity. IGF-II may be the principal somatomedin in the embryo and fetus.[6] Currently, the generic terms "insulin-like growth factor" and "somatomedin" are used interchangeably, while the terms IGF-I and IGF-II are in predominant use for the specific peptides.[7]

Somatomedin Hypothesis   Central to an understanding of skeletal growth is the so-called "somatomedin hypothesis," which postulates that the well-known effect of growth hormone on skeletal growth is indirect and mediated by the somatomedins. According to the classic view of the somatomedin hypothesis, growth hormone produced in the pituitary is released into the bloodstream, which transports it to the liver and other tissues. There, it stimulates production of IGF-I,[8] which is, in turn, released into the circulation to act in an endocrine fashion on its target tissues, including the growth plate.

This model is supported by several lines of evidence. In culture studies, cartilage exposed to serum from hypophysectomized (and hence growth hormone deficient) rats incorporated sulfate more slowly than cartilage cultured with serum from normal rats.[5] The addition of growth hormone to the cartilage failed to restore sulfate incorporation to normal. However, when growth hormone was given to hypophysectomized rats and their serum then added to the cultured cartilage, sulfate incorporation was restored.[5] Growth factors such as the IGFs produce their cellular effects by binding to receptor molecules on their target cells. Thus, if the somatomedin hypothesis is correct, the chondrocytes of the growth plate should possess IGF receptors. Such receptors have been identified and characterized.[9-11] Additional lines of evidence in support of this hypothesis are the observations that serum somatomedin concentrations are growth hormone dependent, that IGF-I exerts negative feedback on growth hormone at both the hypothalamus and pituitary, and that IGF administration stimulates longitudinal skeletal growth in hypophysectomized rats.[6]

Not all studies so clearly support such a role for the somatomedins. Seemingly inconsistent with the somatomedin hypothesis are data suggesting that the action of growth hormone on chondrocytes is a direct one, not involving mediation by IGF-I. Growth hormone has been found to enhance the proliferation of rabbit ear and rib chondrocytes in culture[12] and to stimulate proteoglycan synthesis in cultured rat chondrocytes.[13] Specific binding of growth hormone has been observed on rabbit ear and epiphyseal plate chondrocytes, indicating that these cells possess receptors for growth hormones.[14] In vivo studies have also been interpreted as revealing a direct growth hormone effect on cartilage. Growth hormone injected into the growth plate of hypophysectomized rats elicited an increased growth rate at that physis, suggesting a direct action on longitudinal bone growth.[15] Similarly, when growth hormone was administered intra-arterially to one limb of hypophysectomized rats, the growth rate was increased in that limb but not in the contralateral limb.[16] Furthermore, growth hormone administered systemically to hypophysectomized rats was a more effective stimulus of skeletal growth than IGF-I, even when growth hormone was administered at 50-fold lower doses.[17]

This somewhat confusing discrepancy in the literature over the validity of the somatomedin hypothesis is, perhaps, more apparent than real. Reports addressing the ability of growth hormone to stimulate cartilage may be divided into two categories according to whether the studies were carried out in vivo or in vitro. When so divided, such studies also tend to distribute according to the effect of growth hormone. Reports based on in vivo experiments are strikingly uniform in finding stimulation of cartilage by growth hormone. In contrast, results of in vitro studies generally demonstrate lack of direct stimulation by growth hormone. This in vivo–in vitro dichotomy is consistent with the hypothesis that the effects of growth hormone observed in vivo are dependent on mediating substances, such as IGF-I, that are available in vivo, but not available under most in vitro circumstances.

Classically, the IGFs have been viewed as endocrine factors, circulating with their binding proteins and acting on target cells at a distance from their source. Although IGF-I may indeed act in this fashion, more recent data suggest that IGF-I also acts in an autocrine or paracrine fashion at the growth plate. In support of this view is the observation that the stimulatory effect of intra-arterial growth hormone on the growth plate is blocked by the simultaneous administration of an anti-IGF-I antibody.[18] These data suggest that the observed effect of growth hormone on the growth plate is mediated, at least in part, by locally produced IGF-I. Indeed, recent reports suggest that growth hormone stimulates IGF-I synthesis by growth plate chondrocytes in vitro, and increases expression of IGF-I messenger RNA by growth plate chondrocytes in vivo.[6]

Currently, the somatomedin hypothesis appears to be best viewed from both an endocrine and an autocrine perspective. According to this model (Fig. 1, *left*), growth hormone stimulates production of IGF-I by multiple tissues. This IGF-I then either enters the circulation to act in an endocrine fashion or is retained locally to act in an autocrine or paracrine fashion. These two mechanisms are not mutually exclusive. The relative contribution of each to the regulation of cartilage at different sites and different stages of development remains to be established.

Dual Effector Theory An alternative model for the regulation of skeletal growth by growth hormone and IGF-I is the "dual effector" theory of growth hormone action.[19] This theory postulates that growth hormone induces the differentiation of precursor cells, rendering them susceptible to IGF-I, which then stimulates their clonal expansion. The dual effector theory is supported by the observation that growth hormone, but not IGF-I, promoted the differentiation of cultured preadipocytes to adipocytes and that these newly differentiated cells were more sensitive to the mitogenic effect of IGF-I than the precursor cells.[20] The growth plate is an attractive location to apply this model (Fig. 1, *right*). Reserve zone cells represent appropriate putative precursors that, in response to growth hormone, could become susceptible to clonal expression as proliferative zone cells under the influence of IGF-I. Indeed, reserve zone chondrocytes appear to both bind and respond to IGF-I [21,22] less effectively than their

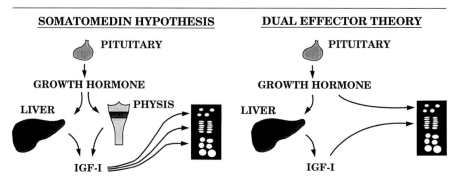

Fig. 1 Left, Somatomedin hypothesis. This model of growth hormone action on skeletal growth postulates that growth hormone stimulates the production of insulin-like growth factor-I (IGF-I) in both nonskeletal tissues (principally the liver) and in skeletal tissues (such as the growth plate). IGF-I then travels through the bloodstream (endocrine mechanism) to local tissues (autocrine/paracrine mechanism) to the chondrocytes to stimulate growth. According to this model, the action of growth hormone is indirect, mediated by IGF-I. **Right**, Dual effector theory. This theory postulates that growth hormone causes immature cells in the reserve zone to differentiate to an IGF-I response state. IGF-I then stimulates cell division in the proliferative zone. According to this model, the actions of growth hormone and IGF-I are sequential.

proliferative zone counterparts. However, any growth hormone dependence of this phenomenon remains to be established.

Further insight into the role of IGF-I in regulating skeletal growth at the growth plate has been provided by studies of transgenic mice. Mice in which an IGF-I gene was inserted under the control of the metallothionein I gene promoter had serum IGF-I levels about 1.5 times higher, and weighed approximately 1.3 times more than their nontransgenic littermates. However, they did not appear to undergo an increase in linear skeletal growth as estimated by radiographs of long bones and by tibial epiphyseal growth over a 10-day period.[23] Transgenic mice have also been developed that overexpress growth hormone. The growth hormone-expressing transgenic animals showed higher IGF-I levels and grew to a larger size than the IGF-I-expressing transgenic mice.[24] Inasmuch as the IGF-I transgenic animals also had normal growth-hormone producing capacity, and because the growth hormone transgenic animals exhibited both elevated growth hormone and elevated IGF-I, these results were not particularly helpful in clarifying the relationships between IGF-I, growth hormone, and skeletal growth. To help distinguish the roles of IGF-I and growth hormone, mice were made transgenic for both the IGF-I gene and for ablation of the cells that express growth hormone. The mice carrying both transgenes (IGF-I and absence of growth hormone) grew larger than their littermates carrying only the growth hormone ablation transgene and exhibited weight and linear growth indistinguishable from that of their normal nontransgenic siblings.[25]

Taken together, these transgene studies indicate that expression of IGF-I alone (in the absence of growth hormone) can generate normal growth, a finding of potential clinical significance for treatment with IGF-I of patients suffering from growth hormone resistance syndromes. These studies also reveal that, in the presence of normal growth hormone secretion, additional chronic expression of IGF-I may not elicit supranormal skeletal growth. Finally, the observation that normal growth is generated by IGF-I in the absence of growth hormone tends to argue against the dual effector theory as it applies to skeletal growth.

Both the somatomedin hypothesis and the dual effector theory are limited by their inclusion of only two substances: growth hormone and IGF-I. Though these may be critical effectors of skeletal growth, considerably more sophisticated models are needed to account for the participation of other regulatory factors.

IGF-II

The contribution of IGF-II to the regulation of skeletal growth appears to be most significant during early development and to become progressively less important during postnatal growth.[6,7] When administered systemically to rats, IGF-II was less potent than IGF-I in stimulating indices of skeletal growth.[26] These results suggest only a limited role for IGF-II in skeletal growth in young rats. However, such studies of IGF-II in postnatal animals may not reflect its true importance in very early skeletal development.

Convincing evidence for a primarily prenatal role of IGF-II in skeletal growth has recently been provided by the development of mice carrying a disrupted IGF-II gene. Chimeric mice possessing one normal and one inactivated IGF-II allele were proportionately smaller than their wild-type littermates, but otherwise appeared normal.[27] Postnatal growth of these heterozygous mice was identical to that of the wild-type animals, suggesting that the IGF-II mutation exerted its influence on the skeleton only during embryonic growth.

Fibroblast Growth Factor

The fibroblast growth factors (FGFs) comprise a family of heparin-binding polypeptides that were originally discovered on the basis of a mitogenic effect on fibroblasts.[28] This group of polypeptides regulates cell functions as diverse as mitogenesis, differentiation, protease production, receptor modulation, and cell maintenance.[29] Basic FGF (bFGF), the first of the FGFs to be identified, was independently discovered in cartilage as cartilage-derived growth factor[30] and in pituitary glands as chondrocyte-stimulating factor.[31]

Several lines of evidence suggest that bFGF plays a role in skeletal growth and development. This peptide has been isolated from cartilage[30] and has been immunolocalized to the proliferative and maturation (but not the hypertrophic) zones of the growth plate.[32] During development of the embryonic mouse skeleton, the highest levels of bFGF transcripts were found in the long bones.[33] Growth plate chondrocytes possess high-affinity receptors for bFGF[29] and may have access to matrix-associated bFGF.[34] Basic FGF is a potent mitogen for chondrocytes,[35,36] including growth plate chondrocytes.[37] In fact, bFGF is both more efficacious and more potent than IGF-I in stimulating bovine growth plate chondrocytes in vitro.[37]

The regulation of cartilage matrix synthesis by bFGF is complex. In contrast to its stimulatory effect on chondrocyte mitotic activity, bFGF has generally been found to exert no effect on, or to inhibit, proteoglycan synthesis by cultured chondrocytes.[37,38] However, in cultures in which chondrocytes were allowed to mature to the hypertrophic stage, bFGF enhanced proteoglycan synthesis.[39] In addition, bFGF appears to inhibit chondrocyte functions associated with differentiation: growth plate chondrocytes cultured with bFGF showed a reduction in alkaline phosphatase,[37,39] and in both calcium deposition and calcium content.[39]

Taken together, these data suggest that bFGF supports an immature chondrocyte phenotype, promoting the proliferation and inhibiting the differentiation of the cells responsible for skeletal growth at the growth plate.

Transforming Growth Factor-Beta

The TGF-β family of polypeptides is composed of at least five molecules (TGF-β1 to TGF-β5) and is itself a member of a superfamily that includes the bone morphogenetic proteins, activins, inhibins, and several other molecules that are morphogenic in early development. Though originally identified because of its ability to promote cellular transformation, TGF-β is now recognized as a multifunctional signaling molecule that can act both as an inhibitor and a stimulator of cell replication.[40,41]

TGF-β is present in multiple skeletal tissues including bone, precartilaginous mesenchyme, articular cartilage, and mineralizing cartilage.[42] However, growth plate chondrocytes, unlike articular chondrocytes and osteocytes, showed no evidence of TGF-β protein in bovine immunohistochemical studies[43] and, unlike osteoblasts and osteoclasts, showed only a low level of TGF-β mRNA in human in situ hybridization studies.[44] The observations that cultured avian growth plate chondrocytes express TGF-β mRNA[45] and secrete the peptide[46] leave open the possibility of an autocrine role for TGF-β in the growth plate.

Although the biologic effect of TGF-β on skeletal tissues has received considerable attention, the results of reported studies are not uniform. TGF-β has been reported both to stimulate[47] and to inhibit[48] DNA synthesis by growth plate chondrocytes. In some experiments, a mitogenic effect of TGF-β was observed at low concentrations, but this effect decreased at higher concentrations.[47] In addition, TGF-β may have different effects on chondrocytes from different anatomic sites. TGF-β has recently been found to stimulate proliferation of fetal human articular, but not costal, chondrocytes[49] in culture.

In vivo studies of TGF-β action confirm a biologic effect on the skeleton, but do not resolve the question of what its role or roles might be. Subperiosteal administration of TGF-β1 or TGF-β2 to newborn rats potently stimulated chondrogenesis, appearing to promote a chondroid phenotype.[50] In contrast, implantation of TGF-β into the developing limb of chick embryos reduced or blocked development of cartilaginous skeletal elements.[51] "Knock-out" of the TGF-β1 gene by homologous recombination in mice yielded homozygous mutants that were phenotypically indistinguishable from their littermates.[52]

Although at times seemingly contradictory, available data suggest that the effects of TGF-β on cells of the developing skeleton are determined in large measure by the cellular environment, by the conversion of latent TGF-β to active form, and, as discussed below, by the presence or absence of other cell signaling factors. Unlike IGF-I and IGF-II, TGF-β1 may not be required for early skeletal growth. Further studies will be required to establish the roles of the various TGF-β isoforms in this process.

Thyroid Hormones

Thyroid hormones play a critical role in skeletal growth and development as evidenced by the profound growth failure that occurs in thyroid hormone insufficiency. This growth failure reflects two distinct skeletal defects: diminished linear growth and delayed ossification. The reduced rate of growth is, at least in part, due to the growth hormone deficiency that occurs in the absence of normal thyroid stimulation of growth hormone production.[7,53] Growth hormone can restore chondrocyte proliferation and cartilage matrix production in thyroidectomized animals, but does not affect the maturation of cartilage leading to replacement by bone.[53] Thyroid hormone administered to thyroid-deficient children is able to accelerate bone growth to an extent sufficient for them to approach normal stature (so-called catch-up growth).[7] However, the observation that catch-up growth is progressively less complete with increasing duration of thyroid hormone insufficiency[54] suggests that there is a developmental window for optimal thyroid hormone effectiveness in the growth plate.

The importance of thyroid hormone to cartilage maturation is exemplified by the results of studies on the thyroidectomized rat. Thyroidectomy at 1 day of age resulted in a failure to increase bone age beyond 20 to 24 days, even if the animals lived to 140 days.[53] Data from in vitro studies have shown that triiodothyronine (T_3) stimulates alkaline phosphatase (an index of chondrocyte maturation) by growth plate cartilage, but not by nongrowth plate cartilage, and specifically increases the width of the zone of hypertrophic chondrocytes in the growth plate.[55] These data suggest an element of cell specificity of thyroid hormone action among different classes of chondrocytes.

Separate mechanisms appear to be involved in the regulation by thyroid hormone of chondrocyte proliferation and of chondrocyte maturation. Incubation of developing chick embryo cartilage with T_3 increased indices of cartilage anabolism (weight and protein synthesis) and also of chondrocyte maturation (alkaline phosphatase). The anabolic effect of T_3, but not its maturational effect, was blocked by an antibody against IGF-I.[56] These data suggest that the enhancement of cartilage growth by T_3 occurs through an IGF-I-related mechanism, whereas that of chondrocyte maturation is through an IGF-I independent mechanism.

Estrogens

The effect of estrogens on skeletal growth is principally one of inhibition. In vivo, estrogen administration reduces longitudinal growth and decreases growth plate width.[7] Interestingly, this inhibition occurs despite an estrogen-associated increase in growth hormone.[57] Estrogen also blocks the stimulatory effect of growth hormone on ^{35}S-sulfate incorporation into cartilage[58] and inhibits the increase in IGF-I produced by growth hormone. These data raise the possibility that the growth hormone–IGF-I axis may be involved in the action of estrogen on the skeleton.[59] The observation that estrogen treatment of young animals renders their growth plates similar to those of older animals has led to the suggestion that estrogen also hastens the aging process in epiphyseal cartilage.[53] The inhibitory or "aging" effect of estrogen on skeletal growth has been used clinically for some time in the treatment of tall girls with pharmacologic doses of estrogen to reduce their final adult height.[60,61] Despite these advances and applications, the mechanism of estrogen action on skeletal growth is not known.

Androgens

In contrast to estrogens, androgens tend to augment skeletal growth. Androgen deficiency causes a delay in growth plate maturation and closure at puberty that is associated with increased numbers of chondrocytes in the maturing zone of the growth plate and a delay in chondrocyte hypertrophy.[53,62] Conversely, androgen administration stimulates chondrocyte proliferation[63] and increases the number of dividing cells in the columnar region of the growth plate.[64] However, large doses of testosterone may reduce the ultimate length of bones and, thus, adult height by accelerating the rate of osseous maturation to a greater degree than the rate of longitudinal growth.[65,66]

The action of androgens on the skeleton, like that of estrogens, appears to involve the participation of growth hormone. Androgen administration in the face of growth hormone deficiency is ineffective in stimulating skeletal growth, but it becomes effective after growth hormone replacement.[7] As is the case for the estrogens, the mechanisms underlying these skeletal responses have not yet been determined.

Vitamin D

Vitamin D deficiency during skeletal development causes classic rickets, a hallmark of which is the disruption of normal endochondral ossification at the growth plate. The physis becomes widened because of the accumulation of hypertrophic chondrocytes and the failure of mineralization. Of the two principal vitamin D metabolites ($1,25$-dihydroxyvitamin D_3 and $24,25$-dihydroxyvitamin D_3), $1,25(OH)_2D_3$ was originally considered to be the active form based on studies of intestinal calcium absorption.[67] Subsequent studies with growth plate chondrocytes demonstrated that $24,25(OH)_2D_3$ could stimulate both DNA synthesis and ^{35}S-sulfate incorporation into proteoglycans by growth plate chondrocytes,[68,69] and recent work[70–73] has established that both metabolites play important roles in growth plate physiology.

One mechanism of vitamin D action on cartilage appears to enlist the participation of phospholipid metabolism and prostaglandin production. The $1,25(OH)_2D_3$ metabolite has recently been shown to stimulate the enzyme, phospholipase A_2, that generates free arachidonic acid and triggers prostaglandin synthesis. In contrast, $24,25(OH)_2D_3$ inhibits this enzyme.[70] It is noteworthy that the above effects were observed in resting zone cells and that neither metabolite influenced growth zone cells. In additional studies, $1,25(OH)_2D_3$ stimulated arachidonic acid turnover in growth zone, but not reserve zone, chondrocytes, whereas $24,25(OH)_2D_3$ stimulated turnover in resting zone cells while inhibiting it in growth zone cells.[71] Thus, these counterbalancing actions of vitamin D metabolites appear to depend on the stage of chondrocyte maturation. The actions of vitamin D extend down the cascade to the prostaglandins themselves. Prostaglandin E_2 production by growth zone cells was stimulated by $1,25(OH)_2D_3$, but unaffected by $24,25(OH)_2D_3$. In contrast, prostaglandin E_2 production by resting zone cells was not influenced by $1,25(OH)_2D_3$ and was inhibited by $24,25(OH)_2D_3$.[72] Another mechanism of vitamin D action may involve chondrocyte differentiation pathways: $1,25(OH)_2D_3$, but not $24,25(OH)_2D_3$, has been found to decrease the alkaline phosphatase activity of growth plate chondrocytes, suggesting an inhibition of differentiation.[73]

Taken together, these data indicate that vitamin D, in its two principal forms, exerts distinct, and at times opposing, actions on the growth of bone. These actions both influence and are themselves influenced by the maturational state of the target chondrocytes.

Retinoids

Vitamin A (retinol) and its congener, retinoic acid, have long been recognized as potent skeletal teratogens, capable of disrupting the pattern of normal skeletal development.[74,75] The extent of this morphogenic influence is exemplified by chick embryo studies in which retinoic acid, applied in vivo at the appropriate developmental stages, caused duplication of segments of the appendicular skeleton.[76] The importance of the retinoids to skeletal development has been emphasized by the recent popularity of vitamin A analogs in the treatment of skin disorders. Consumption of these compounds during pregnancy has resulted in fetal skeletal deformities that include synostoses; syndactylies; and malformations of the hip, ankle, and forearm.[77]

Although these two retinoids (retinol and retinoic acid) differ markedly in their effect on some tissues (eg, retina), both forms restore skeletal growth to vitamin A-deficient animals,[78] and both are similar, although not identical, in their stimulatory effects on DNA synthesis and inhibitory effects on collagen synthesis in calvarial cultures.[79] In cartilage cultures, retinoic acid profoundly influences matrix synthesis by down-regulating the type II collagen gene[80] and type II collagen protein synthesis[81] and by promoting mineralization-related cellular activity.[82]

Although the exact mechanism of retinoic acid action on the formation of the skeleton is uncertain, it is likely to involve a class of patterning genes known as *HOX* genes. The *HOX* gene family is involved in directing the spatial and temporal relationships between cells during development and has been ascribed a role in defining limb structure.[83] Recent studies using transgenic mice to reveal the endogenous expression of *HOX* genes demonstrated that several of them are regulated by retinoic acid in vivo.[84] These data support the view that *HOX* gene products mediate or modulate at least some of the early skeletal effects of the retinols.

Parathyroid Hormone

Although parathyroid hormone (PTH) is best known for its contribution to the regulation of inorganic matrix in mature bone, this hormone also plays a role in chondrocyte function. In vitro PTH stimulated both DNA and proteoglycan synthesis by chondrocytes, including those from the growth plate.[85–87] In vivo, in an immature chick model, PTH deficiency increased the collagen content of tibial epiphyseal cartilage but did not alter the content of the proteoglycan constituents hexosamine, glucosamine, and galactosamine. Treatment with PTH returned the collagen toward normal.[88]

One mechanism of PTH action is through a cascade of reactions involving phosphoinositides, a family of phospholipids that serve as intracellular messengers. PTH binding to its target cell activates the enzyme phospholipase C, which degrades phosphatidyl inositol 4,5-biphosphonate to inositol 1,4,5-triphosphate (IP_3) and diacylglycerol. IP_3 then augments the release of calcium from intracellular stores while diacylglycerol activates another phosphorylating enzyme, protein kinase C. Calcium and protein kinase C both trigger additional incompletely understood pathways to generate cellular responses.[89] Recent studies suggest that this cascade is involved in the regulation of proteoglycan synthesis by PTH in growth plate chondrocytes.[90]

Receptors

All of the cell-signaling molecules discussed above elicit their cellular effects by interacting with receptors on their target cells. Because these receptors are an essential component of the pathways governing cell function, an understanding of them is required for an understanding of cell regulation. A receptor is an information transducer; it converts information carried by a signaling molecule to a form usable by the cell. The presence or absence of a receptor determines whether or not a cell can respond to information in its environment. A receptor may add to the information carried by the signaling molecule by integrating the message with information from the intracellular or extracellular environment. The process of skeletal growth depends heavily on accurate intercellular communication of the information that enables coordinated cellular activities. Transmission of this information is the responsibility of such signaling molecules as growth factors, hormones, and vitamins. The receptors interpret these signals for the cells.

IGF-I Receptor

The IGF-I receptor is a large (>300 kd) complex formed by the disulfide linkage of four subunits. Two of these, termed alpha subunits, are located entirely outside the cell and together bind the IGF-I molecule. The other two subunits (beta subunits) cross the cell membrane. The intracellular portion of the beta subunits possesses tyrosine kinase activity (Fig. 2). This tyrosine kinase initiates a series of incompletely elucidated intracellular reactions that lead to cell activation.

Growth plate chondrocytes have IGF-I receptors[9-11] and respond to IGF-I in accordance with their ability to bind the growth factor.[21,22] Variation in the ability of growth plate chondrocytes from different zones to bind IGF-I[21] suggests that the contribution of IGF-I to the regulation of these cells may be controlled in part at the receptor level and may change during chondrocyte differentiation within the growth plate.

FGF Receptor

To date, four distinct FGF receptor genes have been identified.[91-94] All four receptors share the same general structure, which consists of three immuno-

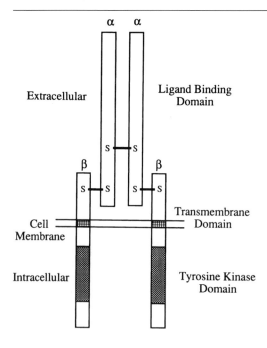

Fig 2 Schematic illustration of the insulin-like growth factor-I (IGF-I) receptor. Two extracellular alpha subunits (α) are linked by disulfide bonds (S-S) and are themselves linked to two beta subunits (β) that traverse the cell membrane (*hatched*). Extracellular IGF-I binds to the alpha subunits, activating the intracellular beta subunit tyrosine kinase (*shaded*) to initiate the cellular response.

globulin-like extracellular domains and an intracellular tyrosine kinase domain that is split by a short nonkinase region (Fig. 3). Thus, like the IGF-I receptor, the FGF receptor family is linked to intracellular pathways by tyrosine kinase activation. With one exception, all four receptors bind to the two major forms of FGF (acidic and basic),[94] but the differences in the biologic effects of these various binding combinations are not yet known.

That such receptors play a role in skeletal development is supported by the demonstration, using affinity labeling techniques, that growth plate chondrocytes possess at least two forms of the high-affinity FGF receptor [29] and that at least one form of FGF receptor is developmentally regulated, decreasing between the proliferative and the hypertrophic stages of chondrocyte maturation.[95]

The FGF receptors may not be the only class of cell-surface binding sites involved in mediating FGF action. Studies of bovine growth plate chondrocytes suggest that these cells bind bFGF not only by means of high affinity classic receptors, but also with a lower affinity, higher capacity class of heparin-like sites on the cell surface.[29] A heparan sulfate proteoglycan enables FGF to bind to its high-affinity receptors on endothelial cells.[96] Although the mechanism underlying this dual-site activation is not clear, it is plausible that the low-affinity site facilitates access of the ligand to its high-affinity receptor.

TGF-β Receptors

Receptors for TGF-β are members of a family that is distinct from the IGF-I and FGF receptor families in part in that it possesses serine and threonine kinase activity rather than tyrosine kinase activity. Thus far, two high-affinity TGF-β receptors have been identified.[97] An important advance in our understanding of the mechanism underlying TGF-β signal transduction is the recent observation that a TGF-β-activated serine/threonine kinase is involved in regulating the retinoblastoma gene product (Rb). The Rb protein is an important negative regulator of cell proliferation; its inhibitory effect is lost when the protein is phosphorylated. This phosphorylation was found to depend on TGF-β-activated serine/threonine kinase.[98] Thus, by blocking its phosphorylation in the early stages of cell division, TGF-β may control the important growth suppressive function of Rb protein. Similarly, Rb may represent a critical component of the TGF-β receptor mechanism of action.

Like the FGFs, the TGF-βs bind to cell surface molecules other than their classic receptors. Among these are a large proteoglycan termed betaglycan and at least four smaller membrane-anchored proteins. Although betaglycan binds well to both the TGF-β1 and TGF-β2 isoforms, binding by the other binding proteins appears to be highly isoform-specific.[97] The biologic roles of these presumably nonsignaling binding sites remain to be determined.

Nuclear Receptors: The Steroid Receptor Superfamily

The cellular actions of the steroid hormones (including the estrogens and androgens), the retinoids, the vitamin D_3 metabolites, and the thyroid hormones are governed by a large group of receptors that were initially distinguished from surface-membrane receptors by their cytoplasmic or nuclear location. The cloning of the genes encoding these receptors has revealed that they share a remarkably similar structure. The generic nuclear receptor consists of a ligand-binding domain, a DNA-binding domain, which is relatively conserved among all members of the superfamily, and a hypervariable region, whose homology among the different members is minimal (Fig. 4).

The presumed mechanism of action of these receptors is a ligand-induced conformational change in the receptor that alters the ability of its DNA-binding domain to interact with DNA. By binding to specific DNA sequences, called hormone response elements, in the regulatory portions of target genes, these receptors can cause either enhancement or inhibition of target gene expression. One example of this mechanism in the regulation of bone formation involves the vitamin D receptor and the osteocalcin gene. Osteocalcin is a protein syn-

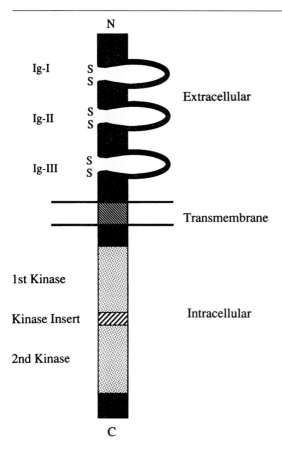

Fig. 3 Schematic representation of a typical FGF receptor. The extracellular region contains three disulfide (S-S) linked domains with structural homology to the immunoglobulins (Ig). The cytoplasmic region contains a kinase domain (*shaded*) that is split by a nonkinase insert.

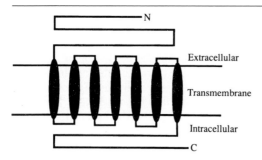

Fig. 4 Prototype of a G-protein-linked receptor. The receptor spans the cell surface membrane seven times, forming three intracellular loops that, with the COOH end (C), bind to intracellular G-proteins. Binding of the ligand (eg, PTH) to the extracellular region initiates the cellular response by catalyzing an intracellular reaction on the receptor-associated G-protein.

thesized by osteoblasts and frequently used as a marker for this cell type. The osteocalcin gene promoter contains a DNA sequence that is specifically recognized by the vitamin D receptor. When the vitamin D receptor binds to this DNA sequence (the vitamin D response element), the promoter is activated to increase osteocalcin gene expression.[99] Thus, the receptors belonging to this superfamily may be viewed as transcription factors that mediate their ligands' signals directly at the level of gene regulation. This bypasses the cascade of intracellular reactions employed by the cell-surface membrane-associated receptors.

The importance of the retinoic acid receptor (RAR) family in determining the development of the skeleton is well illustrated by the recent demonstration that the expression of three of the RAR subtypes correlates closely with the ultimate developmental fate of the tissue.[100] In situ hybridization of RAR transcripts in the mouse fetus revealed that cells expressing the RAR-γ subtype were those in the cartilaginous and skin lineages, those expressing the RAR-β subtype were destined for programmed cell death, and those expressing RAR-α were distributed widely, suggesting a more mundane housekeeping function.[100] These data suggest that the same ligand may exert quite different cellular effects on different cell populations by interacting with differentially expressed receptors.

PTH Receptor

The recent cloning of the PTH receptor[101] identified it as a member of the large family of receptors that transduce their signals through guanyl nucleotide-binding proteins (G-proteins).[102] The structure of this class of receptor differs from that of other membrane-associated peptide hormone receptors in its complex relationship to the cell surface membrane. These receptors are typically long molecules that repeatedly cross the cell membrane, winding their way in and out of the cell seven times between their COOH- and NH$_2$-terminal ends (Fig. 5).

PTH receptors have been de.nonstrated on rabbit costal chondrocytes. The number of receptors per cell was found to be over two times greater on growth cartilage cells than on resting cartilage cells,[103] and this number closely paralleled the synthesis of glycosaminoglycans when the chondrocytes were treated with factors that increased or decreased glycosaminoglycan synthesis.[104] These data are consistent with the hypothesis that the expression of the PTH receptor is, in part, a function of the stage of chondrocyte maturation.

IGF-II/Mannose-6-Phosphate Receptor

Perhaps the most unusual growth factor receptor yet identified in skeletal tissues is that for IGF-II. When the IGF-II receptor was cloned and sequenced, it un-

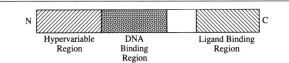

N — Hypervariable Region — DNA Binding Region — Ligand Binding Region — C

Fig. 5 Generic structure of the steroid hormone receptor superfamily. The hypervariable region of the receptors in this superfamily shares little (generally <15%) amino acid sequence homology. In contrast, the DNA binding region is relatively conserved with approximately 40% to 90% homology between receptors. The ligand binding domain occupies the COOH-terminal end (C) of the molecule and is separated by a spacer sequence from the DNA binding region.

expectedly proved to be the same molecule that had been previously identified as the cation-independent mannose-6-phosphate receptor, a molecule that binds and internalizes phosphorylated lysosomal enzymes.[104] The receptor is also used intracellularly to target newly synthesized lysosomal enzymes to lysozomes. This receptor is a large (>260 kd) single-chain molecule, which, on growth plate chondrocytes as well as other cell types, appears to contain intramolecular disulfide bonds, but unlike the IGF-I receptor, is not composed of disulfide linked subunits.[11] This receptor lacks kinase activity. Despite the known presence of IGF-II receptors on many cell types, the biologic role of IGF-II binding to this site has never been established. Although some studies have suggested that IGF-II can stimulate cell activity via its own receptor, most studies of IGF-II biologic effects argue that these effects are mediated by IGF-II binding to the IGF-I receptor.

The receptor has become even more intriguing with the observation that it may be directly linked to G-proteins,[106] The IGF-II receptor may, therefore, function by mediating IGF-II activation of G-protein-linked postreceptor pathways. However, other G-protein-linked receptors identified to date have multiple transmembrane spanning regions (usually seven) making the IGF-II receptor unique in this receptor class. It is also plausible, because the IGF-II receptor is the mannose-6-phosphate receptor, that IGF-II is involved in regulating lysosomal enzyme transport. Although these two seemingly unrelated ligands bind to different sites on the receptor molecule, each is able to modulate the binding of the other. Mannose-6-phosphate may increase IGF-II binding,[107] suggesting a stabilizing effect. However, binding of larger, mannose-6-phosphate-bearing enzymes inhibits IGF-II binding, and vice versa,[108] possibly due to steric hindrance.

Administration of IGF-II to growth plate chondrocytes in culture stimulates ^{3}H-thymidine incorporation into DNA (T Matsumura and associates, unpublished data). However, as with the in vivo effect of IGF-II on growth plate width,[26] the in vitro mitogenic effect of IGF-II on these cells requires relatively high doses of the growth factor to achieve the same effect attained with lower doses of IGF-I. Because IGF-II is able to bind to the growth plate chondrocyte IGF-I receptor, though with a lower affinity than IGF-I,[9-11] these data are consistent with an IGF-II action mediated by the IGF-I receptor. Further studies are needed to define the role of the IGF-II receptor in skeletal tissues.

Signaling Factor Interactions

Given the complexity of skeletal growth and the large number of factors involved in its regulation, there is little chance that these factors act in either temporal or spatial isolation. Therefore, to understand the mechanisms by which growth is regulated, it is necessary to determine if and how the various regulatory factors interact. However influential a factor may appear to be, its action in isolation may have little bearing on its usual role if other factors are present that alter its effect. Conversely, a factor with little evident effect in isolation may be highly significant as a modulator of some other regulating factor or factors. Recent studies focusing on the combined effects of cell regulators have begun to illuminate a wide variety of interactions, only a few of which can be discussed here.

IGF-I and bFGF

Both IGF-I and bFGF, acting individually, are potent mitogens for growth plate chondrocytes.[37] In contrast, IGF-I and bFGF appear to exert differing effects on matrix synthesis. Most studies indicate that IGF-I is much better than bFGF in stimulating sulfate incorporation into glycosaminoglycans.[37] Several studies have been undertaken to determine whether IGF-I interacts with FGF in regulating these chondrocyte functions. With respect to regulation of glycosaminoglycan synthesis, the addition of bFGF reduced the stimulatory effect of IGF-I in rat chondrocytes,[37] whereas in rabbit chondrocytes, the addition of IGF-I partly reversed the inhibition obtained with bFGF.[109] Thus, these factors may, under some circumstances, mitigate each other's effect on glycosaminoglycan synthesis. With respect to mitogenic activity, IGF-I and bFGF appear to have a very different relationship. Both are mitogens for growth plate chondrocytes. When used together, they either exerted no influence on each other[37,109] or were synergistic.[37,110] These studies suggest that IGF-I and bFGF interact to regulate skeletal growth. Such interactions offer a more versatile means of regulating cellular proliferation and matrix synthesis than would be afforded by two factors acting individually.

Thyroid Hormone and Growth Hormone

Both growth hormone and thyroid hormone are essential for normal skeletal growth. However, in animals that are deficient in both hormones, treatment with either growth hormone or thyroid hormone alone stimulates growth minimally, if at all. In contrast, administration of growth hormone and thyroid hormone together markedly augments growth.[7,111] These observations suggest an interdependence between these hormones in regulating development of the skeleton. The mechanism of this interaction is unclear, but appears to be multifactorial. First, thyroid hormone may increase the synthesis and secretion of growth hormone by the pituitary gland.[7] Second, thyroid hormone appears to augment growth hormone-generated increases in serum IGF-I.[111] Third, T_3 enhances the effect of IGF-I on cartilage growth[7] and fourth, T_3 increases IGF-I receptor mRNA levels in epiphyseal chondrocytes,[112] an effect that may account for the ability of T_3 to enhance IGF-I action.

The growth hormone–IGF-I axis and the thyroid hormones may regulate different components of the growth process. IGF-I appears to stimulate predominantly chondrocyte proliferation and matrix synthesis, whereas thyroid hormones appear to stimulate predominantly late chondrocyte maturation.[113] Indeed, T_3 has been found in epiphyseal chondrocytes to inhibit the increase in ^{3}H-thymidine incorporation caused by IGF-I, and IGF-I has been reported to inhibit the stimulatory effect of T_3 on chondrocyte alkaline phosphatase activity.[111] It is evident from these data that the thyroid hormones and growth hormone (with IGF-I) interact at several levels in regulating bone growth, and that these interactions, although not yet fully understood, are probably an essential part of normal growth regulation.

TGF-β and Retinoic Acid

The multifunctional character of TGF-β implies an interplay with other factors that influence its actions. Until such factors are identified, the seemingly contradictory results obtained with this peptide will remain difficult to interpret. For example, TGF-β caused a reduction or absence of skeletal elements when applied to developing chick limbs.[51] Yet, its administration to neonatal rat limbs or the later developing limb in the chick stimulated an excess of cartilage formation.[50,51] This modulation of the action of TGF-β may reflect, in part, the involvement of the retinoids, which, as noted previously, appear to help regulate skeletal morphologic development. The possibility that these factors are jointly involved in this process is supported by several recent studies.[114] Retinoic acid has been shown to increase the expression of TGF-β mRNA and protein in chondrocytes,[115] raising the possibility that some of the actions of retinoic acid may be mediated by TGF-β. In myocytes, this action was reversed: retinoic acid decreased the expression of TGF-β mRNA and TGF-β.[115] These data indicate that this relationship between retinoic acid and TGF-β is cell type-specific.

Although TGF-β and retinoic acid may function coordinately in some circumstances, their actions can also be antagonistic. TGF-β delivered in vivo caused shortening or deletion of skeletal elements during early limb development. In vitro, retinoic acid blocked the stimulation by TGF-β of protein synthesis while TGF-β decreased stimulation by retinoic acid of proteoglycan catabolism in articular cartilage organ cultures.[116]

Taken together, these data strongly suggest an interplay between the TGF-β and retinoic acid families of cell-signaling factors. The data also emphasize, by revealing the variability in the relationship between these substances, that this interplay is itself influenced by other factors.

Summary

Although much has been learned about the mechanisms regulating skeletal development, the understanding of this process is still in its infancy. A wide variety of factors, and something of their effects, are known, but there is little insight into the critically important interrelationships among these factors. Similarly, there has been considerable progress in identification and characterization of the receptors that mediate the cellular actions of these factors, but the postreceptor effector pathways that lead to the cell response remain largely uncharted.

As the knowledge base in these areas grows, it will become increasingly possible, and increasingly challenging, to accurately model the process of bone formation and growth. Existing models used in an attempt to describe relevant cellular control mechanisms (eg, the somatomedin hypothesis or the dual effector theory) are useful because they apply to some regulatory factors, but obviously are limited by their exclusion of other factors. Development of modeling methods and data repositories capable of integrating a body of knowledge that is rapidly becoming simultaneously richer, more dispersed, and more complex may enable therapeutic intervention in the regulation of these mechanisms.

References

1. DeLarco JE, Todaro GJ: Growth factors from murine sarcoma virus-transformed cells. *Proc Natl Acad Sci USA* 1978;75:4001–4005.
2. Seyedin SM, Thomas TC, Thompson AY, et al: Purification and characterization of two cartilage-inducing factors from bovine demineralized bone. *Proc Natl Acad Sci USA* 1985;82:2267–2271.
3. Evans HM, Long JA: The effect of the anterior lobe administered intraperitoneally on growth maturity and oestrous cycles of the rat. *Anat Rec* 1921;21:62–63.
4. Gertner JM, Genel M, Gianfredi SP, et al: Prospective clinical trial of human growth hormone in short children without growth hormone deficiency. *J Pediatr* 1984;104:172–176.
5. Salmon WD, Jr, Daughaday WH: A hormonally controlled serum factor which stimulates sulfate incorporation by cartilage in vitro. *J Lab Clin Med* 1957;49: 825–836.

6. Trippel SB: Role of insulin-like growth factors in the regulation of chondrocytes, in Adolphe M (ed): *Biological Regulation of the Chondrocytes*. Boca Raton, FL, CRC Press, 1992, pp 161–190.

7. Underwood LE, Van Wyk JJ: Normal and aberrant growth, in Wilson JD, Foster DW (eds): *Williams Textbook of Endocrinology*, ed 8. Philadelphia, PA, WB Saunders, 1992, pp 1079–1138.

8. McConaghey P, Sledge CB: Production of "sulphation factor" by the perfused liver. *Nature* 1970;225:1249–1250.

9. Trippel SB, Van Wyk JJ, Foster MB, et al: Characterization of a specific somatomedin-C receptor on isolated bovine growth plate chondrocytes. *Endocrinology* 1983;112:2128–2136.

10. Schalch DS, Sessions CM, Farley AC, et al: Interaction of insulin-like growth factor I/somatomedin-C with cultured rat chondrocytes: Receptor binding and internalization. *Endocrinology* 1986;118:1590–1597.

11. Trippel SB, Chernausek SD, Wan Wyk JJ, et al: Demonstration of type I and type II somatomedin receptors on bovine growth plate chondrocytes. *J Orthop Res* 1988;6:817–826.

12. Madsen K, Friberg U, Ross P, et al: Growth hormone stimulates the proliferation of cultured chondrocytes from rabbit ear and rat rib growth cartilage. *Nature* 1983;304:545–547.

13. Madsen K, Makower A-M, Friberg U, et al: Effect of human growth hormone on proteoglycan synthesis in cultured rat chondrocytes. *Acta Endocrinol* 1985;108: 338–342.

14. Eden S, Isaksson OG, Madsen K, et al: Specific binding of growth hormone to isolated chondrocytes from rabbit ear and epiphyseal plate. *Endocrinology* 1983; 112:1127–1129.

15. Isaksson OG, Jansson J-O, Gause IA: Growth hormone stimulates longitudinal bone growth directly. *Science* 1982;216:1237–1239.

16. Schlechter NL, Russell SM, Greenberg S, et al: A direct growth effect of growth hormone in rat hindlimb shown by arterial infusion. *Am J Physiol* 1986; 250:E231–235.

17. Skottner A, Clark RG, Robinson ICAF, et al: Recombinant human insulin-like growth factor: Testing the somatomedin hypothesis in hypophysectomized rats. *J Endocrinol* 1987;112:123–132.

18. Schlechter NL, Russell SM, Spencer EM, et al: Evidence suggesting that the direct growth-promoting effect of growth hormone on cartilage *in vivo* is mediated by local production of somatomedin. *Proc Natl Acad Sci USA* 1986;83:7932–7934.

19. Green H, Morikawa M, Nixon T: A dual effector theory of growth-hormone action. *Differentiation* 1985;29:195–198.

20. Zezulak KM, Green H: The generation of insulin-like growth factor I-sensitive cells by growth hormone action. *Science* 1986;233:551–553.

21. Trippel SB, Van Wyk JJ, Mankin HJ: Localization of somatomedin-C binding to bovine growth plate chondrocytes *in situ*. *J Bone Joint Surg* 1986;68A:897–903.

22. Trippel SB, Corvol MT, Dumontier MF, et al: Effect of somatomedin-C/insulin-like growth factor I and growth hormone on cultured growth plate and articular chondrocytes. *Pediatr Res* 1989;25:76–82.

23. Mathews LS, Hammer RE, Behringer RR, et al: Growth enhancement of transgenic mice expressing human insulin-like growth factor I. *Endocrinology* 1988; 123:2827–2833.

24. Quaife CJ, Mathews LS, Pinkert CA, et al: Histopathology associated with elevated levels of growth hormone and insulin-like growth factor I in transgenic mice. *Endocrinology* 1989;124:40–48.

25. Behringer RR, Lewin TM, Quaife CJ, et al: Expression of insulin-like growth factor I stimulates normal somatic growth in growth hormone-deficient transgenic mice. *Endocrinology* 1990;127:1033–1040.

26. Schoenle E, Zapf J, Hauri C, et al: Comparison of *in vivo* effects of insulin-like growth factors I and II and of growth hormone in hypophysectomized rats. *Acta Endocrinol* 1985;108:167–174.

27. DeChiara TM, Efstratiadis A, Robertson EJ: A growth-deficiency phenotype in heterozygous mice carrying an insulin-like growth factor II gene disrupted by targeting. *Nature* 1990;345:78–80.

28. Gospodarowicz D: Localisation of a fibroblast growth factor and its effect alone and with hydrocortisone on 3T3 cell growth. *Nature* 1974;249:123–127.

29. Trippel SB, Whelan MC, Klagsbrun M, et al: Interaction of basic fibroblast growth factor with bovine growth plate chondrocytes. *J Orthop Res* 1992;10:638–646.

30. Sullivan R, Klagsbrun M: Purification of cartilage-derived growth factor by heparin affinity chromatography. *J Biol Chem* 1985;260:2399–2403.

31. Kasper S, Friesen HG: Human pituitary tissue secretes a potent growth factor for chondrocyte proliferation. *J Clin Endocrinol Metab* 1986;62:70–76.

32. Gonzalez A-M, Buscaglia M, Ong M, et al: Distribution of basic fibroblast growth factor in the 18-day rat fetus: Localization in the basement membranes of diverse tissues. *J Cell Biol* 1990;110:753–765.

33. Hebert JM, Basilico C, Goldfarb M, et al: Isolation of cDNA's encoding four mouse FGF family members and characterization of their expression patterns during embryogenesis. *Dev Biol* 1990;138:454–463.

34. Bashkin P, Doctrow S, Klagsbrun M, et al: Basic fibroblast growth factor binds to subendothelial extracellular matrix and is released by heparitinase and heparin-like molecules. *Biochemistry* 1989;28:1737–1743.

35. Gospodarowicz D, Mescher AL: A comparison of the responses of cultured myoblasts and chondrocytes to fibroblast and epidermal growth factors. *J Cell Physiol* 1977;93:117–127.

36. Kato Y, Gospodarowicz D: Growth requirements of low-density rabbit costal chondrocyte cultures maintained in serum-free medium. *J Cell Physiol* 1984;120:354–363.

37. Trippel SB, Wroblewski J, Makower A-M, et al: Regulation of growth-plate chondrocytes by insulin-like growth factor I and basic fibroblast growth factor. *J Bone Joint Surg* 1993;75A:177–189.

38. Kato Y, Gospodarowicz D: Sulfated proteoglycan synthesis by confluent cultures of rabbit costal chondrocytes grown in the presence of fibroblast growth factor. *J Cell Biol* 1985;100:477–485.

39. Kato Y, Iwamoto M: Fibroblast growth factor is an inhibitor of chondrocyte terminal differentiation. *J Biol Chem* 1990;265:5903–5909.

40. Sporn MB, Roberts AB: Transforming growth factor-β: Recent progress and new challenges. *J Cell Biol* 1992;119:1017–1021.

41. Massague J, Cheifetz S, Laiho M, et al: Transforming growth factor-β. *Cancer Surv* 1992;12:81–103.

42. Kato Y: Roles of fibroblast growth factor and transforming growth factor-beta families in cartilage formation, in Adolphe M (ed): *Biological Regulation of the Chondrocytes*, Boca Raton, FL, CRC Press, 1992, pp 141–160.

43. Ellingsworth LR, Brennan JE, Fok K, et al: Antibodies to the N-terminal portion of cartilage-inducing factor A and transforming growth factor beta: Immunohistochemical localization and association with differentiating cells. *J Biol Chem* 1986;261:12362–12367.

44. Sandberg M, Vuorio T, Hirvonen H, et al: Enhanced expression of TGF-β and c-fos mRNAs in the growth plates of developing human long bones. *Development* 1988;102:461–470.

45. Crabb ID, Hughes SS, Hicks DG, et al: Non-radioactive *in situ* hybridization using digoxigenin-labeled oligonucleotides: Applications to musculoskeletal tissues. *Am J Pathol* 1992;141:579–589.

46. Gelb DE, Rosier RN, Puzas JE: The production of transforming growth factor-beta by chick growth plate chondrocytes in short term monolayer culture. *Endocrinology* 1990;127:1941–1947.

47. O'Keefe RJ, Puzas JE, Brand JS, et al: Effect of transforming growth factor-beta on DNA synthesis by growth plate chondrocytes: Modulation by factors present in serum. *Calcif Tissue Int* 1988;43:352–358.

48. Hiraki Y, Inoue H, Hirai R, et al: Effect of transforming growth factor-beta on cell proliferation and glycosaminoglycan synthesis by rabbit growth plate chondrocytes in culture. *Biochim Biophys Acta* 1988;969:91–99

49. Brenner RE, Nerlich A, Heinze E, et al: Different regulation of clonal growth by transforming growth factor-beta 1 in human fetal articular and costal chondrocytes. *Pediatr Res* 1993;33:390–393.

50. Joyce ME, Roberts AB, Sporn MB, et al: Transforming growth factor-beta and the initiation of chondrogenesis and osteogenesis in the rat femur. *J Cell Biol* 1990; 110:2195–2207.

51. Hayamizu TF, Sessions SK, Wanek N, et al: Effects of localized application of transforming growth factor-beta 1 on developing chick limbs. *Dev Biol* 1991;145: 164–173.

52. Shull MM, Ormsby I, Kier AB, et al: Targeted disruption of the mouse transforming growth factor-β1 gene results in multifocal inflammatory disease. *Nature* 1992;359:693–699.

53. Lebovitz HE, Eisenbarth GS: Hormonal regulation of cartilage growth and metabolism. *Vitam Horm* 1975;33:575–648.

54. Rivkees SA, Bode HH, Crawford JD: Long-term growth in juvenile acquired hypothyroidism: The failure to achieve normal adult stature. *N Engl J Med* 1988; 318:599–602.

55. Burch WM, Lebovitz HE: Triiodothyronine stimulates maturation of porcine growth plate cartilage *in vitro. J Clin Invest* 1982;70:496–504.

56. Burch WM, Van Wyk JJ: Triiodothyronine stimulates cartilage growth and maturation by different mechanisms. *Am J Physiol* 1987;252:E176–E182.

57. Strickland AL, Sprinz H: Studies of the influence of estradiol and growth hormone on the hypophysectomized immature rat epiphyseal cartilage growth plate. *Am J Obstet Gynecol* 1973;115:471–477

58. Herbai G: Studies on the site and mechanism of action of the growth inhibiting effects of estrogens. *Acta Physiol Scand* 1971;83:77–90.

59. Wiedemann E, Schwartz E: Suppression of growth hormone-dependent human serum sulfation factor by estrogen. *J Clin Endocrinol Metab* 1972;34:51–58.

60. Whitelaw MJ: Experiences in treating excessive height in girls with cyclic oestradiol valerate: A ten year survey. *Acta Endocrinol* 1967;54:473–484.

61. Bartsch O, Weschke B, Weber B: Oestrogen treatment of constitutionally tall girls with 0.1 mg/day ethinyl oestradiol. *Eur J Pediatr* 1988;147:59–63

62. Silberberg M, Silberberg R: Steroid hormones and bone, in Bourne GH (ed): *The Biochemistry and Physiology of Bone*, ed 2. New York, NY, Academic Press, 1971, vol III, pp 401–484.

63. Foss GL: The influence of androgen treatment on ultimate height in males. *Arch Dis Child* 1964;40:66–70.

64. Fahmy A, Lee S, Johnson P: Ultrastructural effects of testosterone on epiphyseal cartilage. *Calcif Tissue Res* 1971;7:12–22.

65. Howard E: Effects of steroids on epiphysiodiaphysial union in prepuberal mice. *Endocrinology* 1963;72:11–18.

66. Kelley VC, Ruvalcaba RHA: Use of anabolic agents in the treatment of short children. *Clin Endocrinol Metab* 1982;11:25–39.

67. Holick M, Schnoes HK, DeLuca HF: Identification of 1,25-dihydroxycholecalciferol, a form of vitamin D_3 metabolically active in the intestine. *Proc Natl Acad Sci USA* 1971;68:803–804.

68. Corvol MT, Dumontier MF, Garabedian M, et al: Vitamin D and cartilage. II. Biological activity of 25-hydroxycholecalciferol and 24,25- and 1,25-dihydroxycholecalciferols on cultured growth plate chondrocytes. *Endocrinology* 1978;102: 1269–1274.

69. Corvol MT, Ulmann A, Garabedian M: Specific nuclear uptake of 24,25-dihydroxycholecalciferol, a vitamin D_3 metabolite biologically active in cartilage. *FEBS Lett* 1980;116:273–276.

70. Schwartz Z, Boyan BD: The effects of vitamin D metabolites on phospholipase A_2 activity of growth zone and resting zone cartilage cells *in vitro*. *Endocrinology* 1988;122:2191–2198.

71. Swain LD, Schwartz Z, Boyan BD: 1,25-$(OH)_2D_3$ and 24,25-$(OH)_2D_3$ regulation of arachidonic acid turnover in chondrocyte cultures is cell maturation-specific and may involve direct effects on phospholipase A_2. *Biochim Biophys Acta* 1992; 1136:45–51.

72. Schwartz Z, Swain LD, Kelly DW, et al: Regulation of prostaglandin E_2 production by vitamin D metabolites in growth zone and resting zone chondrocyte cultures is dependent on cell maturation. *Bone* 1992;13:395–401.

73. Kato Y, Shimazu A, Iwamoto M, et al: Role of 1,25-dihydroxycholecalciferol in growth plate cartilage: Inhibition of terminal differentiation of chondrocytes *in vitro* and *in vivo*. *Proc Natl Acad Sci USA* 1990;87:6522–6526.

74. Cohlan SQ: Excessive intake of vitamin A as cause of congenital anomalies in the rat. *Science* 1953;117:535–536.

75. Kochhar DM: Teratogenic activity of retinoic acid. *APMIS* 1967;70:398–404.

76. Tickle C, Lee J, Eichele G: A quantitative analysis of the effect of all-trans-retinoic acid on the pattern of chick wing development. *Dev Biol* 1985;109:82–95.

77. Aulthouse AL, Carubelli CM, Dow TM, et al: Influence of retinol on human chondrocytes in agarose culture. *Anat Rec* 1992;232:52–59.

78. Dowling JE, Wald G: The role of vitamin A acid. *Vitam Horm* 1960;18:515–541.

79. Dickson IR, Walls J, Webb S: Vitamin A and bone formation: Different responses to retinol and retinoic acid of chick bone cells in organ culture. *Biochim Biophys Acta* 1989;1013:254–258.

80. Horton WE, Yamada Y, Hassell JR: Retinoic acid rapidly reduces cartilage matrix synthesis by altering gene transcription in chondrocytes. *Dev Biol* 1987;123:508–516.

81. Benya PD, Padilla SR: Modulation of the rabbit chondrocyte phenotype by retinoic acid terminates type II collagen synthesis without inducing type I collagen: The modulated phenotype differs from that produced by subculture. *Dev Biol* 1986;118:296–305.

82. Iwamoto M, Shapiro IM, Yagami K, et al: Retinoic acid induces rapid mineralization and expression of mineralization-related genes in chondrocytes. *Exp Cell Res* 1993;207:413–420.

83. Morgan BA, Izpisua-Belmonte J-C, Duboule D, et al: Targeted misexpression of Hox-4.6 in the avian limb bud causes apparent homeotic transformations. *Nature* 1992;358:236–239.

84. Marshall H, Nonchev S, Sham MH, et al: Retinoic acid alters hindbrain Hox code and induces transformation of rhombomeres 2/3 into a 4/5 identity. *Nature* 1992; 360:737–741.

85. Pines M, Hurwitz S: The effect of parathyroid hormone and atrial natriuretic peptide on cyclic nucleotides production and proliferation of avian epiphyseal growth plate chondroprogenitor cells. *Endocrinology* 1988;123:360–365.

86. Takano T, Takigawa M, Shirai E, et al: Effects of synthetic analogs and fragments of bovine parathyroid hormone on adenosine $3',5'$-monophosphate level, ornithine decarboxylase activity, and glycosaminoglycan synthesis in rabbit costal chondrocytes in culture: Structure-activity relations. *Endocrinology* 1985;116: 2536–2542.

87. Koike T, Iwamoto M, Shimazu A, et al: Potent mitogenic effects of parathyroid hormone (PTH) on embryonic chick and rabbit chondrocytes: Differential effects of age on growth, proteoglycan, and cyclic AMP responses of chondrocytes to PTH. *J Clin Invest* 1990;85:626–631.

88. Cipera JD, Cherian AG: Composition of epiphyseal cartilage. VI. Effect of parathyroidectomy and of a parathormone on the epiphyseal cartilage of growing chicks. *Calcif Tissue Res* 1969;3:30–37.

89. Abdel-Latif AA: Calcium-mobilizing receptors, polyphosphoinositides, and the generation of second messengers. *Pharmacol Rev* 1986;38:227–272.

90. Iannotti JP, Brighton CT, Iannotti V, et al: Mechanism of action of parathyroid hormone-induced proteoglycan synthesis in the growth plate chondrocyte. *J Orthop Res* 1990;8:136–145.

91. Lee PL, Johnson DE, Cousens LS, et al: Purification and complementary DNA cloning of a receptor for basic fibroblast growth factor. *Science* 1989;245:57–60.

92. Dionne CA, Crumley G, Bellot F, et al: Cloning and expression of two distinct high-affinity receptors cross-reacting with acidic and basic fibroblast growth factors. *EMBO J* 1990;9:2685–2692.

93. Keegan K, Johnson DE, Williams LT, et al: Isolation of an additional number of the fibroblast growth factor receptor family, FGFR-3. *Proc Natl Acad Sci USA* 1991;88:1095–1099.

94. Partanen J, Makela TP, Eercola E, et al: FGFR-4, a novel acidic fibroblast growth factor receptor with a distinct expression pattern. *EMBO J* 1991;10:1347–1354.

95. Iwamoto M, Shimazu A, Nakashima K, et al: Reduction of basic fibroblasts growth factor receptor is coupled with terminal differentiation of chondrocytes. *J Biol Chem* 1991;266:461–467.

96. Yayon A, Klagsbrun M, Esko JD, et al: Cell surface, heparin-like molecules are required for binding of basic fibroblast growth factor to its high affinity receptor. *Cell* 1991;64:841–848.

97. Massague J, Andres J, Attisano L, et al: TGF-beta receptors. *Mol Reprod Dev* 1992;32:99–104.

98. Ohtsuki M, Massague J: Evidence for the involvement of protein kinase activity in transforming growth factor-beta signal transduction. *Mol Cell Biol* 1992;12: 261–265.

99. Owen TA, Bortell R, Yocum SA, et al: Coordinate occupancy of AP-1 sites in the vitamin D-responsive and CCAAT box elements by Fos-Jun in the osteocalcin gene: Model for phenotype suppression of transcription. *Proc Natl Acad Sci USA* 1990;87:9990–9994.

100. Dolle P, Ruberte E, Kastner P, et al: Differential expression of genes encoding alpha, beta and gamma retinoic acid receptors and CRABP in the developing limbs of the mouse. *Nature* 1989;342:702–705.

101. Juppner H, Abou-Samra A-B, Freeman M, et al: A G protein-linked receptor for parathyroid hormone and parathyroid hormone-related peptide. *Science* 1991; 254:1024–1026.

102. Johnson GL, Dhanasekaran N: The G-protein family and their interaction with receptors. *Endocrine Rev* 1989;10:317–331.

103. Enomoto M, Kinoshita A, Pan H-O, et al: Demonstration of receptors for parathyroid hormone on cultured rabbit costal chondrocytes. *Biochem Biophys Res Comm* 1989;162:1222–1229.

104. Takigawa M, Kinoshita A, Enomoto M, et al: Effects of various growth and differentiation factors on expression of parathyroid hormone receptors on rabbit costal chondrocytes in culture. *Endocrinology* 1991;129:868–876.

105. Morgan DO, Edman JC, Standring DN, et al: Insulin-like growth factor-II receptor as a multifunctional binding protein. *Nature* 1987;329:301–307.

106. Nishimoto I, Murayama Y, Katada T, et al: Possible direct linkage of insulin-like growth factor-II receptor with guanine nucleotide-binding proteins. *J Biol Chem* 1989;264:14029–14038.

107. Roth RA, Stover C, Hari J, et al: Interactions of the receptor for insulin-like growth factor II with mannose-6-phosphate and antibodies to the mannose-6-phosphate receptor. *Biochem Biophys Res Commun* 1987;149:600–606.

108. Kiess W, Thomas CL, Greenstein LA, et al: Insulin-like growth factor-II (IGF-II) inhibits both the cellular uptake of beta-galactosidase and the binding of beta-galactosidase to purified IGF-II/mannose 6-phosphate receptor. *J Biol Chem* 1989; 264:4710–4714.

109. Nataf V, Tsagris L, Dumontier MF, et al: Modulation of sulfated proteoglycan synthesis and collagen gene expression by chondrocytes grown in the presence of bFGF alone or combined with IGF-I. *Reprod Nutr Dev* 1990;30:331–342.

110. Hiraki Y, Inoue H, Kato Y, et al: Combined effects of somatomedin-like growth factors with fibroblast growth factor or epidermal growth factor in DNA synthesis in rabbit chondrocytes. *Mol Cell Biochem* 1987;76:185–193.

111. Wolf M, Ingbar SH, Moses AC: Thyroid hormone and growth hormone interact to regulate insulin-like growth factor-I messenger RNA and circulating levels in the rat. *Endocrinology* 1989;125:2905–2914.

112. Ohlsson C, Nilsson A, Isaksson O, et al: Effects of tri-iodothyronine and insulin-like growth factor-I (IGF-I) on alkaline phosphatase activity, ^{3}H-thymidine incorporation and IGF-I receptor mRNA in cultured rat epiphyseal chondrocytes. *J Endocrinol* 1992;135:115–123.

113. Bohme K, Conscience-Egli M, Tschan T, et al: Induction of proliferation or hypertrophy of chondrocytes in serum-free culture: The role of insulin-like growth factor-I, insulin, or thyroxine. *J Cell Biol* 1992;116:1035–1042.

114. Roberts AB, Sporn MB: Mechanistic interrelationships between two superfamilies: The steroid/retinoid receptors and transforming growth factor-beta. *Cancer Surv* 1992;14:205–220.

115. Jakowlew SB, Cubert J, Danielpour D, et al: Differential regulation of the expression of transforming growth factor-beta mRNAs by growth factors and retinoic acid in chicken embryo chondrocytes, myocytes, and fibroblasts. *J Cell Physiol* 1992;150:377–385.

116. Morales TI, Roberts AB: The interaction between retinoic acid and the transforming growth factors-beta in calf articular cartilage organ cultures. *Arch Biochem Biophys* 1992;293:79–84.

Chapter 5

Physical and Environmental Influences on Bone Formation

Clinton Rubin, PhD
Ted Gross, PhD
Henry Donahue, PhD
Farshid Guilak, PhD
Kenneth McLeod, PhD

Introduction

In the normal adult, the morphology of the skeleton represents a complex interdependent balance between its structural responsibilities (strength), the metabolic advantages inherent in tissue economy (efficiency), and its use as the body's principal mineral reservoir (survival). Ultimately, the structural success of the skeleton can be considered a product of the bone tissue's capacity to recognize some aspect of its physical environment as a stimulus for the formation and retention of tissue in spite of the persistent presence of strong resorptive factors. This formation/resorption optimization process entails a constant struggle between many systemically based osteolytic factors (eg, parathyroid hormone, vitamin D, interleukin-6) aimed at releasing calcium from the skeleton, and biophysical (mechanical/electrical) stimuli acting as potent, local osteogenic factors.

The ability of the skeleton to adapt to its functional demands was formally proposed a century ago, outlined in Julius Wolff's 1892 treatise, which hypothesized that the form and function of bone is a product of alterations in its internal architecture according to "self-ordered" mathematical rules.[1] The basic premise of Wolff's Law, that bone remodeling tends towards optimizing (minimal mass/maximal strength) structural criteria of the skeleton, has gained wide acceptance by bone biologists, bioengineers, physicians, and surgeons. However, controversies abound with regard to identification of those components of the biophysical regimen that mediate the modeling/remodeling process, confounding the potential application of biophysical "growth factors" to the treatment of skeletal disorders.

The search for the osteogenic components of the biophysical milieu has benefited from both qualitative and quantitative observations of the skeleton's response to changes in its functional environment. The sensitivity of the skeleton to physical and environmental stimuli is readily evident in clinically based studies that have shown the skeleton's response to whole body exercise,[2,3] local adaptation to selective exercise,[4,5] reductions in gravitational force,[6,7] bed rest,[8] and remodeling adjacent to implants.[9,10] Although these studies succeed in demonstrating the extreme sensitivity of the skeleton to function, the difficulty in accurately defining the complex loading history of the bone under study makes it essentially impossible to isolate and identify the osteoregulatory component of the physical milieu.

To address these limitations, many experimental and computational models have been developed to study physical influences on bone formation. However, each model supports a specific parameter of the mechanical milieu as responsible for controlling bone morphology. These osteoregulatory factors include strain magnitude,[11-13] the fabric tensor,[14] strain frequency,[15,16] circumferential strain gradients,[17] strain rate,[18,19] electrokinetics,[20] piezoelectricity,[21] fluid flow,[22] strain history,[23] and strain energy density.[24-26] Although many of these models show powerful correlations to site-specific skeletal architecture (eg, transverse sections of the ulna, sagittal section of the proximal femur), none have demonstrated a comprehensive ability to predict and/or control bone morphology. The failure to identify a unifying theory for the biophysical control of bone remodeling may be exacerbated by the presumption that structural efficiency (minimal skeletal strain concomitant with minimal skeletal mass) is the ultimate objective of bone adaptation. Indeed, there is accumulating evidence that minimization of neither bone tissue nor functional strain is achieved.[16,17,26-30] Certainly, for improved understanding of Wolff's Law, it is necessary to consider not only the bioengineering disadvantages of a strained structure, but also the biologic advantages inherent in a tissue exposed to functional levels of strain.

Structural Demands Made on the Skeleton

Even considering the diverse design and function of vertebrates, the primary mechanical role of the skeletal organ is to resist the loads and moments that arise during function. At the level of the tissue these loads and moments result in deformation, which is described using the dimensionless parameter strain. In one dimension, strain is defined by a change in length of an object divided by its original length ($\Delta L/L$). Whether considering a mandible in a macaque, a humerus in a tennis player, a femur in a kangaroo, or a vertebra in a whale, the osteoblast/osteocyte syncytium is exposed to the functionally induced strain in the matrix (eg, chewing, serving, hopping, or swimming). The universal and persistent presence of mechanical strain in the functionally loaded skeleton identifies strain as a reasonable and efficient means of translating the level of activity into a site-specific, generic signal relevant to the cells responsible for osteoregulation (Fig. 1). The increased cortical thickness of the humerus in the serving arm of tennis players[4] or the rapid decline of bone mineral in the postcranial skeleton that parallels bed rest[8] or spaceflight,[6] qualitatively demonstrates the potent influence of biophysical stimuli on the skeleton. To quantitatively address the role of biophysical stimuli in establishing the morphology of the skeleton, it is first important to quantify the type of mechanical signals the skeleton is normally exposed to, a goal achieved by attaching strain gauges directly to a bone in vivo.[31] This technique permits an evaluation of the bone strain at the site to which the gauge is attached; however, a full characterization of the strain "history" can be achieved by using three rosette strain gauges attached around the bone's circumference. This technique permits determination of the distribution of normal and shear strain, as well as the sites of greatest (and least) strains.[32] These in vivo strain gauge measurements have permitted a number of critical observations to be made regarding the structural demands made on the skeleton.

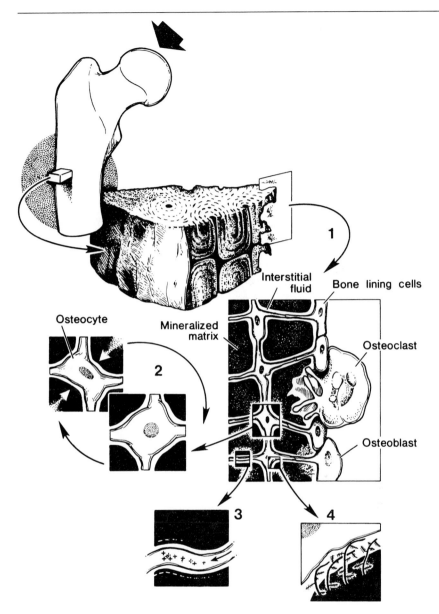

Fig. 1 Possible means of transmitting the functional milieu from the level of the organ to the level of the cell. Regardless of animal, skeletal site, or functional activity, all forces and moments are transduced through the bone organ and perceived at the level of the bone tissue as strain (1). The cell population, consisting of osteocytes (maintenance), osteoblasts (deposition), and osteoclasts (resorption), works to achieve the complex balance between a structurally-appropriate bone morphology and a suitable level of mineral. The mechanism of interaction could occur via (2) strain-induced deformation of the entrapped osteocyte or lining cell; (3) electrokinetic potentials caused by strain-induced flow of charged interstitial fluids past ionic constituents of the mineral phase; or (4) a strain-induced distortion of specific components of the cell/matrix complex (eg, proteoglycan, osteonectin). (Reproduced with permission from Rubin CT, McLeod KJ, Bain SD: Functional strains and cortical bone adaptation: Epigenetic assurance of skeletal integrity. *J Biomech* 1990;23:43–54.)

There is little argument that, for the skeleton to succeed as a structure, bone must avoid approaching the tissue's yield strain of approximately 0.7% (6,800 microstrain, με).[33] Peak strain magnitudes measured in a range of vertebrates, including horse, human, rat, sheep, goose, goat, pig, macaque, turkey, sunfish, lizard, cockerel, and dog, are remarkably similar, ranging in amplitude from 2,000 to 3,500 με (Table 1). This "dynamic strain similarity" suggests that the morphology of the skeleton adjusts in such a way that functional activity elicits a very specific (and perhaps beneficial) level of strain to the bone tissue.[28] Even considering the strong similarity in peak bone strain magnitudes, which presumably is achieved by a common cellular mechanism, any cell embedded within a matrix subject to 2,000 με will be deformed only a very small amount, on the order of angstroms (Fig. 2). Clearly, whatever intra- or intercellular mechanisms are responsible for evaluating and responding to the mechanical milieu of the skeleton must be exceedingly sensitive.

Considering the similarity in peak strain magnitudes across vertebrates, research directed toward defining the bone's overall strain history has focused on correlating bone morphology to the predominant characteristics of the bone's mechanical environment, including peak strain magnitude, peak strain rate, total strain energy density, and number of peak loading cycles. Many theoretical predictions of bone remodeling can accurately describe changes in bone morphology; however, they often are based on a premise of a homogenous strain history across the cortex.[14,24,25,34,35] In other words, over the course of a step or stride each area of the cortex is assumed to be subject to the same strain energy, and, therefore, the same strain stimulus. However, the in vivo strain gauge data show that the distribution of normal and shear strains, as well as strain energy density, are extremely nonuniform.[32]

Table 1 Peak strain magnitudes in vertebrates

Bone	Activity	Peak Strain*	Safety Factor**
Horse radius	Trotting	−2800	2.4
Horse tibia	Galloping	−3200	2.1
Horse metacarpus	Accelerating	−3000	2.3
Dog radius	Trotting	−2400	2.8
Dog tibia	Galloping	−2100	3.2
Goose humerus	Flying	−2800	2.4
Cockerel ulna	Flapping	−2100	3.2
Sheep femur	Trotting	−2200	3.1
Sheep humerus	Trotting	−2200	3.1
Sheep radius	Galloping	−2300	3.0
Sheep tibia	Trotting	−2100	3.2
Pig radius	Trotting	−2400	2.8
Fish hypural	Swimming	−3000	2.3
Macaca mandible	Biting	−2400	2.8
Turkey tibia	Running	−2350	2.0

*Measured by bone-bond strain gauges during the functional activity that elicited the highest record strains.
**Calculated based on a value of 6,800 microstrain for yield tensile strain.[33]
(Adapted with permission from Rubin CT, Lanyon LE: Dynamic strain similarity in vertebrates: An alternative to allometric limb bone scaling. *J Theor Biol* 1984;107: 321–327.)

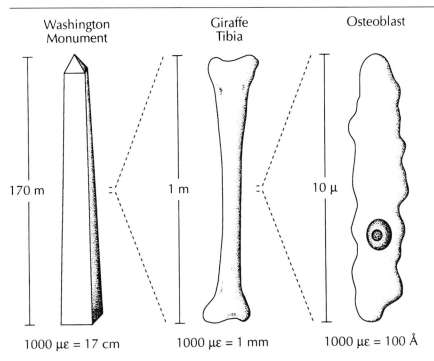

Washington Monument

Giraffe Tibia

Osteoblast

170 m

1 m

10 μ

1000 με = 17 cm

1000 με = 1 mm

1000 με = 100 Å

Fig. 2 Strain is defined as a (load-induced) change in length relative to the structure's original length. In this diagram, 1,000 microstrain (με), or 0.1% strain, is used to represent the amount of strain typically seen in bone tissue during an activity such as walking.[28,36] For a structure such as the 170-m Washington Monument, 1,000 με would represent a 17-cm change in length over the entire structure. In a 1-m giraffe tibia, the same strain would reflect a 1-mm change in the bone's length. At the level of a 10-μm bone lining cell within the periosteum of the giraffe tibia, 1,000 με would result in a dimensional change of 100 Å.

Another persistent presumption of this analytic work is that the tissue will optimize skeletal morphology by simultaneously minimizing peak strains and total bone mass. However, like that of homogenous strain distribution, this assumption is not strongly supported by in vivo data. For example, in the appendicular skeleton, the predominant (>85%) component of strain is generated by bending, although far less bone mass would be required to support the same loads if the bone were loaded axially.[27,36,37] Indeed, a significant portion of the cortex is subject to longitudinal tension, and that area of the cortex near the neutral axis experiences very low strain levels. Nevertheless, bone tissue is retained in these sites far removed from the area of the cortex subject to the peak strains.[17,29]

At one level, these in vivo strain recordings lend support to analytic models that presuppose a common structural objective for the skeleton: to confine the peak strains in the bone tissue to below 4,000 με. However, the high degree of bending and the consistent nonuniformity of the strain distribution contradict such presumptions and, instead, suggest bone cells in different regions of the cortex are differentially sensitive to strain. Some cells strive to 3,000 με in compression; some to 1,500 με in tension; others, near the neutral axis, are content with strains of 50 or 100 με. Alternatively, strain information could be spatially integrated via a cell network facilitated by gap junction intercellular communication,[38] such that the area of the cortex subject to only 100 $\mu\varepsilon$ resists resorption because it receives sufficient homeostatic signals from adjacent areas subject to much higher strain. This "information integration" perspective is supported by the observation that the bone loss that parallels disuse occurs uniformly about the cortex and through the diaphysis, even though the net change in bone strain caused by the absence of function varies widely.[39]

It could also be argued that a uniform strain stimulus is achieved via temporal, rather than spatial, integration of strain information. Such a time-dependent strain memory in bone cell networks has already been demonstrated.[40] A homogenous strain signal could be achieved over the course of time by ensuring all areas of the cortex are subject, at one point or another, to the peak strain milieu.[35] However, this presumption is not consistent with in vivo data, which demonstrate that the inhomogeneity of the strain distribution evident at any given time becomes even more disparate as the strain energy is summed over the course of a stride.[32]

Perhaps the design criteria that drive analytic models of bone adaptation rely too heavily on engineering principles for structural optimization. Because bone is as much a tissue as a structure, it is important to consider the possibility that some biologic benefit may also be derived from biophysical stimuli. Indeed, tissue viability may depend on some aspect of the mechanical milieu that is not rooted in minimal strain/minimal mass criteria, such as strain-dependent perfusion, fluid-mediated electric potentials, or a muscle-induced strain oscillation in the bone tissue. This latter mechanism allows for a single generic strain signal at the level of the cell, regardless of location or intensity of the activity.[15,41] The theory was formulated following the observation of a species-independent band of strain energy in functionally loaded bone. In strain data collected from mammal, bird, and reptile, a "high" frequency, low magnitude strain energy persisted in the functional strain spectra, including those of standing and chewing.[16]

It is clear that the reaction forces due to locomotion give rise to relatively large strains at fundamental frequencies from 1 to 10 Hz; however, spectral analysis of these strain recordings shows that distinct energy components are also evident in the 15 to 50 Hz range. Although the frequencies of the fundamental and harmonics change substantially as a function of speed and gait, these higher frequency strains remain confined to the original, narrow frequency band, independent of the animal, its size, or its speed of travel. In fact, the major change that occurs in this high frequency strain component is an increase in its amplitude as a function of speed. High frequency, low magnitude strains should not be considered a panacea for the control of bone remodeling based simply on their existence in the skeleton; their presence is raised to promote different perspectives on how the skeleton might interpret its functional milieu.

In summary, it is apparent via spaceflight and exercise programs that the skeleton is extremely sensitive to mechanical information. Further, the skeleton is subject to a wide range of mechanical signals, from compressive to tensile strain, and the cortex is subject to a complex, nonuniform distribution of strain history. Finally, it is clear that the cells within the matrix are subject not only to mechanical parameters such as strain and strain energy, but also to derivatives of tissue deformation such as streaming potentials and fluid flow, which may play an important role in mediating an adaptive response. Which specific parameter of this complex biophysical milieu is responsible for communicating with the cell population remains unknown.

Modulation of Bone Tissue by Mechanical Stimuli

One of the most efficient ways to study adaptive remodeling is through animal models in which the mechanical environment can accurately be controlled. Investigations designed to identify those components of the mechanical milieu that regulate skeletal adaptation have involved a number of experimental approaches, including stress protection adjacent to implants of varied stiffness,[42,43] overload caused by osteotomy,[33,44] and externally applied loading.[13,45–47] Although these applied loading experiments have contributed to the understanding of adaptation, they also have distinct limitations, the greatest of which is that the loads are applied for a limited, arbitrarily chosen period of time, and, for the remainder of the day, the animals are able to apply uncontrolled loading to the bone under investigation.

To ensure that the remodeling observed is uniquely the product of those parameters that are applied and to extinguish those strains that occur during the unmonitored activity of the animal, it becomes essential that the bone be exposed to minimal spurious loading events. These requirements have been met through several different animal models, ranging from the loading of cancellous bone in the distal femur of canines,[19] to the loading of tail vertebrae in the rat.[48] In our laboratory, we have studied the adaptation of cortical bone to biophysical stimuli using the functionally isolated avian ulna.[29] The advantage of this model is that the bone tissue is subject only to the mechanical or electrical regimen prescribed by the investigators, with no aberrant biophysical signals entering the preparation. In this model, the left ulna of the adult male turkey is functionally isolated by proximal and distal epiphyseal osteotomies, leaving the entire diaphyseal shaft undisturbed. Caps filled with methylmethacrylate are placed over the ends of the bones, and percutaneous transfixing pins are placed through the caps.

This model has demonstrated that 8 weeks of functional isolation alone will consistently result in a 10% to 15% loss of bone, whereas an externally applied mechanical strain regimen, physiologic in strain magnitude, will lead to significant increases in cross-sectional bone area. More specifically, alterations in bone mass, turnover, and internal replacement are sensitive to changes in the magnitude,[49] distribution,[26] and rate of strain[15] generated within the bone tissue. Further, a loading regimen must be dynamic (intermittent) in nature; static loads do not influence bone morphology.[50] However, the full osteogenic potential of a large amplitude (2,000 $\mu\varepsilon$) regimen is realized following only an extremely short exposure to this stimulus.[51] Moreover, the cells that regulate bone morphology appear able to differentiate hydrostatic from deviatoric stresses, ie, normal and shear strains have distinct osteoregulatory roles.[52] The immediate response of bone to extremely osteogenic signals is generation of woven bone; however, if the signal persists, this disorganized, hypercellular bone will remodel into lamellar bone (Fig. 3).[53] Although it is commonly dismissed as an aberrant pathologic response,[11,12] the generation of woven bone appears to be a timely and effective strategy to rapidly accommodate a new loading milieu. Finally, systemic distress such as age,[54] calcium deficiency,[55] or endocrine imbalance[56] will dramatically compromise the osteogenic nature of a mechanical stimulus (Fig. 4).

Strain levels that are homeostatic in one location induce adaptive remodeling in other locations,[26,29] supporting the hypothesis that each region of each bone is genetically programmed to accept a particular amount and pattern of strain as normal. Deviation from this optimal strain environment stimulates changes

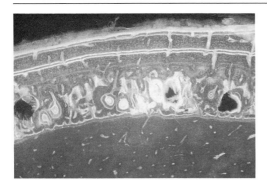

Fig. 3 Fluorescent photomicrograph showing the periosteal surface of a turkey ulna diaphysis after 16 weeks of a mechanical regimen sufficient to cause a peak of 2,000 microstrain. Remnants of the original woven response can be seen serving as interstitial elements of primary and secondarily remodeled bone. In this case, at least, the woven bone response serves as a strategic stage in the achievement of a structurally appropriate increase in bone mass. (Reproduced with permission from Rubin CT, Gross TS, McLeod KJ, et al: Morphologic stages in lamellar bone formation stimulated by potent osteogenic stimuli. *J Bone Miner Res*, in press.)

in the bone's remodeling balance, resulting in an adaptive increase or decrease in its mass. It is not yet clear whether the discrepancy in strain is picked up at the level of each individual osteocyte, which would then manipulate its own interactions with the matrix immediately adjacent to it, or whether the osteocyte network somehow spatially integrates the load information across the cortex, allowing tissue in low loaded regions to retain its mass despite the minimal stimulus. What is clear is that the complexity of the mechanical milieu, even in these carefully controlled animal models, may preclude the identification of the osteogenic component of the biophysical realm.

Mediating Bone Formation with Electrical Signals

The mechanical data described above demonstrate a distinct relationship of function to form, but they do not suggest the means by which the physical signal is interpreted and transformed by the cell into the adaptive process. From one perspective, it may well be the actual deformation of the cell that regulates the response,[57] but considering that, in bone at least, these deformations are on the order of a few angstroms, it seems wise to consider alternatives to strain of the cell per se. One possible mechanism for the coupling of mechanical deformation to cellular activity is strain-induced movement of interstitial fluid in the bone, similar to the water flow through a sponge caused either by stretching or squeezing. While strain-induced fluid flow certainly will contribute to increased nutrient and metabolite transport, this fluid movement also will cause an electrokinetic interaction with the bone tissue.

The potential role of electricity in the regulation of bone tissue was first considered 40 years ago with the report of electrical currents being generated with the loading of dry bone.[58] The discovery of load-induced piezoelectric potentials in bone provided a means by which stress or strain could intrinsically alter the biophysical environment of the bone cell and, thus, influence proliferation and differentiation.[21] This hypothesis became even more attractive when it was demonstrated that, in wet bone, two sources of electrical current existed in parallel: piezoelectric currents, induced by the deformation of collagen, and the relatively large electrokinetic currents (streaming potentials),

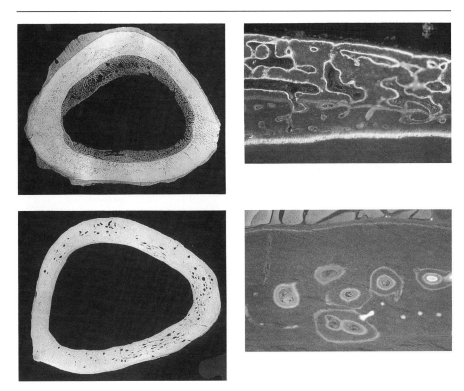

Fig. 4 Top left, Microradiograph of the osteogenic response of the ulna from a 1-year-old skeletally mature turkey (epiphyses fused) following 8 weeks of an applied mechanical regimen sufficient to cause peak normal strains of 3,000 microstrain. Substantial bone formation has been stimulated on both the periosteal and endosteal surfaces, while the intracortical response (porosis) is minimal. **Top right**, Fluorescent photomicrograph of the periosteal surface shows active deposition of bone on the surface, with essentially no intracortical turnover. **Bottom left**, Microradiograph showing lack of response to identical load regimen in a 3-year-old animal. **Bottom right**, Fluorescent photomicrograph of 3-year-old animal, taken from the same area as that of the 1-year-old animal, shows essentially no periosteal response but demonstrates active intracortical turnover. (Reproduced with permission from Rubin CT, Bain SD, McLeod KJ: Suppression of the osteogenic response in the aging skeleton. *Calcif Tissue Int* 1992;50:306–313.)

produced by the strain-induced flow of charged constituents of extracellular fluids flowing past the mineral phase of the matrix.[59,60]

Measurement of the electric potentials generated by functional levels of strain shows the average field intensities in bone are quite small, on the order of 1 microvolt per microstrain (1 $\mu V/\mu\epsilon$).[61] The adult skeleton is seldom subject to strains exceeding 4,000 $\mu\epsilon$;[28,62] therefore, if endogenous fields are to influence bone morphology they must do so at field intensities below 4mV/cm. This field intensity, in and of itself, is certainly sufficient to perturb a membrane potential of an osteoblast to the point of having some biologic effect.[63] However, a large percentage of bone tissue is rarely subject to strains greater than 500 $\mu\epsilon$,[32] yet bone mass is retained in these areas. Therefore, if each cell at each site of the bone is responsible for its own assessment of the physical milieu in its adjacent matrix, fields of 500 $\mu V/cm$, 50% below the 1mV/cm threshold often considered the low end of biologic "relevance," must represent some regulatory role.

The most efficient means of examining the potential influence of electric fields on bone formation is to begin with the electrical signals used for human skeletal disorders.

Since 1975, electrical signals have been used in the clinic for the treatment of delayed unions.[64] The majority of the signals used for pseudoarthroses, delayed union, and even osteonecrosis are complex pulsed electromagnetic fields (PEMFs), which exogenously induce electrical energy into tissue over a broad frequency range (1 to $> 10^6$ Hz).[65] It is important to emphasize that the use of electricity in the clinic remains extremely controversial, with physician camps strongly in support of its use and many who remain unconvinced of its benefit.[66] Principal issues in the pro/con electricity feud include inconsistent efficacy, weak scientific arguments justifying the use of a complex waveform, and, at the level of the cell, the poor experimental support for any of the proposed mechanisms of field interaction.

With the goal of identifying the osteogenic components of the PEMF, we investigated how changes in PEMF characteristics would affect a skeletal remodeling response. In the first series of experiments, electromagnetic fields were induced in the turkey ulna model of disuse osteopenia using Helmholtz coil pairs strapped to the wing of the animal.[67] While keeping the peak intensity of the magnetic fields constant and varying the rise time of the waves, both the PEMF waveshape and, correspondingly, the power of the induced electric field were changed. Exposing the turkey ulna preparation to 1 h/day of subtle variations of the clinical PEMF waveforms established a dose:response curve of bone formation versus the power of the induced electric field. The maximum osteogenic effect was seen at field induction levels between 0.01 and 0.04 Tesla^2/s. In contrast to the 11% loss of bone caused by 8 weeks of disuse, these waveforms stimulated an increase in bone area reaching 12%; this is a net benefit over disuse exceeding 20%. Power levels above or below this range were less effective in generating bone formation and, in some cases, even were incapable of inhibiting bone loss. This dose:response "window" emphasizes that electricity, like any other prophylaxis, must be used with great caution; simply applying a "field" is sufficient neither to stimulate a response nor to justify its use in the clinic.

The wide range of bone tissue responses to slight variations of the PEMF signal (all of which kept the magnetic field constant) suggested that some temporal component of the electric field was responsible for modulating the adaptive response. Spectral analysis of the PEMF signals indicated that, even though the frequencies of the PEMFs ranged from 1 Hz to 250 kHz, the component of the field that correlated most strongly with the PEMF's ability to stimulate new bone formation was the field energy induced at frequencies below 75 Hz.[41] The osteogenic preference for this low-frequency bandwidth was evident even though less than 0.1% of the total PEMF energy was contained in this region. This analytically defined low-frequency affinity was experimentally validated in subsequent studies, with a sinusoidal field induced at 15 Hz appearing to be the most potently osteogenic.[68] Even though this signal was induced at the fundamental frequency (first energy as a function of frequency) of the clinical PEMF and contained one thousandth of its total power, this simple, low frequency (15 Hz) signal was fully 50% more effective in stimulating new bone formation (20.4% versus 13.6% increase). Indeed, electric fields < 100 µV/cm were osteogenic if confined to this frequency domain. At frequencies below 15 Hz (and thus more aptly associated with locomotion), the osteogenic potential decreased dramatically, with induced fields at 5 Hz and below incapable even of preventing disuse bone loss.[69] However, the fact that field intensities in this

10 to 100 Hz range would be on the order of 10 to 100 μV/cm[61] implies that strains on the order of 10 to 100 $\mu\varepsilon$, if induced in this frequency band, could play an important role in mediating bone remodeling.

These findings suggest that bone tissue is most sensitive to a very specific band of electric energy (between 10 and 100 Hz) and imply that the amplitude of the induced electric field used in the clinic could be greatly reduced by eliminating the distribution of power for PEMF signals which occur above 100 Hz. The strong frequency selectivity of bone tissue may suggest a mechanism whereby electric fields, and perhaps biophysical stimuli in general, interact with the skeleton.[69,70] Even if bone tissue is most sensitive to frequencies between 10 and 100 Hz, the physiologic relevance of such a preference is questionable because more than 99% of functional strain energy is contained in frequencies below 15 Hz.[71] However, a "high" frequency band of skeletal strain energy has been shown to persist in the functional domain, between 10 and 50 Hz. Although small (< 10%) when compared to the fundamental of the strain energy (< 3 Hz), this band is present during activities such as standing and speaking.[16] To determine if mechanical energy induced in the optimal electric frequency range is also preferentially osteogenic, we investigated the frequency and strain magnitude dependence of bone remodeling in response to mechanical loads.[72]

As in the case of electric energy, the ability of mechanical strains to stimulate new bone formation was highly frequency dependent, with the osteogenic potential increasing with frequency up through at least 60 Hz. For example, a 0.5-Hz regimen required 2,000 $\mu\varepsilon$ to maintain bone mass, but the load had to be applied for only 8 s/day.[51] A 1-Hz sinusoidal loading regimen at 1,000 $\mu\varepsilon$ had to be applied for 100 s/day to maintain bone mass,[49] while 10 minutes of load with a peak of 800 $\mu\varepsilon$ could maintain bone mass. Over the same 10-min/day regimen, a load of only 200 $\mu\varepsilon$ was necessary to maintain bone mass if the strain was applied in the range of 30 to 60 Hz. These data suggest that the mechanisms responsible for the control of bone remodeling do not necessarily depend on any one factor, but instead represent a complex interdependence on factors such as duration, intensity, and frequency, with extremely small strains induced over long periods of time being as important as large magnitude strains seen only occasionally.

Clinical Significance

Strains less than 500 $\mu\varepsilon$ fall far below those strain levels that jeopardize the structural attributes of bone (>3,000 $\mu\varepsilon$); however, if these low-magnitude strains are induced in the proper frequency domain they become potently osteogenic. This osteogenicity potentiates the use of low-magnitude strains as a novel prophylaxis for the prevention of bone loss associated with disuse, age, or menopause. The use of biophysical stimuli as potent growth factors also has great potential for application to more acute musculoskeletal disorders. One such condition is the enhancement of bone ingrowth into noncemented prosthetic components. Unfortunately, the long-term outcome of this joint replacement procedure is somewhat compromised by inconsistent bony ingrowth into the implant.[9,10] To enhance the osteoconductance and improve fixation, investigators have focused on bioengineering improvements such as component design[73,74] and material modulus,[75,76] as well as organically mediating the response via surface application of growth factors[77,78] and hydroxyapatite.[79,80]

The strong osteogenic nature of biophysical stimuli led us to evaluate the potential of the low-magnitude, high-frequency strains in the promotion of bony ingrowth into a simple, porous-coated, cylindric implant press fit across the turkey ulna midshaft.[81] Ulna preparations were exposed to 8 weeks of either disuse alone, or disuse plus 100 s/day of a 1- or 20-Hz mechanical load sufficient to induce peak strains of less than 150 $\mu\epsilon$ at the site of the bone/implant interface. In the case of disuse, bone resorbed away from the implants, leaving a fibrous membrane between bone and implant (Fig. 5, *top*). However, the extremely low magnitude 1-Hz loading resulted in almost 30% of the available porous implant area being filled with new bone, emphasizing that at least some strain energy is important to initiate the formation process into the implant. When the frequency was raised to 20 Hz, almost 70% of the porous space was filled with new bone (Fig. 5, *bottom*).

These preliminary results suggest that low-level, high-frequency dynamic loading has great clinical potential for the efficacious control of bone formation. These low-level biophysical stimuli may provide a means of rapid stabilization of noncemented implants while avoiding destructive levels of strain energy at the bone/implant interface. Moreover, as the ingrowth becomes established, the mechanical signal itself will diminish to the point at which the strain signals native to the bone may maintain an effective implant/bone interface. The ease and safety with which such low-amplitude strains can be focally induced into bone tissue suggest other clinical situations in which bone loss may be prevented or new bone stimulated, including the acceleration of fracture healing, the inhibition of osteonecrosis, or the enhancement of bony transport.

Summary

The role of biophysical stimuli in the achievement and maintenance of a structurally appropriate bone mass is clear. These factors, which are so critical to retaining an effective skeletal structure, have begun to be applied clinically.[65,82] In contrast to systemic, pharmaceutical intervention such as estrogens, bisphosphonates, calcitonin, or calcium, the attributes of such biophysical prophylaxes are that they are native to the bone tissue, safe at low intensities, and ultimately will induce lamellar bone; moreover, the relative amplitude of the signal will subside as formation persists. However, the widespread use of biophysical stimuli in the treatment of skeletal disorders will undoubtedly be delayed until there is a better understanding of how these signals interact at the cellular and subcellular levels.

In the work presented here, we have concentrated on the organ and tissue level sensitivity of bone to mechanical and electrical stimuli. Although the means by which the bone cells interpret and integrate physical stimuli is beyond the scope of this chapter, much elegant work has begun to address these important issues.[83–96] Much more work must be performed to fully harness the clinical potential of these biophysical signals. However, existing studies emphasize that bone may no longer be perceived as an inert engineering structure.

In summary, at the organ level, biophysical signals exist as a normal, physiologic component of the functional milieu; strain energy appears on the occipital ridge of the macaque, the femur of the lizard, and the metacarpal of the horse. In addition to the large amplitude strains typically associated with functional activity, a species independent strain signal, 50 to 200 $\mu\epsilon$ in amplitude, appears in the frequency band of 10 to 100 Hz. This signal is present in the cranial, axial, and appendicular skeleton and exists at all times, including during passive actions such as standing and speaking.

The osteoregulatory relevance of these high-frequency, low-magnitude strain energies has been evaluated at the tissue level. Although mechanical signals of 500 $\mu\epsilon$ are not influential if induced around 1 Hz, they become extremely

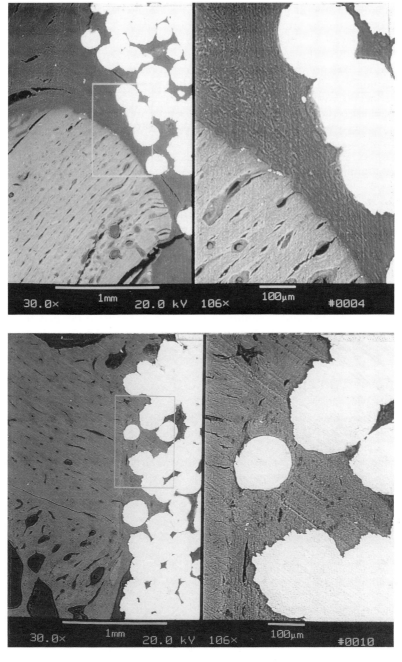

Fig. 5 Backscatter electron microscope photomicrographs of the bone/implant interface following 8 weeks of disuse (**top**) and 8 weeks of 100 seconds per day of a 20-Hz mechanical regimen sufficient to cause 150 microstrain at the interface (**bottom**). In each photomicrograph, the left side is magnified 30 times, while the right side magnifies the highlighted region 106 fold. (Reproduced with permission from Rubin CT, McLeod KJ: Promotion of bony ingrowth by frequency specific, low amplitude mechanical strain. *Clin Orthop* 1994;298:165–174.)

osteogenic if applied between 10 and 60 Hz. The frequency selectivity of bone to biophysical stimuli persists even when the energy is induced electrically. Electric fields on the order of 1 to 10 µV/cm, while ineffective below 5 Hz, are strongly osteogenic if induced between 15 and 50 Hz.

At the level of the cell, the ability of electric fields to modulate bone cell activity depends not only on the frequency and intensity of the signal, but also on the biophysical state of the cell and/or cell population.[94] Fields of 6 µV/cm induced at 30 Hz will enhance alkaline phosphatase activity in osteoblasts at intermediate cell densities ($200,000/cm^2$), yet do not affect phenotypic expression in either sparse ($70,000/cm^2$) or highly confluent cultures ($500,000/cm^2$). Moreover, the osteoregulatory impact of these fields is not specific to osteoblasts; in a murine marrow culture system, 4 days of low-magnitude field exposure inhibited osteoclast recruitment by 40%.[93] These responses have been interpreted to indicate that the effectiveness of the biophysical signal is critically dependent on the size and shape of the cell.

The predominant perception of biophysical modulation of bone physiology is that the signals must be large to have any morphologic impact. However, work at the level of both organ and tissue, and supported by work at the level of the cell, has demonstrated that low magnitude mechanical or electrical signals can be extremely osteogenic if induced in an appropriate frequency domain. Although the basic tenets of Wolff's Law remain intact, we must expand our perception of bone to appreciate the complex biology of the tissue; ie, even though the principal responsibility of the skeleton is structural, it is the bone cell population that is ultimately responsible for the regulation and optimization of skeletal morphology.

Acknowledgments

This work has been supported by grants from The National Institutes of Health (#AR39278, AR41011, & AR41040), The Whitaker Foundation, and The National Science Foundation (PYI 865105). The authors would also like to thank Anne Dusatko and Gail Trocchio for their secretarial support, as well as Tracy O'Hara and Peter Haralabatos for their technical assistance. Finally, thanks go to Steven Bain for his help with the histomorphometry.

References

1. Wolff J: *The Law of Bone Remodelling* (Das Gesetz der Transformation der Knochen). Originally published by Verlag von August Hirshwald, Berlin, 1892. English translation by Maquet P, Furlong, R, published by Springer Verlag, Berlin, 1986.
2. Lane NE, Bloch DA, Jones HH, et al: Long-distance running, bone density and osteoarthritis. *JAMA* 1986;255:1147–1151.
3. Talmage RV, Stinnett SS, Landwehr JT, et al: Age related loss of bone mineral density in non-athletic and athletic women. *Bone Miner* 1986;1:115–125.
4. Jones HH, Priest JD, Hayes WC, et al: Humeral hypertrophy in response to exercise. *J Bone Joint Surg* 1977;59A:204–208.
5. Huddleston AL, Rockwell D, Kulund DN, et al: Bone mass in lifetime tennis athletes. *JAMA* 1980;244:1107–1109.
6. Tilton FE, Degioanni JJ, Schneider VS: Long-term follow-up of Skylab bone demineralization. *Aviat Space Environ Med* 1980;51:1209–1213.
7. Simmons DJ, Russell JE, Winter F, et al: Space flight and the non-weight bearing bones of the rat skeleton (Cosmos 1129). *Trans Orthop Res Soc* 1981;6:65.

8. LeBlanc AD, Schneider VS, Evans HJ, et al: Bone mineral loss and recovery after 17 weeks of bed rest. *J Bone Miner Res* 1990;5:843–850.
9. Engh CA, Massin P, Suthers KE: Roentgenographic assessment of the biologic fixation of porous-surfaced femoral components. *Clin Orthop* 1990;257:107–128.
10. Callaghan JJ: The clinical results and basic science of total hip arthroplasty with porous-coated prostheses. *J Bone Joint Surg* 1993;75A:299–310.
11. Frost HM: Skeletal structural adaptations to mechanical usage (SATMU): 1. Redefining Wolff's Law: The bone modeling problem. *Anat Rec* 1990;226:403–413.
12. Frost HM: Perspectives: Bone's mechanical usage windows. *Bone Miner* 1992;19: 257–271.
13. Akhter MP, Raab DM, Turner CH, et al: Characterization of *in vivo* strain in the rat tibia during external application of a four-point bending load. *J Biomech* 1992; 25:1241–1246.
14. Cowin SC: Bone remodeling of diaphyseal surfaces by torsional loads: Theoretical predictions. *J Biomech* 1987;20:1111–1120.
15. Rubin CT, McLeod KJ: Biologic modulation of mechanical influences in bone remodeling, in Mow VC, Ratcliffe A, Woo SLY (eds): *Biomechanics of Diarthrodial Joints.* New York, NY, Springer-Verlag, 1990, vol 2, pp 97–118.
16. McLeod K, Rubin C: Strain oscillations in the appendicular and axial skeleton: A species independent component of functional loading. *J Biomech*, in press.
17. Gross TS, Rubin CT: Gradients of strain as a powerful predictor of skeletal adaptation. *Trans Orthop Res Soc* 1993;18:125.
18. O'Connor JA, Lanyon LE, MacFie H: The influence of strain rate on adaptive bone remodeling. *J Biomech* 1982;15:767–781.
19. Goldstein SA, Matthews LS, Kuhn JL, et al: Trabecular bone remodeling: An experimental model. *J Biomech* 1991;24(suppl):135–150.
20. Berretta DA, Pollack SR: Ion concentration effects on the zeta potential of bone. *J Orthop Res* 1986;4:337–345.
21. Bassett C: Biologic significance of piezoelectricity. *Calcif Tissue Int* 1968;1:252–272.
22. Weinbaum S, Cowin SC, Zeng Y: Fluid shear stress excitation of osteocytes, in Bidez M (ed): *Advances in Bioengineering.* New York, NY, American Society of Mechanical Engineers, 1992, vol 22, pp 25–28.
23. Hart RT: A theoretical study of the influence of bone maturation rate on surface remodeling predictions: Idealized models. *J Biomech* 1990;23:241–257.
24. Fyhrie DP, Carter DR: A unifying principle relating stress to trabecular bone morphology. *J Orthop Res* 1986;4:304–331.
25. Huiskes R, Weinans H, Grootenboer HJ, et al: Adaptive bone remodeling theory applied to prosthetic-design analysis. *J Biomech* 1987;20:1135–1150.
26. Brown TD, Pedersen DR, Gray ML, et al: Toward an identification of mechanical parameters initiating periosteal remodeling: A combined experimental and analytic approach. *J Biomech* 1990;23:893–905.
27. Rubin CT: Skeletal strain and the functional significance of bone architecture. *Calcif Tissue Int* 1984;36(suppl 1):S11–S18.
28. Rubin CT, Lanyon LE: Dynamic strain similarity in vertebrates: An alternative to allometric limb bone scaling. *J Theor Biol* 1984;107:321–327.
29. Rubin CT, Lanyon LE: Osteoregulatory nature of mechanical stimuli: Function as a determinant for adaptive remodeling in bone. *J Orthop Res* 1987;5:300–310.
30. Rubin CT, McLeod KJ, Bain SD: Functional strains and cortical bone adaptation: Epigenetic assurance of skeletal integrity. *J Biomech* 1990;23:43–54.
31. Lanyon LE, Smith RN: Bone strain in the tibia during normal quadrupedal locomotion. *Acta Orthop Scand* 1970;41:238–248.
32. Gross TS, McLeod KJ, Rubin CT: Characterizing bone strain distributions in vivo using three triple rosette strain gauges. *J Biomech* 1992;25:1081–1087.
33. Carter DR, Harris WH, Vasu R, et al: The mechanical and biological response of cortical bone to in vivo strain histories, in Cowin S (ed): *Mechanical Properties of Bone: Presented at the Joint ASME-ASCE Applied Mechanics, Fluid Engineering,*

and Bioengineering Conference, Boulder, CO, June 22–24, 1981. New York, NY, American Society of Mechanical Engineers, 1981, vol 45, p 81.

34. Beaupre GS, Orr TE, Carter DR: An approach for time-dependent bone modeling and remodeling: Theoretical development. *J Orthop Res* 1990;8:651–661.
35. Van Der Meulen MC, Beaupre GS, Carter DR: Mechano-biologic influences in long bone cross-sectional growth. *Bone* 1993;14:635–642.
36. Rubin CT, Lanyon LE: Limb mechanics as a function of speed and gait: A study of functional strains in the radius and tibia of horse and dog. *J Exp Biol* 1982;101:187–211.
37. Biewener AA: Biomechanics of mammalian terrestrial locomotion. *Science* 1990;250:1097–1103.
38. Donahue HJ, McLeod KJ, Mase CA, et al: Cell to cell communication in osteoblastic networks: Distribution, expression and hormonal regulation of connexin 43. *Trans Orthop Res Soc* 1993;18:73.
39. Gross TS, Rubin CT: The organ response of bone to the removal of functional stimuli. *Trans Am Soc Biomech* 1990;14:49–50.
40. Skerry TM, Suswillo R, El Haj AJ, et al: Load-induced proteoglycan orientation in bone tissue in vivo and in vitro. *Calcif Tissue Int* 1990;46:318–326.
41. McLeod KJ, Rubin CT: Frequency specific modulation of bone adaptation by induced electric fields. *J Theor Biol* 1990;145:385–396.
42. Woo SL, Akeson WH, Coutts RD, et al: A comparison of cortical bone atrophy secondary to fixation with plates with large differences in bending stiffness. *J Bone Joint Surg* 1976;58A:190–195.
43. Carter DR, Vasu R, Spengler DM, et al: Stress fields in the unplated and plated canine femur calculated from in vivo strain measurements. *J Biomech* 1981;14:63–70.
44. Lanyon LE, Goodship AE, Pye CJ, et al: Mechanically adaptive bone remodelling. *J Biomech* 1982;15:141–154.
45. Hert J, Liskova M, Landa J: Reaction of bone to mechanical stimuli: 1. Continuous and intermittent loading of tibia in rabbit. *Folia Morphol (Prague)* 1971;19:290–300.
46. Churches AE, Howlett CR, Waldron K, et al: The response of living bone to controlled time-varying loading: Method and preliminary results. *J Biomech* 1979;12:35–45.
47. Turner CH, Akhter MP, Raab DM, et al: A noninvasive, *in vivo* model for studying strain adaptive bone modeling. *Bone* 1991;12:73–79.
48. Chambers TJ, Evans M, Gardner TN, et al: Induction of bone formation in rat tail vertebrae by mechanical loading. *Bone Miner* 1993;20:167–178.
49. Rubin CT, Lanyon LE: Regulation of bone mass by mechanical strain magnitude. *Calcif Tissue Int* 1985;37:411–417.
50. Lanyon LE, Rubin CT: Static versus dynamic loads as an influence on bone remodelling. *J Biomech* 1984;17:897–905.
51. Rubin CT, Lanyon LE: Regulation of bone formation by applied dynamic loads. *J Bone Joint Surg* 1984;66A:397–402.
52. Rubin C, Gross T, Guilak F, et al: Differentiation of the intracortical remodeling response to axial and torsional loading. *Trans Orthop Res Soc* 1994;19:34.
53. Rubin C, Bain S, Gross T, et al: Stimulation of periosteal bone formation by potent osteogenic stimuli: Morphologic stages in the achievement of lamellar bone. *J Bone Miner Res*, in press.
54. Rubin CT, Bain SD, McLeod KJ: Suppression of the osteogenic response in the aging skeleton. *Calcif Tissue Int* 1992;50:306–313.
55. Lanyon LE, Rubin CT, Baust G: Modulation of bone loss during calcium insufficiency by controlled dynamic loading. *Calcif Tiss Int* 1986;38:209–216.
56. Bain SD, Rubin CT: Metabolic modulation of disuse osteopenia: Endocrine-dependent site specificity of bone remodeling. *J Bone Miner Res* 1990;5:1069–1075.
57. Wang N, Butler JP, Ingber DE: Mechanotransduction across the cell surface and through the cytoskeleton. *Science* 1993;260:1124–1127.

58. Yasuda I: Piezoelectric activity of bone. *J Japanese Orthop Surg Soc* 1954;28:267–269.

59. Lavine LS, Grodzinsky AJ: Electrical stimulation of repair of bone. *J Bone Joint Surg* 1987;69A:626–630.

60. Hastings GW, Mahmud FA: Electrical effects in bone. *J Biomed Eng* 1988;10:515–521.

61. Otter MW, Palmieri VR, Wu DD, et al: A comparative analysis of streaming potentials in vivo and in vitro. *J Orthop Res* 1992;10:710–719.

62. Nunamaker DM, Butterweck DM, Provost MT: Fatigue fractures in thoroughbred racehorses: Relationships with age, peak bone strain, and training. *J Orthop Res* 1990;8:604–611.

63. McLeod KJ, Donahue HJ, Levin PE, et al: Electric fields modulate bone cell function in a density-dependent manner. *J Bone Miner Res* 1993;8:977–984.

64. Brighton CT, McCluskey WP: Cellular response and mechanisms of action of electrically induced osteogenesis, in Peck WA (ed): *Bone and Mineral Research: 4.* New York, NY, Elsevier Science Publishers, 1986, pp 213–254.

65. Bassett CA: Beneficial effects of electromagnetic fields. *J Cell Biochem* 1993;51:387–393.

66. Bassett CA: Fundamental and practical aspects of therapeutic uses of pulsed electromagnetic fields (PEMFs). *Crit Rev Biomed Eng* 1989;17:451–529.

67. Rubin CT, McLeod KJ, Lanyon LE: Prevention of osteoporosis by pulsed electromagnetic fields. *J Bone Joint Surg* 1989;71A:411–417.

68. McLeod KJ, Rubin CT: The effect of low-frequency electrical fields on osteogenesis. *J Bone Joint Surg* 1992;74A:920–929.

69. McLeod K, Rubin C: Frequency and dose dependent responses of bone tissue to exogenous electromagnetic field exposure. *Trans Bioelectr Rep Growth Soc* 1988;8:18.

70. Rubin C, Donahue H, Rubin J, et al: Optimization of electric field parameters for the control of bone remodeling: Exploitation of an indigenous mechanism for the prevention of osteopenia. *J Bone Miner Res* 1993;8:573–581.

71. Antonsson EK, Mann RW: The frequency content of gait. *J Biomech* 1985;18:39–47.

72. McLeod KJ, Rubin CT: The interdependence of strain frequency, duration and amplitude in the control of bone remodeling activity. *Trans Orthop Res Soc* 1994;19:564.

73. Callaghan JJ, Fulghum CS, Glisson RR, et al: The effect of femoral stem geometry on interface motion in uncemented porous-coated total hip prostheses: Comparison of straight-stem and curved-stem designs. *J Bone Joint Surg* 1992;74A:839–848.

74. Huiskes R: The various stress patterns of press-fit ingrown and cemented femoral stems. *Clin Orthop* 1990;261:27–38.

75. Galante JO, Lemons J, Spector M, et al: The biologic effects of implant materials. *J Orthop Res* 1991;9:760–775.

76. Kang JD, McKernan DJ, Druger M, et al: Ingrowth and formation of bone in defects in an uncemented fiber-metal total hip replacement model in dogs. *J Bone Joint Surg* 1991;73A:93–105.

77. Downes S, Kayser MV, Blunn G, et al: An electron microscopical study of the interaction of bone with growth hormone loaded bone cement. *Cells Materials* 1991;1:171–176.

78. Kotani S, Yamamuro T, Nakamura T, et al: Enhancement of bone bonding to bioactive ceramics by demineralized bone powder. *Clin Orthop* 1992;278:226–234.

79. Turner TM, Urban RM, Sumner DR, et al: Revision, without cement, of aseptically loose, cemented total hip prostheses: Quantitative comparison of the effects of four types of medullary treatment on bone ingrowth in a canine model. *J Bone Joint Surg* 1993;75A:845–862.

80. Soballe K, Hansen ES, Brockstedt-Rasmussen H, et al: Tissue ingrowth into titanium and hydroxyapatite-coated implants during stable and unstable mechanical conditions. *J Orthop Res* 1992;10:285–299.

81. Rubin CT, McLeod KJ: Promotion of bony ingrowth by frequency-specific, low-amplitude mechanical strain. *Clin Orthop* 1994;298:165–174.
82. Heckman JD, Ryaby JP, McCabe J, et al: Acceleration of tibial fracture healing by noninvasive low intensity ultrasound. *J Bone Joint Surg* 1994;76A:26–34.
83. McLeod K, Lee RC, Ehrlich HP: Frequency dependence of electric field modulation of fibroblast protein synthesis. *Science* 1987;236:1465–1469.
84. Duncan R, Misler S: Voltage-activated and stretch-activated Ba^{2+} conducting channels in an osteoblast-like cell line (UMR 106). *FEBS Lett* 1989;251:17–21.
85. Skerry TM, Bitensky L, Chayen J, et al: Early strain-related changes in enzyme activity in osteocytes following bone loading in vivo. *J Bone Miner Res* 1989;4:783–788.
86. Vandenburgh H: Mechanical forces and their second messengers in stimulating cell growth in vitro, in *World Congress of Biomechanics: Abstracts of the First International Biomech Congress*. La Jolla, CA, First World Congress of Biomechanics, 1990.
87. Brighton CT, Strafford B, Gross SB, et al: The proliferative and synthetic response of isolated calvarial bone cells of rats to cyclic biaxial mechanical strain. *J Bone Joint Surg* 1991;73A:320–331.
88. Jones DB, Nolte H, Scholubbers JG, et al: Biochemical signal transduction of mechanical strain in osteoblast-like cells. *Biomaterials* 1991;12:101–110.
89. Burger EH, Klein-Nulend J, Veldhuijzen JP: Modulation of osteogenesis in fetal bone rudiments by mechanical stress *in vitro*. *J Biomech* 1991;24(suppl 1):101–109.
90. Buckley MJ, Banes AJ, Levin LG, et al: Osteoblasts increase their rate of division and align in response to cyclic, mechanical tension in vitro. *Bone Miner* 1988;4:225–236.
91. Brighton CT, Sennett BJ, Farmer JC, et al: The inositol phosphate pathway as a mediator in the proliferative response of rat calvarial bone cells to cyclical biaxial mechanical strain. *J Orthop Res* 1992;10:385–393.
92. Fitzsimmons RJ, Strong DD, Mohan S, et al: Low-amplitude, low-frequency electric field-stimulated bone cell proliferation may in part be mediated by increased IGF-II release. *J Cell Physiol* 1992;150:84–89.
93. Rubin J, McLeod K, Nanes M, et al: Extremely low frequency electric fields attenuate osteoclast-like cell recruitment in marrow culture. *Trans Orthop Res Soc* 1993;18:180.
94. McLeod K, Rubin C, Donahue H, et al: The role of polarization forces in mediating the interaction of low frequency electric fields with living tissue, in Blank M (ed): *Electricity & Magnetism in Biology & Medicine*. San Francisco, CA, San Francisco Press, 1993.
95. Juliano RL, Haskill S: Signal transduction from the extracellular matrix. *J Cell Biol* 1993;120:577–585.
96. Guilak F, Donahue HJ, McLeod KJ, et al: Intracellular and intercellular propagation of deformation-induced calcium transients in articular chondrocytes. *Trans Orthop Res Soc* 1994;19:259.

Chapter 6

Heterotopic Ossification

Gregory V. Hahn, MD
Frederick S. Kaplan, MD

Definition

Normal bone formation is a vital component of skeletal growth, repair, and regeneration. Heterotopic ossification is characterized by the formation of normal bone at ectopic soft-tissue locations and comprises a wide variety of disorders of the spatial regulation of osteogenesis. Orthotopic ossification (the formation of extra bone at skeletal sites) and amorphous soft tissue calcification will not be considered in this chapter.

Pathogenesis

Factors involved in the regulation of normal osteogenesis have been implicated in the regulation of heterotopic ossification.[1-9] Regardless of the etiology, the pathogenesis of heterotopic ossification involves three requisite conditions: (1) an inductive morphogenetic agent or agents; (2) a population of inducible osteoprogenitor mesenchymal cells; and (3) a heterotopic environment conducive and permissive to osteogenesis.[10-14]

Much has been written about the myriad causes of heterotopic ossification including trauma, burns, infections, neoplasia, seronegative spondyloarthropathies, neurologic diseases, postsurgical trauma, chronic venous insufficiency, and heritable disease (Outline 1),[12,13,15,16] but to date no definitive inductive factor has been identified in any of the naturally occurring forms of heterotopic ossification. The recent identification and successful cloning of the bone morphogenetic proteins (BMPs),[3,4,6-9] as well as the recognition of other morphogen-like molecules, such as the *fos* and *jun* nuclear regulatory proteins[17] and retinoic acid,[1] suggest likely candidate molecules in the early induction pathways of heterotopic ossification.

A population of inducible osteoprogenitor mesenchymal cells that can respond to an inductive signal and orchestrate a highly regulated pathway of tissue morphogenesis is a second requirement for heterotopic ossification.[9,12,13] To date, the clonal identity of inducible osteoprogenitor cells is uncertain, but recent experimental data point to osteoprogenitor cells within local mesenchyme, stem cells within marrow stroma, or fixed tissue vascular cells, such as the perivascular cell or endothelial cell, as possible candidates.[10,18]

Finally, the biochemical, cellular, histologic, and microvascular environments must be permissive to the ossification pathways at all stages of osteogenesis, from the earliest putative inductive event through remodeling of mature lamellar bone.

79

Outline 1 Etiologies of heterotopic ossification

I.   Injury
   A. Central Nervous System
      1. Brain
         a. Closed head trauma with coma
         b. Cerebrovascular accident with hemiplegia
      2. Spinal Cord
         a. Paraplegia
         b. Quadriplegia
      3. Lower Motor Neuron (poliomyelitis)
   B. Soft Tissue
      1. Blunt Trauma
         a. Muscle hematoma
         b. Joint dislocation
      2. Postsurgical
         a. Following total hip arthroplasty
         b. Surgical scars
      3. Osteoma Cutis
         a. Burns
         b. Nevi
         c. Idiopathic
II. Vascular
   A. Chronic Vascular Insufficiency
   B. Aortic Insufficiency
III. Arthropathies
   A. Ankylosing Spondylitis
   B. Psoriatic Arthritis
   C. Seronegative Arthropathies
   D. Diffuse Idiopathic Skeletal Hyperostosis
IV. Genetic—Developmental
   A. Fibrodysplasia Ossificans Progressiva (FOP)
   B. Progressive Osseous Heteroplasia (POH)
   C. Albright's Hereditary Osteodystrophy (AHO)
   D. Tracheopathia Osteoplastica (TO)

Etiology

Acquired Forms of Heterotopic Ossification

Commonly noted causes of heterotopic ossification include trauma, scars, burns, paraplegia, cerebral injury, poliomyelitis, surgical trauma, and arthropathies.[12,13,15,16]

Myositis ossificans traumatica often develops following muscular hematoma resulting from sports-related injuries. The ossification process is predominantly endochondral in nature, and in some cases the ossification may resemble extraosseous osteosarcomas.[12,13]

Heterotopic ossification is commonly seen following neurologic problems, such as paraplegia, quadriplegia, cerebral injuries, or poliomyelitis. Paralyzed muscle is susceptible to ossification below the level of the paralysis. Local factors such as stasis, edema, swelling, and prolonged immobilization are often cited as contributing factors. Heterotopic ossification following neurologic injuries such as spinal cord trauma or closed head injuries is often seen within 1 to 4 months of the accident. Attempts to isolate local or systemic factors that could stimulate inducible osteogenic precursor cells have not been fruitful.[12,13,16]

Intravascular heterotopic ossification has been noted in areas of calcified aortic plaques.[18] Although local pathogenetic factors have not been identified, BMP2 expression has been identified in the pericyte-like cells of the aortic wall. BMP2 was found in calcified atherosclerotic plaque. It thus appears that arterial ossification is a regulated process, which possibly is mediated by pericyte-like cells.[18]

Surgical trauma is a common cause of heterotopic ossification, especially following total hip replacement. Occurrence of heterotopic ossification ranges from 8% to 12% following total hip arthroplasty, with estimates as high as 20%. Clinically significant (limiting motion) heterotopic ossification following total hip arthroplasty is seen in 1% to 3% of cases. Commonly cited contributing factors include male gender, osteoarthritis, or ankylosing spondylitis.[12,13,16]

Ossification of spinal ligaments is commonly seen in patients with seronegative spondyloarthropathies including ankylosing spondylitis, Reiter's syndrome, psoriatic arthritis, and arthritis associated with inflammatory bowel disease. Ossification of the longitudinal ligaments of the spine is also commonly seen in association with diffuse idiopathic skeletal hyperostosis. The pathogenesis of ossification is unknown in all of these conditions.[12,13,16]

Genetic and Developmental Forms of Heterotopic Ossification

In addition to the many acquired forms of heterotopic ossification, there are several rare genetic and developmental etiologies (Table 1). In all of these forms, the heterotopic ossification appears to be genetically programmed, and it often develops with no predisposing insult or injury to the soft tissues. In some forms, however, external factors such as blunt trauma appear to promote disease progression.

Fibrodysplasia Ossificans Progressiva (FOP) FOP is a progressively disabling genetic disorder characterized by congenital skeletal malformations and progressive heterotopic ossification.[19–27] It is an exceedingly rare condition, with a point prevalence estimated at 0.6×10^{-6} based on a study from the United Kingdom.[21] Most cases of FOP appear to arise by spontaneous mutation and no sex, race, or ethnic predilection has been observed. Although reproductive fitness is low, and several large series of patients failed to report any familial transmission, autosomal dominant transmission has been documented recently.[21,24–26]

Nearly all patients who have FOP have congenital malformations of the great toes.[20] The most common malformation is a shortened great toe with a single phalanx. Other, more variable congenital malformations include short broad femoral necks, bilateral clinodactyly, and abnormal cervical vertebrae with small bodies, large pedicles, and large spinous processes.[20,25,26] Progressive heterotopic ossification begins early in childhood, often during infancy, and first appears in the posterior cervical region. The ectopic bone formation progresses throughout life and results in ankylosis of the major joints. Most patients are completely immobilized and confined to wheelchairs by the fourth decade of life.[19,20,25,27] In a study of 44 patients, ectopic ossification was noted to progress in several regular patterns or gradients.[19] Ossification appears proximally before distally, axially before appendicularly, cranially before caudally,

Table 1 Developmental disorders of heterotopic ossification

	Fibrodysplasia Ossificans Progressiva	Albright's Hereditary Osteodystrophy	Progressive Osseous Heteroplasia	Tracheopathia Osteoplastica
Gender distribution	M = F	F > M	F > M	M = F
Congenital papular rash	No	No	Yes	No
Congenital malformation of great toes	Yes	No	No	No
Brachydactyly, short stature, obesity, round facies, and mental retardation	No	Yes	No	No
Cutaneous ossification	No	Yes	Yes	No
Extensive heterotopic ossification of deep connective tissue	Yes	No	Yes	No
Predominant mechanism of ossification	Endochondral	Noninflammatory osseous heteroplasia	Noninflammatory osseous heteroplasia	Endochondral
Presence of hematopoietic marrow in mature heterotopic bone	Yes	No	No	Yes
Stringent developmental patterns of progressive ossification	Yes	No	No	No
Exacerbation by trauma	Yes	No	No	No
Hypocalcemia; hyperphosphatemia; and ↓ urinary cAMP response to PTH	No	Yes (Pseudohypoparathyroidism) No (Pseudopseudohypoparathyroidism)	No	No
Serum alkaline phosphatase	Usually elevated	Usually normal	Variable	Normal
Serum parathyroid hormone level	Normal	Elevated	Normal	Normal
Pathogenesis	Unknown	Inherited defect in stimulatory Gs protein of adenylate cyclase	Unknown	Unknown

and dorsally before ventrally.[19] The paraspinal muscles are involved early in life with subsequent progression to the shoulder and hip regions. The ankles, wrists, and jaw are affected later.[19] Other variable clinical features associated with FOP include deafness, baldness, and amenorrhea.[20,25]

Impending ossification at any site is heralded by painful nodules of noninflammatory fibroproliferative tissue involving tendons, ligaments, and connective tissue of skeletal tissue. These nodules rarely regress spontaneously; most often, they mature rapidly through an endochondral sequence to form normal lamellar bone that rigidly immobilizes the joints of the axial and appendicular skeleton.[20] The mature heterotopic bone in FOP is indistinguishable from mature skeletal bone.[23] Bone formation can be triggered by blunt trauma but most often occurs spontaneously. Excision of heterotopic bone is futile, because surgical trauma predictably leads to the stimulation of new heterotopic ossification at the operative site. The diaphragm, extra-ocular muscles, heart, and smooth muscles are characteristically spared.[20] Untimely death often results from respiratory failure due to restrictive movement of the chest wall or from inanition due to ankylosis of the jaw.[20]

The genetic mutation and pathogenesis of the disorder are unknown.[21,23,26] However, the array of developmental gradients seen in FOP is similar to developmental anomalies induced by pleiotropic mutations of the decapentaplegic (dpp) locus in *Drosophila melanogaster*.[22] Intriguingly, the protein encoded by dpp shares a 75% sequence homology with BMP2 and BMP4 and is the *Drosophila* homolog of these BMPs.[9,22] The recent demonstration that human BMP4 sequences can confer normal dorsal-ventral patterning in the *Drosophila* embryo suggests that the BMP gene family has the capacity to regulate pattern formation as well as tissue morphogenesis.[28] BMPs are the only biomolecules discovered thus far that are capable of inducing endochondral ossification at a heterotopic site. FOP is a disorder characterized by a disturbed developmental expression of the endochondral ossification program and may represent a mutation resulting in a dominant gain of function.[22] The developmental similarities between dpp in the fly and FOP in man suggest a useful model for the study of FOP and implicate the BMPs as plausible candidate genes in genetic disorders of heterotopic ossification.[22]

There is currently no effective treatment for FOP. Corticosteroids, diphosphonates, physiotherapy, and surgical excision have all been tried without any objective benefit.[20,25,27] Patients who have FOP should be instructed to avoid precipitating factors such as blunt muscle trauma, intramuscular injections, and surgical attempts to excise ectopic bone.

Progressive Osseous Heteroplasia (POH) POH is another rare developmental disorder of heterotopic ossification in children; it is characterized by focal dermal ossification in infancy with progressive intramembranous ossification of subcutaneous fat and deep connective tissue.[29–34] The first signs of the disease are cutaneous plaques of ossification that coalesce and eventually progress to involve the adjacent connective tissues. This extensive ossification of the deep tissues often results in ankylosis of affected joints and focal growth retardation of involved limbs. Etiology and pathogenesis of the disorder are unknown.[33] To date there are only nine reported cases, seven are females. Two of the previously reported cases of POH appeared to be sporadic, while two were familial. One POH patient had numerous male and female relatives in two generations who were affected with clinically insignificant dermal ossification. Clinical observations in that family support a dominant mode of inheritance for the trivial osteoma cutis lesions.[32] Gardner and associates[32] postulated that the patient's local severe disease arose from an early somatic conversion to homozygosity (analogous to retinoblastoma). Such a conversion would lead predictably to somatic cell mosaicism with severe localized disease in tissues containing the homozygous mutant alleles.[32]

A curious feature of POH is the predominant female involvement.[33] Although the finding may be a coincidence of the small number of cases to date, it may alternatively prove to be an important biologic clue. The paucity of male cases suggests male lethality in utero, and the possibility of X-linkage must be considered. Although most, but not all, X-borne loci are, following lyonization, functionally monoallelic, the possibility exists that the putative abnormal gene resides on the X-chromosome and leads to a mild gain of function rather than loss of function mutation. Somatic conversion to homozygosity prior to lyonization might account for a more severe phenotype in females. An autosomal location with sex limitation also remains possible.[33]

The anatomic distribution of lesions in POH suggests that the pathogenesis may involve a mesenchymal cell destined for widespread mosaic distribution. Although dermal fibroblasts and internal limb structures arise embryonically from limb bud mesenchyme, the fate map of the blastoderm mammalian embryo suggests that given cell types, such as muscle or bone, are of polyclonal origin. Conversely, in the mature organism, a single cell such as a hematopoietic stem cell or connective tissue stem cell can, under various conditions, generate a wide variety of cell types. At present, little is known about the molecular mechanisms of the signal and response system of mesodermal induction, and the clonal nature of lesions in POH remains a mystery.[33]

The heterotopic ossification in POH occurs predominantly by an intramembranous pathway. Intramembranous ossification was observed exclusively on the initial biopsy in five of the six patients.[33] Although the predominant pathway of intramembranous heterotopic osteogenesis seen in POH is similar to that observed in Albright's hereditary osteodystrophy (AHO), the lesions in AHO are limited to the skin, whereas those in POH also involve the deeper tissues. Furthermore, no patient with POH had the morphologic or endocrine disturbances characteristically seen with AHO. The heterotopic ossification in POH appears to be the only manifestation of the disease. The patients thus far all have normal intelligence, normal developmental milestones, and no biochemical or endocrine abnormalities, except for transient elevations in serum alkaline phosphatase.[33]

The long-term prognosis of patients who have POH is uncertain; only one of the six cases has been followed beyond adolescence. At present, there is no definitive prevention or treatment available for children with POH. In children with FOP, heterotopic ossification recurs predictably at the site of excision. In children with POH, the prognosis following surgical excision is less certain. The extensive coalescence of ossified skin plaques and the relentless progressive ossification of deep tissues pose perplexing therapeutic dilemmas.[33]

Albright's Hereditary Osteodystrophy AHO was first described in 1942, in three patients with an unusual constellation of findings including hypocalcemia, hyperphosphatemia, and clinical features of hypoparathyroidism.[35] The patients also exhibited obesity, short stature, round faces, brachydactyly, and subcutaneous ossifications. They were unresponsive to parathyroid extract and, thus, were labeled as having pseudohypoparathyroidism (PHP). In 1952, Albright[36] described a similar case in which the patient had the clinical features of PHP with normal calcium and phosphorus levels. This syndrome was named pseudopseudohypoparathyroidism (PPHP). It is clear that the two syndromes are variable expressions of the same disease, because there are kindreds of AHO in which several members have hormonal resistance (PHP) while others do not (PPHP). In addition, many individuals exhibit only transient hormonal resistance.

The genetics of AHO remained unclear until recently. Autosomal dominant transmission has been proven with the detection of several defects in the alpha subunit of the Gs-protein encoded on human chromosome 20.[37,38]

The clinical spectrum of AHO is quite variable. The most commonly reported signs are rounded facies, short neck, and early onset obesity. Mental retardation is also present in approximately 54% of cases. The most common skeletal manifestations are ectopic subcutaneous ossifications, brachydactyly, and generalized osteoporosis.[33] Histopathologic studies of the subcutaneous ossifications have shown that the heterotopic bone in AHO develops by an intramembranous pathway.[33] Most patients exhibit PHP type Ia, which is characterized by end-organ resistance to hormones, such as parathyroid hormone, that act by stimulating adenylate cyclase activity. However, some patients do not have end-organ resistance despite reduced adenylate cyclase activity (PPHP).

In the original report,[35] Albright and associates were unable to explain the connection between the biochemical abnormalities and the unusual physical features in AHO, and this confusion persists. The recent discovery of several mutations in the alpha subunit of one hormone-sensitive, adenyl-cyclase linked Gs protein explains the hormonal resistance seen in some patients. However, this discovery does not adequately account for those patients without hormonal resistance nor does it explain why any of the patients develop the characteristic morphologic anomalies. An etiologic link between the alpha subunit of the Gs protein and the signal transduction pathways leading to bone formation has not been established.[37,38]

Currently, treatment in AHO is aimed at controlling the endocrine disturbances with Vitamin D and calcium supplementation. In marked contrast to FOP, the heterotopic bone in AHO can be successfully excised. Although most of the ectopic foci are small and painless, on rare occasions they may coalesce into large masses.[33]

Tracheopathia Osteoplastica (TPO) TPO, also known as tracheobronchopathia osteochondroplastica, is an unusual disease of unknown etiology.[39] The disease is characterized by multiple osseous or cartilaginous nodules projecting into the tracheobronchial lumen. These projections most often arise from the anterolateral walls of the distal trachea and proximal mainstem bronchi. The disease is usually asymptomatic; however, it may cause dyspnea, stridor, hoarseness, cough, hemoptysis, or pneumonitis. In severe cases, marked deformity of the tracheobronchial tree may result, and death from TPO has been reported.

Most cases of TPO are reported as incidental findings during autopsy; however, computed tomography and bronchoscopy often aid in earlier diagnosis in patients suspected of having the disorder. The prevalence of the disease may be underestimated given its indolent and asymptomatic nature. The disease has no gender predilection, and most cases appear to arise spontaneously, although one case of familial transmission (mother to daughter) has been reported.

Histologic examination of the nodules demonstrates islands of cartilage and lamellar bone surrounded by hematopoietic marrow.[39] Fibrous tissue bands bridge the islands of bone and separate the ectopic bone from the hyaline cartilage rings of the trachea. There is no evidence of amyloid, granuloma, or tumor in the histologic sections. The pathogenesis of TPO is unknown, and hypotheses have included a congenital malformation, infection, metaplasia of elastic tissue, ecchondrosis, exostosis, or degenerative disease. There is little evidence to support any of these theories. There is no established medical treatment, and laser therapy is not beneficial.

Experimental Models

Despite many clinical varieties of heterotopic ossification, little is known about the inductive process in any form of heterotopic ossification. During the past century, experimental induction of heterotopic ossification has become a valuable tool in understanding this complex process.[12,13,40] The discovery and molecular characterization of the BMPs and the nuclear regulatory proteins such as *fos* and *jun* have provided some insight into bone induction. However, these accomplishments represent only the first step in understanding the mechanisms that initiate and regulate heterotopic osteogenesis.

The earliest experimental models of heterotopic ossification focused on such traumatic insults to extraskeletal sites as repeated blunt trauma to tendon and muscle tissue, forced joint manipulation following prolonged immobilization, and intramuscular injection of chemical irritants such as calcium chloride, ethanol, or quinine.[40,41] Later experiments illustrated the osteogenic potential of different cell types. In the classic experiments of Huggins,[42] heterotopic bone formation was induced by autotransplantation of bladder transitional epithelium into the rectus abdominis sheaths of dogs. The bone formed in these experiments developed directly from the mesenchymal tissue without cartilage precursors. These experiments revealed the significance of a conducive environment, because bone was not formed when the epithelium was transplanted into liver, kidney, or spleen.[42] Similar experiments showed gallbladder epithelium and human amniotic tissue to be osteogenic as well. Skeletal tissue grafts, such as whole bone, cartilage, and bone marrow have also induced heterotopic ossification. The significance of these experiments is debated, however, because it is difficult to distinguish between the induction of new bone and osteoconduction from the graft itself.[40]

In the late 1940s, alcohol extracts of rabbit bone were shown to induce heterotopic ossification when injected into a muscle.[12] This work was pursued vigorously by Urist, who in 1965[14] demonstrated that demineralized bone matrix could induce new bone formation when injected intramuscularly or subcutaneously into rodents or rabbits. Urist termed this osteoinductive factor BMP. This model has been studied extensively.[43] Unlike the earlier models of bone induced by transitional epithelium, Reddi[44] described the sequence of histologic events as proceeding through chondrogenesis. Following implantation, the bone matrix stimulates the migration of mesenchymal stem cells, which subsequently differentiate into cartilage and bone forming cells.[11] Within 1 week, cartilage formation is present and calcification of the cartilage begins. Ossification and the development of a bone marrow result in a fully functioning ossicle of mature heterotopic bone.

Although the osteoinductive properties of BMP were clearly reproducible, the precise composition of proteins and their corresponding gene structures remained elusive until recently. In pioneering work, investigators isolated and characterized seven unique BMPs.[3,4,6,9] The protein coding regions for these seven polypeptides have been cloned and termed BMP1 through BMP7. BMP2 through BMP7 are closely related to each other and are members of the transforming growth factor-beta superfamily based on their amino acid sequence homology and stringent conservation of seven cysteine residues. BMP2 through BMP7 all exhibit chondrogenic and osteogenic properties in a rat ectopic bone assay system.

Recombinant technology has provided a basis for testing the osteoinductive properties of individual human BMPs (rhBMPs).[8] This work has shown that rhBMP2 or rhBMP4, when reconstituted with a collagenous matrix, can independently induce the entire cascade of endochondral ossification at an extraskeletal site in vivo.[8,9] In a unique rat model, Khouri and associates[45] demonstrated that muscle flaps injected with purified BMP3, coated with demineralized bone matrix, and placed in molds could be transformed into mature cancellous bone that matched the exact shape of the molds. Further analysis of the molecular organization and regulation of the BMP genes will enhance understanding of their role in normal and heterotopic bone induction.

The prostaglandins (PGs) are another group of molecules that has been implicated in bone formation.[2,5,13] Retrospective studies on infants receiving continuous PGE_2 infusions for patent ductus arteriosus have shown that the children have increased intramembranous bone formation. They have a periostitis with periosteal elevation and cortical hyperostosis. There appears to be a PG-induced rapid formation of primitive woven bone that is completely reversible with cessation of the PGE_2 infusion. The influence of PGE_2 infusions on skeletal tissues has also been studied in rats.[2,5,13] In these studies, the rats undergo an initial period of decreasing periosteal and endosteal bone formation, which is subsequently followed by a late increase in endosteal and trabecular bone formation. The net result is an increase in proximal tibial metaphyseal hard tissue mass with a significant dose-dependent effect on cortical-endosteal bone formation. These studies provide the basis for nonsteroidal anti-inflammatory drug therapy in the prevention of heterotopic ossification.

The most recent model for studying heterotopic ossification involves the overexpression of a proto-oncogene, c-fos,[17] which is a nuclear transcription factor that is expressed during growth, development, and differentiation of various tissues in response to growth factors. Recent studies using transgenic mice have shown exogenous fos to be restricted to developing bone, cartilage, and hematopoietic tissues. In situ hybridization reveals that c-fos expression is restricted to the perichondral growth regions of the cartilage skeleton and web-forming cells of digits. In addition, deregulated fos expression in transgenic mice interferes with normal bone development resulting in hyperplasia and increased bone formation. In a study by Wang and associates,[17] ectopic c-fos expression during embryonic development in embryonic stem-cell chimeras led to postnatal formation of paravertebral and periarticular osteochondral tumors. This work suggests that a population of inducible osteoprogenitor cells is transformed by fos, and it provides a basis for further investigation of disorders such as FOP.[17]

Further work with transgenic animal models and the development of new models will inevitably lead to a greater understanding of normal and abnormal bone induction. This understanding will, in turn, allow investigators to develop rational diagnostic and treatment strategies for a wide range of developmental and acquired disorders of heterotopic ossification.

Physical Features and Laboratory Findings

The symptoms, signs, and laboratory findings are similar in most forms of heterotopic ossification and, thereby, permit a generic description. Heterotopic ossification, regardless of the cause, is associated with local symptoms including pain, swelling, and decreased mobility of adjacent joints (Table 2).[12,13,46] The early lesions often appear inflammatory and may be mistaken for cellulitis, infection, thrombophlebitis, tumor, or soft-tissue amorphous nonosseous calcification. A detailed medical history will often reveal distinguishing clues that help in confirming or excluding disorders unrelated to heterotopic ossification. Serum calcium and phosphorus levels are normal in all forms of heterotopic ossification, and are abnormal in metastatic calcification. Serum alkaline phosphatase levels will be elevated early in the course of heterotopic ossification, but will return to normal as the maturation proceeds. Radionuclide bone scans, which are sensitive but nonspecific, show dramatic increased uptake early in the evolution of heterotopic ossification before mineralization is apparent on plain roentgenograms. Biopsy may be helpful in excluding an ossifying soft-tissue tumor. However, open biopsy often exacerbates heterotopic ossification, especially in patients with some genetic forms of the disorder.[23]

Treatment

Numerous pharmacologic and physical modalities such as diphosphonates,[27,47–49] nonsteroidal anti-inflammatory drugs (NSAIDs),[47,50] radiotherapy,[47,51,52] physiotherapy,[53,54] and surgical resection[55–58] have been proposed for the treatment of heterotopic ossification (Figure 1). These modalities have enjoyed some success in the prevention of various forms of heterotopic ossification, but at present there are no generally accepted preventive measures.

For many years, ethane hydroxy diphosphonate enjoyed great popularity in the prevention of heterotopic ossification. However, recent data indicate that brief courses of diphosphonates merely delay the mineralization of osteoid matrix and are ineffective in the long-term inhibition of osteoid matrix formation.[47–49] When diphosphonate therapy is discontinued, mineralization proceeds. It appears that diphosphonates, even at high doses, are not effective in inhibiting clinically significant heterotopic ossification.

Various NSAIDs have been successful in preventing some forms of heterotopic ossification, especially following total hip arthroplasty.[47,50] The mechanism of action of NSAIDs in the prevention of heterotopic ossification remains unclear. However, it is well known that some prostaglandins enhance ossifi-

Table 2 Clinical and laboratory manifestations of heterotopic ossification

Approximate Times (Weeks)	Symptoms	Signs*	Alkaline Phosphatase	Histo-pathology	Radionuclide Bone Scan	Radiographic Findings
Early (0–4)	↑ Pain, swelling, and stiffness	Erythema Warmth Induration Tenderness Decreasing ROM	Elevated	Mesenchymal metaplasia	Positive phase I and II	None Soft-tissue swelling
Intermediate (5–15)	Same	Further decreasing ROM	Elevated and plateaus	Osseous or chondro-osseous dif-ferentiation	Positive phase III	Early osteoge-nesis
Late (16–25)	↓ Pain and swelling	Decreased ROM Possible ankylosis	Returns to normal	Bone	Decreasing phase III	Late osteo-genesis with re-modeling

* ROM = range of motion

Inducer:
Morphogen, Growth Factor,
Proto-oncogene, ?BMP, ? Fos,
?Retinoic Acid
$\Downarrow$ 1, 2
Primordial
Mesenchymal Cell
$\Downarrow$ 1, 2
Osseous or Chondro-osseous
Progenitor Cell
$\Downarrow$?2
Osteoblast
$\Downarrow$?4
Matrix Production
$\Downarrow$ 3, ?4
Mineralization
$\Downarrow$
Mature Bone
5

Fig. 1 Effect of inhibitors on mechanistic pathways of heterotopic ossification. 1 = radiation; 2 = nonsteroidal anti-inflammatory medication; 3 = ethane-hydroxy diphosphonate, 4 = physical therapy; and 5 = surgical excision.

cation. The NSAIDs are thought to act by inhibiting prostaglandin synthesis. Indomethacin, the most widely studied of the NSAIDs for the prevention of heterotopic ossification, is ineffective in inhibiting ossification once it has begun.

Radiation therapy has been used widely since 1981 in the prevention of recurrent heterotopic ossification in high-risk patients who have an acquired form of the disorder and who have undergone resection of a mature lesion.[47,51,52] Coventry and Scanlon[59] recommended 2,000 rads in each of 10 doses within 10 days to 2 weeks following resection of a mature heterotopic ossified lesion. However, new protocols recommend lower doses of 700 to 800 rads within 1 to 4 days postoperatively and for no more than two doses.[52] These lower doses, directed to the site of ossification within several days of surgical excision, appear to be as effective as the higher dose longer-duration regimen. The theoretical target of radiation therapy is the localized pool of inducible osteoprogenitor cells.

Physical therapy has remained controversial as a preventive and treatment modality for heterotopic ossification.[53,54] Aggressive stretching of spastic limbs has been implicated as a causative factor in heterotopic ossification. Michelsson and associates[60] developed a rabbit model in which forcible joint manipulation induces heterotopic ossification. Reports on early studies of physiotherapy following heterotopic ossification described worsening of the ossification, which resulted in complete joint ankylosis in some cases. Subsequent reports have shown that passive range of motion exercises may be beneficial in heterotopic ossification of neurogenic etiology. Neither the beneficial nor the adverse effects of physical therapy are understood.

Surgical excision of heterotopic ossification would appear to be the most definitive and beneficial treatment; however, surgical excision has resulted in numerous complications including infection, hemorrhage, and recurrence of ossification.[55–58] Surgical intervention should be restricted to patients who have advanced symptomatology or ankylosis, and it must be delayed until the heterotopic bone is mature, as determined by radiographic and radionuclide studies. The etiology of the heterotopic ossification may be the most important factor when considering surgical management. Although surgical resection has been proven beneficial in some cases, such as heterotopic ossification resulting from neurologic and thermal injuries, it is ineffective and even detrimental in others. In FOP, surgical intervention is absolutely contraindicated except in the most emergent circumstances, because surgery invariably results in recurrence of ossification and often causes extensive progression of the disease.[23]

References

1. Campbell JT, Kaplan FS: The role of morphogens in endochondral ossification. *Calcif Tissue Int* 1992;50:283–289.
2. Canalis E, McCarthy T, Centrella M: Growth factors and the regulation of bone remodeling. *J Clin Invest* 1988;81:277–281.
3. Celeste AJ, Iannazzi JA, Taylor RC, et al: Identification of transforming growth factor β family members present in bone-inductive protein purified from bovine bone. *Proc Natl Acad Sci USA* 1990;87:9843–9847.
4. Luyten FP, Cunningham NS, Ma S, et al: Purification and partial amino acid sequence of osteogenin, a protein initiating bone differentiation. *J Biol Chem* 1989; 264:13377–13380.
5. Mohan S, Baylink DJ: Bone growth factors. *Clin Orthop* 1991;263:30–48.
6. Ozkaynak E, Rueger DC, Drier EA, et al: OP-1 cDNA encodes an osteogenic protein in the TGF-β family. *EMBO J* 1990;9:2085–2093.
7. Urist MR, DeLange RJ, Finerman GA: Bone cell differentiation and growth factors. *Science* 1983;220:680–686.
8. Wang EA, Rosen V, D'Alessandro JS, et al: Recombinant human bone morphogenetic protein induces bone formation. *Proc Natl Acad Sci USA* 1990;87:2220–2224.
9. Wozney JM, Rosen V, Celeste AJ, et al: Novel regulators of bone formation: Molecular clones and activities. *Science* 1988;242:1528–1534.
10. Caplan AI: Mesenchymal stem cells. *J Orthop Res* 1991;9:641–650.
11. Muthukumaran N, Reddi AH: Bone matrix-induced local bone induction. *Clin Orthop* 1985;200:159–164.
12. Puzas JE, Miller MD, Rosier RN: Pathologic bone formation. *Clin Orthop* 1989; 245:269–281.
13. Sawyer JR, Myers MA, Rosier RN, et al: Heterotopic ossification: Clinical and cellular aspects. *Calcif Tissue Int* 1991;49:208–215.
14. Urist MR: Bone: Formation by autoinduction. *Science* 1965;150:893–899.
15. Bravo-Payno P, Esclarin A, Arzoz T, et al: Incidence and risk factors in the appearance of heterotopic ossification in spinal cord injury. *Paraplegia* 1992;30:740–745.
16. Garland DE: A clinical perspective on common forms of acquired heterotopic ossification. *Clin Orthop* 1991;263:13–29.
17. Wang ZQ, Grigoriadis AE, Mohle-Steinlein U, et al: A novel target cell for c-fos-induced oncogenesis: Development of chondrogenic tumours in embryonic stem cell chimeras. *EMBO J* 1991;10:2437–2450.
18. Bostrom K, Watson KE, Horn S, et al: Bone morphogenetic protein expression in human atherosclerotic lesions. *J Clin Invest* 1993;91:1800–1809.
19. Cohen RB, Hahn GV, Tabas JA, et al: The natural history of heterotopic ossification in patients who have fibrodysplasia ossificans progressiva: A study of forty-four patients. *J Bone Joint Surg* 1993;75A:215–219.
20. Connor JM, Evans DAP: Fibrodysplasia ossificans progressiva: The clinical features and natural history of 34 patients. *J Bone Joint Surg* 1982;64B:76–83.
21. Connor JM, Evans DAP: Genetic aspects of fibrodysplasia ossificans progressiva. *J Med Genet* 1982;19:35–39.

22. Kaplan FS, Tabas JA, Zasloff MA: Fibrodysplasia ossificans progressiva: A clue from the fly? *Calcif Tissue Int* 1990;47:117–125.

23. Kaplan FS, Tabas JA, Gannon FH, et al: The histopathology of fibrodysplasia ossificans progressiva: An endochondral process. *J Bone Joint Surg* 1993;75A:220–230.

24. Kaplan FS, McCluskey W, Hahn GV, et al: Genetic transmission of fibrodysplasia ossificans progressiva: Report of a family. *J Bone Joint Surg* 1993;75A:1214–1220.

25. McKusick VA: *Heritable Disorders of Connective Tissue*, ed 4. St. Louis, MO, CV Mosby, 1972, pp 687–706.

26. McKusick VA: 13510. Fibrodysplasia ossificans progressiva (FOP), in McKusick VA (ed): *Mendelian Inheritance in Man. Cataloges of Autosomal Dominant, Autosomal Recessive, and X-linked Phenotypes*, ed 10. Baltimore, MD, The Johns Hopkins University Press, 1992, p 392.

27. Rogers JG, Geho WB: Fibrodysplasia ossificans progressiva: A survey of 42 cases. *J Bone Joint Surg* 1979;61A:909–914.

28. Padgett RW, Wozney JM, Gelbart WM: Human BMP sequences can confer normal dorsal-ventral patterning in the *Drosophila* embryo. *Proc Natl Acad Sci USA* 1993;90:2905–2909.

29. Brook CGD, Valman HB: Osteoma cutis and Albright's hereditary osteodystrophy. *Br J Dermatol* 1971;85:471–475.

30. Edmonds HW, Coe HE, Tabrah FL: Bone formation in skin and muscle: Localized tissue malformation or heterotopia. *J Pediatr* 1948;33:618–623.

31. Foster CM, Levin S, Levin M, et al: Limited dermal ossification: Clinical features and natural history. *J Pediatr* 1986;109:71–76.

32. Gardner RJM, Yun K, Craw SM: Familial ectopic ossification. *J Med Genet* 1988;25:113–117.

33. Kaplan FS, Craver R, MacEwen GD, et al: Progressive osseous heteroplasia: A distinct developmental disorder of heterotopic ossification. *J Bone Joint Surg* 1994;76A:425–436.

34. Lim MO, Mukherjee AB, Hansen JW: Dysplastic cutaneous osteomatosis: A unique case of true osteoma. *Arch Dermatol* 1981;117:797–799.

35. Albright F, Burnett CH, Smith PH, et al: Pseudo-hypoparathyroidism—an example of "Seabright-Bantam Syndrome": Report of three cases. *Endocrinology* 1942;30:922–932.

36. Albright F, Forbes AP, Henneman PH: Pseudo-pseudohypoparathyroidism. *Trans Assoc Am Physicians* 1952;65:337–350.

37. Patten JL, Johns DR, Valle D, et al: Mutation in the gene encoding the stimulatory G protein of adenylate cyclase in Albright's hereditary osteodystrophy. *N Engl J Med* 1990;322:1412–1419.

38. Weinstein LS, Gejman PV, Friedman E, et al: Mutations of the Gs alpha-subunit gene in Albright hereditary osteodystrophy detected by denaturing gradient gel electrophoresis. *Proc Natl Acad Sci USA* 1990;87:8287–8290.

39. Prakash UB, McCullough AE, Edell ES, et al: Tracheopathia osteoplastica: Familial occurrence. *Mayo Clin Proc* 1989;64:1091–1096.

40. Ekelund A, Brosjo O, Nilsson OS: Experimental induction of heterotopic bone. *Clin Orthop* 1991;263:102–112.

41. Michelsson JE, Rauschning W: Pathogenesis of experimental heterotopic bone formation following temporary forcible exercising of immobilized limbs. *Clin Orthop* 1983;176:265–272.

42. Huggins CB: Formation of bone under the influence of epithelium of the urinary tract. *Arch Surg* 1931;22:377–408.

43. Urist MR: Bone morphogenetic protein, bone regeneration, heterotopic ossification and the bone marrow consortium, in Peck WA (ed): *Bone and Mineral Research*. New York, NY, Elsevier Science Publishers, 1989, pp 6–57.

44. Reddi AH: Cell biology and biochemistry of endochondral bone development. *Collagen and Related Research* 1981;1:209–226.

45. Khouri RK, Koudsi B, Reddi AH: Tissue transformation into bone in vivo: A potential practical application. *JAMA* 1991;266:1953–1955.

46. Connor JM: *Soft Tissue Ossification.* Berlin, Springer-Verlag, 1983.

47. Ahrengart L, Lindgren U, Reinholt FP: Comparative study of the effects of radiation, indomethacin, prednisolone, and ethane-1-hydroxy-1,1-diphosphonate (EHDP) in the prevention of ectopic bone formation. *Clin Orthop* 1988;229:265–273.

48. Francis MD, Russell RGG, Fleisch H: Diphosphonates inhibit formation of calcium phosphate crystals *in vitro* and pathological calcification *in vivo. Science* 1969;165:1264–1266.

49. Hu HP, Kuijpers W, Slooff TJ, et al: The effect of biphosphonate on induced heterotopic bone. *Clin Orthop* 1991;272:259–267.

50. DiCesare PE, Nimni ME, Peng L, et al: Effects of indomethacin on demineralized bone-induced heterotopic ossification in the rat. *J Orthop Res* 1991;9:855–861.

51. Ayers DC, Pellegrini VD Jr, Evarts CM: Prevention of heterotopic ossification in high-risk patients by radiation therapy. *Clin Orthop* 1991;263:87–93.

52. Pellegrini VD Jr, Konski AA, Gastel JA, et al: Prevention of heterotopic ossification with irradiation after total hip arthroplasty: Radiation therapy with a single dose of eight hundred centrigray administered to a limited field. *J Bone Joint Surg* 1992;74A:186–200.

53. Crawford CM, Varghese G, Mani MM, et al: Heterotopic ossification: Are range of motion exercises contraindicated? *J Burn Care Rehabil* 1986;7:323–327.

54. Garland DE, Razza BE, Waters RL: Forceful joint manipulation in head-injured adults with heterotopic ossification. *Clin Orthop* 1982;169:133–138.

55. Ahrengart L: Periarticular heterotopic ossification after total hip arthroplasty: Risk factors and consequences. *Clin Orthop* 1991;263: 49–58.

56. Garland DE, Orwin JF: Resection of heterotopic ossification in patients with spinal cord injuries. *Clin Orthop* 1989;242:169–76.

57. Garland DE: Surgical approaches for resection of heterotopic ossification in traumatic brain-injured adults. *Clin Orthop* 1991; 263:59–70.

58. Stover SL, Niemann KM, Tulloss JR: Experience with surgical resection of heterotopic bone in spinal cord injury patients. *Clin Orthop* 1991;263:71–77.

59. Coventry MB, Scanlon PW: The use of radiation to discourage ectopic bone: A nine-year study in surgery about the hip. *J Bone Joint Surg* 1981;63A:201–208.

60. Michelsson JE, Granroth G, Andersson LC: Myositis ossificans following forcible manipulation of the leg: A rabbit model for the study of heterotopic bone formation. *J Bone Joint Surg* 1980; 62A:811–815.

Chapter 7

Sarcomatous Bone Formation

Randy Rosier, MD, PhD
David G. Hicks, MD

Introduction

Sarcomatous bone formation is specific to osteosarcomas, which are malignant neoplasms derived from osteoblastic cells. The hallmark of these tumors is the elaboration of bone matrix, or osteoid, which usually undergoes mineralization. This property of matrix production is shared by benign bone-forming tumors, including osteoid osteoma and osteoblastoma. The phenotype of the neoplastic cells in osteosarcoma is varied, and these cells can include areas of chondroblastic and fibroblastic elements in addition to osteoblasts. In addition, the degree of matrix production and cellular differentiation varies widely among these tumors. This heterogeneity forms the basis for the subclassification of osteosarcomas into distinct clinical and histologic subtypes. True bone formation within sarcomas of other histogenesis is extremely rare, although calcifications are common in many types of soft-tissue sarcoma, such as synovial sarcoma.[1] Histologically these calcifications generally do not resemble bone or show evidence of osteoid.

Despite the production of mineralizing osteoid by tumors, the microstructure of neoplastic bone differs from that of normal bone. Neoplastic bone remains as woven bone and does not remodel into lamellar bone, thus providing an essential means of differentiating neoplastic bone from injury and repair processes. Osteosarcoma is an unusual example of an aggressive, highly proliferative malignancy that retains many features of differentiated cellular function.

Types of Osteosarcoma

Osteosarcoma is the most common primary bony malignancy apart from multiple myeloma, and it generally affects individuals in the second and third decades of life. The most common form is the classic, metaphyseal, high-grade, bone-producing tumor of long bones. Numerous variants have been described, including chondroblastic and fibroblastic osteosarcomas, small-cell osteosarcoma, periosteal osteosarcoma, parosteal osteosarcoma, well-differentiated osteosarcoma, telangiectatic osteosarcoma, and secondary osteosarcoma.[2] Small-cell osteosarcomas are characterized by a high nuclear-to-cytoplasmic ratio, primitive cells, and sparse osteoid production.[3] Periosteal, parosteal, and intraosseus well-differentiated osteosarcomas all have a less aggressive biologic behavior than classic high-grade osteosarcoma, as well as a decreased tendency to metastasize.

Periosteal osteosarcomas originate beneath the periosteum and often have a chondroblastic predominance. In contrast, parosteal osteosarcoma is thought to arise outside the periosteum, most often in the distal femur, and it usually exhibits well-differentiated cellular morphology with osteoblastic and fibroblastic elements, and, occasionally, cartilage. The trabecular organization of parosteal osteosarcoma tends to be better defined and resembles normal bone more than that of other variants, occasionally making diagnosis difficult. Telangiectatic osteosarcoma is a high-grade variant, which histologically and grossly resembles an aneurysmal bone cyst containing large blood-filled cavities. However, malignant osteoid-producing stromal cells are found within the fibrous septae, frequently showing marked nuclear pleomorphism. Secondary osteosarcomas arise characteristically in preexisting lesions, including Paget disease, fibrous dysplasia, chronic osteomyelitis, and following radiation treatment. Pagetic and postradiation osteosarcomas are the more common types. Secondary osteosarcomas are always high-grade, aggressive tumors, are associated with a poor prognosis, and usually occur in an older age group.[4]

The treatment of all high-grade types of osteosarcoma involves surgical excision of the lesion with limb reconstruction or amputation and with wide to radical surgical margins. Adjuvant chemotherapy, usually with drugs such as doxorubicin, methotrexate, Cytoxan, and vincristine, is an essential component of the therapy and significantly reduces the incidence of metastases.[5] Lower-grade osteosarcomas, such as well-differentiated intraosseus and parosteal variants, may be managed with wide to radical surgical resection alone. Most osteosarcomas are resistant to radiation, and radiotherapy is generally not recommended as a part of the treatment program. The overall disease-free 5-year survival for high-grade lesions ranges from 50% to 75% in different series.[6,7]

Histologic Features

Sarcomas other than osteosarcoma can exhibit some of the histologic features of osteosarcoma. For example, chondrosarcomas contain malignant cartilaginous tissue, and fibrosarcomas contain malignant fibrous tissue. However, the presence of any osteoid production by the cells of a tumor (in the absence of pathologic fracture) defines it as an osteosarcoma. The most important feature of neoplastic bone is its persistence in a woven or nonlamellar form. Although woven bone is a prominent feature of injury and repair processes, including myositis ossificans, fracture healing, and reactive bone formation, these lesions demonstrate a transition from woven to lamellar bone that is a key to pathologic differential diagnosis. Endochondral calcification of cartilaginous areas of osteosarcoma can occur, but it occurs without the smooth transition from calcified matrix to lamellar bone formation observed with injury and repair.

Tissue Organization

The overall organization of the various histologic elements found in osteosarcoma also differs in an important way from that in physiologic processes. The least differentiated and most aggressive regions of a malignant neoplasm are at the periphery of the lesion, farthest from the site of origin or "field" in which the tumor arose. In reparative processes, such as myositis ossificans, the most cellular and least differentiated areas are central, with progressive maturation toward the periphery (zonation) where lamellar bone formation usually is apparent. Central regions of osteosarcomas may exhibit necrosis, and bone formation in these areas demonstrates increased mineralization as well as a tendency for "normalization" of the malignant osteoblasts entrapped in matrix, with a decrease in nuclear atypia and other cellular features of malignancy.

Similarly, the malignant property of invasiveness is most obvious at the peripheral interface with the host tissue. One other interface that is important in evaluating these lesions is the periosteum adjacent to the lesion. The invading tumor frequently elevates the periosteum and induces reactive bone formation by the periosteum itself. The layer of bone formed by the elevated periosteum can be visualized radiographically and is called Codman's triangle. The "hair-on-end" or "sunburst" periosteal bone formations that have been described in association with Codman's triangle consist of parallel streamers or rays of reactive bone that are oriented perpendicular to the longitudinal axis of the cortex. These periosteal bone formations consist of both woven and lamellar bone and must be recognized as a reactive phenomenon, because they represent one of only two circumstances under which lamellar bone forms in conjunction with osteosarcoma. The other is in fracture callus in rare cases associated with pathologic fracture.

Microscopic Structure

The microscopic structure of sarcomatous bone differs in a number of ways from that of normal bone. Usually, neoplastic bone is more cellular and the size and shape of its cells and its degree of calcification are variable. Osteoblastic rimming of neoplastic trabeculae is observed in benign tumors, such as osteoid osteoma and osteoblastoma, but is absent in most osteosarcomas. The overall trabecular organization is poor, with decreased connectivity and smaller trabeculae. Marrow elements may be entrapped by malignant osteoid, as are normal bony trabeculae, with effacement of both in some areas. Areas of necrosis are common in osteosarcoma.

Malignant osteoid may be deposited directly on existing trabecular host bone and often has a more basophilic appearance under routine hematoxylin and eosin staining (Fig. 1, *left*). The poorly organized woven quality of the malignant bone deposition is further delineated under polarized light. The orderly orthogonal orientation of the collagen fibrils in successive lamellae of normal bone shows a distinct linear pattern, whereas the random orientation of fibrils in the malignant woven bone matrix does not (Fig. 1, *right*). The undeveloped trabeculae of osteosarcoma can appear as a lace-like pattern of osteoid, which is readily seen with a reticulin stain (Fig. 2). This stain highlights smaller diameter collagen fibrils, including type III collagen and immature type I collagen, which have been shown to be increased in osteosarcoma.[8]

Although resorption of normal host bone by both tumor and osteoclastic cells is common, osteoclastic resorption of sarcomatous bone does not appear to occur. Osteoclastic resorption of tumor bone is absent even in areas of spontaneous necrosis or necrosis secondary to chemotherapy, whereas adjacent spicules of necrotic normal lamellar bone may undergo active osteoclastic resorption (DGH, personal observation). Thus, the normal local coupling of bone resorption and formation is absent in osteosarcoma, and probably accounts for the inability of malignant bone to remodel. It is not known whether sarcomatous bone can respond to mechanical forces, but this seems unlikely given the apparent lack of local coupling in this tissue and its disorganization and poor trabecular connectivity. Malignant osteoid is usually less fully calcified than normal bone (Fig. 3). However, as it is in normal bone, the mineral form in osteosarcomatous bone is hydroxyapatite.[9]

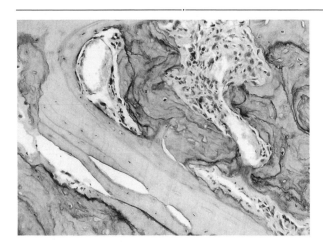

Fig. 1 Top, Human osteosarcoma with deposition of woven bone on host lamellar bony trabeculae. Note the darker (more basophilic) staining of the tumor bone (hematoxylin and eosin, × 100). **Bottom,** Human osteosarcoma viewed under polarized light. Note the bright linear patterns within the lamellar host bone which are absent in the sarcomatous woven bone (× 100).

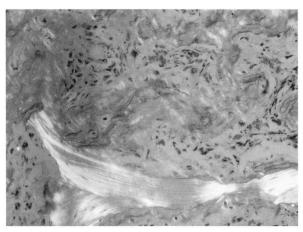

Ultrastructure

Ultrastructural studies have demonstrated similarities between the bone formation in osteosarcoma and in embryonic bone. These similarities include the random orientation of the collagen fibers, some cytologic features, and the incomplete degree of calcification. The collagen fibrils are randomly oriented along the cell surface, although the normal 640 Å periodicity has been observed in most studies.[9] The fibril diameter is 30 to 90 nm, which is smaller than in normal bone, and the collagen composition has been found to be 65% type I, 25% type III, and 10% type V as compared with almost entirely type I in normal bone.[8] In addition, there is an abnormally high ratio of $\alpha 1(I)$ to $\alpha 2(I)$ chains, which suggests that part of the type I collagen expressed in osteosarcomas is present as type I trimer collagen $[\alpha 1(I)]_3$, which normally is prominent only during early development.[8] The hydroxylysine content of the collagen is also increased.[8] Cytologically, osteosarcoma cells exhibit an overabundance of dilated rough endoplasmic reticulum cisternae, irregular nuclei that are more central and larger than normal, moderate numbers of mitochondria, and dense chromatin.[9-11] The various cellular phenotypes represented in osteosarcoma—osteoblasts, fibroblasts, and chondroblasts—appear similar to each other in

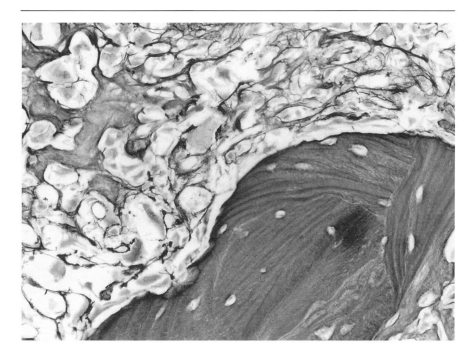

Fig. 2 Human osteosarcoma stained with reticulin. There is homogeneous staining of the host lamellar bone without an identifiable fibrillar pattern but the lace-like pattern of the collagen fibrils in the woven neoplastic bone is readily apparent (× 200).

these cytologic features.[9,11] The formation of hydroxyapatite crystals along the collagen fibrils is haphazard.[9] Matrix vesicles have been reported in calcifying osteoid of both osteosarcoma and normal bone, but their role and any differences between normal and abnormal tissue remain unclear.[12–14]

Matrix Composition

Several studies have examined the expression of various matrix components in osteosarcoma. The majority of these studies have focused on the use of osteosarcoma cell models in tissue culture, as will be discussed later. In general, most proteins, including growth factors, known to be present in normal bone have been identified in osteosarcoma bone matrix or in cultures of osteosarcoma cells. As in normal mineralizing bone and cartilage, the bone-forming cells in osteosarcoma contain very high levels of alkaline phosphatase.[15,16] The role of alkaline phosphatase is unclear, but it is thought to facilitate mineral deposition, possibly by providing high local concentrations of phosphate. Serum levels of alkaline phosphatase are often elevated in patients with osteosarcoma, making serum alkaline phosphatase one of the few biochemical indicators of musculoskeletal malignancy. Alkaline phosphatase levels may decrease with chemotherapy, and progressive mineralization of the osteoid and cellular necrosis are usually observed.[17] Alkaline phosphatase activity has also been studied in cultured osteosarcoma cells, and resembles that in cultured normal osteoblasts, both in level of expression and in regulation by growth factors.[18]

Although some studies have indicated that demineralized bone matrix from osteosarcoma is less osteogenic than normal bone matrix,[19] both osteogenic

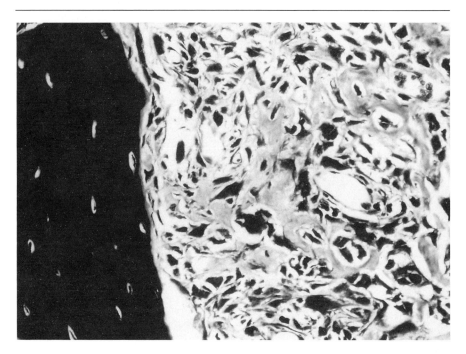

Fig. 3 Osteosarcoma stained with Gomori's trichrome (demineralized section). Collagen in-cluding osteoid appears blue in color with this stain but fully mineralized tissue appears dark red in these sections. The red stain here is represented by the dark areas. The fully mineralized host bone is readily differentiated from the incompletely mineralized osteoid of the osteosarcoma matrix ($\times$ 200).

activity and bone morphogenetic proteins (BMPs) have been found in tumor bone.[20–23] The induction of bone and cartilage formation by in vivo implantation of killed osteosarcoma cells[24] or of BMP extracted from osteosarcoma cells[20,21,23] is qualitatively normal and similar to that by implantation of BMP extracted from normal bone. Immunohistochemically, BMP has been localized along collagen fibrils and in mesenchymal, marrow stromal, and periosteal cells in normal bone, which have the potential under the right circumstances to generate new bone. Minimal staining was present in normal bone cells or cal-cified bone matrix with the antibody used in these studies. However, in human embryos BMP was localized in immature bone matrix, osteoblasts, and bone cell, but not in calcified matrix.[22] The neoplastic osteoblasts of osteosarcoma were found to contain abundant BMP.[22] Thus, the distribution or quantities of some of these proteins may be abnormal in tumor bone. Transforming growth factor-beta (TGF-ß) is also produced by osteosarcoma cells,[25] but the amount in sarcomatous bone matrix relative to normal bone is unknown.

The presence of bone-specific proteins, such as osteocalcin and osteopontin, has also been demonstrated immunohistochemically in bone-forming tumors. Osteocalcin is a vitamin K-dependent, glutamic acid-containing glycoprotein constituent of normal bone matrix that binds calcium. Its function is unknown, but several lines of evidence implicate osteocalcin as important in enabling bone resorption.[26,27] Osteocalcin-deficient bone matrix from vitamin K-depleted rats is poorly resorbed when implanted as compared with normal bone matrix.[26] Furthermore, hydroxyapatite or mixtures of hydroxyapatite with albumin or type I collagen are similarly resistant to resorption, whereas hydroxyapatite/ osteocalcin mixtures readily induce osteoclastic resorption of the material.[28] Immunolocalization of osteocalcin in bone demonstrates diffuse weak staining of the bone matrix with increased staining concentrated along cement lines between lamellae and in osteocytes (Fig. 4, *left* and *center*). In contrast, in osteosarcoma, the tumor cells stain intensely for osteocalcin, but the matrix generally does not (Fig. 4, *right*). Similar findings have been reported in osteoid osteoma.[29] Thus, while osteocalcin appears to be produced by osteogenic tumors, it apparently is either not secreted or not incorporated into the bone matrix. This may explain the observed inability of neoplastic bone to undergo normal resorption and remodeling.

Cell Biology

Osteosarcoma Cell Models

Numerous cell lines have been produced from both animal and human osteosarcomas by clonal isolation or cellular transformation. These have been used extensively to study bone-cell behavior and regulation of phenotypic expression. Some of the more commonly used cell lines include ROS 17/2.8 (rat), UMR 106 (rat), SAOS2 (human), MG-63 (human), MC3T3 (murine), and TE-85 (human). In general, the literature has tended to emphasize the characteristics of these cell models, which are similar to normal osteoblasts, although many differences have also been reported both between normal and osteosarcoma cells and among the different osteosarcoma cell types. Essentially, every growth factor and matrix component identified in normal osteoblasts has been identified in one or another of these osteosarcoma cell lines, demonstrating some degree of qualitative similarity between osteosarcoma and normal osteoblasts. These proteins include type I collagen, osteopontin, osteonectin, insulin-like growth factor-I (IGF-I), interleukins, osteocalcin, TGF-β, BMPs, protein-derived growth factor (PDGF), bone-specific proteoglycans, β2-microglobulin, protein S, and matrix Gla protein.[30–39] Little is known about the relative production of these components in normal versus sarcomatous cells, because few comparative studies have been reported. TGF-β is expressed at similar mRNA and protein levels in osteosarcoma and normal fetal osteoblasts, although the responses of these cells to exogenous TGF-β are qualitatively different.[25] TGF-β also has chemotactic properties toward both cell types.[40,41] In other studies, similar responses were found to parathyroid hormone (PTH) and vitamin D metabolites in both normal and transformed osteoblasts. These responses include stimulation of collagenase and other matrix metalloproteinases by PTH and stimulation of osteocalcin by 1,25-dihydroxyvitamin D_3.[42,43] Both normal and osteosarcoma cells also produce mineralizing nodules in confluent cultures when supplemented with ascorbate and β-glycerol phosphate.[44] However, these mineralizing nodules do not resemble trabecular bone histologically in either model, suggesting that the participation of other cell populations or factors present in vivo may regulate the architecture of deposited bony matrices.

Matrix Metalloproteinases

The three major categories of matrix metalloproteinases (MMPs) include type I (collagenases), type II (gelatinases or type IV collagenase), and type III (stromelysins). These enzymes are secreted by both chondrocytes and osteoblasts, and are thought to be important in normal matrix remodeling. Other neutral

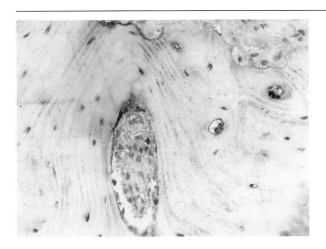

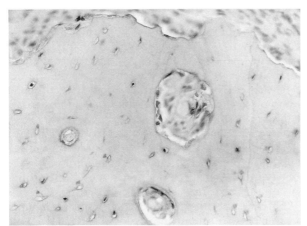

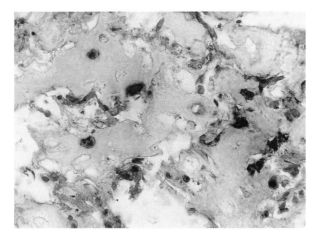

Fig. 4 Top, Normal lamellar bone stained using immunoperoxidase technique to localize osteocalcin. Note the staining within osteocytes and along the cement lines of the lamellae (× 100). **Center**, This is a negative control of the same specimen (primary antiosteocalcin antibody omitted) (× 100). **Bottom**, Osteocalcin immunohistochemistry in a human osteosarcoma. There is intense staining within the malignant osteoblasts throughout but no staining of the neoplastic matrix (× 200).

proteases such as cathepsins have been identified in both osteoblasts and osteoclasts.[45] In addition, two forms of a natural inhibitor of MMP activity, tissue inhibitors of metalloproteinase (TIMP), are also produced by osteoblasts and appear to function to maintain a balance between matrix production and breakdown. MMP production in both normal and malignant phenotypes of osteoblastic cells is regulated similarly by calcitropic hormones.[42,43] However, excessive secretion of gelatinase in cultured osteosarcoma cells has been reported,[32] and it may play a role in the invasive and metastatic properties of the tumor. Elevated MMP activity resulting from abnormal secretion of MMPs or deficient production of TIMPs may also account for the frequently observed erosion or destruction of normal host trabeculae by osteoblastic tumor cells in osteosarcoma.

Cell Adhesion Factors

Recently, abnormalities of β1 integrin and corresponding ligand expression have been identified in osteosarcoma.[46] Although osteosarcomas express abundant type I collagen, cells from these tumors have been found, unlike cells from normal connective tissues, to lack the collagen receptor. In addition, expression of laminin and the laminin receptor is diminished in osteosarcoma matrix, although there is strong expression of the α4 and α5 fibronectin receptors and abundant expression of fibronectin. The abnormalities of expression of the integrins and ligands may have some relevance to the ability of osteosarcoma to metastasize. Therapeutic use of integrin ligands has inhibited metastasis in animal models,[47] and overexpression of an integrin subunit by a transfected tumor cell line has been shown to enhance its metastatic potential.[48] A recent osteosarcoma animal model has been reported in which injection of malignant cells into nude mice reproducibly caused pulmonary metastases. When explants of lung or isolated lung endothelial cells were implanted subcutaneously in an ectopic location in the mice, metastasis to the ectopic lung tissue or cells as well as to the lung occurred.[49] This phenomenon strongly implicates cellular adhesion factors or regional chemotactic factors in determining the site specificity of metastatic disease.

Osteoclasts

Osteoclast-like giant cells are frequently observed in bone forming tumors, although questions remain as to their function. Osteoclastic resorption of tumor bone is almost never observed; this lack of resorption may relate to the previously mentioned abnormality of osteocalcin distribution in neoplastic bone. Osteocalcin has been suggested to induce preosteoclast differentiation.[27,28] In histochemical assessment, tartrate-resistant acid phosphatase, a marker of normal bone resorptive cells, was found in the osteoclast-like cells of osteosarcoma and osteoblastoma. However, carbonic anhydrase, also present in normal osteoclasts, was found to be absent, suggesting that the giant cells observed in these bone tumors may not represent fully functional resorptive cells.[50]

Pathogenesis

Although the cause of osteosarcoma is unknown, a number of predisposing factors have been identified. Osteosarcoma most commonly arises in adolescence during maximal growth and near the most active growth plates in the long bones (distal femur and proximal tibia), suggesting a derangement of normal growth and remodeling processes. Because long bone growth depends on growth hormone stimulation of local IGF-I, it has been hypothesized that this growth factor, which is produced in the growth plate and in bone, may be involved in the development of osteosarcoma.[51–53] Hypophysectomy in animal models has slowed growth of osteosarcoma and decreased metastases,[52] and IGF-I responsiveness and production have been demonstrated in both human and murine osteosarcoma cells in culture.[51] Furthermore, osteosarcoma has been shown to express more IGF-I receptors than other types of sarcoma.[53] Thus IGF-I stimulation may play a role in the development or progression of osteosarcoma.

A considerable amount of evidence has accumulated that implicates tumor suppressor genes as important in the pathogenesis of osteosarcoma. Two suppressor genes in particular, p53 and the RB gene, have been studied in this regard. The RB gene encodes a 105-kd nuclear phosphoprotein that is thought to be a transcription factor involved in regulation of the cell cycle. This unphosphorylated form appears to prevent entry into S phase of the cell cycle, while the phosphorylated form of the protein is permissive for cell cycle progression.[54–57] Abnormalities of the RB gene were initially noted in retinoblastoma, and over 40% of patients with retinoblastoma exhibit germline mutations in one allele. Conversely, patients with RB germline mutations have a 95% risk of developing retinoblastoma, and a familial recessive inheritance of the disease.[54] The action of suppressor genes is generally not an all or none phenomenon; if one allele is normal some growth suppressing activity is retained, and homozygosity for the defective gene is required for oncogenesis.[56,58]

An association of retinoblastoma and osteosarcoma has been observed, and patients with germline RB mutations have a 15% risk of developing osteosarcoma. Germline mutations strongly predispose to malignancy because only a single additional somatic mutation of the other allele is necessary to result in loss of suppressor function of the gene. Most osteosarcomas that have been studied exhibit loss or abnormality of the protein encoded by the RB gene. Additionally, sarcomas with RB mutations tend to be more aggressive biologically than those with normal RB expression.[57] Thus, abnormalities of the RB gene may provide one mechanism of oncogenesis in osteosarcoma.

The p53 tumor suppressor gene, located on the short arm of chromosome 17, is the most frequently mutated gene described in human cancers.[58–65] This gene, which under normal circumstances associates to form tetramers, is a nuclear protein that inhibits cell growth. Recently, binding of p53 to specific DNA sequences has been demonstrated, supporting its role as a putative transcription factor.[66] Germline mutations of p53 involving gene rearrangement have been identified in the Li-Fraumeni syndrome, in which there is a high familial incidence of sarcomas and other cancers in young adults.[67–69] Mutations of p53 also include deletions and point mutations, with some form of abnormality identified in approximately 70% to 75% of osteosarcomas.[54,56,59,70] The effect of a given mutation on the p53 protein is variable and ranges from absence of expression to normal or elevated levels of dysfunctional protein.[59] The half-life of p53 is short (20 to 30 minutes), and elevated levels of expression may result from defective degradation of some mutant forms of the protein. Mutations of p53 also have been reported in many other types of cancers, including soft-tissue sarcoma, carcinomas, and leukemias.[65] In one series of multifocal osteosarcomas, all four patients studied exhibited germline or somatic p53 mutations.[71] In SAOS2 osteosarcoma cells, which lack the p53 gene, transfection with a normal p53 gene inhibited tumorigenesis while transfection with mutant p53 did not. Transfection of both normal and mutant p53 resulted in a nontumorigenic phenotype, indicating dominance of the wild type (nonmutant) suppressor protein.[58] Most osteosarcomas exhibit loss or abnormalities of the p53 suppressor in addition to loss of the RB suppressor. This indicates the usual requirement for multiple mutations in order for full expression of the malignant phenotype to occur. This "multiple hit" theory of oncogenesis also explains the inheritable predispositions to certain sarcomas.[56]

Another mechanism of regulation of p53 suppressor function has been identified recently. A murine tumor cell line containing amplified DNA sequences in the form of double minutes (small acentromeric extrachromosomal nuclear inclusions) was analyzed for the amplified sequences, and the corresponding protein was identified as murine double minute 2 (MDM2). The MDM2 was found to bind p53 proteins, inhibiting their transcriptional function.[70,72–74] Thus, overexpression of MDM2 provides another mechanism by which p53 dysfunction can contribute to oncogenesis. Recently, amplification of the human homolog of MDM2 has been identified in approximately 15% of a series of osteosarcomas.[70]

Tumor suppressor mutations may influence the biologic behavior of a particular tumor in other ways. Approximately 30% to 50% of osteosarcomas express P-glycoprotein, the protein gene product of the multiple drug resistance gene 1 (MDR1).[75,76] The P-glycoprotein, which functions as a plasma membrane adenosine triphosphatase, actively pumps a wide variety of chemotherapeutic agents out of the tumor cells, thereby maintaining sublethal intracellular levels, and it is one of the known mechanisms of multiple drug resistance in tumors. In addition, chemotherapy increases its expression, and levels of P-glycoprotein expression correlate inversely with both long-term survival and tumor response to chemotherapy.[75–79] Mutant forms of p53 have recently been found to stimulate the MDR1 promoter, while normal p53 is inhibitory.[80] Therefore, some osteosarcomas with p53 abnormalities may exhibit resistance to chemotherapy and, correspondingly, more aggressive clinical behavior as a result of the suppressor mutation.

Other oncogenes have also been implicated in the pathogenesis of osteosarcoma. The oncogene c-*fos* codes for a nuclear transcription factor that, when overexpressed in transgenic mice, leads to osteosarcomas and chondrosarcomas.[81,82] Moreover, c-*fos* has been found to be overexpressed in human osteosarcomas.[83] Another oncogene, c-*myc*, has been found to be amplified in some osteosarcomas,[84] and may play some role in the transformation to the malignant phenotype. The importance of these oncogenes in the biogenesis of osteosarcoma and their relationship to the tumor suppressor genes await further study.

Conclusions

The composition of osteosarcoma and normal bone matrix is qualitatively similar, although some significant differences in the amounts and types of collagen have been identified. Whether various other components of the matrix are quantitatively present in differing amounts remains unknown. The most obvious histologic abnormalities in osteosarcomatous bone include the disorganization of the trabecular structure and the persistence of the bone in a woven form that does not appear to have the capacity to remodel into lamellar bone. Defective incorporation of osteocalcin in the sarcomatous matrix may play a role in this observed remodeling defect.

Numerous osteosarcoma cell models have provided a large amount of information regarding the production of growth factors, proteases, and matrix components, as well as the response patterns and mechanisms of action of hormones and cytokines on bone cells. In general, most of these cell types behave similarly to normal bone cells. However, numerous differences do exist, as do differences among the more commonly used osteosarcoma cell lines.

Significant progress has been made over the past decade in understanding the molecular biologic mechanisms responsible for the malignant transformation in osteosarcoma. Mutations in two tumor suppressor genes, the RB gene and p53, appear to play an essential role in this process. Germline transmission of some of these mutations may explain familial syndromes of cancer susceptibility, and identification of these lesions may provide a method of predicting this susceptibility clinically. Oncogenes have also been implicated in the pathogenesis of osteosarcoma, but their importance relative to suppressor gene mutations remains unknown.

References

1. Enzinger FM, Weiss SW: *Soft Tissue Tumors*. St. Louis, MO, CV Mosby, 1983, pp 519–549.
2. Mirra JM, Picci P, Gold R: *Bone Tumors: Clinical, Radiologic, and Pathologic Correlations*. Philadelphia, PA, Lea & Febiger, 1989.
3. Dickersin GR, Rosenberg AE: The ultrastructure of small-cell osteosarcoma, with a review of the light microscopy and differential diagnosis. *Hum Pathol* 1991;22: 267–275.
4. Healey JH, Buss D: Radiation and pagetic osteogenic sarcomas. *Clin Orthop* 1991; 270:128–134.
5. Rosen G, Caparros B, Huvos AG, et al: Preoperative chemotherapy for osteogenic sarcoma: Selection of postoperative adjuvant chemotherapy based on the response of the primary tumor to preoperative chemotherapy. *Cancer* 1982;49:1221–1223.
6. Simon MA: Limb salvage for osteosarcoma. *J Bone Joint Surg* 1988;70A:307–310.
7. Yasko AW, Lane JM: Chemotherapy for bone and soft-tissue sarcomas of the extremities. *J Bone Joint Surg* 1991;73A:1263–1271.
8. Shapiro FD, Eyre DR: Collagen polymorphism in extracellular matrix of human osteosarcoma. *J Natl Cancer Inst* 1982;69:1009–1016.
9. Williams AH, Schwinn CP, Parker JW: The ultrastructure of osteosarcoma: A review of twenty cases. *Cancer* 1976;37:1293–1301.
10. Sela J, Boyde A: Further observations on the relationship between the matrix and the calcifying fronts in osteosarcoma. *Virchows Arch A Pathol Anat* 1977;376: 175–180.
11. Paschall HA, Paschall MM: Electron microscopic observations of 20 human osteosarcomas. *Clin Orthop* 1975;111:42–56.
12. Morris DC, Masuhara K, Takaoka K, et al: Immunolocalization of alkaline phosphatase in osteoblasts and matrix vesicles of human fetal bone. *Bone Miner* 1992; 19:287–298.
13. Bonewald LF, Schwartz Z, Swain LD, et al: Stimulation of matrix vesicle enzyme activity in osteoblast-like cells by 1,25(OH)2D3 and transforming growth factor beta (TGF beta). *Bone Miner* 1992;17:139–144.
14. Fedde KN: Human osteosarcoma cells spontaneously release matrix-vesicle-like structures with the capacity to mineralize. *Bone Miner* 1992;17:145–151.
15. Timmer J, Hadders HN, Hardonk MJ, et al: An experimental investigation into the development of callus and induced bone tumours in mice studies by histological and enzyme histochemical methods. *Br J Cancer* 1968;22:422–436.
16. Jeffree GM: Enzymes in fibroblastic lesions: A histochemical and quantitative survey of alkaline and acid phosphatase, beta glucuronidase, non-specific esterase and leucine aminopeptidase in benign and malignant fibroblastic lesions of bone and soft tissue. *J Bone Joint Surg* 1972;54B:535–546.

17. Delling G, Krumme H, Salzer-Kuntschik M: Morphological changes in osteosarcoma after chemotherapy—COSS 80. *J Cancer Res Clin Oncol* 1983;106(suppl): 32–37.

18. Randall JC, Morris DC, Zeiger S, et al: Presence and activity of alkaline phosphatase in two human osteosarcoma cell lines. *J Histochem Cytochem* 1989;37:1069–1074.

19. Muthukumaran N, Reddi AH: Bone matrix-induced local bone induction. *Clin Orthop* 1985;200:159–164.

20. Hanamura H, Higuchi Y, Nakagawa M, et al: Solubilized bone morphogenetic protein (BMP) from mouse osteosarcoma and rat demineralized bone matrix. *Clin Orthop* 1980;148:281–290.

21. Kubler N, Urist MR: Cell differentiation in response to partially purified osteosarcoma-derived bone morphogenetic protein in vivo and in vitro. *Clin Orthop* 1993; 292:321–328.

22. Yang LJ, Jin Y: Immunohistochemical observations on bone morphogenetic protein in normal and abnormal conditions. *Clin Orthop* 1990;257:249–256.

23. Nogami H, Oohira A: Postnatal new bone formation. *Clin Orthop* 1984;184:106–113.

24. Hanamura H, Urist MR: Osteogenesis and chondrogenesis in transplants of Dunn and Ridgway osteosarcoma cell cultures. *Am J Pathol* 1978;91:277–298.

25. Robey PG, Young MF, Flanders KC, et al: Osteoblasts synthesize and respond to transforming growth factor-type beta (TGF-beta) in vitro. *J Cell Biol* 1987;105: 457–463.

26. Glowacki J, Lian JB: Impaired recruitment and differentiation of osteoclast progenitors by osteocalcin-deplete bone implants. *Cell Growth Differ* 1987;21:247–254.

27. Lian JB, Marks SC Jr: Osteopetrosis in the rat: Coexistence of reductions in osteocalcin and bone resorption. *Endocrinology* 1990;126:955–962.

28. Glowacki J, Rey C, Glimcher MJ, et al: A role for osteocalcin in osteoclast differentiation. *J Cell Biochem* 1991;45:292–302.

29. Vermeulen AH, Vermeer C, Bosman FT: Histochemical detection of osteocalcin in normal and pathological human bone. *J Histochem Cytochem* 1989;37:1503–1508.

30. Kubota T, Yamauchi M, Onozaki J, et al: Influence of an intermittent compressive force on matrix protein expression by ROS 17/2.8 cells with selective stimulation of osteopontin. *Arch Oral Biol* 1993;38:23–30.

31. Tornehave D, Teisner B, Rasmussen HB, et al: Fetal antigen 2 (FA2) in human fetal osteoblasts cultured osteoblasts and osteogenic osteosarcoma cells. *Anat Embryol* 1992;186:271–274.

32. Johansen JS, Williamson MK, Rice JS, et al: Identification of proteins secreted by human osteoblastic cells in culture. *J Bone Miner Res* 1992;7:501–512.

33. Maillard C, Berruyer M, Serre CM, et al: Protein-S, a vitamin K-dependent protein, is a bone matrix component synthesized and secreted by osteoblasts. *Endocrinology* 1992;130:1599–1604.

34. Noda M, Rodan GA: Type beta transforming growth factor regulates expression of genes encoding bone matrix proteins. *Connect Tissue Res* 1989;21:71–75.

35. Kream BE, Rowe D, Smith MD, et al: Hormonal regulation of collagen synthesis in a clonal rat osteosarcoma cell line. *Endocrinology* 1986;119:1922–1928.

36. Oldberg A, Franzen A, Heinegård D, et al: Identification of a bone sialoprotein receptor in osteosarcoma cells. *J Biol Chem* 1988;263:19433–19436.

37. Fraser JD, Otawara Y, Price PA: 1,25-Dihydroxyvitamin D3 stimulates the synthesis of matrix gamma-carboxyglutamic acid protein by osteosarcoma cells: Mutually exclusive expression of vitamin K-dependent bone proteins by clonal osteoblastic cell lines. *J Biol Chem* 1988;263:911–916.

38. Kaplan GC, Eilon G, Poser JW, et al: Constitutive biosynthesis of bone Gla protein in a human osteosarcoma cell line. *Endocrinology* 1985;117:1235–1238.

39. Bosse A, Schwarz K, Vollmer E, et al: Divergent and co-localization of the two small proteoglycans decorin and proteoglycan-100 in human skeletal tissues and tumors. *J Histochem Cytochem* 1993;41:13–19.
40. Pfeilschifter J, Wolf O, Naumann A, et al: Chemotactic response of osteoblastlike cells to transforming growth factor beta. *J Bone Miner Res* 1990;5:825–830.
41. Lucas PA: Chemotactic response of osteoblast-like cells to transforming growth factor beta. *Bone* 1989;10:459–463.
42. Einhorn TA, Majeska RJ: Neutral proteases in regenerating bone. *Clin Orthop* 1991;262:286–297.
43. Civitelli R, Hruska KA, Jeffrey JJ, et al: Second messenger signaling in the regulation of collagenase production by osteogenic sarcoma cells. *Endocrinology* 1989;124:2928–2934.
44. Guo JZ, Friesen HG: The osteoblastic properties of human osteogenic sarcoma cell line HOS TE85 characterized by morphological, histochemical and molecular biological studies. *J Bone Miner Res* 1991;6(suppl 1):S203.
45. Freimert C, Closs EI, Silbermann M, et al: Isolation of a cathepsin B-encoding cDNA from murine osteogenic cells. *Gene* 1991;103:259–261.
46. Kawaguchi S, Uede T: Distribution of integrins and their matrix ligands in osteogenic sarcomas. *J Orthop Res* 1993;11:386–395.
47. Humphries MJ, Olden K, Yamada KM: A synthetic peptide from fibronectin inhibits experimental metastasis of murine melanoma cells. *Science* 1986;233:467–470.
48. Chan BMC, Matsuura N, Takada Y, et al: In vitro and in vivo consequences of VLA-2 expression on rhabdomyosarcoma cells. *Science* 1991;251:1600–1602.
49. Kuratsu S, Uchida A, Araki N: Mechanism of organ selectivity in the determination of metastatic patterns of Dunn osteosarcoma. *Trans Orthop Res Soc* 1992;17:196.
50. Toyosawa S, Ogawa Y, Chang CK, et al: Histochemistry of tartrate-resistant acid phosphatase and carbonic anhydrase isoenzyme II in osteoclast-like giant cells in bone tumours. *Virchows Arch A Pathol Anat Histopathol* 1991;418:255–261.
51. Sem A, Bell RS, Pollak M, et al: IGF-responsiveness in human and murine osteosarcoma. *Trans Orthop Res Soc* 1992;17:226.
52. Pollak M, Sem AW, Richard M, et al: Inhibition of metastatic behavior of murine osteosarcoma by hypophysectomy. *J Natl Cancer Inst* 1992;84:966–971.
53. Sekyi-Otu A, Ohashi C, Bell RS, et al: IGF-receptors in sarcomas. *Trans Orthop Res Soc* 1993;18:594.
54. Knudson AG Jr: Pediatric molecular oncology: Past as prologue to the future. *Cancer* 1993;71(10 suppl):3320–3324.
55. Weinberg RA: Tumor suppressor genes. *Science* 1991;254:1138–1146.
56. Hansen MF: Molecular genetic considerations in osteosarcoma. *Clin Orthop* 1991;270:237–246.
57. Cance WG, Brennan MF, Dudas ME, et al: Altered expression of the retinoblastoma gene product in human sarcomas. *N Engl J Med* 1990;323:1457–1462.
58. Chen PL, Chen YM, Bookstein R, et al: Genetic mechanisms of tumor suppression by the human p53 gene. *Science* 1990;250:1576–1580.
59. Andreassen A, Oyjord T, Hovig E, et al: p53 abnormalities in different subtypes of human sarcomas. *Cancer Res* 1993;53:468–471.
60. Ueda Y, Dockhorn-Dworniczak B, Blasius S, et al: Analysis of mutant P53 protein in osteosarcomas and other malignant and benign lesions of bone. *J Cancer Res Clin Oncol* 1993;119:172–178.
61. Toguchida J, Yamaguchi T, Dayton SH, et al: Prevalence and spectrum of germline mutations of the p53 gene among patients with sarcoma. *N Engl J Med* 1992;326:1301–1308.
62. Chandar N, Billig B, McMaster J, et al: Inactivation of p53 gene in human and murine osteosarcoma cells. *Br J Cancer* 1992;65:208–214.
63. Masuda H, Miller C, Koeffler HP, et al: Rearrangement of the p53 gene in human osteogenic sarcomas. *Proc Natl Acad Sci USA* 1987;84:7716–7719.
64. Vogelstein B, Kinzler KW: p53 function and dysfunction. *Cell* 1992;70:523–526.

65. Hollstein M, Sidransky D, Vogelstein B, et al: p53 mutations in human cancers. *Science* 1991;253:49–53.

66. Kern SE, Kinzler KW, Bruskin A, et al: Identification of p53 as a sequence-specific DNA-binding protein. *Science* 1991;252:1708–1711.

67. Li FP, Fraumeni JF Jr, Mulvihill JJ, et al: A cancer family syndrome in 24 kindreds. *Cancer Res* 1988;48:5358–5362.

68. Porter DE, Holden ST, Steel CM, et al: A significant proportion of patients with osteosarcoma may belong to Li-Fraumeni cancer families. *J Bone Joint Surg* 1992; 74B:883–886.

69. Malkin D, Li FP, Strong LC, et al: Germ line p53 mutations in a familial syndrome of breast cancer, sarcomas, and other neoplasms. *Science* 1990;250:1233–1238.

70. Ladanyi M, Cha C, Lewis R, et al: MDM2 gene amplification in metastatic osteosarcoma. *Cancer Res* 1993;53:16–18.

71. Iavarone A, Matthay KK, Steinkirchner TM, et al: Germ-line and somatic p53 gene mutations in multifocal osteogenic sarcoma. *Proc Natl Acad Sci USA* 1992;89:4207–4209.

72. Fakharzadeh SS, Trusko SP, George DL: Tumorigenic potential associated with enhanced expression of a gene that is amplified in a mouse tumor cell line. *EMBO J* 1991;10:1565–1569.

73. Oliner JD, Kinzler KW, Meltzer PS, et al: Amplification of a gene encoding a p53-associated protein in human sarcomas. *Nature* 1992;358:80–83.

74. Momand J, Zambetti GP, Olson DC, et al: The mdm-2 oncogene product forms a complex with the p53 protein and inhibits p53-mediated transactivation. *Cell* 1992; 69:1237–1245.

75. Wunder JS, Bell RS, Wold L, et al: Expression of the multidrug resistance gene in osteosarcoma: A pilot study. *J Orthop Res* 1993;11:396–403.

76. Rosier RN, Hicks DG, Sickel JZ, et al: Immunohistochemical detection of a multiple drug resistance gene product (MDR1) in osteosarcoma. *Trans Orthop Res Soc* 1992;17:253.

77. Weinstein RS, Kuszak JR, Kluskens LF, et al: P-glycoproteins in pathology: The multidrug resistance gene family in humans. *Hum Pathol* 1990;21:34–48.

78. Gerlach JH, Bell DR, Karakousis C, et al: P-glycoprotein in human sarcoma: Evidence for multidrug resistance. *J Clin Oncol* 1987;5:1452–1460.

79. Chan HSL, Thorner PS, Haddad G, et al: Immunohistochemical detection of P-glycoprotein: Prognostic correlation in soft tissue sarcoma of childhood. *J Clin Oncol* 1990;8:689–704.

80. Chin KV, Ueda K, Pastan I, et al: Modulation of activity of the promoter of the human MDR1 gene by Ras and p53. *Science* 1992;255:459–462.

81. Grigoriadis AE, Schellander K, Wang ZQ, et al: Osteoblasts are target cells for transformation in c-fos transgenic mice. *J Cell Biol* 1993;122:685–701.

82. Ruther U, Komitowski D, Schubert FR, et al: c-fos expression induces bone tumors in transgenic mice. *Oncogene* 1989;4:861–865.

83. Wu JX, Carpenter PM, Gresens C, et al: The proto-oncogene c-fos is over-expressed in the majority of human osteosarcomas. *Oncogene* 1990;5:989–1000.

84. Healey JH, Ladanyi M, Park CK, et al: myc oncogene alterations in osteogenic sarcoma. *Trans Orthop Res Soc* 1993;18:598.

Section 1

Future Research Directions

Study human diseases and develop animal models to understand the key regulatory steps in bone formation.

William Harvey, the discoverer of the circulatory system, wrote in 1657, "Nature is nowhere accustomed more openly to display her secret mysteries than in cases where she shows traces of her workings apart from the beaten path." Much human misery arises from disabling skeletal disorders. These afflictions range from the very common to the very rare. Although all disabling skeletal diseases need solutions, many of these naturally-occurring conditions and their associated animal models provide a rare opportunity for in vivo study of specific genes, their protein products, and key regulatory steps involved in skeletogenesis and bone remodeling.

The study of naturally occurring human diseases and animal models to elucidate key regulatory steps in bone formation involves first the clear identification of disease characteristics or clinical phenotypes as well as variability within the study population. An example of this approach can be seen in the expanding number of reports of collagen gene anomalies. Although this strategy is not limited to a particular type of disorder, it finds a natural application in the study of genetic diseases. At times, a specific gene product abnormality may be known, and research efforts can proceed to functional cloning of the gene with subsequent identification of the structural or regulatory defect in the specific patient population or animal model. An example of this approach was the identification of collagen gene anomalies in osteogenesis imperfecta.

In other cases, a candidate gene approach in association with genetic linkage analysis will provide the most direct means of elucidating the genetic defect and associated structural or regulatory anomaly. The identification of the fibrillin gene in the Marfan Syndrome is an example that used this approach. In yet other cases, the location of a putative gene will be known on the basis of an abnormal karyotype, and cloning of the unknown gene can proceed on the basis of its chromosomal location. A related example of this latter approach was the identification of the dystrophin gene in children who have Duchenne muscular dystrophy. Many naturally occurring genetic diseases in animals are amenable to the same approach and can provide parallel opportunities for the study of relevant genetic diseases of the skeleton.

Common obstacles to progress include lack of availability of naturally occurring animal models and erroneous identification of disease phenotype. The development of transgenic animal models following the successful cloning of a gene by either functional or positional methods can provide additional insight into the complex regulation of skeletal development and bone remodeling. These basic genetic strategies provide powerful in vivo tools to dissect the complex regulatory pathways of normal and disordered bone formation and remodeling. Such approaches will inevitably lead to a more fundamental understanding of osteogenesis and to a more rational and therapeutic approach to a wide variety of disorders involving the regulation of bone formation in humans.

What are the key signaling systems controlling the physiology and pathophysiology of bone formation?

The mechanisms that regulate the formation and maintenance of the skeleton are not well understood. It is evident, however, that cell-signaling molecules and their receptors play critical roles in these processes. These molecules are remarkable for their number, diversity, and complexity. They include hormones, growth factors, cytokines, oncogene products, morphogens, vitamins, ions, and other bioactive molecules that determine the normal, or abnormal, form and function of the skeleton. Better understanding of these substances may ultimately contribute to the therapeutic regulation of bone growth and homeostasis.

In vitro and in vivo studies are needed to define the specific actions of cell-signaling molecules at a physiologic and cell biologic level. Biochemical and molecular biologic methods are needed to define the underlying mechanisms by which these signals are transduced. These studies will include (1) an analysis of the effects of cell-signaling molecules on cell proliferation, differentiation, and synthesis of matrix constituents; (2) the characterization of the receptors that mediate these actions; and (3) identification of the postreceptor effector pathways by which the cellular response is generated. Such data may permit the establishment of defined roles for cell-signaling molecules in skeletal function and provide insight into abnormalities in these mechanisms that may be responsible for skeletal disease.

What are the structural and nonstructural roles of bone matrix proteins involved in regulating osteogenesis? Which of the bone matrix proteins are essential for regulation of mineralization? How does extracellular matrix composition and architecture control cell shape and function?

The noncollagenous proteins produced by skeletal cells may serve multiple roles: in cell adhesion, modulation of cell shape, matrix organization, cell signaling, matrix turnover, initiation of mineralization, regulation of mineral crystal size, regulation of mineral turnover, etc. Because most extracellullar matrix proteins bind to apatite, it will be necessary to distinguish those proteins that accumulate passively from those that directly affect mineralization. Knowledge of the functions of the matrix proteins is essential for the development of therapies for conditions in which osteogenesis is aberrant (impaired or excessive) and for the design of synthetic or composite materials for bone repair.

These problems can be approached in the following ways: (1) Develop in vitro (cell-mediated and cell-free) systems for functional analyses, which include interaction of multiple matrix proteins and altered matrix protein composition. (2) Analyze alteration of matrix protein gene expression, protein composition, and structural organization of different types of bones in patients with diseases of osteogenesis. (3) Develop and analyze animal models with altered matrix protein composition. (4) Develop in vivo (transgenic animals) and in vitro (antisense treatment or stable transfection) models for analyses of function. (5) Develop new methods to modify matrix protein synthesis and modification. (6) Determine the effects of physiologic and chemical modification of matrix proteins on the proteins' in vitro and in situ functions. (7) Develop new systems for evaluating the effects of matrix proteins on physiologic mineral deposition.

How do physical factors modulate bone cell biology?

There is extensive qualitative evidence that physical factors (mechanical, electrical, gravitational) are potent determinants of bone-cell metabolism and skeletal morphology. However, there are few quantitative data that isolate and identify specific parameters of the physical regimen that mediate the cell response. Furthermore, we do not know what specific intracellular, intercellular, and/or cell-matrix mechanisms transduce the physical stimulus to a biochemical response. If we are to better understand the means by which physical factors influence normal bone biology, as well as how disruptions in these processes are etiologically linked to pathologies such as osteopenia and delayed unions, it is important to identify the specific mechanism of interaction of mechanical and electrical stimuli on bone cell metabolism.

In vitro and in vivo protocols must be developed in which the biophysical "input" can be rigorously controlled and the biochemical/histologic response accurately assayed. These approaches would include mechanical and electrical stimulation of bone cells in tissue or organ cultures, the development of animal models, and the study of clinical conditions (eg, type I osteopenia). Critical issues to address would be differentiating the response of amplitude, duration, and frequency of events, as well as determining the downstream sequences in which these osteogenic responses occur. Further, comparing the response of normal bone to physical stimuli with the response that occurs in metabolic bone diseases may help identify the mechanisms by which osteogenesis occurs. Real-time assays, such as fluorescent analysis of variation in cell calcium, scanning confocal laser microscopic analysis of changes in cell shape or composition, and atomic force microscopic analysis of protein mineral or cell-protein interactions, may well expedite the optimization of the osteogenic components of these exogenous signals.

How do the various cell modulating systems interact?

Given the complexity of skeletal development and homeostasis, and given the large number of factors involved in the regulation of these processes, there is little chance that the various agents act in either temporal or spatial isolation. Therefore, to understand the mechanisms by which bone is regulated, it is necessary to determine if and how the various regulating factors interact. However influential an individual factor may be, its action in isolation may have little bearing on its usual role if other factors are present that alter its effect. Conversely, a factor with little evident activity in isolation may be highly significant as a modulator of some other regulating factor or factors.

The ability of individual cell-signaling molecules to modulate each other's action on the processes of bone formation and homeostasis requires elucidation in both in vitro and in vivo models. The mechanisms of interaction may then be explained by further studies employing cell biologic and molecular biologic methods. Such interactions extend beyond the interplay between signal molecule-receptor-gene activation systems. Of equal importance are the relationships between signal transduction by physical forces and by cell-signaling molecules, the role of the extracellular matrix in modulating cell behavior, and the influence of direct cell-cell contacts. With such data, it may ultimately be possible to model the complex, integrated pathways by which the many aspects of bone formation are controlled.

How do vascularity and angiogenesis relate to bone structure and function?

a. How does angiogenesis relate to bone formation?

Close observation of bone formation during development, either via the intramembranous or endochondral replacement pathway, reveals that it occurs in intimate association with angiogenesis. What is not clear is: (1) whether cells in the osteoblastic lineage influence ingrowth of the vasculature (as is suggested by production of vascular endothelial growth factor [VEGF] by osteoblastic cells); (2) whether full osteoblastic maturation requires the presence of vascular cells (endothelium, pericytes, etc) as exemplified by the fact that the most osteogenic cultures are usually the most heterogeneous; or (3) whether both patterns of influence are required. It has been postulated that osteogenic precursors are intimately associated with invading capillaries (and perhaps are even pericytes themselves) and thereby provide a stem cell precursor pool that repopulates an area that is excavated by osteoclasts.

b. How does vascularity direct bone structure and function?

The process by which different types of bone (cortical vs trabecular) are established during late development and remodeling has not been well established. Because the pattern of bone formation by cells in the osteoblastic lineage is fairly uniform from one type of bone to another, it is possible that the differences are established by other associated cell types, in particular, the cells of the vasculature. Factors produced by these cell types, as well as other associated tissues such as periosteal tissue or marrow tissue, perhaps in response to physical forces, may influence the ultrastructural and architectural organization of the matrix laid down by bone-forming cells.

Study of the influence of vasculature on osteoblastic metabolism, and vice versa, will depend on the development of in vitro and in vivo model systems. Critical questions to be answered that can be addressed experimentally are whether cell contact is required or whether modulation of metabolism is mediated by soluble factors. There are a number of endothelial cell culture systems available that could be used directly in co-culture with osteoblastic cells, either in direct cell contact or separated by a membrane, to determine the nature of the interaction. In addition, incubation of endothelial cells with certain basement membrane type matrices has been reported to induce tubes (capillary-like structures). It is possible that these three-dimensional structures may exhibit more physiologic properties. Alternatively, intact blood vessels could be obtained by digestion of developing tissue with various enzymes. Although this approach has not been successfully applied to developing bone, such structures have been formed from the retina in the eye. In vivo, osteoblastic cells could be implanted on the chorioallantoic membrane of developing chicken eggs, and the resulting angiogenesis dissected biochemically through the use of in situ hybridization and immunochemistry. These types of studies should be quite informative in determining the interrelatedness of the two essential processes of osteogenesis and angiogenesis.

What is/are the origin(s) of osteoblasts? What are the functional differences among osteoblasts, and what is the basis for this variability? Does the normal adult organism rely primarily on precommitted osteoprogenitor cells or pluripotential stem cells for bone formation associated with normal bone remodeling and fracture repair?

During development, bone is formed from embryonic mesenchyme via one of two pathways, intramembranous or endochondral; regardless of the pathway, initial stages must involve commitment to an osteo (or osteo/chondro) progenitor lineage. During adult life, the body requires a constant supply of osteoblasts, which might be derived either from resident local osteoprogenitor cells or from less committed stem cells. Identifying the origin of these cells is important for understanding embryonic bone development as well as normal and abnormal bone formation in the adult. It has recently become apparent that differentiated osteoblasts differ in their biosynthetic and morphologic characteristics. The basis for these differences may reside in specific bone function, tissue architecture, local microenvironment, age, cell origin, or phase in the cell cycle. Maintenance of osteoblast variability is likely to be important for normal bone function, and understanding the mechanism underlying such variability should contribute to maintenance or restoration of normal bone function.

To identify the regulatory factors governing osteogenic and chondrogenic differentiation of skeletal mesenchymal cells, it will be important to trace lineage by (1) marking stem cells, (2) inactivating stem cells, (3) interfering with stages of osteoprogenitor maturation, and (4) analyzing systems with specific gene defects that result in abnormal bone formation. Criteria should be established for assessing the variability among osteoblasts, including (1) extracellular matrix gene expression, (2) type, density, and distribution of cell-surface receptors, (3) mineralization capacity, and (4) response to calciotropic factors. Having established these criteria, it will be possible to examine the basis for osteoblast variability. This examination can be approached by correlating phenotype with growth factors and osteoactive factors, presence of other cell types, composition and organization of the matrix, proximity to the vasculature, and physical forces acting on the cells.

Develop an interactive database in bone cell biology.

The knowledge base in the field of bone formation and regeneration is becoming more rich, complex, diverse, and dispersed. As this process continues, it will become increasingly challenging to access and integrate all the available data relevant to any particular aspect of bone biology. This problem will be of particular importance as contributions from multiple disciplines are focused on the same aspects of bone biology.

Build a database, compiled from the literature of the various disciplines (orthopaedics, endocrinology, cell biology, molecular biology, engineering, rheumatology, biochemistry, etc.), that contributes to the field of bone biology and is structured so as to permit integration of data pertaining to general and specific parameters of value to researchers in the field. This database will facilitate the interdisciplinary approach to the mechanisms of bone formation and regeneration that is required for the elucidation of function.

Section 2

Bone Regeneration and Repair

Section Editors:
Carl T. Brighton, MD, PhD
Gideon A. Rodan, MD, PhD

Mark E. Bolander, MD
Harold Brem, MD
Carl T. Brighton, MD, PhD
James T. Bronk
Thomas A. Einhorn, MD

Judah Folkman, MD
Ernst B. Hunziker, MD
Patrick J. Kelly, MD
A. Hari Reddi, PhD
Robert K. Schenk, MD

Chapter 8

Histologic and Ultrastructural Features of Fracture Healing

Robert K. Schenk, MD
Ernst B. Hunziker, MD

Introduction

Ham and Harris[1] introduced the first edition of their famous article, "Repair and Transplantation of Bone," with the following words:

> "The succession of histological changes that occur in and about a fracture, and which eventually result in its healing, are described in almost every textbook of pathology and surgery. It might be expected that by this time the accounts of bone repair in these books would be as uniform, simple, and accurate as, for example, the accounts they contain of the process of acute inflammation. But the accounts of bone repair are not uniform; indeed, many are bewilderingly involved, being attempts to reconcile the many (and often irreconcilable) controversies that have arisen in this field over the last one hundred years. Accordingly, in a book such as this, some attempt should be made to explain the reasons for the present-day confusion about this important matter as well as to deal with the process of bone repair in a fairly comprehensive fashion."

The basis for this introductory statement resided in the ongoing discussion about the role of the blood clot and its organization by granulation tissue, as well as in speculation about the origin of various cells involved in fracture repair. A similar dilemma now exists in attempts to fit recently gained insights into the role and nature of activation factors and regulators to the complex processes governing fracture healing. A fruitful discussion of the roles, effects, and interplay of such local regulators under physiologic and pathologic conditions in vivo requires a precise knowledge of the structural and topographic relationships in this process and of the cells and tissues involved. It is the purpose of this article to supply such a morphologic basis.

Types of Bone Tissue

Once activated, bone formation depends on two fundamental prerequisites: ample blood supply and a mechanically solid surface for bone deposition, because osteoblasts can function only in the neighborhood of capillaries, and bone matrix deposition and mineralization occur only under mechanically stable conditions. The solid surface required for bone matrix deposition may be provided by preexisting bone surfaces, or by the elaboration of calcified cartilage or calcified fibrous tissue. During physiologic development, growth, and repair of bone, various types of bone tissue evolve. In addition to woven and lamellar bone, a third and intermediate type, parallel-fibered (finely-bundled) bone, is of particular importance in bone repair processes. This classification of bone tissue dates back to Weidenreich[2] and has recently been redescribed by Palumbo and associates.[3] Woven bone tissue is structurally characterized by the random orientation of its collagen fibrils, the presence of numerous and irregularly-shaped osteocytes, and its capacity to form rapidly outgrowing beams and plates (trabeculae), which are preferentially located between and around blood vessels. Parallel-fibered bone is formed exclusively by apposition on preexisting bone surfaces. Its fibrils run parallel to the underlying surface, with osteocytes flattened in the same direction and less numerous than in woven bone.[1] In lamellar bone, collagen fibers are organized into parallel, 2- to 3-μm wide layers, with alternating courses from one lamella to another. This interpretation is, however, somewhat controversial, and on the basis of recent scanning electron microscope (SEM) studies, it has been modified.[4,5] Marotti and Muglia[4,5] suggest the lamellar pattern is due to differences in density rather than to changes in the course of collagen fibrils.

Both parallel-fibered and lamellar bone are formed exclusively by apposition. Fluorochrome labeling reveals a band-like pattern in each case, with the latter having a somewhat higher rate of deposition; in contrast, the extremely rapid mineralizing capacity of woven bone leads to a diffuse uptake of fluorochromes, which is reflected in the labeling pattern.

A microscopic differentiation between these three types of bone tissue is based on differences in matrix compartment organization. However, because such an analysis can be difficult to make, it is often neglected in histologic studies of fracture repair. The stains commonly used for both decalcified and undecalcified microtome sections obscure the specific characteristics and boundaries of these bone-type specific matrix compartments, thus rendering distinctions difficult. Polarized light microscopy might be used to achieve a reliable identification. In microradiographs, woven bone can frequently be identified by its higher mineral density. In our hands, plastic-embedded ground sections, polished and superficially stained, offer the best basis for identifying bone tissue types.[6] The great potential of this histologic method is now illustrated in the context of guided bone regeneration experiments.

Repair of Cortical Bone Defects

The repair of experimental cortical bone defects exemplifies the sequences of cell and tissue differentiation in a model that is not subjected to mechanical instability. In this case, direct (or primary) bone formation takes place.[7-10]

Repair of Small Cortical Bone Defects

Drilling of burr holes per se leads to activation of osteogenic cells in the periosteal, endosteal, and endocortical envelope, in which the cells rapidly proliferate, differentiate, and form bone (Fig. 1). Topographically, these processes begin along the walls of the holes within a couple of days (in the rabbit model). At the end of the first week, "small" holes (ie, <1 mm in diameter) may already be bridged by a primary scaffold of woven bone. The trabeculae are randomly oriented, and the intertrabecular compartments measure about 200 μm in diameter; they contain granulation tissue with numerous blood vessels. Subsequently, a continuous layer of osteoblasts is built up along the surface of the primary (trabecular) scaffold, and these cells begin to deposit parallel-fibered and, occasionally, lamellar bone in concentric layers on the walls of the intertrabecular spaces. This filling process leads to a narrowing of the holes, which,

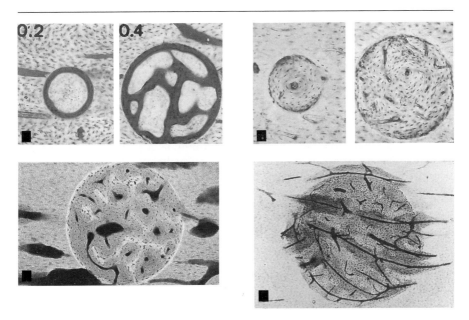

Fig. 1 Bone repair in small burr holes made in rabbit tibial cortex. **Top left,** 0.2- and 0.4 mm diameter holes 1 week after creation. **Top right,** 0.2- and 0.4-mm diameter holes 4 weeks after creation. Note the size-dependent differences in healing pattern. Sections stained with basic fuchsin. **Bottom left,** 0.6-mm hole at 6-week stage. The initially-formed woven bone appears brighter in the microradiograph owing to its higher mineral density. **Bottom right,** After 6 months, most of the originally-formed bony filling has been substituted by newly-formed osteons, thus restoring the original architecture of the cortex. Microradiograph; same magnification as bottom left. (Reproduced with permission from Johner R: Zur Knockenheilung in Abhängigkeit von der Defektgrösse. *Helv Chir Acta* 1972;39:409–411.)

by the end of the first month, are not larger than the cortical bone vascular channels. Completion of the filling process does not imply that the defects have fully healed; the structure of the filling material differs markedly from the surrounding cortical bone. However, in the subsequent months, the primary cortical repair tissue undergoes extensive remodeling and substitution, and after a couple of months, such defects are barely distinguishable microscopically and can be considered fully healed.[7]

Four important conclusions can be drawn from these rather simple experiments: (1) Creation of small bone defects under mechanically stable conditions leads to activation of bone-forming cells and direct bone formation. A pathway via cartilage tissue formation, and thus endochondral ossification, does not appear. (2) Bone tissue is always deposited on a solid surface, which is provided either by the defect wall itself, onto which the primary scaffold of woven bone is anchored or, later, by the surfaces of the woven bone trabeculae. (3) No osteoclasts are present during the initial period of defect filling. They appear only after 3 to 4 weeks, at the onset of cortical bone remodeling: first within the avascular cortical rim of the burr hole, and from there advancing into the regenerated tissue along the tips of the remodeling units. (4) Because no osteoclasts are present within the first weeks, there is no coupling of resorption with formation, and all factors (signaling substances) involved in the cell activation mechanisms must have a primary (or direct) influence on osteoblasts and their precursor cells.[11–18] Other cell types, such as endothelium and marrow-derived cells,[19] may also be involved in bone formation (cell activation, differentiation, and regulation mechanisms).

Healing of Large Cortical or Corticocancellous Bone Defects

The healing pattern of bone defects is size-dependent. In rabbit cortical bone, up to 1-mm wide defects are almost instantly bridged, or, in other words, intramembranous bone formation starts simultaneously across the entire defect space. Filling of larger holes (eg, after removal of bone screws) takes considerably longer. A further increase in diameter may lead to a critical dimension at which defects persist permanently. Such critical-size defects, however, are determined not only by their respective size, but also by their location and other environmental conditions.

In all these defects, continuity of the surrounding bone is maintained, in contrast to segmental defects in which bone continuity is interrupted by a fracture or osteotomy. Repair of segmental defects, therefore, falls into the category of fracture healing and depends primarily on mechanical stabilization and other therapeutic measures.

Repair of critical size defects requires promotion of bony callus formation. Such promotion can be obtained, essentially, by four different principles: osteoinduction (or osteogenic transfer), osteoconduction, callus distraction, and guided bone regeneration. Among these four principles, osteoinduction and osteoconduction are well known from vast experience gained in the field of bone transplantation. Callus distraction will be extensively discussed in separate chapters of this book. In the following paragraphs, some histologic aspects of guided bone regeneration will be presented, because this process gives important insights into bone regeneration in general.

Promotion of Callus Formation by Barrier Membranes

A phenomenon associated with the repair of critical-size defects that recently has attracted considerable attention is the competition between activated bone precursor cells and ingrowing, less differentiated cells, which originate from surrounding tissues. This competition leads, sometimes temporarily, but often permanently, to occupation of the defect areas by nonboneforming cells. As a result of this, the defects become only partially filled with bone tissue.

The idea of using cell-occluding "barrier membranes" to prevent the ingrowth of more primitive "scar tissue" into healing bone defects is not new.[20–26] However, during the last couple of years, this method has again attracted attention. Oral surgeons used this method for the treatment of periodontal disease and for alveolar ridge augmentation. It is now commonly referred to as guided tissue regeneration (GTR) or, more specifically, guided bone regeneration (GBR).[25,27–30] In view of its considerable importance for the biology of fracture repair, we will briefly summarize some of its histophysiologic features.

Repair of Corticocancellous Bone Defects Beneath Barrier Membranes

A recent histologic study of the repair of surgically created corticocancellous defects in the canine mandible was described.[31] The premolar teeth were extracted and 3 months allotted for healing of the extraction sockets. Then 12- to 15-mm wide and 10- to 12-mm deep defects were created in the alveolar crest and re-covered with the mucoperiosteal flap. The defect space was filled with a blood clot.

In the control defects, bone formation was activated along the defect margins and, within 2 months, succeeded in closing the surgically created openings of the marrow cavity (Fig. 2). There was, however, no further ingrowth of bone into the defect area, and a deep indentation, filled with the collapsed mucosa, persisted in the contour of the alveolar crest. No further reduction in size of the bony defect was noted at 4 months, indicating that this lesion falls into the category of critical-size defects.

Test defects, of identical size and position, were covered by partially cell-occlusive membranes. To achieve a homogeneous coagulum, remnants of air in the membrane-covered space were removed by injection of intravenously aspirated blood. The membranes were tightly adapted to the bony margins and fixed with miniscrews. After 2 months, the membranes had almost completely prevented the ingrowth of undifferentiated cells and blood vessels from the external soft tissues (Fig. 3). The hematoma was invaded by granulation tissue originating from the bone marrow space. The ingrowing tissue was extremely well vascularized, and direct woven bone formation began from all the bony surfaces present at the margin of the defects or exposed at the borderline of the surrounding marrow space (Fig. 4). The woven bone tissue advanced rapidly into the space beneath the membrane, forming a primary scaffold that extended from the bottom and the mesial and distal walls toward the center of the defect. The bony scaffold formed had a structure similar to that described in the section on repair of small cortical defects. The initial bone volume density of this spongework was about 50%, and the mean diameter of the intertrabecular spaces measured 200 to 400 μm. The trabeculae observed had no preferential orientation pattern; they surrounded the numerous blood vessels and were covered by continuous layers of osteoblasts, which increased trabecular width by deposition of parallel-fibered bone tissue. The architecture of the primary scaffold appeared to be governed primarily by the ingrowing vascular network, which precedes organization of the original blood clot in the membrane-protected cavity.

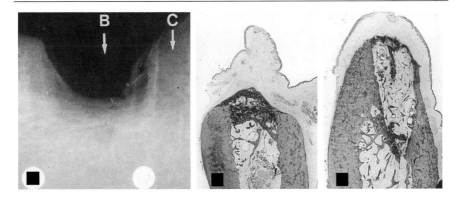

Fig. 2 Guided bone regeneration; control defect at 2 months. **Left,** Radiograph of a control defect at 2 months. Bone formation is restricted to defect margins. Arrows indicate the location of center and right sections. **Center,** Buccolingual section through the middle part of the defect. Newly-formed bone covers the surgically-created opening of the marrow space. **Right,** Section through the distal wall (with extraction socket) of the defect illustrating the outline of the original alveolar crest. (Reproduced with permission from Schenk RK, Buser D, Hardwick WR, et al: Healing pattern of bone regeneration in membrane-protected defects: A histologic study in the canine mandible. *Int J Oral Maxillofac Implants* 1994;9:13–29.)

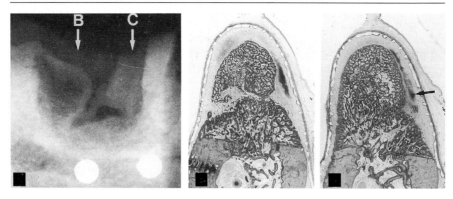

Fig. 3 Bone formation beneath a barrier membrane at 2 months. **Left,** Radiograph. Three bony caps, originating from the walls of the defect, grow into the middle portion and have partially fused. Arrows indicate the positions of center and right sections. **Center,** Section through mesial part of the defect. The tangentially cut tip of the mesial cap is separated from the bony cover at the bottom by fibrous bone marrow. Toluidine blue surface stain. **Right,** Toward the distal wall, the bony cover at the bottom and the distal cap have fused. On the lingual side, remnants of the original hematoma are still visible beneath the membrane (arrow). Toluidine blue surface stain. (Reproduced with permission from Schenk RK, Buser D, Hardwick WR, et al: Healing pattern of bone regeneration in membrane-protected defects: A histologic study in the canine mandible. *Int J Oral Maxillofac Implants* 1994;9:13–29.)

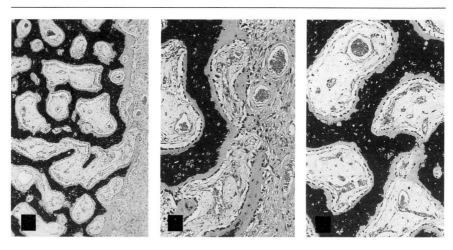

Fig. 4 Formation of primary spongiosa. The 5-μm thick microtome sections are stained with von Kossa and MacNeal's tetrachrome. **Left,** Along the borderline with the former hematoma, intramembranous bone formation advances towards the membrane from left to right. **Center,** Along the ossification front, trabeculae, consisting solely of osteoid, emerge and proliferate into the granulation tissue, which contains numerous blood vessels. **Right,** The primary spongiosa is comprised of plate-like trabeculae, which consist mainly of woven bone, and the surrounding intertrabecular spaces, which contain well vascularized primitive bone marrow. The trabeculae are lined by a continuous layer of osteoid and osteoblasts.

During the subsequent weeks, filling of the secluded defect continued, and the bone structure was further elaborated. At 4 months, the rather uniform scaffold of primary bone trabeculae was transformed into a cortical layer surrounding a marrow space that was subdivided by cancellous bone trabeculae (Fig. 5). The rather compact layer of cortical bone was formed by the filling-in of the former intertrabecular spaces with parallel-fibered bone and, later, by lamellar bone. These activities result in the formation of primary osteons around small vascular canals. The formation of the cortical bone layer is not based on remodeling activities; no osteoclastic resorption is involved. Moreover, the original framework of woven bone, now buried in parallel-fibered and/or lamellar bone, is still identifiable in adequately prepared histologic sections (Fig. 6, *top left* and *right* and *bottom left*).

Osteoclasts do not appear on the scene until haversian remodeling begins, ie, when the primary cortical bone is replaced by secondary osteons. This step has occurred by 4 months in some locations, where resorption canals and secondary osteons are present in various stages of completion (Fig. 6, *bottom right*). In the marrow space, however, osteoclastic resorption begins earlier. At 4 months, the volume density of cancellous bone is already reduced, and the trabeculae of the secondary spongiosa consist of a mixture of primary scaffold remnants, supplemented and substituted by lamellar bone tissue (Fig. 5, *right*).

Role of the Barrier Membrane and Surrounding Soft Tissue

The term guided bone regeneration might be somewhat misleading. The membrane does not provide a guide structure for the outgrowing bone tissue. Instead, it forms a "barrier" that protects the bone-forming elements within a membrane-secluded space against the ingrowth of competing soft-tissue

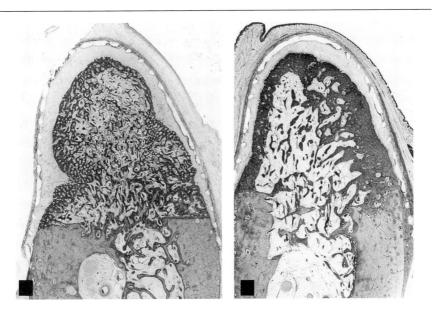

Fig. 5 Maturation of primary spongiosa. **Left,** Orofacial section through the distal portion of a defect at 2 months. The primary spongiosa fills most of the space delimited by the membrane. Ground section, surface-stained with toluidine blue and basic fuchsin. **Right,** Corresponding section at 4 months, illustrating the elaboration of a cortical layer around the secondary spongiosa in the marrow space. (Reproduced with permission from Schenk RK, Buser D, Hardwick WR, et al: Healing pattern of bone regeneration in membrane-protected defects: A histologic study in the canine mandible. *Int J Oral Maxillofac Implants* 1994;9:13–29.)

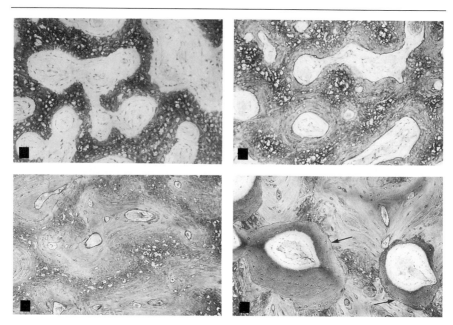

Fig. 6 Corticalization of primary spongiosa. Ground sections, surface-stained with toluidine blue. **Top left,** At 2 months, the newly-formed primary spongiosa consists of woven bone lined by osteoid seams and osteoblasts. Note the numerous, densely-packed osteocytes. **Top right,** The initially-formed woven bone is covered by more regularly structured, parallel-fibered bone and, in places, by lamellar bone. Bone deposition is still in progress. **Bottom left,** At 4 months, corticalization has led to formation of primary osteons. Their wall consists of parallel-fibered and lamellar bone. The original woven bone is still recognizable and fills the space between the primary osteons. **Bottom right,** Substitution of the primary cortical bone by haversian remodeling has begun at 4 months. Two evolving secondary osteons at different stages of completion are delimited by cement lines (arrows). Note remnants of woven bone and primary osteons. (Reproduced with permission from Schenk RK, Buser D, Hardwick WR, et al: Healing pattern of bone regeneration in membrane-protected defects: A histologic study in the canine mandible. *Int J Oral Maxillofac Implants* 1994;9:13–29.)

elements. The cell-occlusive parts of the membrane completely separate the granulation tissue, which arises from bone marrow elements, from the more rapidly proliferating fibrous tissues of the gingival lamina propria. Other parts of the barrier membrane have a porous structure and allow, to a certain extent, an ingrowth of cells and tissue elements. The intramembranous interstices of these parts are preferentially invaded by marrow elements. Bone develops within such parts of the membrane only at sites where newly-formed bone has established direct contact by ongrowth on the inner leaflet of the membrane.

In view of the ongoing discussion about a possible contribution of external soft tissues to fracture repair,[32,33] the tissue differentiation occurring outside the barrier membrane is also of some interest. This compartment consists of a rather dense fibrous tissue, practically identical to the gingival lamina propria. In some instances, bone tissue is deposited on the external surface of the membrane. This ossification remains strictly localized, and it most likely arises from remnants of the periosteum detached from the bone surface during surgery and accidentally placed on the membrane. It is unlikely that this ossification represents "transfilter bone induction." [34]

It is possible to argue that the competition between alveolar crest bone and oral mucosa tissue represents a special situation, and that these observations should not be generalized. However, preliminary results relating to the use of barrier membranes in the healing of segmental defects in long bones confirm the beneficial effects of membrane protection on bone repair under conditions in which a contribution from extraosseal vessels and soft-tissue elements is practically excluded.[35–37]

Fracture Healing

In contrast to stable cortical bone defect models, a bone fracture or an osteotomy destroys the anatomic continuity of the bone and, thus, leads to mechanical instability between the fragment ends. The first priority of fracture repair, therefore, is to restore continuity and mechanical stability. Restoration can be achieved by open reduction and stable internal fixation (ORIF) or by biologic means after partial immobilization or in spontaneously healing fractures.

In the event that internal fixation results in perfect stability, viz, prevents any interfragmentary motion, healing, ie, bony reunion, is achieved mainly by direct or primary bone formation. In this situation, bone union is achieved without any intermediate fibrous tissue or cartilage formation in the fracture gaps. Indirect (or secondary) healing under unstable conditions is characterized by more or less prominent callus formation and, as the decisive criterion, by indirect bone formation, ie, fibrocartilage formation and endochondral ossification in the interfragmentary area.

Direct (Primary) Fracture Healing

A direct fracture healing pattern originally was described in shaft fractures after fixation with compression plates, and was defined by its radiographic appearance: gradual disappearance of the fracture line and lack of external callus formation (Fig. 7).[38,39] Histologically, direct healing was characterized by direct bone formation in the fracture gap, followed by intensive cortical remodeling at the fragment ends, which also unite interfragmentary contact areas by traversing secondary osteons. The original observations by Schenk and Willenegger[8,40–43] have since been confirmed by numerous authors.

In the light of knowledge relating to cortical bone defect healing, this pattern of direct fracture healing is by no means surprising. Exact anatomic reduction and stable fixation create conditions that are almost identical to the burr hole case or any other stable defect model. However, even after very meticulous reposition, a full congruency between the fragment ends is never achieved. Contact follows compression only in circumscribed zones (or points); these are separated by large areas in which small gaps between the fragment ends are present. Adjacent contact sites protect these gaps against mechanical deformation as long as the static preload applied exceeds the dynamic forces created by muscle activity or weightbearing.

The pattern of gap healing follows the same sequence of events observed for the filling of cortical bone defects. An initial scaffold of woven bone is formed, followed by reinforcement by parallel-fibered and/or lamellar bone; and, after a lag of some weeks, haversian remodeling of both the avascular areas at the fragment ends and the newly-formed tissue in the fracture gap (Figs. 8, 9). The numerous activated regenerating osteons provide a good basis for the histologic

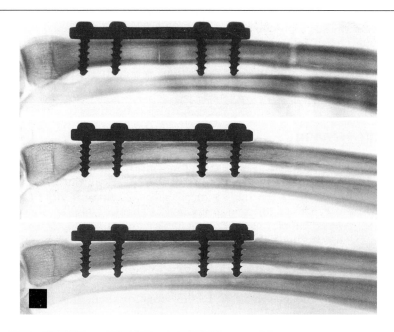

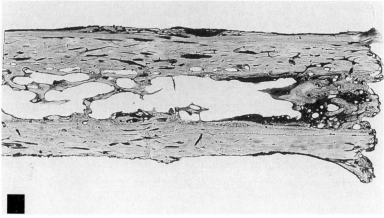

Fig. 7 Direct bone healing of a transverse osteotomy in dog radius. **Top,** In radiographs, no external callus formation is seen; the osteotomy line disappears within 5 to 6 weeks. **Bottom,** A longitudinal ground section at 10 weeks confirms minimal callus formation around the osteotomy site, but considerable bone deposition around the thread of the screw. (Reproduced with permission from Schenk R, Willenegger H: Zum histologischen Bild der sogenannten Primaerheilung der Knochenkompakta nach experimentellen Osteotomien am Hund. *Experientia* 1963;19:593–595.)

description of cortical bone remodeling, and also for an analysis of the remodeling dynamics at the cell and tissue levels.[8,43]

Gap healing occurs in two phases, namely initial bone filling followed by remodeling; whereas in contact healing, contact areas remain unchanged during the activation period, and consolidation of these sites depends on bridging by evolving secondary osteons, which can, in fact, cross the interface between fragments as readily as the restored bony bridges in the gaps (Fig. 10). The

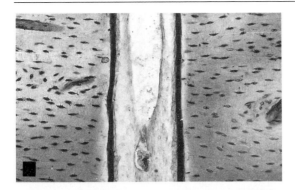

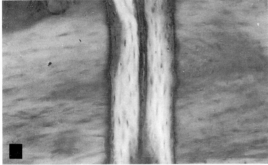

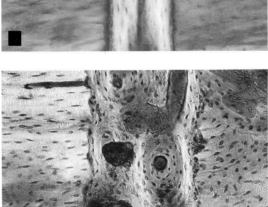

Fig. 8 Gap healing in dog radii, first stage. Application of straight compression plates produces small gaps in the cortex opposite the plate. **Top,** A 0.2-mm wide gap, 1 week after osteotomy. Blood vessels and mesenchymal cells have invaded the gap, and osteoblasts have begun to deposit bone on the surface of the fragment ends. **Center,** After 4 weeks, a 0.2-mm gap has been completely filled by lamellar bone. **Bottom,** Six weeks postoperation, a 0.4-mm gap has been filled directly by bone with a more complicated pattern (compare with Fig. 1, *bottom left*). (Reproduced with permission from Schenk RK: Cytodynamics and histodynamics of primary bone repair, in Lane JM (ed): *Fracture Healing.* New York, NY, Churchill Livingstone, 1987, pp 23–32.)

impressive appearance of contact healing at the histologic level, especially in the large contact areas directly beneath compression plates after transverse osteotomies, might be one of the reasons why its importance has been overestimated in many papers. Moreover, direct fracture healing is sometimes confused with contact healing.[44] Even in accurately reduced and compressed fractures, the gap healing processes (direct ossification) clearly dominate the scene quantitatively in interfragmentary healing mechanisms, and contact healing (in contact areas) occurs relatively rarely. Thus, gap healing affords the most important contribution to the consolidation of a rigidly-fixed fracture, and its first and essential phase of direct bone formation is, as with cortical-bone-defect filling, a fast and effective one.

Clinical fracture management by ORIF certainly has its pitfalls and risks. From a microscopic and biologic point of view, the disturbance or interruption

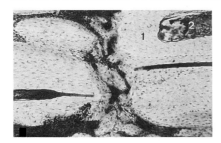

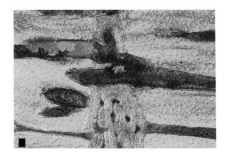

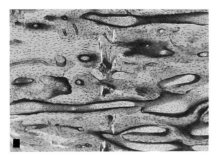

Fig. 9 Gap healing in dog radii, second stage. **Top left,** Six weeks postoperation, cortex in the fragment ends reveals areas of extensive devitalization (1). This bone, as well as the newly-formed bone in the gap, has been substituted by activation of bone remodeling units (BMU) based on haversian remodeling (2). **Top right,** Six weeks postoperation, the osteoclastic cutter cone in the tip of a BMU has just crossed the former osteotomy gap. **Bottom,** After 10 weeks, a considerable part of the osteotomy site has been replaced by newly-reconstructed cortical bone. (Reproduced with permission from Schenk R, Willenegger H: Zum histologischen Bild der sogenannten Primaerheilung der Knochenkompakta nach experimentellen Osteotomien am Hund. *Experientia* 1963;19: 593–595.)

of blood supply associated with surgical intervention and exposure of the bone fragments, as well as by the insertion of implant materials, is the most obvious pitfall. Plates, for example, generally compromise the periosteal vessels, screws create local avascular areas within the cortex, and intramedullary devices destroy the blood supply in the marrow cavity, leading to extensive cell death (necrosis) within the inner layers of the cortex. All such compromised bone sites need to be revascularized and substituted, and it may take years until full vitality is restored. Numerous attempts are therefore undertaken to reduce the extent of vascular damage by an appropriate design of the implant materials,[45-47] as well as by modifications in surgical procedure, such as indirect reduction techniques and more biologic fixation.[48,49]

Spontaneous (Indirect, Secondary) Fracture Healing

Fracture of a bone means loss of mechanical integrity and continuity. In addition, it is accompanied by lesions (or ruptures) of blood vessels, leading to localized avascularity of fragment ends, which may, moreover, have become displaced. The natural (or spontaneous) course of fracture healing begins with (1) interfragmentary stabilization by callus formation and by interfragmentary fibrocartilage differentiation; (2) restoration of continuity and bone union by intramembranous and endochondral ossification; and (3) substitution of avascular and necrotic areas by bone remodeling. At the same time, malalignment of fragments may be corrected to a certain extent by (1) modeling processes at

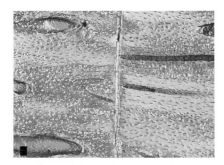
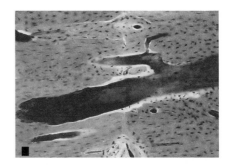

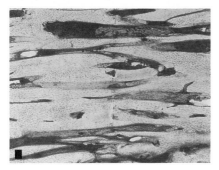

Fig. 10 Contact healing in dog radii. **Top left,** Contact interface beneath plate, 1 week postoperation. **Top right,** Tetracycline-labeled bone remodeling unit crossing the contact interface. Note branching with formation of a Volkmann's canal. **Bottom,** Contact healing, 6 weeks postoperation. Numerous newly-formed osteons have crossed the contact interface. Note the branching osteons. (Reproduced with permission from Schenk R, Willenegger H: Zum histologischen Bild der sogenannten Primaerheilung der Knochenkompakta nach experimentellen Osteotomien am Hund. *Experientia* 1963;19:593–595.)

the fracture site; (2) functional adaptation; and (3) complete substitution of repair bone tissue by lamellar bone for integration in the original bone structural arrangement. In principle, this healing pattern also is effective after external fixation by conservative means and in many instances in which open or closed surgical reduction does not result in rigid fixation. This healing pattern is often referred to as secondary or indirect healing, mainly because intermediate connective tissue or fibrocartilage is initially formed within the fracture gaps and replaced secondarily by bone tissue.[1,50–52]

The decisive step in spontaneous fracture healing is biologic stabilization. It is based on callus formation and tissue differentiation within the fracture gap, in which deformable tissues become gradually replaced by mechanically more resistant ones, and finally with tissue types characterized by solid intercellular matrices.

Biologic Stabilization by Callus Formation

Callus formation is the response of determined osteoprogenitor cells, principally in the periosteum and endosteum, to a number of activating factors released from freshly injured bone tissue.[32,33,51,53–55] Callus formation also occurs, usually to a minor degree, along the free cortical bone tissue fracture surfaces and trabeculae in bone marrow spaces. In these spaces, determined osteoprogenitor cells originate either from perivascular cells or from bone marrow stroma cells.[19] This type of response is generally fast; bone formation starts within a few days, and its promptness depends mainly on the state (or restitution) of the blood supply in the fracture area. Histologically, callus formation occurs predominantly by appositional, direct bone formation, and its main sites of occurrence, ie, the outer and inner surfaces of the fragment ends, serve as a solid base on which new bone tissue is deposited (Fig. 11).

Initially, woven bone is formed; its trabeculae surround wide vascular channels that are concentrically narrowed by apposition of parallel-fibered and lamellar bone. Haversian remodeling starts only after 3 to 4 weeks. The classic periosteal callus forms a conical cuff around the fragment ends, with the cuff's largest diameter facing the fracture plane. The degree of periosteal callus formation reflects somewhat the degree of instability or interfragmentary movement, provided that vascularization remains intact. The mechanical role of callus formation is obvious; it gradually enlarges the diameter of the fragment ends and, thereby, the cross-sectional area of the fragment site.[56] That is, the physiologically narrow bone is enlarged by materials of similar mechanical properties, resulting in a significant gain in bending strength. At the same time, the localized increase in bone diameter afforded by the callus formation reduces the mobility of the fragments and possible unwanted strain at the fracture site.[57,58]

Tissue Differentiation in the Fracture Gap

Tissue differentiation in fracture gaps is influenced strongly by mechanical forces acting on the various cell populations and by the blood supply.[59] Interfragmentary tissue differentiation is initiated by the invasion of granulation tissue into the hematoma. The cell differentiation processes that follow lead to the regional formation of vascularized connective tissue and fibrocartilage. The appearance of these tissue types and their local distribution within the fracture gap vary considerably, as would be anticipated from the large differences in the width and shape of the fracture area and in the local mechanical and blood supply conditions. Granulation and loose connective tissue are well vascularized and rich in fixed and mobile cells of high differentiation potential. The fine collagen fibrils of the granulation tissue are randomly oriented and barely contribute to interfragmentary mechanical stability. Connective tissue contains more and thicker collagen fibrils, which are organized into bundles and frequently anchored in the bony fragment ends. The course of these bundles often appears to reflect the main direction of tensile stress produced by interfragmentary motion forces.

Fibrocartilage tissue, which is a composite of connective tissue and cartilage, deserves special attention because of its particular mechanical and metabolic properties. The chondrocytes, surrounded by a cartilaginous matrix, are distributed as small cartilaginous islands in a meshwork of connective tissue fibers. In fibrocartilage, the fibrous component consists primarily of unmasked bundles of type I collagen. The cartilaginous portion contains type II collagen fibrils, is rich in proteoglycans (aggrecans), and has the general capacity of cartilage to withstand and survive avascular or anaerobic metabolic conditions. In cases of delayed healing or when hypertrophic nonunions develop, more and more of the interfragmentary tissue transforms into fibrocartilage, which ultimately fills the whole fracture gap. This mechanism makes the interfragmentary tissue space considerably stiffer and more resistant to deformation caused by motion of fragment ends.[10,60,61]

Origin of Fibrocartilage in Fracture Gaps The occurrence of cartilage differentiation within the fracture gaps has led to a number of different explanations and hypotheses. The classic ones pertain to a direct influence of mechanical forces (instability). Others are related to environmental conditions (lack of

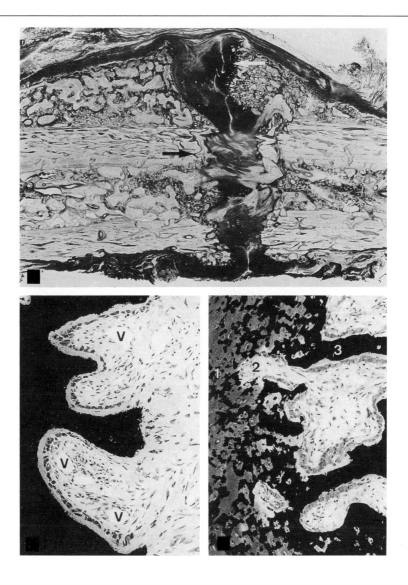

Fig. 11 Spontaneous fracture healing in dog radii after transverse defect-osteotomy without external fixation. **Top,** Longitudinal section 14 weeks postoperation shows extensive bony callus formation along the periosteal surface and within the marrow cavity. The black arrow indicates the area depicted *bottom left*, and the white arrow, *bottom right*. Ground section stained with basic fuchsin. **Bottom left,** The central part of the fracture gap contains fibrous tissue that is sufficiently vascularized and permits intramembranous ossfication. The fragment ends are lined by osteoblasts and osteoid seams, indicating ongoing bone deposition. V = blood vessels. Von Kossa and acid fuchsin stains. **Bottom right,** Fibrocartilage (to the left) has to mineralize (1) before undergoing resorption and vascular invasion (2). As at other sites of endochondral ossification, bone is deposited on persisting calcified cartilage cores (3). Von Kossa and acid fuchsin stains. (Reproduced with permission from Schenk R, Willenegger H: Zum histologischen Bild der sogenannten Primaerheilung der Knochenkompakta nach experimentellen Osteotomien am Hund. *Experientia* 1963;19:593–595.)

blood vascular supply) or induction principles (presence of cartilage-inducing factors). The nature and competence of available cell pools (stem cell potential, degree of commitment, etc) have also been held responsible.

Modulation of Tissue Differentiation by Mechanical Forces A direct dependence of cell and tissue differentiation on mechanical conditions acting at the fracture site has been postulated by numerous authors. Krompecher,[62] and later on, Pauwels[63,64] attempted to correlate the differentiation processes of supporting tissues to the dominating forces at the sites of tissue formation. According to Pauwels,[64] unidirectional (vectorial) forces (such as tension, compression, and shear stresses), which probably cause cell shape deformation, lead to connective tissue formation, whereas uniform (ie, nondirectional or hydrostatic) compression forces stimulate cartilage formation. Bone formation was believed to result from small deformations in a preexisting scaffold. These concepts and theories were derived from clinical observations and animal experiments in which accurate control and monitoring of the local mechanical force conditions frequently were not possible. They thus remain largely hypothetical in nature. It is now well known that a number of alternative local factors, such as streaming potentials, dynamic deformation pattern (micromotion), static compressive load patterns, ionic conditions, pH variation, and genetic and endocrine factors, may play key roles.[33,55,65–70] Nevertheless, the older, simplified theories still provide a useful concept for a general understanding of some of the tissue reactions in fracture repair (and around metal implants in bone tissue).

Role of the Inductive Principle A typical and reproducible cascade of cell differentiation steps that run from connective tissue through cartilage tissue to endochondral ossification has been documented in numerous experiments relating to ectopic bone formation processes.[71] The principles governing these events have been related to fracture repair mechanisms, although a straightforward analogy is questionable because of the overwhelming dominance of direct bone formation processes during fracture healing under mechanically stable conditions, which usually are assured clinically by conventional and surgical treatment measures. Whether pathways of ossification are direct or indirect appears to depend on the nature of the stem cells available and activated.[12,72] Heterotopic induction factors act primarily on inducible osteoprogenitor cells (IOPCs);[18,73] the response to these factors is cartilage formation followed by endochondral (indirect) ossification. In fracture repair processes, mainly determined osteoprogenitor cells (DOPCs) in the bone itself and in its "envelopes" are activated, and direct (or intramembranous) ossification, without any intermediate cartilage formation, results.

If cell and tissue induction phenomena are assumed to occur heterotopically, ie, by an indirect ossification mechanism, then invading cells must be recruited from the surrounding soft-tissue compartments. External (extraosseous) soft-tissue participation in callus formation and its major role in biologic stabilization are discussed extensively and analyzed by Ham and Harris,[1] and McKibbin.[74] Such tissues have free access to the defect site and are exposed to activating and inducing factors released from the bony fragment ends.[75,76] This is especially true of fractures characterized by a torn periosteum. The ingrowth of blood vessels into the external callus from extraosseous sources is a well-documented phenomenon. The origin and fate of perivascular fibroblast-like cells are, however, less well understood.[11–13,15,17] These cells might belong to the population of IOCPs and react to inducers such as bone morphogenetic proteins (BMPs), thus resulting in differentiation pathways to cartilage and endochondral ossification. However, recent experience gained from studies using barrier membranes raises serious doubts about the role and overall importance of these cells during fracture healing.

Activation of Various Stem Cell Types Growth factors and other signaling substances liberated at the fracture site will not act exclusively on angiogenic and osteogenic cells; these substances also will act on a number of other cell lines. Thus, various precursor cells of fibroblasts, chondroblasts, and osteoblasts could be stimulated and recruited simultaneously, and local metabolic and mechanical conditions could favor (or impede) their further proliferation and differentiation.[77-79] Two important parameters affected by these environmental conditions are strain tolerance and oxygen supply.[25,80-82] For example, osteoblasts differentiate and function only in the vicinity of capillaries, whereas chondrocytes are able to survive in a cartilaginous matrix that delivers nutrients by diffusion over considerable distances. In addition, the strain tolerance of various tissues varies widely: granulation tissue tolerates elongation up to 100%, connective tissue from 5% to 17%, fibrocartilage from 10% to 13%, and bone from 1% to 2%.[83] Therefore, until the mechanical and metabolic conditions necessary for bone formation are established, biologic stabilization processes must gradually build up a tissue structure and tissue properties that are able to reduce the strain on interfragmentary cells. Another factor affecting tissue formation is oxygen supply; for discussion, see chapter 10.

Modulation of Osteogenic Activity Osteogenic cells themselves also may be the source of chondroblasts; that is, their differentiation direction can be modulated by the above described environmental conditions. Ham and Harris[1] concluded that low oxygen tension, resulting from the rapid proliferative activities of precursor cells, was responsible for the change in the cells' gene expression, leading to formation of cartilage tissue instead of bone. This hypothesis was supported by earlier tissue culture experiments.[84] Low oxygen tension may also result from local alterations in blood supply due to compression or destruction of vessels in the interfragmentary area as a result of insufficient mechanical stabilization and micromotion.

Contribution of Fibrocartilage to Biologic Stabilization

Cartilage has unique mechanical properties; its intrinsic swelling pressure provides its viscoelastic properties and renders the cartilage resistant to compression and shear forces. These forces depend on the proteoglycan content. Chemical analysis and biochemical characterization of proteoglycan macromolecules have substantially contributed to the understanding of their mechanical roles. Aggrecan molecules and, in particular, their numerous and long glycosaminoglycans (mainly chondroitin sulfate and keratan sulfate chains), have a high fixed anionic charge density. This density is afforded by carboxyl and sulfate groups, which are negatively charged under physiologic conditions,[85-87] and results in the formation of large aqueous domains. Because proteoglycans are secreted by chondrocytes in an underhydrated state, a continually high swelling pressure is maintained in cartilage. The network of collagen fibrils confines the interfibrillar spaces available for proteoglycans to about one fifth of the volume that would pertain in free solution,[86] and this confinement creates an intrinsic pressure in the range of two to three atmospheres.[88] An alternative way of explaining these relationships and physicochemical tissue properties is by osmotic pressure effects and/or electrostatic forces.[65,66,89-93]

Mechanical Role of Proteoglycan Production Fibrocartilage tissue within the fracture gap develops preferentially at locations subject to variable compression forces. Continuous or intermittent compression is detrimental to the blood supply and promotes the formation of tissue types capable of living under anaerobic conditions. For example, in in vitro tests, cyclic loading increased cell activity in bovine articular cartilage,[90,94,95] chondrocyte cultures,[90] and tendon fibrocartilage tissue.[96] It may be assumed that the resistance of such tissues to deformation forces will increase continuously, thereby reducing instability conditions, provided that the chondrocytes continue to extrude proteoglycan molecules into the extracellular matrix. A steady increase in proteoglycan concentration has been suggested indirectly by the steady rise in such areas' affinity for cationic dyes. Therefore, the fibrocartilage tissue contributes mechanically to biologic stabilization of fracture sites by increasing the intrinsic pressure and the elastic modulus of the fracture callus.

Fibrocartilage Mineralization and Endochondral Ossification Continuous proteoglycan synthesis and increasing proteoglycan concentration in fibrocartilage contribute to the stiffening of the interfragmentary space; however, some elasticity will always remain. A prerequisite for the final substitution and replacement of fibrocartilage by bone tissue is fibrocartilage mineralization. As in the growth plate, mineralization does not occur uniformly, but the calcifying compartments are even less clearly defined and mineral is deposited in clusters around groups of chondrocytes.

Electron microscopy of the mineralized parts of fibrocartilage reveals structurally (and, thus, also functionally) intact cells that are well equipped with rough endoplasmic reticulum and mitochondria, and often contain lipid droplets.[97-100] The chondrocytes always remain separated from the mineralized matrix parts by a pericellular layer of unmineralized matrix. Ruthenium red staining reveals this compartment to be very rich in precipitated proteoglycans (Fig. 12). The hypothesis that fibrocartilage mineralization is initiated and controlled by chondrocytes is indirectly supported by the presence of matrix vesicles at locations where freshly deposited apatite crystals are found.[101,102] Numerous cytoplasmic processes protrude over short distances into the surrounding matrix, and these most likely play a role in the generation of the matrix vesicles, perhaps by a budding-off mechanism.[103] Chondrocytes in these areas disintegrate very rarely and, therefore, matrix vesicle formation by cell fragmentation appears to be an unlikely mechanism.

The additional steps of bony substitution at the fracture site closely resemble endochondral ossification processes. Vascular invasion of fibrocartilage occurs and is coupled with resorption of mineralized matrix by multinucleated chondroclasts and degradation of nonmineralized matrix compartments by macrophages/endothelial cells (Fig. 11, *bottom right*; Fig. 13, *top*). Blood vessels, accompanied by perivascular mesenchymal-like cells, ie, osteoblastic precursor cells, as well as osteoblasts, follow the resorbing front. Calcified fibrocartilage compartments are, however, only partially resorbed. Their remnants are freed from adhering nonmineralized matrix before osteoblasts begin using them as a solid scaffold for new bone matrix deposition. In a similar way to the primary spongiosa in growing bone metaphyses, newly-formed bone trabeculae are easily recognized by the enclosed core of calcified fibrocartilage.[50,98] The analogy to growth plate histophysiology is further supported by the fact that any disturbance of fibrocartilage mineralization leads to inhibition of vascular ingrowth and bony substitution of the interfragmentary fibrocartilage site, which are common findings in delayed unions and nonunions.

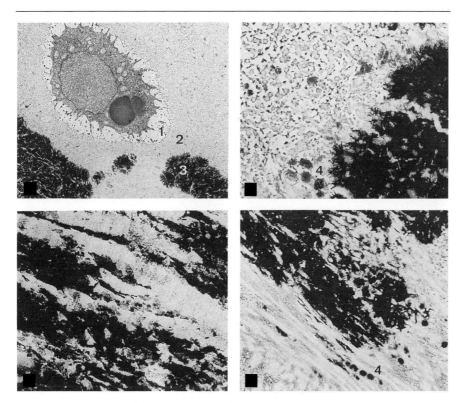

Fig. 12 Mineralization of fibrocartilage and fibrous tissue. **Top left,** Fibrochondrocyte surrounded by proteoglycans (1), cartilaginous matrix (2), and islands of calcification (3). **Top right,** Matrix vesicles (4) are regularly found along the borderline between mineralized and nonmineralized fibrocartilaginous matrix. **Bottom left,** Mineralized fibrous tissue closely resembles bone but lacks the close association between apatite crystals and cross striations of type I collagen fibrils ($\times$ 62,000). **Bottom right,** Again, matrix vesicles are present along the mineralization front of the connective tissue ($\times$ 40,000). (Reproduced with permission from Schenk R, Willenegger H: Zum histologischen Bild der sogenannten Primaerheilung der Knochenkompakta nach experimentellen Osteotomien am Hund. *Experientia* 1963;19:593–595.)

The arrest of fibrocartilage mineralization is one of the main features characterizing viable, biologically active nonunions[8,60,61] and is believed to be related to persisting instability conditions. Because cyclic mechanical loading patterns stimulate proteoglycan synthesis by chondrocytes[95] and these molecules may be capable of inhibiting calcification,[104–107] the imbalance between proteoglycan production and degradation could be an explanation for the lack of mineralization under these circumstances.

Mineralization and Substitution of Connective Tissue The interfragmentary space is not homogeneously filled by fibrocartilage, but it also contains areas of loose and dense fibrous tissue. Provided that local vascularity is sufficiently intact and mechanical protection by adjacent fibrocartilaginous buttresses is adequate, such parts can unite by appositional bone formation of the desmal or intramembranous (direct) type (Fig. 11, *bottom left*). Occasionally, a bone tissue formation pattern, which resembles that occurring at sites of ligament or tendon insertion in growing bones,[8,60,108,109] may also be seen. Densely packed,

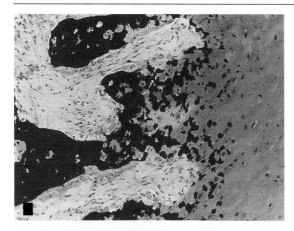

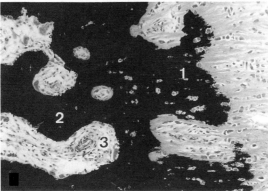

Fig. 13 Two types of secondary (indirect) bone formation in fracture gaps. **Top,** Bony substitution of fibrocartilage (compare with Fig. 11, *bottom right*). Von Kossa and acid fuchsin stains. **Bottom,** Bony substitution of dense fibrous tissue. Fibrous tissue undergoes mineralization (1), and is subsequently resorbed and substituted by bone (2) and bone remodeling unit-like elements (3). Von Kossa and acid fuchsin stains. (Reproduced with permission from Schenk R, Willenegger H: Zum histologischen Bild der sogenannten Primaerheilung der Knochenkompakta nach experimentellen Osteotomien am Hund. *Experientia* 1963;19:593–595.)

parallel-oriented collagen fibrils are mineralized and, by this effect, become morphologically almost indistinguishable from bone tissue (Fig. 13, *bottom*). The encapsulated fibrocytes, however, do not have long cell processes communicating via canaliculi.

In the electron microscope, mineralized fibrous tissue exhibits rather thick collagen fibrils (mainly type I) with a 64-nm periodicity (Fig. 12, *bottom left* and *right*). The apatite crystals often form plates rather than needles[110] and preferentially occupy interfibrillar spaces. Calcification seems to be associated with the presence of matrix vesicles.[111,112] Mineralized fibrous tissue is subsequently replaced by osteoclastic resorption followed by bone formation, in analogy to the ossification pattern and remodeling of tendons.[8,113]

Modeling and Remodeling at the Fracture Site

The outline and the internal structure of a consolidated fracture differ markedly from those of the original bone, especially after secondary healing, when union is achieved by callus formation, fibrocartilage differentiation, and endochondral ossification. Bone tissue forming the callus and uniting the fragments is of a rather primitive type, which fulfills mechanical requirements only by its excess production. Avascular and necrotic areas also persist along the fragment ends. The fracture site as a whole, therefore, needs to be subjected to extensive modeling and remodeling until the original shape and internal structure of the bone are restored. This reconstruction phase is a feature common to all types of fracture repair and may continue over years.

In cortical bone, modeling is based on shape-deforming resorptive and formative activities of the periosteal and endosteal envelopes. Stabilization via periosteal callus formation results in the formation of a double-cone. Periosteal bone resorption gradually smooths it out to a spindle form, and, ultimately, the cylindrical contour of the original shaft is restored. At the same time, the marrow space reappears, and a compact cortical wall is reconstructed. In addition, the fracture site as a whole is subjected to extensive remodeling until the original osteonal structure is restored.

Remodeling During Cortical Bone Defect Healing and Fracture Repair Bone remodeling activity always represents a final stage in bone repair, regardless of whether defect healing or direct or indirect fracture healing are involved. Remodeling means bone substitution, and this process originates with osteoclastic resorption followed by lamellar bone formation. Resorption and formation are coupled both in space and time, and they occur in topographically discrete bone remodeling units (Fig. 14). On the grounds of their considerable importance in the pathogenesis of various metabolic bone diseases, such remodeling units were designated by Frost[114,115] as "bone multicellular units" or "bone metabolizing units," or, simply as BMU. A single BMU forms a "bone structural unit" or BSU. In cortical bone, BSUs are identical to secondary osteons; in cancellous bone, they are also referred to as packets. BSUs are always delimited from the adjacent matrix compartments by a cement line of the reversal type. Reversal lines appear at the level where osteoclastic resorption ceases and bone formation resumes.

The microscopic structure of cortical remodeling units, as well as their dynamics at the cellular level, is well known.[116] In adult canine bone, the osteoclastic resorption rate is about 50 to 60 μm/day, the daily lamellar bone apposition rate about 1.5 to 2 μm. Filling of the osteonal cross section takes 6 to 8 weeks (in human bone 3 to 4 months). Another interesting phenomenon is the coupling between resorption and formation. This coupling seems to be regulated by a variety of factors, which also control the balance between the matrix volumes turned over by the resorptive and formative activities operative in the remodeling process. (These aspects will be discussed in another chapter of this book.)

In the context of bone repair, the recruitment (or activation) of BMUs, especially during cortical remodeling, is of particular interest. The activation itself is due not so much to the exposure of fractured bone matrix surfaces, as to the local interruption of vascular supply within the fragment ends.[1,74] This interruption deprives the osteocytes within the canaliculolacunar network of their source of nutrients, and, consequently, they die. Although the osteocytes' possible survival time is not known, the interruption of the blood circulation that accompanies a fracture obviously lasts long enough to cause quite extensive necrotic areas in the affected cortex.

Revascularization and Substitution of Avascular Cortical Bone Before the onset of remodeling, the avascular cortex needs to be revascularized. This process originates from surrounding cortical vascular channels that still have an intact circulation, or from persisting or regenerated vessels in the periosteal and endosteal envelopes. Some disconnected, persisting vessels may be linked to the still-functioning vascular net by end-to-end anastomosis and be recanalyzed, or new vascular sprouts may grow into the preformed and anastomizing cor-

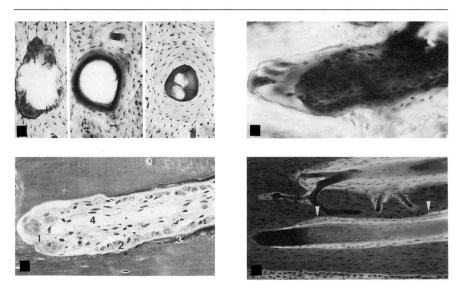

Fig. 14 Cortical bone remodeling (micrographs taken from studies of fracture repair in dogs). **Top left,** Transverse section, from left to right: resorption canal, forming and completed secondary osteon. (Reproduced with permission from Schenk RK: Biology of fracture repair, in Browner BD, Jupiter JB, Levine AM, et al (eds): *Skeletal Trauma.* Philadelphia, PA, WB Saunders, 1992, pp 31–75.) **Top right,** A 90-μm thick ground section demonstrating the osteoclastic cutter cone. (Reproduced with permission from Schenk R, Willenegger H: Zum histologischen Bild der sogenannten Primaerheilung der Knochenkompakta nach experimentellen Osteotomien am Hund. *Experientia* 1963;19:593–595.) **Bottom left,** Goldner-stained, 5-μm thin microtome section illustrating osteoclasts (1), osteoblasts (2), osteoid (3), and blood vessels (4) associated with perivascular (osteoprecursor) cells. (Reproduced with permission from Schenk R, Willenegger H: Zur Histologie der primaeren Knochenheilung. *Langenbecks Arch Klin Chir* 1964;308:440–452.) **Bottom right,** Sequential labeling allows calculation of osteoclastic resorption rates by measurement of the distance between the tips of individual labels (arrowheads). (Reproduced with permission from Schenk R, Willenegger H: Morphological findings in primary fracture healing, in Krompecher S, Kerner E: *Symposia Biologica Hungarica v. 7: Callus Formation Symposium on the Biology of Fracture Healing.* Budapest, Akadémiai Kiado, 1967, pp 75–86.)

tical canals. Such vessels are often accompanied by osteoprogenitor cells, which may become activated and deposit a tiny (wallpaper-like) layer of new bone on the inner wall of the otherwise devitalized osteon (Fig. 15).

In other sites, the haversian canals are widened by osteoclastic resorption before bone deposition on the remaining necrotic wall of the osteon leads to its partial substitution. Full-sized bone remodeling units result in the formation of regular secondary osteons having outer diameters of 150 to 200 μm and a wall thickness of 60 to 80 μm. Moreover, the regular osteoclastic cutter cones rarely follow the course of preexisting channels; instead, they form independent new resorption cavities, which quite often ramify or anastomose with neighboring haversian systems (Fig. 10). Revascularization and substitution, therefore, are not firmly coupled, and there is quite a variation, ranging from simple restoration of the blood circulation via vascular ingrowth and partial substitution of devitalized bone to the full reconstruction of regular secondary osteons.

Activation and Dynamics of Cortical Bone Remodeling Osteoclastic reaming of resorption cavities begins only after the delay that follows the arrest of local

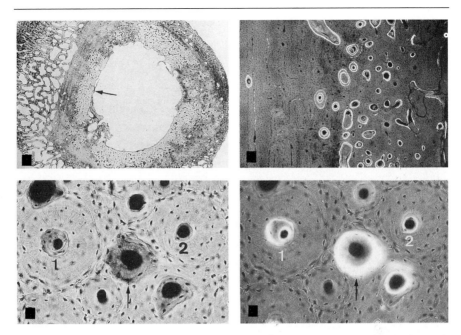

Fig. 15 Revascularization and substitution of cortical bone 8 weeks after intramedullary nailing in a canine tibia. **Top left,** Low magnification of a cross section stained with basic fuchsin. Devitalized areas are less intensely stained by fuchsin (arrow indicates position of *top right*). (Reproduced with permission from Eitel F, Schenk RK, Schweiberer L: Corticale revitalisierung nach marknagelung an der hundetibia. *Hefte Unfall* 1979;83:202–207.) **Top right,** Sequential labeling with fluorochromes demonstrates intense remodeling of the inner half of the lateral cortex, which became avascular and devitalized. **Bottom left** and **right,** Although almost all haversian canals are revascularized, substitution of the devitalized bone is still incomplete after 8 weeks. Small osteons at the center have been completely substituted (arrow). Partial substitution (1) or coating of a preformed haversian canal with a thin layer of new bone (2) causes the persistence of large devitalized areas still awaiting substitution. (Reproduced with permission from Schenk RK: Biology of fracture repair, in Browner BD, Jupiter JB, Levine AM, et al (eds): *Skeletal Trauma*. Philadelphia, PA, Saunders, 1992, pp 31–75.)

blood circulation. This delay lasts for a few weeks, and its duration probably is species-specific. On the basis of sequential fluorochrome labeling experiments, Schenk[8] proposed an activation profile for the remodeling intensity in rigidly fixed canine radii osteotomies (Fig. 16). These observations recently have been confirmed by another, as yet unpublished, experiment. In canine femora, the medullary vessels were destroyed by curettage of the marrow space through a small proximal opening to produce rather extensive avascular areas in the inner half of the cortex over almost the whole length of the diaphysis.

Subsequent systematic polychrome labeling allows both classification of BMUs according to their "birthdate," and determination of the complete haversian remodeling activation profile, which is stimulated without a direct mechanical insult/trauma to the bone. In the dog, the lag period lasts 2 to 3 weeks. It is followed by an increase in remodeling activity that reaches its climax after about 6 weeks. Thereafter, the "birthrate" of new BMUs begins to decrease; it again approaches physiologic levels after approximately 3 to 4 months. This activation/deactivation curve represents the effect of one single activation insult, restricted in time to a single procedure. In a healing fracture, and especially

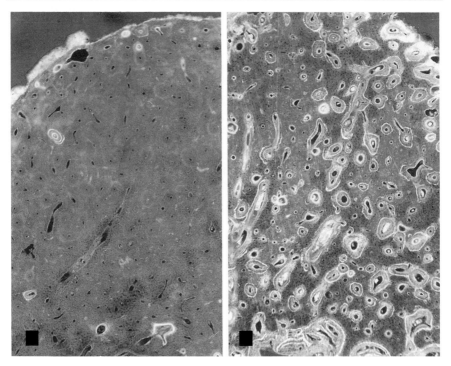

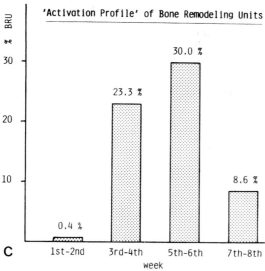

Fig. 16 Activation of cortical remodeling by transverse osteotomies in canine radii. Tetracycline sequential labeling. **Top left,** Control radius, 2.5% of the osteons are in the remodeling state. **Top right,** Transverse section near the osteotomy. After 8 weeks, 62.5% of the osteons have been replaced or are in the formative phase of renewal. **Bottom,** Activation profile confirms the lag phase of 2 to 3 weeks between activation and onset of remodeling and the peak of bone remodeling unit recruitment in the second month. (Reproduced with permission from Schenk R, Willenegger H: Zur Histologie der pimaeren Knochenheilung. *Langenbecks Arch Klin Chir* 1964;308:440–452.)

under unstable healing conditions, multiple vascular lesions will usually follow the initial dramatic event, and, thus, a repetitious activation pattern will tend to prolong the remodeling period.

In the above model, remodeling processes always begin along the demarcation line/interface between the intact periosteal and the interrupted medullary cortical circulatory domains. Thus, the observed lag period cannot be interpreted as the interval necessary for restoration of the blood supply. This period seems more likely to represent the time required for the mobilization and release of activating factors (signaling substances) from disintegrating osteocytes or their surrounding bone matrix and for the delivery/transport of such factors via the lacunocanalicular system[117–119] to the cell population of the endocortical (haversian) envelope that has an intact circulation. This lag period also plays an important role in the delivery of osteoclast precursor cells.[120–122] Furthermore, the "signals" inducing remodeling or substitution appear to expire with time, over a period of months rather than weeks. Avascular bone tissue that has not been revascularized within this period will lose its capacity to activate its cell pools for remodeling and, thus, gradually turn into necrotic bone, finally becoming a sequester. This feature and the fact that osteoclastic resorption processes are always activated first illustrate the existence of regulatory relationships that are important for the understanding of physiologic bone remodeling processes.

References

1. Ham AW, Harris WR: Repair and transplantation of bone, in Bourne GH (ed): *The Biochemistry and Physiology of Bone. Development and Growth*, ed 2. New York, NY, Academic Press, 1971, vol 3, pp 337–399.
2. Weidenreich F: Das Knochengewebe, in von Möllendorff W (ed): *Handbuch der Mikroskopischen Anatomie des Menschen*. Berlin, Springer-Verlag, 1930, vol 2, part 2, pp 391–520.
3. Palumbo C, Palazzini S, Zaffe D, et al: Osteocyte differentiation in the tibia of newborn rabbit: An ultrastructural study of the formation of cytoplasmic processes. *Acta Anat (Basel)* 1990;137:350–358.
4. Marotti G: A new theory of bone lamellation. *Calcif Tissue Int* (Suppl) 1993; 53:S47–S56.
5. Marotti G, Muglia MA: A scanning electron microscope study of human bony lamellae: Proposal for a new model of collagen lamellar organization. *Arch Ital Anat Embriol* 1988;93:163–175.
6. Schenk RK, Olah AJ, Herrmann W: Preparation of calcified tissues for light microscopy, in Dickson GR (ed): *Methods of Calcified Tissue Preparation*. Amsterdam, Elsevier Science Publishers, 1984, pp 1–56.
7. Johner R: Zur Knochenheilung in Abhängigkeit von der Defektgrösse. *Helv Chir Acta* 1972;39:409–411.
8. Schenk RK: Biology of fracture repair, in Browner BD, Jupiter JB, Levine AM, et al (eds): *Skeletal Trauma*. Philadelphia, PA, WB Saunders, 1992, pp 31–75.
9. Schenk RK, Willenegger HR: Histology of primary bone healing: Modifications and limits of recovery of gaps in relation to extent of the defect. *Unfallheilkunde* 1977;80:155–160.
10. Shapiro F: Cortical bone repair: The relationship of the lacunar-canalicular system and intercellular gap junctions to the repair process. *J Bone Joint Surg* 1988;70A: 1067–1081.
11. Beresford JN: Osteogenic stem cells and the stromal system of bone and marrow. *Clin Orthop* 1989;240:270–280.
12. Friedenstein AJ: Precursor cells of mechanocytes. *Int Rev Cytol* 1976;47:327–359.
13. Krompecher S: Die Entwicklung der Knochenzellen und die Bildung der knochengrund-substanz bei der knorpelig und bindegewebig vorgebildeten sowie der primaeren reinen Knochen-bildung. *Verhandl Anat Gesellsch* 1934;42:34–53.
14. Maximow AA: Morphology of mesenchymal reactions. *Arch Pathol Lab Med* 1927;4:557–606.
15. Owen M: Marrow stromal stem cells. *J Cell Sci Suppl* 1988;10:63–76.

16. Owen M, Friedenstein AJ: Stromal stem cells: Marrow-derived osteogenic precursors, in Evered D, Harnett S (eds): *Cell and Molecular Biology of Vertebrate Hard Tissues*. Ciba Foundation Symposium No. 136. Chichester, England, John Wiley & Sons, 1988, pp 42–60.

17. Rouget C: Mémoire sur le développement, la structure et les propriétés physiologiques des capillaires sanguins et lymphatiques. *Arch Physiol Norm Pathol* 1873; 5:603–663.

18. Scutt A, Mayer H, Wingender E: New perspectives in the differentiation of bone-forming cells. *Biofactors* 1992;4:1-13.

19. Brighton CT, Hunt RM: Early histological and ultrastructural changes in medullary fracture callus. *J Bone Joint Surg* 1991;73A:832–847.

20. Bassett CAL: Contributions of endosteum, cortex, and soft tissues to osteogenesis. *Surg Gynecol Obstet* 1961;112:145–152.

21. Bassett CA: Environmental and cellular factors regulating osteogenesis, in Frost H (ed): *Bone Biodynamics*. Boston, MA, Little Brown, 1966, pp 233–244.

22. Boyne PJ: Regeneration of alveolar bone beneath cellulose acetate filter implants. *J Dent Res* 1964;43:827.

23. Boyne PJ, Mikels TE: Restoration of alveolar ridges by intramandibular transposition osseous grafting. *J Oral Surg* 1968;26:569–576.

24. Boyne PJ: Restoration of osseous defects in maxillofacial casualties. *J Am Dent Assoc* 1969;78:767–776.

25. Hurley LA, Stinchfield FE, Bassett AL, et al: The role of soft tissues in osteogenesis: An experimental study of canine spine fusions. *J Bone Joint Surg* 1959;41A:1243–1254.

26. Ruedi TP, Bassett CAL: Repair and remodeling in millipore-isolated defects in cortical bone. *Acta Anat* 1967;68:509–531.

27. Dahlin C, Alberius P, Linde A: Osteopromotion for cranioplasty: An experimental study in rats using a membrane technique. *J Neurosurg* 1991;74:487–491.

28. Dahlin C, Gottlow J, Linde A, et al: Healing of maxillary and mandibular bone defects using a membrane technique: An experimental study in monkeys. *Scand J Plast Reconstr Hand Surg* 1990;24:13–19.

29. Dahlin C, Linde A, Gottlow J, et al: Healing of bone defects by guided tissue regeneration. *Plast Reconstr Surg* 1988;81:672–676.

30. Nyman S, Lindhe J, Karring T: Reattachment: New attachment, in Lindhe J (ed): *Textbook of Clinical Periodontology*, ed 2. Copenhagen, Munksgaard, 1989, pp 450–476.

31. Schenk RK, Buser D, Hardwick WR, et al: Healing pattern of bone regeneration in membrane-protected defects: A histologic study in the canine mandible. *Int J Oral Maxillofac Implants* 1994;9:13–29.

32. Einhorn TA: Bone remodeling in fracture repair. *Triangle* 1992;31:89–98.

33. Einhorn TA: Clinical applications of recombinant gene technology: Bone and cartilage repair. *Cell Mater* 1992;2:1-11.

34. Buring K, Urist MR: Transfilter bone induction. *Clin Orthop* 1967;54:235–242.

35. Buser DK, Dula U, Belser HP, et al: Localized ridge augmentation using guided bone regeneration: I. Surgical procedure in the maxilla. *Int J Periodont Rest Dent* 1993;13:29–45.

36. Farso Nielsen F, Karring T, Gogolewski S: Biodegradable guide for bone regeneration: Polyurethane membranes tested in rabbit radius defects. *Acta Orthop Scand* 1992;63:66–69.

37. Nyman S: Bone regeneration using the principle of guided tissue regeneration. *J Clin Periodontol* 1991;18:494–498.

38. Danis R: *Theorie et Pratique de l'Ostosynthese*. Paris, Masson & Cie, 1949.

39. Layton TB: Lane WA: *An Enquiry into the Mind and Influence of a Surgeon*. Edinburgh, Livingstone, 1956.

40. Schenk R, Willenegger H: Zum histologischen Bild der sogenannten Primaerheilung der Knochenkompakta nach experimentellen Osteotomien am Hund. *Experientia* 1963;19:593–595.

41. Schenk R, Willenegger H: Zur Histologie der primaeren Knochenheilung. *Langenbecks Arch Klin Chir* 1964;308:440–452.
42. Schenk R, Willenegger H: Morphological findings in primary fracture healing, in Krompecher S, Kerner E: Symposia Biologica Hungarica v. 7: Callus Formation Symposium on the Biology of Fracture Healing. Budapest, Akadémiai Kiado, 1967, pp 75–86.
43. Schenk RK: Cytodynamics and histodynamics of primary bone repair, in Lane JM (ed): *Fracture Healing.* New York, NY, Churchill Livingstone. 1987, pp 23–32.
44. Woo SL-Y, Akeson WH: Appropriate design criteria for less rigid plates, in Lane JM (ed): *Fracture Healing.* New York, NY, Churchill Livingstone, 1987, pp 159–172.
45. Hontzsch D, Perren SM, Weller S: Das biologische Konzept der LC-DCP aus Titan. Dynamische Kompressionsplatte mit limitiertem Kontakt. *OP Journal* 1992;8:47–50.
46. Klein MPM, Rahn BA, Frigg R: Reaming versus non-reaming in medullary nailing: Interference with cortical circulation of the canine tibia. *Arch Orthop Trauma Surg* 1990;109:314–316.
47. Perren SM, Klaue K, Pohler O, et al: The limited contact dynamic compression plate (LC-DCP). *Arch Orthop Trauma Surg* 1990;109:304–310.
48. Gerber C, Mast JW, Ganz R: Biological internal fixation of fractures. *Arch Orthop Trauma Surg* 1990;109:295–303.
49. Mast J, Jakob RP, Ganz R: *Planning and Reduction Technique in Fracture Surgery.* Berlin, Springer-Verlag, 1989.
50. Aho AJ: Electron microscopic and histological observations on fracture repair in young and old rats. *Acta Pathol Microbiol Scand Suppl* 1966;184:1-95.
51. Simmons DJ: Fracture healing perspectives. *Clin Orthop* 1985;200:100–113.
52. Willenegger H, Perren SM, Schenk R: Primary and secondary healing of bone fractures. *Chirurg* 1971;42:241–252.
53. Jingushi S, Joyce ME, Bolander ME: Genetic expression of extracellular matrix proteins correlates with histologic changes during fracture repair. *J Bone Miner Res* 1992;7:1045–1055.
54. Rosen V, Thies RS: The BMP proteins in bone formation and repair. *Trends Genet* 1992;8:97–102.
55. Sandberg MM, Aro HT, Vuorio EI: Gene expression during bone repair. *Clin Orthop* 1993;289:292–312.
56. Rahn BA: Bone healing: Histologic and physiologic, in Sumner Smith G (ed): *Bone in Clinical Orthopaedics: A Study in Comparative Osteology.* Philadelphia, PA, WB Saunders, 1982, pp 335–386.
57. Perren SM: Physical and biological aspects of fracture healing with special reference to internal fixation. *Clin Orthop* 1979;138:175–196.
58. White AA III, Panjabi MM, Southwick WO: The four biomechanical stages of fracture repair. *J Bone Joint Surg* 1977;59A:188–192.
59. Rhinelander FW: Tibial blood supply in relation to fracture healing. *Clin Orthop* 1974;105:34–81.
60. Schenk R, Muller J: Histologie des pseudoarthroses, in Boitzy A (ed): *Periarthrite de l'epaule, Osteogenese Compression: Travaux divers.* Bern, Hans Huber Verlag, 1972, pp 174–185.
61. Schenk RK, Muller J, Willenegger H: Experimentell-histologischer Beitrag zur Entstehung und Behandlung von Pseudarthrosen. *Hefte Unfallheilkd* 1968;94:15–24.
62. Krompecher S: *Die Knochenbildung.* Jena, Germany, G Fischer, 1937.
63. Pauwels F: Grundriss einer Biomechanik der Frakturheilung. *Verh Dtsch Orthop Ges* 1940;34:62–108.
64. Pauwels F: Eine neue Theorie ueber den Einfluss mechanischer Reize auf die Differenzierung der Stuetzgewebe. *Z Anat Entwicklungsgesch* 1960;121:478–515.
65. Frank EH, Grodzinsky AJ: Cartilage electromechanics: I. Electrokinetic transduction and the effects of electrolyte pH and ionic strength. *J Biomech* 1987;20:615–627.

66. Frank EH, Grodzinsky AJ: Cartilage electromechanics: II. A continuum model of cartilage electrokinetics and correlation with experiments. *J Biomech* 1987;20: 629–639.

67. Gray ML, Pizzanelli AM, Lee RC, et al: Kinetics of the chondrocyte biosynthetic response to compressive load and release. *Biochim Biophys Acta* 1989;991:415–425.

68. Lavine LS, Grodzinsky AJ: Electrical stimulation of repair of bone. *J Bone Joint Surg* 1987;69A:626–630.

69. MacGinitie LA, Wu DD, Cochran GVB: Streaming potentials in healing, remodeling, and intact cortical bone. *J Bone Miner Res* 1993;8:1323–1335.

70. Mundy GR: Cytokines and local factors which affect osteoclast function. *Int J Cell Cloning* 1992;10:215–222.

71. Reddi AH: Cell biology and biochemistry of endochondral bone development. *Coll Relat Res* 1981;1:209–226.

72. Friedenstein AJ: Determined and inducible osteogenic precursor cells, in Elliott K, Fitzsimmons DW (eds): *Hard Tissue Growth, Repair, and Remineralization.* Ciba Foundation Symposium No. 11. Amsterdam, Elsevier, 1973, pp 169–185.

73. Abe YA, Akamine A, Aida Y, et al: Differentiation and mineralization in osteogenic precursor cells derived from fetal rat mandibular bone. *Calcif Tissue Int* 1993;52:365–371.

74. McKibbin BM: The biology of fracture healing in long bones. *J Bone Joint Surg* 1978;60B:150–162.

75. Tanaka T, Taniguchi Y, Gotoh K, et al: Morphological study of recombinant human transforming growth factor beta 1-induced intramembranous ossification in neonatal rat parietal bone. *Bone* 1993;14:117–123.

76. Taniguchi Y, Tanaka T, Gotoh K, et al: Transforming growth factor beta 1-induced cellular heterogeneity in the periosteum of rat parietal bones. *Calcif Tissue Int* 1993;53:122–126.

77. Joyce ME, Roberts AB, Sporn MB, et al: Transforming growth factor-beta and the initiation of chondrogenesis and osteogenesis in the rat femur. *J Cell Biol* 1990; 110:2195–2207.

78. Sporn MB, Roberts AB: *Peptide Growth Factors and Their Receptors I.* New York, NY, Springer-Verlag, 1990.

79. Sporn MB, Roberts AB: Regulation of cell differentiation and proliferation by retinoids and transforming growth factor β, in Burger MM, Sordat B, Zinkernagel RM (eds): *Cell to Cell Interaction: International Symposium.* Basel, Karger, 1990, pp 2–15.

80. Perren SM, Boitzy A: Cellular differentiation and bone biomechanics during consolidation of a fracture. *Anat Clin* 1978;1:13–28.

81. Perren SM, Cordey J: The concept of interfragmentary strain, in, Uhthoff HK (ed): *Current Concepts of Internal Fixation of Fractures.* Berlin, Springer-Verlag, 1980, pp 63–77.

82. Brighton CT, Schaffer JL, Shapiro DB, et al: Proliferation and macromolecular synthesis by rat calvarial bone cells grown in various oxygen tensions. *J Orthop Res* 1991;9:847–854.

83. Yamada H, Evans FG: *Strength of Biological Materials.* Baltimore, MD, Williams & Wilkins, 1970.

84. Bassett CAL, Herrmann I: Influence of oxygen concentration and mechanical factors on differentiation of connective tissues in vitro. *Nature* 1961;190:460–461.

85. Hardingham TE, Fosang AJ: Proteoglycans: Many forms and many functions. *FASEB J* 1992;6:861–870.

86. Hascall VC: Interaction of cartilage proteoglycans with hyaluronic acid. *J Supramol Struct* 1977;7:101–120.

87. Poole AR: Proteoglycans in health and disease: Structures and functions. *Biochem J* 1986;236:1–14.

88. Maroudas A, Urban JPG: Swelling pressures of cartilaginous tissues, in Maroudas A, Holborow EJ (eds): *Studies in Joint Disease.* Massachusetts, Pitman Publications, 1980, pp 87–116.

89. Basser PJ, Grodzinsky AJ: The Donnan model derived from microstructure. *Biophys Chem* 1993;46:57–68.

90. Buschmann MD, Grodzinsky AJ: A molecular model of proteoglycan-associated electrostatic forces in cartilage mechanics. *J Biomech Eng*, in press.

91. Eisenberg SR, Grodzinsky AJ: Swelling of articular cartilage and other connective tissues: Electromechanochemical forces. *J Orthop Res* 1985;3:148–159.

92. Eisenberg SR, Grodzinsky AJ: Electrokinetic micromodel of extracellular matrix and other polyelectrolyte networks. *Phys Chem Hydrodyn* 1988;10:517–539.

93. Mow VC, Holmes MH, Lai WM: Fluid transport and mechanical properties of articular cartilage: A review. *J Biomech* 1984;17:377–394.

94. Larsson T, Aspden RM, Heinegard D: Effects of mechanical load on cartilage matrix biosynthesis in vitro. *Matrix* 1991;11:388–394.

95. Sah RL, Kim YJ, Doong JY, et al: Biosynthetic response of cartilage explants to dynamic compression. *J Orthop Res* 1989;7:619–636.

96. Koob TJ, Clark PE, Hernandez DJ, et al: Compression loading in vitro regulates proteoglycan synthesis by tendon fibrocartilage. *Arch Biochem Biophys* 1992; 298:303–312.

97. Chai BF, Tang XM: Ultrastructural investigation of experimental fracture healing: I. Electron microscopic observation of cellular activity. *Chin Med J (Engl)* 1979; 92:530–535.

98. Gothlin G: Electron microscopic observations on fracture repair in the rat. *Acta Pathol Microbiol Scand (A)* 1973;81:507–522.

99. Prasad GC, Udupa KN: Studies on ultrastructural pattern of osteogenic cells during bone repair. *Acta Orthop Scand* 1972;43:163–175.

100. Tang XM, Chai BF: Ultrastructural investigation of experimental fracture healing: IV. Electron microscopic observation on transformation and fate of fibroblasts and chondrocytes. *Chin Med J (Engl)* 1981;94:291–300.

101. Amir D, Schwartz Z, Weinberg H, et al: The distribution of extracellular matrix vesicles in healing of rat tibial bone three days after intramedullary injury. *Arch Orthop Trauma Surg* 1988;107:1–6.

102. Ketenjian AY, Arsenis C: Morphological and biochemical studies during differentiation and calcification of fracture callus cartilage. *Clin Orthop* 1975;107:266–273.

103. Bonucci E: Fine structure of early cartilage calcification. *J Ultrastruct Res* 1967; 20:33–50.

104. Chen CC, Boskey AL: Mechanisms of proteoglycan inhibition of hydroxyapatite growth. *Calcif Tissue Int* 1985;37:395–400.

105. Chen CC, Boskey AL, Rosenberg LC: The inhibitory effect of cartilage proteoglycans on hydroxyapatite growth. *Calcif Tissue Int* 1984;36:285–290.

106. Dziewiatkowski DD, Majznerski LL: Role of proteoglycans in endochondral ossification: Inhibition of calcification. *Calcif Tissue Int* 1985;37:560–564.

107. Howell DS, Pita JC: Calcification of growth plate cartilage with special reference to studies on micropuncture fluids. *Clin Orthop* 1976;118:208–229.

108. Arsenault AL: Structural and chemical analyses of mineralization using the turkey leg tendon as a model tissue. *Bone Miner* 1992;17:253–256.

109. Christoffersen J, Landis WJ: A contribution with review to the description of mineralization of bone and other calcified tissues in vivo. *Anat Rec* 1991;230:435–450.

110. Arsenault AL, Grynpas MD: Crystals in calcified epiphyseal cartilage and cortical bone of the rat. *Calcif Tissue Int* 1988;43:219–225.

111. Boskey AL: Models of matrix vesicle calcification. *Inorg Perspect Biol Med* 1978; 2:51–92.

112. Boskey AL: Mineral-matrix interactions in bone and cartilage. *Clin Orthop* 1992; 281:244–274.

113. Schenk RK: Die Histologie der primaeren Knochenheilung im Lichte neuer Konzeptionen ueber den Knochenumbau. *Unfallheilkunde* 1978;81:219–227.

114. Frost HM: *Bone Remodelling Dynamics*. Springfield, IL, CC Thomas, 1963.

115. Frost HM: *Bone Dynamics in Osteoporosis and Osteomalacia.* Springfield, IL, CC Thomas, 1966.

116. Frost HM: Editorial: Suggested fundamental concepts in skeletal physiology. *Calcif Tissue Int* 1993;52:1–4.

117. Doty SB: Morphological evidence of gap junctions between bone cells. *Calcif Tissue Int* 1981;33:509–512.

118. Jeansonne BG, Feagin FF, McMinn RW, et al: Cell-to-cell communication of osteoblasts. *J Dent Res* 1979;58:1415–1423.

119. Piekarski K, Munro M: Transport mechanism operating between blood supply and osteocytes in long bones. *Nature* 1977;269:80–82.

120. Blair HC, Schlesinger PH, Ross FP, et al: Recent advances toward understanding osteoclast physiology. *Clin Orthop* 1993;294:7–22.

121. Prallet B, Male P, Neff L, et al: Identification of a functional mononuclear precursor of the osteoclast in chicken medullary bone marrow cultures. *J Bone Miner Res* 1992;7:405–414.

122. Zaidi M, Alam ASMT, Shankar VS, et al: Cellular biology of bone resorption. *Biol Rev Camb Philos Soc* 1993;68:197–264.

Chapter 9
Endochondral Bone Development Is a Cascade

A. Hari Reddi, PhD

Introduction

The remarkable regenerative potential of the vertebrate skeletal system is common knowledge. Repair and regeneration, in general, recapitulate embryonic development. For example, the sequence of events in limb regeneration in newts and salamanders and the stages of fracture healing in mammals recapitulate the sequential stages of limb development and morphogenesis. The operational dissection of the fracture repair into sequential stages has immense implications for fracture management in orthopaedic surgery. This chapter provides a description of the cascade of endochondral bone development and emphasizes the parallels between the fracture-healing sequence and limb morphogenesis. This discussion will include the identification, purification, cloning, and expression of bone morphogenetic proteins (BMPs), which are involved in initiating, promoting, and maintaining endochondral bone development.[1,2]

Bone Development Is a Cascade

A cellular and molecular approach to the investigation of endochondral bone development during limb morphogenesis, epiphyseal growth plate development, and fracture repair is inherently difficult because of asynchrony and developmental heterogeneity. The potential obstacles to the cellular analysis of endochondral bone development can be overcome in part by the judicious use of a matrix-induced bone morphogenesis model.[3-5]

Subcutaneous or intramuscular implantation of demineralized extracellular matrix of bone results in sequential cartilage and bone development that is reminiscent of endochondral bone morphogenesis in the epiphyseal growth plate. The development of the long bones occurs via proliferation of mesenchymal cells, differentiation and hypertrophy of chondrocytes, and calcification of cartilage matrices before their replacement by bone in the metaphyses. The spatial and temporal problems in the study of epiphyseal growth plate or of fracture callus can be avoided by the matrix-induced bone morphogenetic cascade model.

Implantation of demineralized diaphyseal bone matrix in a subcutaneous site results in hemostasis and formation of a blood clot around the implant, as in the fracture-healing sequence. By 24 hours after implantation of demineralized bone matrix the implant is discrete and is a button-like planoconvex plaque that consists of implanted collagenous extracellular matrix and a fibrin meshwork with enmeshed polymorphonuclear leukocytes. By day 3, the im-

147

plant consists of mesenchymal cells and monocyte-macrophages. The first chondroblasts appear on day 5 and chondrocytes are maximal on days 7 and 8. On day 9, the hypertrophic cartilage matrix undergoes calcification and the onset of angiogenesis and vascular invasion is observed. On days 10 to 11, basophilic osteogenic precursors and osteoblasts are observed in the vicinity of invading capillaries. Bone remodeling is evident on days 12 to 18, resulting in selective dissolution of the implanted matrix and the formation of an ossicle replete with bone marrow by day 21. Outline 1 summarizes the key steps in the cascade of endochondral bone development.[4,5]

Cellular and Molecular Aspects of the Cascade

The sequential cascade of histologic changes during bone development is accompanied by attendant changes in the various molecular components. Figure 1 demonstrates the sequential transitions in $^{35}SO_4$ incorporation into proteoglycans, ^{45}Ca incorporation into bone mineral, and ^{59}Fe incorporation into heme during hematopoiesis. There is a key increase in alkaline phosphatase activity prior to mineralization. It is noteworthy that transforming growth factor-beta 1 (TGF-β1) accumulates in the newly mineralized cartilage and bone matrix.[6] Although numerous in vitro experiments have implicated TGF-β1 in bone development, its detection in vivo during endochondral bone development is significant.[6] The developmental appearance, accumulation, and compartmentation of this cytokine and growth modulator raise additional questions regarding its metabolic disposition and regulation. In order for TGF-β to have a regulatory role, its activity in bone must be precisely controlled.

Both extractions and immunohistochemical analysis of bone indicate that TGF-β is bound to the mineralized matrix. This compartmentation may explain its sequestration in bone and its activation during bone remodeling. Plasminogen activators and acidic environment have been implicated in the processing of TGF-β1. Both TGF-β isoforms, β1 and β2, appear to increase coordinately during bone development, which implies they have a critical role in this process.[6] Recent work with TGF-β1 gene-knockout mice revealed bone development proceeds normally; however, the mice succumb because of a deficit in immune regulation.

Gene Expression During Bone Morphogenesis

Temporal changes in gene expression were monitored by determining steady-state levels of messenger RNA (mRNA) for various extracellular matrix (ECM) components.[7] Figure 2 summarizes the quantitative changes in expression of ECM genes. Type I collagen gradually increased until it reached a peak at day 18. The steady-state level of type II collagen mRNA increased on day 5, peaked

---

Outline 1   Endochondral bone development is a sequential cascade

1. Chemotaxis of progenitor cells
2. Proliferation of mesenchymal cells
3. Differentiation of chondrocytes
4. Calcification of cartilage matrix
5. Angiogenesis and vascular invasion
6. Bone differentiation and mineralization
7. Bone remodeling and marrow differentiation

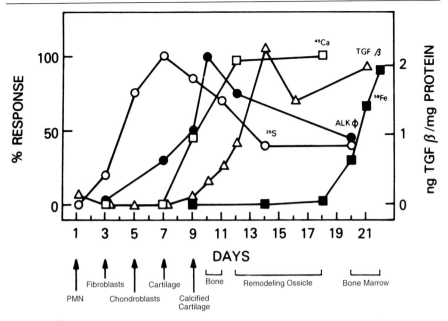

Fig. 1 Cascade of endochondral bone development induced by bone morphogenetic proteins present in the extracellular matrix of bone. Demineralized diaphyseal bone matrix was implanted subcutaneously over the ventral thoracic region on day 0. On day 1 the implant consisted of polymorphonuclear leukocytes. By days 2 to 3 monocyte-macrophages and mesenchymal fibroblast-like cells are present in the vicinity of the implanted bone matrix. By days 5 to 7 chondrogenesis is evident with maximal $^{35}SO_4$ incorporation into proteoglycans on day 7. ^{45}Ca incorporation begins to increase on day 9 during cartilage calcification and increases more on day 11, with mineralization of bone. The newly formed bone is remodeled and is the site of hematopoietic differentiation including erythropoiesis as indicated by ^{59}Fe incorporation into heme. The changes in accumulation of transforming growth factor-β are also plotted.

on day 7, and declined by day 9. Type IX collagen expression was maximal on day 9. A similar pattern was observed for proteoglycan aggrecan core protein and link protein. Fibronectin expression was detectable throughout the bone development cascade and was maximal on day 1 during matrix-cell interactions. The $\beta1$ subunit of integrin appeared to be expressed at a constant level in the bone development sequence.[6] The expression of TGF-$\beta1$ was observed throughout bone development, but was higher during early chondrogenesis on day 5 and initial osteogenesis on day 9 (Fig. 3). Both diaphysis and hematopoietic marrow exhibited TGF-β expression.

Pyrophosphatase and Bone

Inhibitors of calcium phosphate crystallization, such as pyrophosphate, must be removed before calcification can occur.[8] Thus, it is likely that pyrophosphatase hydrolyzes pyrophosphate at sites of mineralization. Pyrophosphatase activity was assayed during the endochondral bone morphogenetic cascade and found to be maximal on days 9 to 11 during peak mineralization (Fig. 4).[9] These data support the notion that pyrophosphatase and alkaline phosphatase may play a role in biologic mineralization of developing bone.

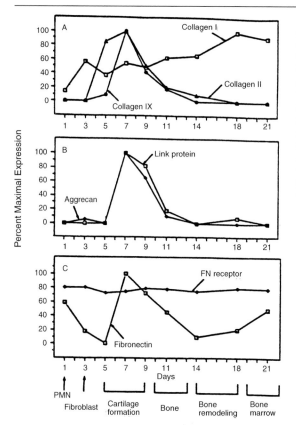

Fig. 2 Northern blot analysis of steady-state levels of mRNA for extracellular matrix genes during the cascade of endochondral bone formation. The blots were quantitated by scanning densitometry and the results plotted relative to the maximal expression of each transcript. **Top,** mRNA levels of types I, II, and IX collagens. **Center,** Expression of aggrecan and link protein. **Bottom,** Levels of expression of fibronectin and fibronectin receptor integrin β1 subunit.

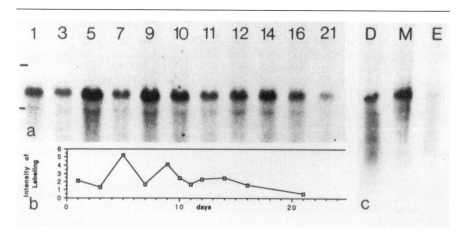

Fig. 3 Changes in the expression of steady-state levels of TGF-β1 as revealed by Northern blot analysis. **a,** RNA from matrix-induced implants of bone development cascade were analyzed. **b,** Graphic representation of the densitometric scans of the blot in **a. c,** Northern blots of diaphysis (D), bone marrow (M), and epiphysis (E).

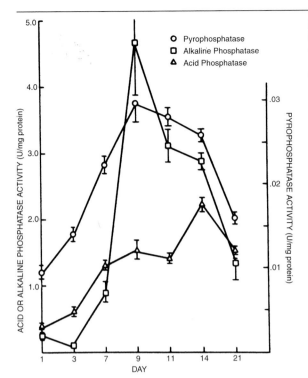

Changes in DNA, RNA, and Polyamines

It is axiomatic that cell proliferation precedes cell differentiation during development. In view of this, the changes in DNA, RNA, and polyamine biosynthesis were studied during endochondral bone development.[10] Cell proliferation was investigated by determining [3H]-thymidine incorporation using autoradiography and measurement of acid-precipitable radioactivity. The autoradiographs demonstrate incorporation during mesenchymal proliferation, early bone formation, and marrow proliferation (Fig. 5). On day 3, numerous labeled mesenchymal cells were in the vicinity of the implanted matrix (Fig. 5, *top left*). On day 8, perivascular osteoprogenitor cells in the vicinity of hypertrophic chondrocytes were intensely labeled (Fig. 5, *top right*); however, differentiated chondrocytes were devoid of the thymidine label. On day 11, during osteogenic cell proliferation, numerous labeled cells were in juxtaposition to the hypertrophic cartilage (Fig. 5, *center*). Numerous hematopoietic precursor cells were labelled with [3H]-thymidine during bone marrow differentiation on days 15 to 19 (Fig. 5, *bottom*). Figure 6 demonstrates the changes in [3H]-thymidine incorporation into acid-precipitable material. Maximal synthesis occurred on days 3, 9 to 11, and 19. These peaks correspond to cell proliferation peaks prior to chondrogenesis, osteogenesis, and hematopoiesis, respectively.

RNA synthesis was investigated by [3H]-uridine incorporation into acid-precipitable material. There were three peaks of incorporation corresponding to chondrogenesis, osteogenesis, and hematopoiesis on days 5, 11, and 19, respectively (Fig. 7).

The aliphatic polyamines—putrescine, spermidine, and spermine—and associated biosynthetic enzymes are known to be present in rapidly dividing tis-

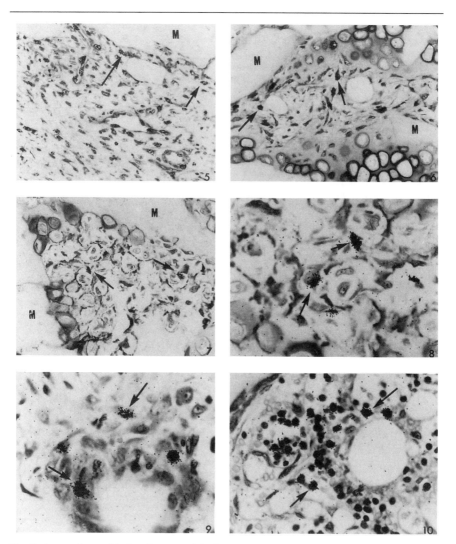

Fig. 5 Autoradiographic localization of [³H]-thymidine incorporation during the matrix-induced endochondral bone development cascade. Plastic sections stained with toluidine blue M, implanted bone matrix. **Top left,** Day 3. Labeled mesenchymal cells (arrows) in the vicinity of the implanted matrix (m) (× 260). **Top right,** Day 8. [³H]-Thymidine labeling is present in perivascular mesenchymal cells (arrows) (× 260). **Center left,** Day 11. The [³H]-thymidine label is restricted to presumptive osteoprogenitor cells (arrows) (× 260). **Center right,** Day 11. Same as *center left.* Arrows point to presumptive progenitor cells (× 690). **Bottom left,** Day 15. Labeling of extravascular islands of hemocytoblasts during early stages of hematopoiesis (× 690). **Bottom right,** Day 19. Intense labeling of erythropoietic colonies in the ossicle (× 690).

sues.[11-13] Figure 8 depicts the transitions in S-adenosylmethionine decarboxylase (SAM decarboxylase) and ornithine decarboxylase (ODC), a rate-limiting enzyme in the biosynthesis of putrescine. The levels of both enzymes peaked on day 3 during mesenchymal progenitor cell proliferation. A smaller, but reproducible peak for ODC occurred on days 8 and 9 and fell abruptly. The concentrations of all the polyamines—putrescine, spermidine, and spermine—

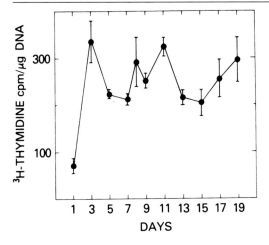

Fig. 6 Changes in the incorporation of [³H]-thymidine in acid-precipitable DNA as an index of cell proliferation during the matrix-induced cascade of endochondral bone development. Each point is a mean of eight observations from four rats. The bars represent the standard error of the mean.

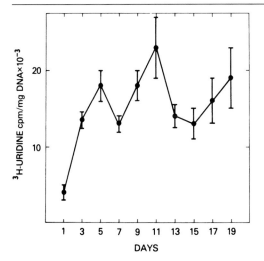

Fig. 7 Changes in the incorporation of [³H] uridine into acid-precipitable RNA during the matrix-induced cascade of endochondral bone development. Each point is a mean of eight observations from four rats. The bars represent the standard error of the mean.

were low on day 1, increased to maximal values on day 2 during bone morphogenesis, and declined thereafter (Fig. 9). Putrescine, but not spermidine and spermine, had a small, but broad peak on days 3 to 7 during mesenchymal progenitor cell proliferation and chondrogenesis.

The concentration of proline biosynthetic and degradative enzymes is relatively high in collagenous tissues such as cartilage and bone. Proline can be synthesized from either glutamic acid or ornithine via the formation of a pyrroline-5-carboxylate intermediate; it can be degraded to glutamic acid by proline oxidase and pyrroline-5-carboxylate dehydrogenase. Proline metabolizing enzymes in developing cartilage and bone have been characterized.[14] Ornithine aminotransferase and pyrroline-5-carboxylate reductase are maximal during type II collagen biosynthesis in cartilage and in bone formation (Fig. 10). In contrast, levels of proline oxidase and pyrroline-5-carboxylate dehydrogenase are low. Arginase, which catalyzes ornithine biosynthesis from arginine, is maximal on day 3 during mesenchymal cell proliferation, and then it declines.

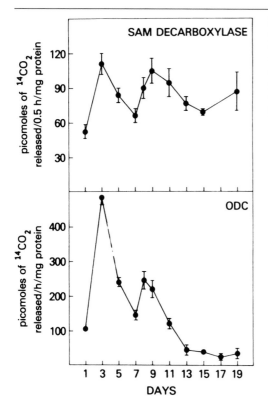

Fig. 8 Changes in ornithine decarboxylase (ODC) and S-adenosylmethionine decarboxylase (SAM-decarboxylase) during the matrix-induced cascade of endochondral bone development. Each point is a mean of eight samples from four rats. The bars represent the standard error of the mean.

Fibronectin and Integrins

Fibronectin is a cell-surface glycoprotein involved in cell-ECM and cell-cell interactions.[15–17] A structurally related and immunologically cross-reactive protein, plasma fibronectin, is present in the blood plasma and was previously known as cold insoluble globulin. Despite numerous in vitro studies of fibronectin, there are major gaps in the understanding of its role in vivo.

The matrix-induced endochondral bone development cascade has been used as a model for the study of the role of fibronectin.[18,19] Indirect immunofluorescence was used to locate fibronectin during endochondral bone development. Plasma fibronectin was bound by implanted collagenous demineralized bone matrix before and during mesenchymal cell proliferation. In addition, newly recruited mesenchymal cells exhibited prominent biosynthesis of fibronectin. The newly synthesized fibronectin consisted of a fibrillar meshwork. During chondrogenesis, the cartilage matrix included fibronectin; however, it required prior treatment with hyaluronidase to unmask the staining. Proteoglycan aggregates probably masked endogenous fibronectin. Fibronectin was present in the fibrillar network in the vicinity of osteoblasts and osteoprogenitor cells, and the hematopoietic colonies were associated with the fibronectin. Thus, fibronectin is present throughout endochondral bone development.

The immunolocalization of fibronectin in articular cartilage of growing rats (6 to 8 weeks of age) was informative. High reactivity for fibronectin was observed in the perichondrium and chondrocyte cell surface. The ECM of cartilage

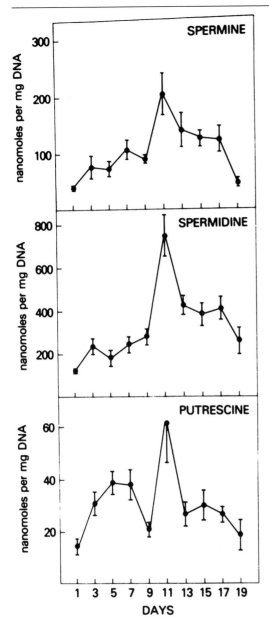

Fig. 9 Changes in the concentration of putrescine, spermidine, and spermine during the matrix-induced cascade of endochondral bone development. Each point represents eight samples from four rats. The bars represent the standard error of the mean.

was devoid of immunofluorescence; however, treatment of sections with hyaluronidase revealed intense fibronectin staining, which suggests the fibronectin was masked by proteoglycan aggregates.

In the epiphyseal growth plate, endochondral bone formation occurs in a continuum. Figure 11 depicts a section of the epiphyseal growth plate treated with hyaluronidase and stained for fibronectin. Hyaluronidase unmasked the staining in cartilage matrix. Hypertrophic chondrocytes accumulated fibronectin in the pericellular zone, and the transverse septa of the hypertrophic chon-

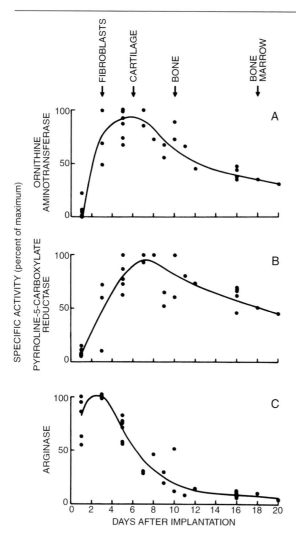

Fig. 10 Transitions in the specific activity of proline synthetic enzymes in the matrix-induced cascade of endochondral bone development. Each point represents a separate determination. Activities in µm/h/mg DNA are expressed as a percent of maximum to correct for differences between experiments.

drocyte zone reacted positively to fibronectin. A lacy meshwork of fibronectin surrounded the osteoblasts in the endosteal surface of cancellous bone. The β1 subunit of integrin, the fibronectin receptor, is expressed throughout bone development.

The foregoing description of the association of fibronectin during endochondral bone development as demonstrated by biosynthesis and immunolocalization allows the formulation of a hypothetical model for the role of fibronectin. Initially, plasma fibronectin binds to demineralized ECM of bone. A similar step may occur during initial stages of fracture repair. This step may be conducive to cell attachment and chemotaxis of progenitor cells. During mesenchymal cell proliferation, fibronectin is present in a cottony array; during chondrogenesis it is associated with the pericellular zone of chondrocytes. During chondrolysis, loss of proteoglycans unmasks the fibronectin in the hypertrophic cartilage matrix. This "exposed" fibronectin then may serve as a nidus for osteoprogenitor cell attachment and differentiation into osteoblasts.

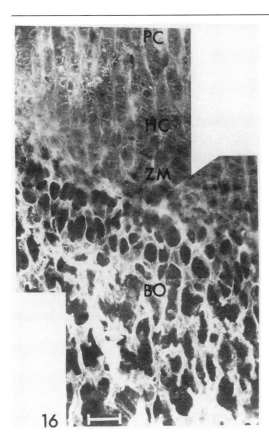

Fig. 11 Immunofluorescent localization of fibronectin in a frozen section of rat epiphyseal growth plate. Section was pretreated with hyaluronidase to unmask fibronectin. PC, proliferation chondrocytes; HC, hypertrophic chondrocytes; ZM, zone of provisional mineralization; BO, bone formation on the surface of calcified cartilage spicules ($\times$ 400).

Enzyme Changes

Although the precise role of alkaline phosphatase (pH 9.3) in mineralization is far from clear, alkaline phosphatase is a useful marker enzyme for new bone differentiation and mineralization. As already described in Figure 1, the increase in alkaline phosphatase precedes the upswing in ^{45}Ca incorporation into bone mineral.

Lactic and malic dehydrogenase are pyridine nucleotide-linked enzymes. Lactic dehydrogenase (LDH) is useful for monitoring chondrogenesis because the levels of this anaerobic glycolytic enzyme are high in avascular cartilage[20] and during matrix-induced cartilage development (Fig. 12). Malic dehydrogenase (MDH) levels are uniform throughout endochondral bone development. The ratio of LDH to MDH can be expressed as a quotient that is greater than one during the cartilage phase of endochondral bone development and declines during bone formation (Fig. 13).

Because cartilage is degraded and replaced by bone during endochondral bone formation, considerable attention has been focused on lysomal enzymes and their role in cartilage degradation.[21–23] Correlative changes in acid phosphatase, β-glucuronidase, and arylsulfatase have been investigated using combined biochemical and histochemical techniques.[24] Levels of these enzymes increase during chondrogenesis and rise even higher during bone remodeling. It

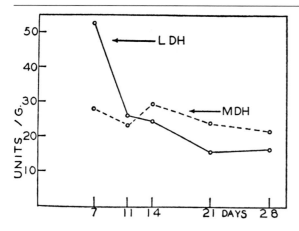

Fig. 12 Changes in the levels of lactic dehydrogenase (LDH) and malic dehydrogenase (MDH) during the matrix-induced cascade of endochondral bone development. Highest levels of LDH are found during chondrogenesis on day 7, and the activity declines on day 11 during bone formation.

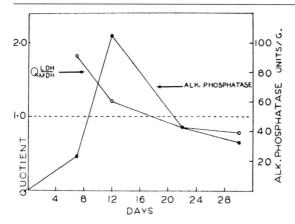

Fig. 13 Changes in the quotient of LDH/MDH during the matrix-induced cascade of endochondral bone development. Also depicted are changes in alkaline phosphomonoesterase (alkaline phosphatase).

is noteworthy that arylsulfatase is a useful marker of bone resorption and re-modeling.

Proteoglycans in Transition

Proteoglycans and collagens are the two major classes of macromolecules in skeletal tissues, such as cartilage and bone. The proteoglycans of hyaline cartilage have been well characterized according to their polydispersity and their ability to interact with hyaluronic acid via a hyaluronic acid binding domain of the core protein.[25,26] This interaction is stabilized by the link protein and results in the formation of high molecular weight proteoglycan aggregates.

The biosynthesis of proteoglycans, which were labeled in vivo at various stages of the bone development cascade, was studied.[27] On day 7, during maximal chondrogenesis, the elution profile demonstrated proteoglycan aggregates in the void volume of the Sepharose 2B column (Fig. 14). There is a decline in cartilage proteoglycan synthesis during calcification of cartilage matrix on day 9. Bone formation is accompanied by the appearance of smaller bone proteoglycans. The cartilage proteoglycans and link protein persist in the calcified cartilage spicules during cartilage mineralization.[28]

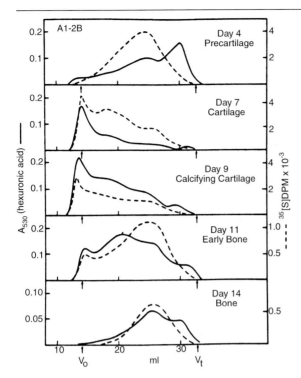

Fig. 14 Changes in the biosynthesis of proteoglycan aggregates prepared by direct associative extraction of matrix-induced implants. Chromatography was performed on Sepharose-2B columns. The solid line represents hexuronic acid, and indicates accumulated proteoglycans. The dashed line depicts $^{35}SO_4$ incorporation into newly synthesized proteoglycans.

The metabolic fate of newly synthesized cartilage proteoglycans was systematically studied.[29] Analysis of proteoglycan profiles revealed two major components (peaks I and II) of 0.28 and 0.68 kd, respectively. After the onset of osteogenesis, a mineral-associated bone proteoglycan was prominent[29] with a half-life of 7 days.

γ-Carboxyglutamic Acid Containing Proteins

Gamma-carboxyglutamic acid (Gla) is a critical amino acid in vitamin K-dependent blood coagulation proteins such as prothrombin. By virtue of the vicinal carboxyl group on the γ-carbon atom of glutamic acid, Gla proteins are ideally poised to interact with divalent cations such as calcium. Therefore, the occurrence of Gla acid in bone was investigated, and Gla was found in ethylenediaminetetra-acetic acid (EDTA) extracts.[30,31] Bone Gla protein (BGP) can be quantitated by a radioimmunoassay. Changes in BGP during the matrix-induced cascade of endochondral bone development indicate that BGP increases only after the initial mineralization (Fig. 15). These results raise the prospect that BGP may indicate bone remodeling and turnover rather than the onset of mineralization.[32]

Prostaglandins and Bone Formation

Prostaglandins (PGs) are derivatives of 20-carbon unsaturated fatty acids with ubiquitous distribution. Although the effects of PGs on bone resorption are well known, their effects on bone formation have been appreciated only recently.[33] The initial reports of new bone formation in response to PG were based

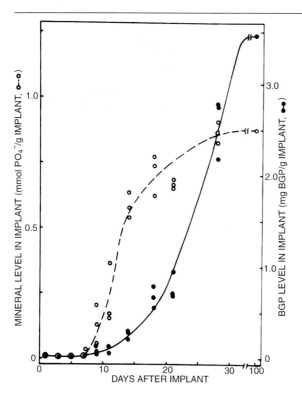

Fig. 15   Developmental changes of vitamin K-dependent bone Gla protein (BGP, also know as osteocalcin) in relation to inorganic phosphate in the matrix-induced cascade of endochondral bone development.

on infants with cardiovascular complications who were given PGE_1 to maintain patency of the ductus arteriosus. The treatment is, of course, based on the well-known vasodilatory actions of PGE_1. The changes in PG levels were examined during the matrix-induced cascade of bone development.[34] During mesenchymal cell proliferation there was a rise in endogenous thromboxane B_2. $PGF_{2\alpha}$ levels were maximal during chondrolysis. During bone formation, PGE_2, thromboxane B_2, and 6-keto $PGF_{1\alpha}$ were elevated (Fig. 16). PGE_2 and $PGF_{2}\alpha$ are increased during hematopoiesis.

Isolation of Molecular Signals: The BMPs

Given the fact that the demineralized bone matrix can initiate the cascade of endochondral bone development, a search for the molecular signals that initiate this process was undertaken. Because bone matrix is insoluble, chaotropic reagents were employed to solubilize matrix components.[35,36] A reconstitution assay was used to quantitate the bioactivity of the dissociative extracts.[35] The BMPs were purified to homogeneity.[37] The BMPs have been cloned by recombinant DNA methods and have been expressed and found to be osteoinductive.[38–42]

The recombinant BMPs are pleiotropic in their actions. Pleiotropy may be defined as the property of a gene or gene product to act in a multiplicity of ways. BMPs can initiate chemotaxis, mitosis, and differentiation of mesenchymal cells. Recombinant BMP-2B (also known as BMP-4) and purified BMP-3 (osteogenin) are the most potent (Fig. 17) chemoattractants to human monocytes.[43] Recall that chemotaxis of polymorphonuclear leukocytes and mono-

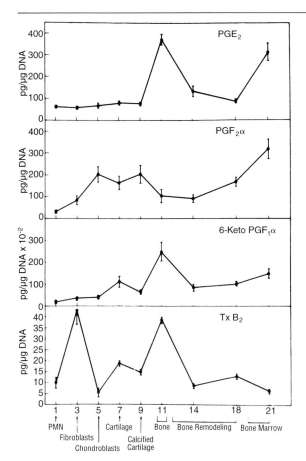

Fig. 16 Changes in tissue concentration of prostaglandin E_2 (PGE_2), $PGF_{2\alpha}$, 6-keto $PGF_{1\alpha}$, and thromboxane B2 during matrix-induced endochondral bone development. Note the massive accumulation of PGE_2 during new bone formation and the decline during bone resorption and remodeling.

cytes is the first step in the cascade of matrix-induced bone development. It has been hypothesized that monocytes attracted to the site may secrete additional cytokines, including TGF-β and basic fibroblast growth factor (bFGF), to promote differentiation of mesenchymal progenitor cells to cartilage and bone.

Angiogenesis and Osteogenesis

Angiogenesis and vascular invasion are prerequisites for bone formation.[44,45] The developing osteoprogenitor cells and osteoblasts are in contact with the basement membrane of the invading capillaries. The ECM around invading capillaries may interact with BMPs. Basement membrane components such as laminin, type IV collagen, and factor VIII antigen are localized around invading capillaries.[45] During experiments on the interactions of BMPs with ECM, it unexpectedly was found that BMP-3 and recombinant BMP-4 avidly bound to type IV collagen.[46–48] BMP-3 also binds to types I and IX collagens. The binding is pH- and time-dependent. Because BMP-3 is a member of the TGF-β supergene family, the binding of TGF-β1 to type IV collagen was also tested. TGF-β1 also bound avidly to type IV collagen.

Type IV collagen is characteristic of basement membranes. The other components of basement membranes include laminin, heparan sulfate proteogly-

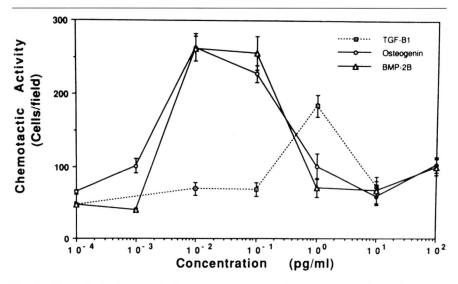

Fig. 17 Chemotaxis of monocytes in response to osteogenin and bone morphogenic protein-2B (BMP-2B) present in demineralized bone matrix. TGF-β1 is transforming growth factor-beta 1.

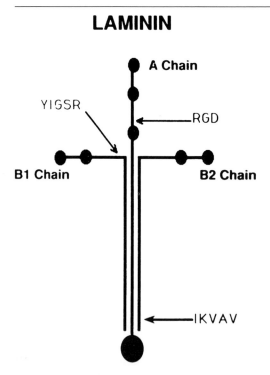

Fig. 18 Molecular domains in laminin with special reference to molecular motifs of RGD (arginine-glycine-aspartic acid) in the A chain, YIGSR (tyrosine-isoleucine-glycine-serine-arginine) in the B1 chain, and IKVAV (isoleucine-lysine-valine-alanine-valine) in the B2 chain.

can, and nidogen/entactin. These observations and the binding of BMPs to type IV collagen served as an impetus for the examination of the influence of basement membrane components on bone-cell phenotype in vitro. Both primary

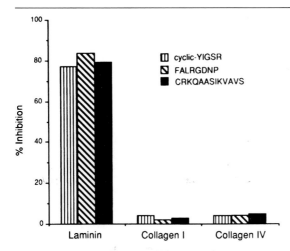

Fig. 19 Inhibition of adhesion to laminin, type I collagen, and type IV collagen. Attachment of osteoblastic MC3T3-E1 cells to laminin coating (100 mg/well) was assayed in the presence of exogenous peptides (200 mg/ml). All three peptides with YIGSR (tyrosine-isoleucine-glycine-serine-arginine), RGD (arginine-glycine-aspartic acid), and IKVAV (isoleucine-lysine-valine-alanine-valine) motifs inhibited cell adhesion to laminin substratum. However, cell attachment to types I and IV collagens was not blocked by laminin-specific molecular domains.

osteoblasts and the osteoblastic cell line MC3T3-E1 demonstrated profound phenotypic alterations when in contact with type IV collagen or laminin.[47] The phenotypic hallmark of these cells is the formation of canalicular cell processes reminiscent of terminally differentiated osteocytes.[47] Antibodies to laminin and the exogenous addition of a synthetic peptide with a YIGSR (tyrosine, isoleucine, glycine, serine, arginine) motif blocked canalicular cell process formation (Figs. 18 and 19). Although osteocytes are not in contact with basement membranes, they may retain the "memory" of their initial contact with laminin. Osteons in the haversian system consist of a central capillary with concentric circles of osteoblasts, implying that the initial capillary basement membrane-osteoprogenitor interaction governs the geometry of the lamellar bone.

These advances in the cascade of endochondral development and the attendant isolation of BMPs have far-reaching implications for orthopaedics, oral surgery, plastic and reconstructive surgery, and the emerging discipline of "tissue engineering" of new bone.[49,50]

Acknowledgments

This work is supported by the Virginia M. and William A. Percy Chair in Orthopaedic Science and grants from the National Institutes of Health. I thank Ms. Brenda Ludgood for superb assistance in the preparation of this manuscript.

References

1. Reddi AH: Cell biology and biochemistry of endochondral bone development. *Coll Relat Res* 1981;1:209–226.
2. Reddi AH: Regulation of cartilage and bone differentiation by bone morphogenetic proteins. *Curr Opin Cell Biol* 1992;4:850–855.
3. Urist MR: Bone: Formation by autoinduction. *Science* 1965;150:893–899.
4. Reddi AH, Huggins C: Biochemical sequences in the transformation of normal fibroblasts in adolescent rats. *Proc Natl Acad Sci USA* 1972;69:1601–1605.
5. Reddi AH, Anderson WA: Collagenous bone matrix-induced endochondral ossification and hemopoiesis. *J Cell Biol* 1976;69:557–572.

6. Carrington JL, Roberts AB, Flanders KC, et al: Accumulation, localization and compartmentation of transforming growth factor beta during endochondral bone development. *J Cell Biol* 1988;107:1969–1975.

7. Yu YM, Becvar R, Yamada Y, et al: Changes in the gene expression of collagens, fibronectin, integrin, and proteoglycans during matrix-induced bone morphogenesis. *Biochem Biophys Res Commun* 1991;177:427–432.

8. Glimcher MJ: Composition, structure and organization of bone and other mineralized tissues and the mechanism of calcification, in Geiger SR, Aurbach GD, Greep RO, et al (eds): *Handbook of Physiology: Section 7: Endocrinology; Volume VII: Parathyroid Gland.* Washington, DC, American Physiological Society, 1976, pp 25–116.

9. Meyer JL, Reddi AH: Changes in pyrophosphatase activity during the *de novo* mineralization associated with cartilage and bone formation. *Arch Biochem Biophys* 1985;242:532–539.

10. Rath NC, Reddi AH: Changes in polyamines, RNA synthesis, and cell proliferation during matrix-induced cartilage, bone and bone marrow development. *Dev Biol* 1981;82:211–216.

11. Tabor CW, Tabor H: 1,4 Diaminobutane (putrescine), spermidine, and spermine. *Annu Rev Biochem* 1976;45:285–306.

12. Rath NC, Reddi AH: Changes in ornithine decarboxylase activity during matrix-induced cartilage, bone and bone marrow differentiation. *Biochem Biophys Res Commun* 1978;81:106–113.

13. Takigawa M, Watanabe R, Ishida H, et al: Induction by parathyroid hormone of ornithine decarboxylase in rabbit costal chondrocytes in culture. *J Biochem* (Tokyo) 1979;85:311–314.

14. Smith RJ, Reddi AH, Phang JM: Changes in proline-synthetic and degradative enzymes during matrix-induced cartilage and bone formation. *Calcif Tissue Int* 1979; 27:275–279.

15. Ruoslahti E, Pierschbacher MD: New perspectives in cell adhesion: RGD and integrins. *Science* 1987;238:491–497.

16. Hynes RO: Integrins: A family of cell surface receptors. *Cell* 1987;48:549–554.

17. Yamada KM: Adhesive recognition sequences. *J Biol Chem* 1991;266:12809–12812.

18. Weiss RE, Reddi AH: Synthesis and localization of fibronectin during collagenous matrix-mesenchymal cell interaction and differentiation of cartilage and bone in vivo. *Proc Natl Acad Sci USA* 1980;77:2074–2078.

19. Weiss RE, Reddi AH: Appearance of fibronectin during the differentiation of cartilage, bone, and bone marrow. *J Cell Biol* 1981;88:630–636.

20. Reddi AH, Huggins C: Lactic-malic dehydrogenase quotients during transformation of fibroblasts into cartilage and bone. *Proc Soc Exp Biol Med* 1971;137:127–129.

21. Dean RT (ed): *Lysosomes.* London, Edward Arnold, 1977.

22. Doty SB, Schofield BH: Enzyme histochemistry of bone and cartilage cells. *Prog Histochem Cytochem* 1976;8:1–38.

23. Thyberg J, Friberg U: The lysosomal system in endochondral growth. *Prog Histochem Cytochem* 1978;10:1–46.

24. Rath NC, Hand AR, Reddi AH: Activity and distribution of lysosomal enzymes during collagenous matrix-induced cartilage, bone, and bone marrow development. *Dev Biol* 1981;85:89–98.

25. Heinegård D, Oldberg A: Structure and biology of cartilage and bone matrix noncollagenous macromolecules. *FASEB J* 1989;3:2042–2051.

26. Heinegård D, Paulsson M: Structure and metabolism of proteoglycans, in Piez KA, Reddi AH (eds): *Extracellular Matrix Biochemistry.* New York, NY, Elsevier, 1984, pp 277–328.

27. Reddi AH, Hascall VC, Hascall GK: Changes in proteoglycan types during matrix-induced cartilage and bone development. *J Biol Chem* 1978;253:2429–2436.

28. Poole AR, Reddi AH, Rosenberg LC: Persistence of cartilage proteoglycan and link protein during matrix-induced endochondral bone development: An immunofluorescent study. *Dev Biol* 1982;89:532–539.

29. Tian MY, Yanagishita M, Hascall VC, et al: Biosynthesis and fate of proteoglycans in cartilage and bone during development and mineralization. *Arch Biochem Biophys* 1986;247:221–232.

30. Hauschka PV, Lian JB, Gallop PM: Direct identification of the calcium binding amino acid, gamma-carboxyglutamate, in mineralized tissue. *Proc Natl Acad Sci USA* 1975;72:3925–3929.

31. Price PA: GLA-containing proteins of mineralized tissues, in Slavkin H, Price P (eds): *Chemistry and Biology of Mineralized Tissues*. Amsterdam, Elsevier Science Publishers, 1992, pp 169–176.

32. Price PA, Lothringer JW, Baukol SA, et al: Developmental appearance of the vitamin K-dependent protein of bone during calcification: Analysis of mineralizing tissues in human, calf, and rat. *J Biol Chem* 1981;256:3781–3784.

33. Marks SC, Miller SC: Prostaglandins and the skeleton: The legacy and challenges of two decades of research. *Endocrine J* 1993;1:337–344.

34. Wientroub S, Wahl LM, Feuerstein N, et al: Changes in tissue concentration of prostaglandins during endochondral bone differentiation. *Biochem Biophys Res Commun* 1983;117:746–750.

35. Sampath TK, Reddi AH: Dissociative extraction and reconstitution of extracellular matrix components involved in local bone differentiation. *Proc Natl Acad Sci USA* 1981;78:7599–7603.

36. Sampath TK, Reddi AH: Homology of bone-inductive proteins from human, monkey, bovine, and rat extracellular matrix. *Proc Natl Acad Sci USA* 1983;80:6591–6595.

37. Luyten FP, Cunningham NS, Ma S, et al: Purification and partial amino acid sequence of osteogenin, a protein initiating bone differentiation. *J Biol Chem* 1989;264:13377–13380.

38. Wozney JM, Rosen V, Celeste AJ, et al: Novel regulators of bone formation: Molecular clones and activities. *Science* 1988;242:1528–1534.

39. Ozkaynak E, Rueger DC, Drier EA, et al: OP-1 cDNA encodes an osteogenic protein in the TGF-beta family. *EMBO J* 1990;9:2085–2093.

40. Wang EA, Rosen V, D'Alessandro JS, et al: Recombinant human bone morphogenetic protein induces bone formation. *Proc Natl Acad Sci USA* 1990;87:2220–2224.

41. Hammonds RG Jr, Schwall R, Dudley A, et al: Bone-inducing activity of mature BMP-2b produced from a hybrid BMP-2a/2b precursor. *Mol Endocrinol* 1991;5:149–155.

42. Reddi AH, Chao EYS, Stauffer RN: Skeletal regeneration: Reality for orthopaedic practices of the twenty-first century. *Adv Operative Orthopaedics* 1993;1:23–37.

43. Cunningham NS, Paralkar V, Reddi AH: Osteogenin and recombinant bone morphogenetic protein 2B are chemotactic for human monocytes and stimulate transforming growth factor beta 1 mRNA expression. *Proc Natl Acad Sci USA* 1992;89:11740–11744.

44. Trueta J: The role of the vessels in osteogenesis. *J Bone Joint Surg* 1963;45B:402–418.

45. Foidart JM, Reddi AH: Immunofluorescent localization of type IV collagen and laminin during endochondral bone differentiation and regulation by pituitary growth hormone. *Dev Biol* 1980;75:130–136.

46. Paralkar VM, Nandedkar AK, Pointer RH, et al: Interaction of osteogenin, a heparin binding bone morphogenetic protein, with type IV collagen. *J Biol Chem* 1990;265:17281–17284.

47. Vukicevic S, Luyten FP, Kleinman HK, et al: Differentiation of canalicular cell processes in bone cells by basement membrane matrix components: Regulation by discrete domains of laminin. *Cell* 1990;63:437–445.

48. Paralkar VM, Vukicevic S, Reddi AH: Transforming growth factor beta type I binds to collagen IV of basement membrane matrix: Implications for development. *Dev Biol* 1991;143:303–308.
49. Ripamonti U, Reddi H: Growth and morphogenetic factors in bone induction: Role of osteogenin and related bone morphogenetic proteins in craniofacial and periodontal bone repair. *Crit Rev Oral Biol Med* 1992;3:1–14.
50. Khouri RK, Koudsi B, Reddi AH: Tissue transformation into bone in vivo: A potential practical application. *JAMA* 1991;266:1953–1955.

Chapter 10
Fracture Callus Metabolism

Carl T. Brighton, MD, PhD

Introduction

Definition of Metabolism

Metabolism is the sum of the processes by which cells maintain themselves in their environment. More specifically, metabolism embraces the ways in which cells extract energy from their environment and the ways in which cells synthesize macromolecules. This chapter will be concerned exclusively with energy metabolism, or the ways in which fracture callus cells extract energy from the microenvironment. A succeeding chapter will deal specifically with the ways in which fracture callus cells synthesize macromolecules.

Growth Plate Studies Versus Fracture Callus Studies

Knowledge of the energy metabolism of hard tissue in general and fracture callus in particular has lagged behind that of soft tissue for many reasons.[1] The physical nature of bone and fracture callus makes the study of cellular metabolism in such tissue technically difficult. The fracture callus contains a heterogeneous cell population in which there is not a consistent spatial relationship between callus regions. In addition, the cell population in the fracture callus changes with time, and the spatial relationships between callus regions also change with time. Finally, it is difficult to study the fracture callus in situ, and it is especially difficult to study the energy metabolism of the cells within the callus.

For these reasons, researchers who wish to study endochondral ossification frequently turn to the growth plate, a structure that is morphologically stratified such that different regions or zones are relatively easy to identify. In addition, the cells within each zone of the growth plate represent a relatively homogeneous population. Fortunately, as will be brought out in detail below, the metabolism of the growth plate appears to be very similar to that of the fracture callus. In this chapter, data from metabolic studies of the fracture callus, when available, will be presented and compared to data from similar studies of the growth plate. When data are not available for the fracture callus but are available for the growth plate, those data will be presented as indirect evidence of the energy metabolism of the fracture callus.

How Cells Extract Energy From Substrate Molecules: A Brief Overview

Stages In Extraction of Energy From Substrates

Cells metabolize substrates in three stages.[2] In stage one, large molecules are hydrolyzed to smaller molecules: proteins are hydrolyzed to amino acids, carbohydrates to simple sugars, and fats to glycerol and fatty acids (Fig. 1). No energy is generated in stage one. In stage two, the small molecules produced during stage one are degraded further to form acetyl coenzyme A (CoA): amino acids are transaminated to acetyl CoA, glucose forms acetyl CoA through glycolysis, and glycerol and fatty acids form acetyl CoA by oxidative degradation through the sequential removal of two-carbon atoms. A small amount of adenosine triphosphate (ATP) is generated in stage two. In stage three, the large majority of ATP is generated by the cell through the citric acid cycle and oxidative phosphorylation.

Glycolysis

The highlights of glycolysis are presented to help the reader understand more fully the implications of the studies to be discussed later in this chapter. Glycolysis occurs in the cytosol. It is the sequence of biochemical reactions that converts one molecule of glucose into two molecules of pyruvate if the Po_2 is ample, or into two molecules of lactate if the Po_2 is greatly diminished, as in hypoxia or anoxia. In the process of converting one molecule of glucose to two molecules of pyruvate or lactate, two ATP molecules are formed. ATP is the cells' source of free energy; when ATP is hydrolyzed to adenosine diphosphate (ADP) and orthophosphate (Pi), free energy is released equal to 12 Kcal/mol of ATP. This released free energy is harnessed to drive biologic reactions. In fact, the ATP-ADP cycle is the dominant manner of energy exchange in biologic systems.

In the glycolytic cycle, the oxidized form of nicotinamide adenine dinucleotide (NAD^+) is continuously being reduced to the reduced form of nicotinamide adenine dinucleotide (NADH). NAD^+ accepts a hydrogen ion and two electrons in its conversion to NADH. Thus, NAD^+ is a major electron acceptor and NADH a major electron carrier in the oxidation of substrate molecules. In order for glycolysis to continue, NAD^+ must be in plentiful supply (Fig. 2).

In the aerobic state, when the supply of O_2 is plentiful, pyruvate enters the mitochondrial matrix, where, by means of the citric acid cycle and oxidative

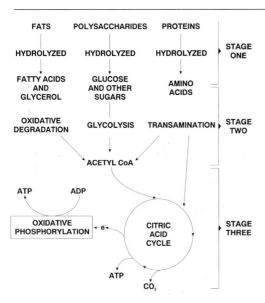

Fig. 1 Stages in the extraction of energy from substrates. (Adapted with permission from Stryer L: *Biochemistry*, ed 3. New York, NY, W.H. Freeman and Co, 1988, p 325.)

phosphorylation in the electron transport chain, NAD$^+$ is regenerated to allow glycolysis to continue. If O$_2$ is in short supply, the citric acid cycle and electron transport chain are not operational, and no NAD$^+$ is regenerated to allow glycolysis to continue. In such a condition of low PO$_2$, pyruvate does not enter the mitochondria; instead it is reduced by NADH to form lactate plus NAD$^+$ (Fig. 3).

The NAD$^+$ produced when pyruvate is reduced to lactate is used to sustain glycolysis under anaerobic conditions. The reduction of pyruvate to lactate is catalyzed by lactate dehydrogenase (LDH). LDH is a tetramer containing two kinds of subunits, an H type that is found predominantly in the heart and an M type that is found predominantly in muscle and liver. These subunits form five types of tetramers: H4 or LDH1, H3H2 or LDH2, H2M2 or LDH3, H1M3 or LDH4, and M4 or LDH5. The LDH1 isozyme oxidizes lactate to pyruvate in the heart under conditions of aerobic metabolism. The LDH5 isozyme converts pyruvate to lactate to allow glycolysis to proceed under anaerobic conditions.

Kreb Cycle and Oxidative Phosphorylation

The reactions of the Kreb citric acid cycle and oxidative phosphorylation occur in the mitochondria, whereas glycolysis occurs in the cytosol. Pyruvate enters the mitochondrial matrix where it is oxidatively decarboxylated to form acetyl CoA. To start the cycle, acetyl CoA, a two-carbon unit, joins with oxaloacetate, a four-carbon unit, to form citrate, a six-carbon unit. Through two separate oxidative decarboxylations, citrate yields a four-carbon compound, succinate, from which oxaloacetate is regenerated to renew the cycle. In the process, three molecules of NADH, one molecule of the reduced state of flavin adenine dinucleotide (FADH$_2$), two molecules of CO$_2$, and one molecule of ATP are formed (Fig. 4). NADH and FADH$_2$ are the major electron carriers in the oxidation of substrates that fuel the cell. Each molecule of these electron carriers carries a pair of electrons into the electron transport chain.

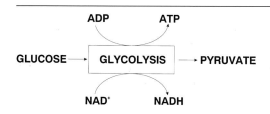

Fig. 2 In the conversion of glucose to pyruvate, NAD$^+$ is reduced to NADH. In order for glycolysis to continue, NAD$^+$ must be continuously supplied to the reaction.

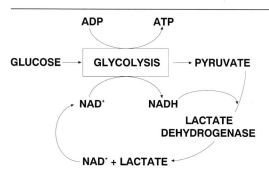

Fig. 3 Under anaerobic conditions, pyruvate is reduced by NADH to form lactate and NAD$^+$. The NAD$^+$ generated is used to sustain glycolysis under low PO$_2$ conditions.

Whereas the reactions of the citric acid cycle occur in the mitochondrial matrix, oxidative phosphorylation occurs in the electron transport chain (respiratory chain) located in the inner membranes of mitochondria. NADH and $FADH_2$ carry electron pairs to the respiratory chain, where the electrons are transferred by a series of electron carriers to oxygen (Fig. 5). Oxygen is the final electron acceptor in the electron transport chain. Oxygen is completely reduced to H_2O. Concomitantly, four protons are pumped from the mitochondrial matrix to the opposite side of the inner mitochondrial membrane, forming a transmembrane proton gradient. Thus, mitochondrial electron transfer and ATP synthesis are linked by a transmembrane proton gradient. Proton gradients, in turn, power a variety of energy-requiring reactions such as active Ca^{2+} transport by mitochondria.

Net Yield of ATP per Molecule of Glucose Versus Pathway

The dominant purpose of energy metabolism is to generate ATP molecules for fuel for the cell. ATP is continuously formed and consumed; it is not stored.

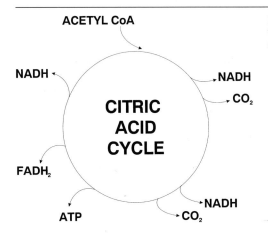

Fig. 4 The citric acid cycle generates three molecules of NADH and one molecule of $FADH_2$.

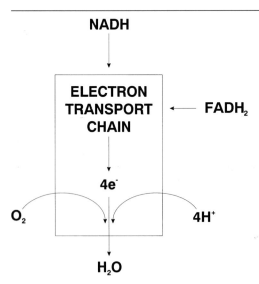

Fig. 5 Electron pairs are transferred from NADH and $FADH_2$ to O_2 by a series of electron carriers in the electron transport, or respiratory, chain.

Each molecule of ATP releases free energy (12 Kcal per molecule of ATP) when it is hydrolyzed to ADP. This free energy is harnessed to drive cellular reactions. The net ATP molecules formed per molecule of glucose consumed in the metabolic pathways described above are given in Table 1.

Under aerobic conditions, 36 ATP molecules per molecule of glucose, or 17 ATP molecules per molecule of pyruvate (glycolysis yields two pyruvate molecules per one glucose molecule consumed), are formed. Under anaerobic conditions, wherein the O_2 supply is so limited that the electron transport chain and the citric acid cycle become inoperative, only 2 ATP molecules are formed for each molecule of glucose consumed. Obviously, energy metabolism under hypoxic or anoxic conditions is much less efficient than under conditions of ample O_2 supply.

Glycerol Phosphate Shuttle

To maintain glycolysis, NAD^+ must be continuously regenerated (Fig. 2). To do this, cytoplasmic NADH must be oxidized to NAD^+. However, the mitochondrial membrane is impermeable to both NAD^+ and NADH, so NADH cannot be oxidized directly by the respiratory chain. Instead, electrons from NADH are shuttled by carriers that readily cross the mitochondrial membrane. Two shuttles exist, the glycerol phosphate shuttle and the malate-aspartate shuttle. Because the malate-aspartate shuttle has been described only in heart and liver, it will not be discussed further here. In the glycerol phosphate shuttle, electrons are carried across the mitochondrial membrane by glycerol 3-phosphate, which readily penetrates the outer mitochondrial membrane. In the cytosol, NADH is oxidized by dihydroxyacetone phosphate to form NAD^+ and glycerol 3-phosphate (Fig. 6). This reaction is catalyzed by glycerol 3-phosphate dehydrogenase (G3-PDH).

Glycerol 3-phosphate penetrates the mitochondrial membrane and is reoxidized to dihydroxyacetone phosphate on the inner mitochondrial membrane. An electron pair is transferred to $FADH_2$ in the process. Dihydroxyacetone

Table 1 Net ATP molecules formed per molecule of glucose metabolized in various metabolic pathways

Pathway	Molecules of ATP
Glycolysis	2
Citric acid cycle	2
Oxidative phosphorylation (Respiratory chain; electron transport chain)	32
Total	36

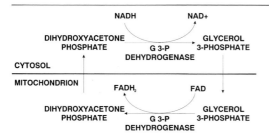

Fig. 6 Glycerol 3-phosphate (G 3-P) shuttles electrons from NADH in the cytosol to $FADH_2$ in the mitochondrion. This is an important shuttle because NADH cannot itself penetrate the mitochondrial membrane and, hence, cannot otherwise be oxidized to regenerate NAD^+ and maintain glycolysis. See also Figure 2.

phosphate then diffuses back into the cytosol to complete the shuttle. The G3-PDH in the mitochondria differs from G3-PDH in the cytosol in that mitochondrial G3-PDH uses flavin adenine dinucleotide (FAD) rather than NAD+ as the electron acceptor. The glycerol phosphate shuttle is important because without it NADH cannot be oxidized to regenerate NAD+ and maintain glycolysis.

Pentose Phosphate Shunt

In most biosynthetic reactions, the precursors are more oxidized (have lost hydrogen or one or more electrons) than their final end products. Hence, reductive power, or the ability to reduce precursor molecules (that is, to add hydrogen or one or more electrons), is required in addition to ATP. The major electron donor in reductive biosynthesis is nicotinamide adenine dinucleotide phosphate (NADPH). NADPH is used primarily for reductive biosynthesis, whereas NADH is used primarily for the generation of ATP. The main source of NADPH is the pentose phosphate shunt, which occurs in the cytosol and generates NADPH and ribose 5-phosphate, a five carbon (pentose) sugar. The pentose phosphate shunt begins with the dehydrogenation of glucose 6-phosphate (G 6-P) by glucose 6-phosphate dehydrogenase. (This is not to be confused with glycolysis, which begins with the conversion of G 6-P to fructose 6-phosphate by phosphoglucose isomerase.) Through a series of three reactions, G 6-P is converted into two molecules of NADPH and one molecule of ribose 5-phosphate (Fig. 7). This is the oxidative branch of the pentose phosphate shunt.

The fascinating aspect of the pentose phosphate shunt is that the ribose 5-phosphate can be converted back to G 6-P by transketolase and to fructose 6-phosphate by transaldolase. These nonoxidative branches of the pentose phosphate shunt create a reversible link between the shunt and glycolysis. The interplay of glycolysis and the pentose phosphate shunt enables the cell to adjust the levels of NADPH, ATP, and building blocks, such as ribose 5-phosphate, as needed.

This brief discussion of cellular energy metabolism covered only the salient features of that complex subject; ie, those features that will be useful in appreciating more fully how fracture callus cells extract energy from substrate molecules. For a more detailed description of energy metabolism, the reader is referred to Stryer[3] or Devlin.[4]

Microenvironment of the Fracture Callus

It is quite obvious from the brief review of energy metabolism presented above that the local microenvironment, especially the local Po_2, can affect the efficiency by which cells extract energy from substrate molecules. A cell in an hypoxic environment must follow predominantly the much less efficient glycolytic pathway rather than the much more efficient citric acid cycle and elec-

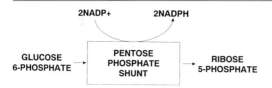

Fig. 7 The oxidative branch of the pentose phosphate shunt produces two molecules of NADPH and one molecule of ribose 5-phosphate.

tron transport chain. Therefore, the microenvironment of the fracture callus will now be discussed.

Blood Supply

Many studies have demonstrated a gradual-to-rapid increase in blood flow and vascularity in the fractured bone and fracture callus during the repair process.[5-14] The blood flow studies obviously could not correlate flow with the various regions of the fracture callus, such as the medullary callus, the interfragmentary callus, the periosteal callus, or the external callus. The vascular studies, especially those in which microangiographs were used,[15-19] have correlated, to some extent, vascularity, time postfracture, and region of callus. Figure 8 shows diagrammatically the regions of a typical fracture callus.

The interfragmentary callus, initially the fracture hematoma, remains avascular for a number of days following the fracture. The medullary callus has been described as consisting of two regions: a region of high cell density adjacent to the interfragmentary callus and one of low cell density adjacent to the normal marrow.[19] The region of high cell density contains predominantly polymorphic mesenchymal cells. With light and electron microscopy, no vessels have been seen in this region, for at least the first 48 hours following fracture. The region of low cell density in the medullary callus contains small blood vessels, but frequently the endothelial cells appear enlarged and ultrastructurally changed toward a more primitive cell. These changes suggest that perhaps the endothelial cell is dedifferentiating into a primitive osteoblast precursor cell.[19] If this is the case, the small vessels of the region of low cell density in the medullary callus, at least early in the healing process, may not be delivering nutrients and O_2 to this region. The periosteal callus shows an extensive microvasculature from early in the healing process. The external callus, however, may be relatively avascular for several days after fracture. In fact, the fully developed external callus contains chondrocytes predominantly, with those cells at the periphery of the external callus appearing as proliferating chondroblasts and those cells toward the center appearing as hypertrophic chon-

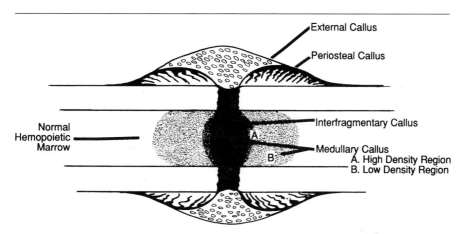

Fig. 8 Drawing depicting the regions of a typical fracture callus. (Reproduced with permission from Brighton CT, Hunt RM: Early histological and ultrastructural changes in medullary fracture callus. *J Bone Joint Surg* 1991;73A:832–847.)

drocytes. This central region of the external callus is avascular, similar to that of the hypertrophic zone in the growth plate.

From the above studies, limited though they may be, it is apparent that the microvascularity of the fracture callus is not homogeneous and that some regions of the callus may have an ample blood supply while others may be relatively avascular. Time is also an important factor in evaluating fracture callus vascularity. Those regions in the callus that are relatively avascular early in the healing process must become fully vascularized later.

Local Po$_2$

It has been well documented that soft-tissue wounds normally heal under a condition of relative hypoxia.[20-24] There is a large Po$_2$ gradient across a soft-tissue wound; it ranges from 50 to 60 mm Hg at the terminal capillary to 5 to 6 mm Hg at the wound margin.[23] This large oxygen gradient is gradually abolished during the healing phase. Two separate studies have measured the oxygen tension during fracture repair.[25,26] In one study,[25] a tonometer system was used to measure the Po$_2$ in healing bone defects in the ribs of dogs. Oxygen tensions of 8 mm Hg were recorded at 3 days, 32 $\pm$ 2 mm Hg at 3 weeks, and 46 $\pm$ 2 mm Hg at 6 weeks postdefect. Arterial Po$_2$ was recorded at 102 $\pm$ 14.2 mm Hg. Oxygen consumption measurements made at the same time failed to reveal an increase in consumption above normal levels. It was concluded that the low Po$_2$ found in a healing bone defect was due not to an increase in O$_2$ consumption but to a decrease in delivery of O$_2$ to the fracture site.[25]

In the second study,[26] platinum microelectrodes were used to measure the oxygen tension in various tissues in the callus of the rabbit fibula at various postfracture time intervals. Oxygen tensions were lowest in fiber bone (22.1 to 39.6 mm Hg) and cartilage (28.9 to 37.2 mm Hg) and highest in fibrous tissue (64.2 to 70.9 mm Hg) and diaphyseal or cortical bone (89.5 to 109.1 mm Hg).[26] Surprisingly, the oxygen tensions did not vary greatly within the above tissue groups from day 4 postfracture to day 25 postfracture, at which time mechanical testing indicated the fractures were healed. It is quite likely that the Po$_2$ in the cartilage and fiber bone prior to the fourth postfracture day would have been even lower than those given above, if those measurements had been made. No attempt was made in this study to correlate the oxygen tension measurements with the region of the callus from which the measurements were taken, that is, measurements taken from cartilage could have been from cartilage in the external callus, the subperiosteal callus, and so forth. The same microelectrode system used in the above study was used to measure the Po$_2$ in well-established nonunions in fractured femora of the rabbit.[27] The oxygen tension was significantly higher in cartilage and fiber bone in nonunion than it was in the control, healing fractures until union occurred in the latter group.

The oxygen tensions in the various zones of the in vivo growth plate have also been measured and correlate well with the oxygen tension measurements from the fracture callus. In the growth plate, Po$_2$ in the proliferative zone, which is supplied by the epiphyseal artery, was relatively high (57.0 $\pm$ 5.8 mm Hg), while the oxygen tension in the hypertrophic zone and the fiber bone in the metaphysis were significantly lower (24.3 $\pm$ 2.4 mm Hg and 19.8 $\pm$ 3.2 mm Hg, respectively).[28]

Diffusion Coefficient

All tissues in the fracture callus depend on the diffusion to the cells of oxygen and nutrients from adjacent capillaries in order to maintain viability. Calcification of the matrix between the cells, which occurs in those callus regions containing cartilage, might adversely affect such diffusion. Unfortunately, the diffusion coefficients of the various tissues in the different regions of the fracture callus have not been determined. However, the diffusion coefficients of the various zones of the growth plate have been determined, and, perhaps, those data can be extrapolated to the fracture callus.

A desorption technique using [³H] inulin and [¹⁴C] sucrose, two relatively low-molecular-weight, extracellular, nonionic substances, demonstrated that the diffusion coefficient in the normal growth plate of the rabbit was lowest in the zone of hypertrophic cells and increased progressively through the proliferative zone, the reserve zone, and hyaline cartilage.[29] In the rachitic rat growth plate, the diffusion coefficient in the hypertrophic zone was significantly greater than that in the normal rat, and it decreased rapidly with healing of the rickets. The ash content, or the amount of mineral present, was the one parameter that correlated best with the diffusion coefficients. It was concluded from these studies that calcification of the cartilage matrix in the growth plate significantly inhibits diffusion of nutrients, including oxygen, to the chondrocytes.[29] It seems likely that this same phenomenon is also operational in the cartilaginous tissues of the fracture callus.

How Fracture Callus Cells Extract Energy From Substrate Molecules: Evidence for Dominance of Anaerobic Metabolism

From the above description of the microenvironment of the fracture callus, it is clear that the various cells in the different regions of the fracture callus are exposed to different states of vascularity. It is to be expected, therefore, that both glycolysis and the citric acid/oxidative phosphorylation pathways are active in the fracture callus. This activity has been demonstrated in several studies in which the enzymes catalyzing various steps of glycolysis, the citric acid cycle, and oxidative phosphorylation in the electron transport chain have been demonstrated.[30–32] Two of these studies indicated that anaerobic glycolysis was dominant early in the course of fracture healing, whereas aerobic metabolism was dominant toward the end of fracture healing.[31,32] In another study, Dunham and associates[33] measured G3-PDH, an enzyme active in the glycolytic pathway, and LDH, an enzyme that catalyzes the conversion of pyruvate to lactate under anaerobic conditions (Fig. 3), in the fracture callus of the rat. They found that G3-PDH was highest in cellular granulation tissue of the callus, decreased as cartilage calcified, and was relatively low in osteoblasts. They found that LDH activity was relatively high in chondrocytes, cellular granulation tissue, and bone cells, and that LDH decreased as cartilage calcified.

Other authors showed that the dominant metabolic pathway in the fracture callus through the greater part of the healing process was anaerobic glycolysis.[34–36] Lenart and associates[34] found that LDH activity was high at day 7 postfracture in the rat tibia, and was even higher at day 14 postfracture. Penttinen[35] measured lactate production in the callus of rat tibial fractures and found it highest on day 9 postfracture, a time when glycosaminoglycan synthesis was maximum. He concluded that the energy metabolism of the fracture callus was anaerobic. Gudmundson and Semb[36] found lactate dehydrogenase isoenzymes in callus tissue typical of anaerobic tissue. They found the activity of LDH5, the M type LDH, to be much higher in the rat femoral fracture callus at 7 and 15 weeks postfracture than that present in normal bone. They concluded that a more anaerobic metabolism was present in the fracture callus than in normal bone. Finally, Shapiro and associates[37] demonstrated in growth plate slices from the chick tibiae and fibulae that the NADH/NAD$^+$ ratio in the hypertrophic zone was comparable to that found in hypoxic and anoxic tissues. Although this was a study of endochondral bone formation in the growth plate, it is reasonable to expect comparable NADH/NAD$^+$ ratios in the hypertrophic chondrocytes in the endochondral bone formation occurring in the fracture callus.

Thus, the preponderance of evidence indicates that the dominant energy pathway followed by cells in the fracture callus is anaerobic glycolysis. At the very least, anaerobic metabolism appears to predominate early in the course of healing in all cells of the callus, and throughout the healing process in the hypertrophic cartilage cells. From the oxygen tension studies and the LDH isozyme studies described above, it seems most likely that even in the later stages of callus healing, during fiber bone formation, the callus is still following predominantly an anaerobic pathway.

Absence of the Glycerol Phosphate Shuttle

Cartilage slices from the various zones of the rabbit rib growth plate were analyzed for glycerol phosphate dehydrogenase activity, and no activity of this enzyme was found in any zone.[38] This means that NADH generated during glycolysis in the cytosol cannot transfer its electrons to glycerol 3-phosphate and, thereby, be oxidized to NAD$^+$ to maintain glycolysis as it normally does (Figs. 2, 6, and 9, *left*). When the enzyme G3-PDH is absent, instead of being oxidized by glycerol 3-phosphate, NADH is oxidized by pyruvate to form lactate and NAD$^+$. The regeneration of NAD$^+$ by this means maintains glycolysis (Fig. 9, *right*).

Absence of the phosphate shuttle means that the cartilage cell is obliged to follow a much less efficient metabolic pathway: for each molecule of pyruvate that does not enter a mitochondrion but, instead, oxidizes a molecule of NADH to form lactate and NAD$^+$, the chondrocyte is deprived of 17 molecules of ATP.

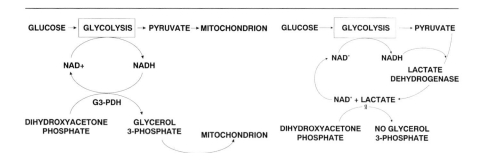

Fig. 9 *Left,* Glycerol phosphate shuttle (see also Figure 6). G3-PDH (glycerol 3-phosphate dehydrogenase) catalyzes the conversion of dihydroxyacetone phosphate to glycerol 3-phosphate. In the process, glycerol 3-phosphate accepts two electrons from NADH and carries them into the mitochondrion. NADH is oxidized to regenerate NAD$^+$, which maintains glycolysis. *Right,* Absence of the enzyme glycerol 3-phosphate dehydrogenase prevents the oxidation of NADH by glycerol 3-phosphate. Instead, NADH is oxidized by pyruvate to form lactate and NAD$^+$, a reaction catalyzed by lactate dehydrogenase.

There is another electron shuttle, the malate-aspartate shuttle, but it is found only in the heart and liver. Therefore, cartilage cells in the growth plate, in the absence of these shuttles, will produce lactate even under aerobic conditions.[39] It also seems most likely that cartilage cells in the fracture callus also would not possess these shuttles. If this is true, then there are two reasons for the high levels of lactate and LDH found in the fracture callus: low oxygen tensions leading to anaerobic glycolysis and the absence of the electron shuttles.

Active Pentose Phosphate Shunt

Several studies have shown that the fracture callus shows high levels of G6-PDH, an enzyme of the pentose phosphate shunt, throughout most of the healing process.[30,32,33,40] The activity of G6-PDH was high in the rabbit femoral midshaft fracture callus in undifferentiated granulation tissue, in proliferative fibrous tissue, in hypertrophic cartilage, and in newly formed bone through day 21 postfracture, the last time period studied.[30] In the healing callus of the rat metatarsal, G6-PDH activity was high in the cellular granulation tissue, in mature cartilage, and in the osteoblasts of new bone formation through day 49 postfracture.[33] G6-PDH was absent or only mildly elevated in calcified cartilage in that same study. G6-PDH was also active in the periosteal cells of the early callus, whereas in normal periosteal cells with no fracture present, G6-PDH was very low.[40] These studies indicate that no matter what metabolic pathway is operative in the fracture callus, anaerobic or aerobic, the pentose phosphate shunt is active. The ability of the pentose phosphate shunt to interplay its oxidative and nonoxidative branches between glycolysis and the shunt enables the fracture callus cell to adjust to the levels of NADPH, ATP, and building blocks such as ribose 5-phosphate that are required at the time and are dictated by the microenvironment.

Energy Metabolism and Calcification of the Fracture Callus

Mitochondrial Ca^{2+}

Energy metabolism may be directly linked to matrix calcification in the growth plate and in the fracture callus. It has been shown that mitochondria of growth plate chondrocytes contain electron-dense granules that reach highest concentration in the hypertrophic zone of the growth plate.[41,42] By direct energy dispersive radiographic analysis, these granules were shown to consist of calcium and phosphorus.[43] Using K-pyroantimonate as a calcium stain at the ultrastructural level, it was shown that mitochondria of growth plate chondrocytes begin to accumulate calcium in the top portion of the hypertrophic zone, begin to lose calcium toward the middle of the hypertrophic zone at the same level in which matrix vesicles in the longitudinal septa begin accumulating calcium, and lose all calcium stainability toward the bottom of the hypertrophic zone as the matrix vesicles show crystal formation typical of hydroxyapatite.[44,45] Further, in a rachitic model in the rat, the mitochondria in the chondrocytes near the bottom of the hypertrophic zone did not lose calcium as did those from the normal, control animals, and matrix calcification did not occur.[46] With the addition of phosphorus to the diet, however, mitochondria at the extreme bottom of the hypertrophic zone rapidly lost calcium, and matrix calcification began.[47]

The above studies in the growth plate were repeated in the fracture callus of the rabbit rib.[48] In those areas of the callus containing cartilage in which the matrix was not mineralized, chondrocyte mitochondria were heavily laden with the calcium; in those areas of cartilage matrix showing early mineralization, the chondrocyte mitochondria showed less calcium; and in those areas of cartilage matrix showing advanced mineralization, the chondrocyte mitochondria were devoid of any stainable calcium. Thus, the fracture callus showed the same mitochondrial calcium/matrix mineralization relationship in cartilage areas as that demonstrated in the hypertrophic zone of the growth plate (Fig. 10).

As discussed above, mitochondrial electron transfer and ATP synthesis are linked by a transmembrane proton gradient. Such proton gradients power a

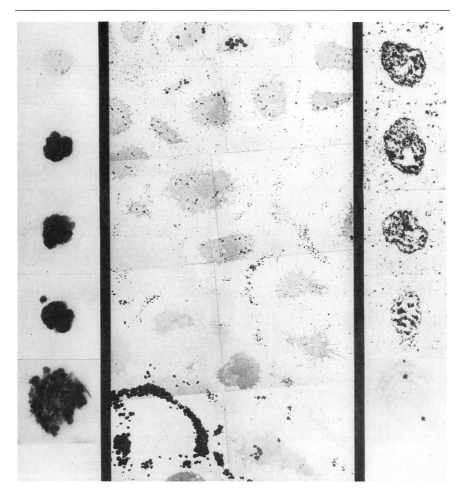

Fig. 10 Montage of electron micrographs from the cartilaginous callus of rabbit rib 5 days postfracture. The calcium-stain complex is predominantly intracellular in areas of little or no matrix mineralization (top of the montage), but becomes progressively more extracellular in areas of beginning-to-advanced mineralization (bottom of the montage). The micrographs on the extreme right ($\times$ 38,000) show mitochondria of chondrocytes at different levels in the callus. The levels of these chondrocytes are shown in the centrally placed micrographs ($\times$ 2100). The micrographs on the extreme left ($\times$ 82,000) show matrix vesicles located at the same levels in the callus as the chondrocytes containing the mitochondria shown on the right. (Reproduced with permission from Brighton CT, Hunt RM: Histochemical localization of calcium in the fracture callus with potassium pyroantimonate: Possible role of chondrocyte mitochondrial calcium in callus calcification. *J Bone Joint Surg* 1986;68A:703–715.)

variety of energy-requiring reactions including Ca^{2+} transport by mitochondria.[49] The accumulation of calcium and the formation of ATP by mitochondria require energy, but both processes cannot occur at the same time in the same locus in the mitochondria.[50] That is, the more mitochondria accumulate calcium, the less ATP they synthesize. Why chondrocyte mitochondria accumulate or store calcium in the hypertrophic zone of the growth plate or in hypertrophic chondrocytes in the fracture callus is not known. However, it is known that glycogen is present in the cytoplasm of chondrocytes in the reserve and proliferative zones, as well as in the top portion of the hypertrophic zone, of the growth plate,[51,52] and in proliferating and enlarging cartilage cells in the fracture callus.[31] In hypertrophic chondrocytes in both the growth plate and fracture callus, glycogen in the cytoplasm abruptly disappears at the same place where matrix calcification begins. Thus, it is hypothesized that chondrocytes in both the growth plate and fracture callus use glycogen to fuel glycolysis and the citric acid cycle/electron transport chain such that enough energy is generated in the mitochondria via proton gradients to accumulate and store calcium. Once the glycogen is depleted, presumably no other substrate is available in these avascular regions to provide energy for the chondrocyte mitochondria to retain calcium. Then, calcium is released, and matrix mineralization begins.

Indirect support for the above hypothesis has been provided by studies dealing with isolated mitochondria from growth plate chondrocytes. In most isolated mitochondria, the addition of ADP causes a several fold increase in the O_2 consumption rate, whereas the addition of Ca^{2+} stimulates a much lower rise in the O_2 consumption rate. In mitochondria isolated from growth plate chondrocytes, the opposite happens; that is, the addition of Ca^{2+} stimulates a higher rise in O_2 consumption than does ADP.[53] In addition, isolated mitochondria from growth plate chondrocytes possess a greater endogenous calcium content, a greater capacity for calcium accumulation, and a larger labile Ca^{2+} pool than do mitochondria of hepatocytes.[54] These results all suggest that chondrocyte mitochondria are specialized for calcium transport and are important in the calcification of the extracellular matrix of the growth plate. It is most likely that the same results and conclusions would be applicable to mitochondria of hypertrophic chondrocytes in the fracture callus.

Vitamin K

The vitamin K cycle not only is involved in the synthesis of prothrombin in the coagulation cascade, but it also is involved in the synthesis of other calcium-binding proteins such as osteocalcin. In the vitamin K cycle, the epoxide form of the vitamin, designated K_2 or $K(0)$, is reduced by NADH or NADPH to the dihydroquinone form of the vitamin, designated K_1, or $K(H_2)$. $K(H_2)$ is then oxidized back to $K(0)$ in a two-step process whereby glutamic acid residues (Glu) are carboxylated to γ-carboxyglutamic acid (Gla) (Fig. 11). Vitamin $K(H_2)$ acts as a hydrogen donor in the reaction.[55,56] The double carboxy group in Gla chelates Ca^{2+}. Osteocalcin, a small calcium-binding peptide, is synthesized in bone, contains Gla residues, and is thought to be important in the mineralization and development of bone.[57,58] Osteocalcin has a cluster of three glutamic acid residues that are converted to the much stronger chelator of Ca^{2+}, Gla, by the vitamin K cycle.

That the vitamin K cycle is important in bone repair stems from two pieces of evidence. One, vitamin K_1 was found to be markedly depressed in the plasma of patients with fractures, and the time required for the plasma K_1 levels to return to normal appeared to be influenced by the severity of the fracture.[56]

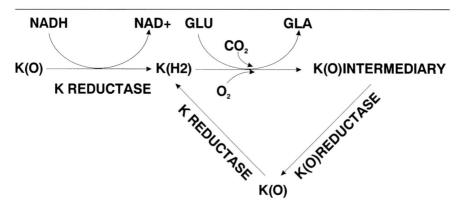

Fig. 11 The vitamin K cycle. When the reduced form of vitamin K, designated K(H)₂, is oxidized to the epoxide form, designated K(0), glutamic acid residues (GLU) are converted to γ-carboxyglutamic acid (Gla), a strong Ca^{2+} chelator.

Two, dicumarol inhibits the vitamin K cycle by blocking the conversion of K(H₂) to the epoxide K(0).[59] When dicumarol was fed to rats in which a closed fracture of the metatarsals had been induced, there was a highly significant decrease in the amount of bone produced.[60] Also, there was a decrease in G6-PDH in the developing fracture callus. G6-PDH is an enzyme in the pentose phosphate shunt. Thus, not only was dicumarol blocking the vitamin K cycle, it also was inhibiting the pentose phosphate shunt so that less NADPH was available for the conversion of K(0) to K(H₂). Again, this demonstrates the interrelation between energy metabolism and calcification in the fracture callus.

Vitamin B₆

It was shown above that vitamin K(H₂) is an intermediate carrier of reducing equivalents in mineralization. It was also shown that an important source of these reducing equivalents, or electron pairs, is NADPH generated from G6-PDH in the pentose phosphate shunt. Another vitamin that appears to be important in energy metabolism as it relates to calcification in the fracture callus is pyridoxine or vitamin B₆. Rats fed a pyridoxine-deficient diet exhibited marked diminution in G6-PDH activity in the developing callus of metatarsal fractures and a significant delay in maturation of the fracture callus and in the time to union.[61] Exactly how vitamin B₆ deficiency diminishes G6-PDH activity in the pentose phosphate shunt is not completely known. However, vitamin B₆ is required for the production of putrescine by orithine decarboxylase, and it has been shown that G6-PDH activity of rat metatarsal osteoblasts may be regulated by putrescine.[62] However vitamin B₆ regulates G6-PDH activity in the pentose phosphate shunt, its effect on the fracture callus is yet another example of the interrelation between energy metabolism and fracture healing.

Summary

The energy metabolism pathway of a cell depends to a large extent on the microenvironment of that cell. If oxygen and substrates are plentiful, the end product of glycolysis, pyruvate, will enter mitochondria and, through the citric acid cycle and oxidative phosphorylation in the electron transport chain, will provide 17 ATP molecules per pyruvate molecule or 36 molecules per glucose molecule. If the Po_2 in the cell's local microenvironment is low, pyruvate will not enter mitochondria but, instead, will be reduced by NADH to form lactate and NAD^+. The NAD^+ so generated sustains glycolysis under low Po_2 conditions. However, under such conditions, only two molecules of ATP are produced per one molecule of glucose consumed.

NAD^+ is also generated by the glycerol phosphate shuttle, in which electron pairs from NADH are carried across the mitochondrial membrane by glycerol 3-phosphate, regenerating NAD^+ in the process to sustain glycolysis in the cytosol.

In most biosynthetic reactions, substrates need to be reduced through the addition of hydrogen or one or more electrons to form the final end products. The major electron donor in reductive biosynthesis is NADPH, which is supplied primarily by the pentose phosphate shunt. The pentose phosphate shunt can follow an oxidative path, in which NADPH and ribose 5-phosphate are formed from glucose 6-phosphate, or a nonoxidative path, in which the ribose 5-phosphate can be converted back to glucose 6-phosphate and fructose 6-phosphate. This choice provides a reversible link between the shunt and glycolysis, which enables the cell to adjust the levels of NADPH, ATP, and building blocks such as ribose 5-phosphate as needed.

The fracture callus consists of a heterogeneous cell population in which the blood supply and Po_2 differ from region to region and with time. Some regions may remain relatively avascular and hypoxic throughout much of the healing process. Metabolically, both glycolysis and the citric acid/oxidative phosphorylation pathways are active in the fracture callus. However, the preponderance of evidence indicates that the dominant energy pathway followed by cells in the fracture callus is anaerobic glycolysis.

The glycerol phosphate shuttle is absent in chondrocytes of the growth plate and most likely in chondrocytes of the fracture callus as well. This means that even if the oxygen supply were ample at the local microenvironment level in the fracture callus, the chondrocytes would still obtain energy predominantly from glycolysis because pyruvate, rather than entering the citric acid cycle in the mitochondria, remains in the cytosol to oxidize NADH to NAD^+ to maintain glycolysis.

The pentose phosphate shunt is active in the fracture callus regardless of what pathway, aerobic or anaerobic, is operative. The ability of the shunt to interplay with glycolysis allows the cells of the fracture callus to adjust NADPH, ATP, and building blocks, such as ribose 5-phosphate, as needed.

The energy metabolism of the fracture callus is directly linked to calcification and fracture healing. Chondrocyte mitochondria in the fracture callus accumulate Ca^{2+} as the cells enlarge, and lose Ca^{2+} from the hypertrophic cells at the level in the callus where matrix calcification begins. Isolated mitochondria from growth plate chondrocytes seem specialized for calcium transport, and it is assumed the same is true for mitochondria from fracture callus chondrocytes. The release of accumulated calcium by callus mitochondria is thought to be due to a depletion of energy substrates.

Vitamin $K(H_2)$ acts as a hydrogen carrier in the conversion of glutamic acid residues to Gla. Osteocalcin contains glutamic acid residues that are converted to Gla, a strong Ca^{2+} chelator, by the vitamin K cycle. Vitamin K levels are markedly depressed in the plasma of patients with fractures. Blocking the vitamin K cycle with dicumarol also inhibits the pentose phosphate shunt in the rat developing fracture callus, demonstrating the interrelation between energy metabolism and fracture healing.

Vitamin B_6 deficiency in rats leads to a marked deficiency in G6-PDH of the pentose phosphate shunt in the developing fracture callus and to a significant delay in both fracture callus maturation and the time to union, again demonstrating the interrelation between energy metabolism and fracture healing.

Acknowledgment

This work was supported in part by NIH grants AM13812, AM18033, and AM07132.

References

1. Dunham J: Metabolism of the fracture callus, in Hall BK (ed): *Bone Fracture Repair and Regeneration*, Boca Raton, FL, CRC Press, 1992, pp 1–31.
2. Krebs HA, Kornberg HL: *Energy Transformation in Living Matter: A Survey*. Berlin, Springer-Verlag, 1957.
3. Stryer L: *Biochemistry*, ed 3. New York, NY, W.H. Freeman, 1988.
4. Devlin TM: *Textbook of Biochemistry With Clinical Correlations*, ed 3. New York, NY, Wiley-Liss, 1992.
5. Laurnen EL, Kelly PJ: Blood flow, oxygen consumption, carbon-dioxide production, and blood-calcium and pH changes in tibial fractures in dogs. *J Bone Joint Surg* 1969;51A:298–308.
6. Paradis GR, Kelly PJ: Blood flow and mineral deposition in canine tibial fractures. *J Bone Joint Surg* 1975;57A:220–226.
7. Cavadias AX, Trueta J: An experimental study of the vascular contribution to the callus of fracture. *Surg Gynecol Obstet* 1965;120:731–747.
8. Gothman L: Vascular reactions in experimental fractures: Microangiographic and radioisotope studies. *Acta Chir Scand Suppl* 1961;284:1–34.
9. Rhinelander FW, Baragry RA: Microangiography in bone healing: I. Undisplaced closed fractures. *J Bone Joint Surg* 1962;44A:1273–1298.
10. Rhinelander FW: The normal microcirculation of diaphyseal cortex and its response to fracture. *J Bone Joint Surg* 1968;50A:784–800.
11. Rhinelander FW, Phillips RS, Steel WM, et al: Microangiography in bone healing: II. Displaced closed fractures. *J Bone Joint Surg* 1966;48A:1015.
12. Wray JB, Lynch CJ: The vascular response to fracture of the tibia in the rat. *J Bone Joint Surg* 1959;41A:1143–1148.
13. Nutton RW, Fitzgerald RH Jr, Kelly PJ: Early dynamic bone-imaging as an indicator of osseous blood flow and factors affecting the uptake of ^{99}mTc hydroxymethylene diphosphonate in healing bone. *J Bone Joint Surg* 1985;67A:763–770.
14. Kelly PJ, Montgomery RJ, Bronk JT: Reaction of the circulatory system to injury and regeneration. *Clin Orthop* 1990;254:275–288.
15. Aho AJ: Electron microscopic and histological observations on fracture repair in young and old rats. *Acta Pathol Microbiol Scand* 1966;184:1–95.
16. Chai BF, Tang XM: Ultrastructural investigation of experimental fracture healing: I. Electron microscopic observation of cellular activity. *Chin Med J* 1979;92:530–535.
17. Gothlin G: Electron microscopic observations on fracture repair in the rat. *Acta Pathol Microbiol Scand* 1973;81:507–522.
18. Tang XM, Chai BF: Light microscopic and electron microscopic observation on experimental fracture healing. *Chin Med J* 1982;95:721–730.
19. Brighton CT, Hunt RM: Early histological and ultrastructural changes in medullary fracture callus. *J Bone Joint Surg* 1991;73A:832–847.
20. Ehrlich HP, Grislis G, Hunt TK: Metabolic and circulatory contributions to oxygen gradients in wounds. *Surgery* 1972;72:578–583.
21. Heppenstall RB, Littooy FN, Fuchs R, et al: Gas tensions in healing tissues of traumatized patients. *Surgery* 1974;75:874–880.

22. Hunt TK, Pai MP: The effect of varying ambient oxygen tensions on wound metabolism and collagen synthesis. *Surg Gynecol Obstet* 1972;135:561–567.
23. Hunt TK, Zederfeldt B, Goldstick TK: Oxygen and healing. *Am J Surg* 1969;118:521–525.
24. Niinikoski J, Hunt TK, Dunphy JE: Oxygen supply in healing tissue. *Am J Surg* 1972;123:247–252.
25. Heppenstall RB, Grislis G, Hunt TK: Tissue gas tensions and oxygen consumption in healing bone defects. *Clin Orthop* 1975;106:357–365.
26. Brighton CT, Krebs AG: Oxygen tension of healing fractures in the rabbit. *J Bone Joint Surg* 1972;54A:323–332.
27. Brighton CT, Krebs AG: Oxygen tension of nonunion of fractured femurs in the rabbit. *Surg Gynecol Obstet* 1972;135:379–385.
28. Brighton CT, Heppenstall RB: Oxygen tension in zones of the epiphyseal plate, the metaphysis, and diaphysis: An in vitro and in vivo study in rats and rabbits. *J Bone Joint Surg* 1971;53A:719–728.
29. Stambaugh JE, Brighton CT: Diffusion in the various zones of the normal and the rachitic growth plate. *J Bone Joint Surg* 1980;62A:740–749.
30. Kuhlman RE, Balowski MJ: The biochemical activity of fracture callus in relation to bone production. *Clin Orthop* 1975;107:258–265.
31. Ketenjian AY, Arsenis C: Morphological and biochemical studies during differentiation and calcification of fracture callus cartilage. *Clin Orthop* 1975;107:266–273.
32. Balogh K Jr, Hajek JV: Oxidative enzymes of intermediary metabolism in healing bone fractures. *Am J Anat* 1965;116:429–448.
33. Dunham J, Catterall A, Bitensky L, et al: Metabolic changes in the cells of the callus during fracture healing in the rat. *Calcif Tissue Int* 1983;35:56–61.
34. Lenart G, Szell V, Csorba E: Comparative investigations on bone and callus enzymes. *Acta Biochim Biophys Hung* 1971;6:243–250.
35. Penttinen R: Biochemical studies on fracture healing in the rat with special reference to the oxygen supply. *Acta Chir Scand Suppl* 1972;432:1–32.
36. Gudmundson C, Semb H: Enzyme studies of fractures with normal and delayed union. *Acta Orthop Scand* 1971;42:18–27.
37. Shapiro IM, Golub EE, Kakuta S, et al: Initiation of endochondral calcification is related to changes in the redox state of hypertrophic chondrocytes. *Science* 1982;217:950–952.
38. Brighton CT, Lackman RD, Cuckler JM: Absence of the glycerol phosphate shuttle in the various zones of the growth plate. *J Bone Joint Surg* 1983;65A:663–666.
39. Dunham J, Dobbs RA, Nahir AM, et al: Aerobic glycolysis of bone and cartilage: The possible involvement of fatty acid oxidation. *Cell Biochem Funct* 1983;1:168–172.
40. Dunham J, Shedden RG, Catterall A, et al: Pentose-shunt oxidation in the periosteal cells in healing fractures. *Calcif Tissue Res* 1977;23:77–81.
41. Martin JH, Matthews JL: Mitochondrial granules in chondrocytes, osteoblasts, and osteocytes: An ultrastructural and microincineration study. *Clin Orthop* 1970;68:273–278.
42. Martin JH, Matthews JL: Mitochondrial granules in chondrocytes. *Calcif Tissue Res* 1969;3:184–193.
43. Suftin LV, Holtrop ME, Ogilvie RE: Microanalysis of individual mitochondrial granules with diameters less than 1000 angstroms. *Science* 1971;174:947–949.
44. Brighton CT, Hunt RM: Mitochondrial calcium and its role in calcification: Histochemical localization of calcium in electron micrographs of the epiphyseal growth plate with k-pyroantimonate. *Clin Orthop* 1974;100:406–416.
45. Brighton CT, Hunt RM: Histochemical localization of calcium in growth plate mitochondria and matrix vesicles. *Fed Proc* 1976;35:143–147.
46. Brighton CT, Hunt RM: Electron microscopic pyroantimonate studies of matrix vesicles and mitochondria in the rachitic growth plate. *Metab Bone Dis Relat Res* 1978;1:199–204.

47. Brighton CT, Hunt RM: The role of mitochondria in growth plate calcification as demonstrated in a rachitic model. *J Bone Joint Surg* 1978;60A:630–639.
48. Brighton CT, Hunt RM: Histochemical localization of calcium in the fracture callus with potassium pyroantimonate: Possible role of chondrocyte mitochondrial calcium in callus calcification. *J Bone Joint Surg* 1986;68A:703–715.
49. Lehninger AL, Carafoli E, Rossi CS: Energy-linked ion movements in mitochondrial systems. *Adv Enzymol Relat Areas Mol Biol* 1967;29:259–320.
50. Lehninger AL: Mitochondria and calcium ion transport. *Biochem J* 1970;119:129–138.
51. Pritchard JJ: A cytological and histochemical study of bone and cartilage formation in the rat. *J Anat* 1952;86:259–277.
52. Brighton CT, Ray RD, Soble LW, et al: In vitro epiphyseal plate growth in various oxygen tensions. *J Bone Joint Surg* 1969;51A:1383–1396.
53. Stambough JL, Brighton CT, Iannotti JP, et al: Characterization of growth plate mitochondria. *J Orthop Res* 1984;2:235–246.
54. Iannotti JP, Brighton CT, Stambough JL, et al: Calcium flux and endogenous calcium content in isolated mammalian growth-plate chondrocytes, hyaline-cartilage chondrocytes, and hepatocytes. *J Bone Joint Surg* 1985;67A:113–120.
55. Vermeer C: γ-carboxyglutamate-containing proteins and the vitamin K-dependent carboxylase. *Biochem J* 1990;266:625–636.
56. Bitensky L, Hart JP, Catterall A, et al: Circulating vitamin K levels in patients with fractures. *J Bone Joint Surg* 1988;70B:663–664.
57. Hauschka PV, Lian JB, Gallop PM: Vitamin K and mineralization. *Trends Biochem Sci* 1978;3:75–78.
58. Price PA, Williamson MK: Primary structure of bovine matrix gla-protein, a new vitamin K-dependent bone protein. *J Biol Chem* 1985;260:14971–14975.
59. Whitlon DS, Sadowski JA, Suttie JW: Mechanism of coumarin action: Significance of vitamin K epoxide reductase inhibition. *Biochemistry* 1978;17:1371–1377.
60. Dodds RA, Catterall A, Bitensky L, et al: Effects on fracture healing of an antagonist of the vitamin K cycle. *Calcif Tissue Int* 1984;36:233–238.
61. Dodds RA, Catterall A, Bitensky L, et al: Abnormalities in fracture healing induced by vitamin B_6-deficiency in rats. *Bone* 1986;7:489–495.
62. Dodds RA, Dunham J, Bitensky L, et al: Putrescine may be a natural stimulator of glucose-6-phosphate dehydrogenase. *FEBS Lett* 1986;201:105–108.

Chapter 11

Regulation of Fracture Repair and Synthesis of Matrix Macromolecules

Mark E. Bolander, MD

Introduction

Fracture repair is accomplished by cell activity in the external callus. Soon after fracture of a long bone, the area becomes acutely inflamed; as inflammation subsides, a firm swelling develops at the fracture site. This hard mass, or callus, persists until the bone is completely united. Histologic evaluation of this callus demonstrates that various cells in this mass complete the membranous bone formation, chondrogenesis, and endochondral ossification required for repair of the fracture.[1,2] Despite the important role of the callus in repair of the fractured bone, the origin of different types of cells in the callus, and the factors responsible for regulating the differentiation, proliferation, and protein synthesis of these cells, are not completely understood. This review will define factors responsible for regulating the progression of cellular events during fracture repair.

Origin of Cartilage in the Fracture Callus

The earliest studies of fractures recognized that cartilage in the callus was important for repair, but the origin of this cartilage tissue has been disputed. Duhamel[3] and Dupuytren[4] maintained that cartilage formed from the periosteum and bone marrow, whereas von Haller[5] and Hunter[6] argued that cartilage was derived from the hematoma and the granulation tissue that replaced it. More recent investigators have noted that cartilage appears only in the external callus, and not in the callus that forms from the osteoprogenitor cells of the periosteum and bone marrow.[7] Despite numerous studies of fracture repair, the origin of the external callus and the cells that give rise to cartilage remains uncertain.

Histology of Fracture Repair

Periosteal Reaction to Fracture: Membranous Bone Formation

Cells in the inner layer of the periosteum respond almost immediately after fracture with an increase in DNA synthesis and cell proliferation.[8] The outer, fibrous layer of the periosteum remains intact except where disrupted by the fracture. In the early callus, proliferating cells are organized into zones or layers; cells in the outer layer continue to proliferate, while cells closer to the cortex secrete an extracellular matrix, or osteoid, which is mineralized and forms bone spicules. Distributed throughout these bone spicules are large spaces that contain vascular channels and undifferentiated cells. Osteoclasts are seen in the callus as soon as the newly formed bone develops. With the progression of healing and osteoclast remodeling, bone spicules are replaced by mature lamellar bone, and the spaces develop mature marrow elements.

Cortical Reaction to Fracture: Increased Bone Remodeling

The vascular spaces and haversian canals of adult cortical bone are lined with flattened osteoblasts and small numbers of osteoclasts. These cells also are activated soon after fracture. The haversian canals become markedly widened and increased in number, leading to a markedly decreased density as the bone is remodeled. Increased remodeling activity continues between the cortex and membranous bone in the subperiosteal regions, obliterating the early distinction between the cortex and the callus. Increased remodeling in a longitudinal direction forms the "cutting cones" that traverse the fracture gap and establish bone continuity in primary bone repair.

Extraperiosteal Reaction to Fracture: Chondrogenesis and Endochondral Ossification

Muscle and other soft tissues outside the periosteum show considerable cellular activity after fracture. Extravasated blood is found in the hematoma, above the periosteum, and between muscle fibers. First, polymorphs and then macrophages are found in regions of extravasated blood. The structure of the overlying muscle changes dramatically with proliferation of cells, fibroblasts or possibly satellite cells, between the muscle fibers and concomitant muscle-fiber degeneration. With fiber loss, the basement membrane around the muscle thickens, then is degraded. Proliferating cells from the muscle add to the cellular mass of the callus, mixing with inflammatory cells and cells from the periosteum. This large cell mass is quickly vascularized; small arterioles with a muscularis layer and large venules are seen in abundance.

A dramatic change occurs in the callus with the development of cartilage adjacent to newly formed membranous bone. In standard animal fracture models, cartilage invariably forms at the juncture between the cortex and subperiosteal bone; in human fractures, where the structure of the callus is more disorganized, cartilage is found adjacent to regions of early bone formation. Cell proliferation decreases, and cells synthesize a basophilic matrix devoid of blood vessels. As this region becomes avascular, lacunae form around the cells, which develop the large nuclei typical of chondrocytes. In animal models, this process continues until the entire space between regions of subperiosteal bone is filled with cartilage. Chondrogenesis progresses in a manner reminiscent of the maturation of the growth plate; after chondrocytes have developed a histologically mature matrix, cells hypertrophy and the matrix calcifies. The calcified cartilage matrix adjacent to the membranous bone is invaded by blood vessels, and, reminiscent of endochondral ossification in the growth plate, forms bone on the mineralized cartilage matrix. These mixed cartilage and bone spicules are remodeled to bone, which is continuous with and indistinguishable from subperiosteal bone formed by membranous ossification.

In humans, the extent of cartilage formation is difficult to document accurately. Random samples obtained from cases of delayed internal fixation suggest extensive cartilage formation, whereas samples from surgical treatment of nonunions suggest minimal cartilage formation (unpublished data). These observations are not controlled for the time after fracture, however, and different healing times could easily explain the observed differences in cartilage. Despite the difficulty in comparing animal models and human fractures, observations of human samples suggest that cartilage formation is a critical, necessary step for fracture repair in long bones. This view is supported by the observation that metabolic conditions known to cause delayed union or nonunion in humans, including diabetes and chemotherapy treatment, are associated with decreased cartilage formation in animal models.[9,10]

Source of Chondrocyte Precursors

Two opposing explanations of the origin of cartilage formation have been put forth in the last 50 years. The commonly accepted theory is reflected in the work of Ham,[7] Ham and Harris,[11] and Owen,[12] who believe the essential feature of fracture repair is the proliferation of osteogenic cells from the periosteum and marrow. According to their view, progenitor cells from the periosteum also form the external cartilage callus, which develops because of an insufficient blood supply and low oxygen content in the rapidly growing callus tissue.[11] Motion of the fracture fragments also promotes formation of cartilage instead of bone.[13]

Other investigators have proposed that the essential feature of repair is the organization of the blood clot by invading fibroblasts. According to these authors, cells that form the external callus and give rise to cartilage are derived from newly sprouting vessels,[13–16] from the surrounding musculature, or from circulating cells in the blood.[17,18]

This latter view, in a sophisticated form, is still with us today in the views of Brighton,[19] Cruess and Dumont,[20] Henricson and associates,[21] and Hulth.[22] For Cruess and Dumont,[20] the essential feature of bone repair is the hematoma and the invading vascular cells described by McLean and Urist.[14] Henricson and associates[21] and Hulth[22] report that chondrogenesis occurs during fracture repair by the influence of inflammatory cells on cells derived from the overlying muscle and attendant vasculature. On the basis of both transmission and electron microscopy, Brighton[19] has suggested that perivascular mesenchymal cells are induced to differentiate into chondroblasts. With further development of the callus, these cells undergo endochondral ossification.

Comparison of fracture repair in different bones and in different models indicates that rival opinions about the origin of cartilage in the callus are supported by subtle variations in the histologic patterns of repair. Periosteally derived osteoblasts and the osteoblastic progeny of undifferentiated circulating precursor cells, muscle satellite cells, or perivascular cells appear to be present in every fracture. The relative expression of these cells and the significance of their contribution to fracture repair change with the type of injury and the age of the patient, probably precluding a histologic answer to the question of cartilage origin. Modern molecular techniques for investigating cell lineage hold promise for determining cartilage origin. The central importance of cartilage formation in normal fracture repair and the absence of cartilage in conditions where healing is impaired, such as diabetes[9] and after chemotherapy treatment (unpublished data), demonstrate the need to identify chondrocyte precursors in the callus and to characterize the factors that regulate their differentiated function.

Regulation of Cell Activity

Multiple factors determine the progression of cellular events during fracture repair. The callus formed during fracture repair is a complex histologic structure that includes cells from the periosteum, invading blood vessels, and overlying muscle. In a standard animal fracture model, in which mechanical variables associated with the force of injury and biologic variables that differ from one individual to the next are controlled, cells are seen to undergo membranous bone formation, chondrogenesis, and endochondral ossification.[1] The predictable nature of these cellular activities, their sequence, and their location suggest that cell activity in the callus is highly regulated.

Current literature suggests that the differentiation of mature osteoblasts and chondrocytes from precursor cells, the synthesis of extracellular matrix by these differentiated cells, and other cellular events are affected by powerful systemic and local influences, including hormones from the endocrine system, local regulating factors, or growth factors, synthesized in the callus, and mechanical forces acting at the fracture site.[23]

Local Regulation of Fracture Repair by Polypeptide Growth Factors

Although cells in the callus differ in their tissue of origin, they share several underlying events that are subject to regulation. These include cell proliferation and differentiation, chemotaxis, and the synthesis of extracellular matrix. The current literature presents convincing data that local factors are appreciated as important regulators of fracture repair, but are less well characterized than systemic factors.

Growth Factors Regulate Bone and Cartilage Cell Function

Local regulators of fracture repair could be secreted by both inflammatory and noninflammatory cells. Current investigations indicate that macrophages and other inflammatory cells at sites of injury in nonskeletal tissues secrete cytokines and growth factors that are critical regulators of healing.[23] The presence of inflammatory cells in the fracture callus suggests that these cells also secrete cytokines and growth factors during the initial stages of fracture repair. Current literature on growth factors demonstrates growth factor regulation of chondrocyte, osteoblast, and periosteal cell proliferation; the initiation of chondrocyte differentiation and the expression of type II procollagen in the periosteum; and modulation of extracellular matrix synthesis by chondrocytes and osteoblasts. Because similar cellular events occur in the fracture callus, these studies imply that growth factors also act as regulators of cell differentiation and matrix synthesis in the later stages of fracture repair.[24]

Growth factors could also be synthesized by osteoblasts, macrophages, or chondrocytes within the fracture callus. Alternatively, growth factors may be delivered to the fracture callus by the bloodstream, or, more likely, they could be released by platelets into the fracture hematoma.[25] Growth factors synthesized by macrophages include transforming growth factor-β1 (TGF-β1), the acidic and basic fibroblast growth factors (aFGF and bFGF), as well as interleukins and tumor necrosis factors. Platelet degranulation during hematoma formation is also a significant source of growth factors, including TGF-β1, and the platelet-derived growth factor (PDGF).[25] Other sources of growth factors include osteoblasts (FGF, TGF-β1, and PDGF) and chondrocytes (FGF, TGF-β). Bone matrix is a reservoir for growth factors and contains high concentrations of FGF and TGF-β.[26] The number of growth factors likely to have a significant role in the regulation of wound repair, osteogenesis, and chondrogenesis is increasing. A partial list of growth factors that affect healing in the fracture callus is presented in Table 1.

Growth factors in the callus may regulate fracture repair by paracrine or autocrine pathways,[27] and can exert a broad spectrum of activities. Consequently, determination of the precise location of different growth factors is important for elucidating their ultimate role in the callus.

Synthesis and Localization of Growth Factors in the Fracture Callus

The presence of a growth factor within the fracture callus is obviously a prerequisite for the growth factor to exert regulatory actions during fracture heal-

Table 1 Growth factors found in the fracture callus

Growth Factors*	Source	Matrix Location**	Responding Cells	Unique Characteristics
TGF-β	Platelets, inflammatory cells (monocytes, macrophages), osteoblasts, chondrocytes	Bone is the most abundant source of TGF-β in the body	Most cells have TGF-β	Inactive precursor peptide, most potent chemoattractant identified for macrophages, promotes angiogenesis, activates a serine-threonine receptor
BMPs (BMP-2, BMP-4, BMP-5, and BMP-7)	Chondrocytes, urinary bladder, epithelium, brain	BMPs were originally identified in bone, but now are known to be widely distributed throughout the body	Unknown	TGF-β-like structure; may be involved in cartilage formation, important regulator during embryogenesis
Fibroblast Growth Factors (aFGF, bFGF)	Inflammatory cells, osteoblasts, chondrocytes	Binds HSPG in bone and cartilage matrix	Most cells of mesoderm or neuroectoderm origin	Stimulates neovascularization, evidence for an autocrine, intracellular function; stimulates type IV collagenase
Platelet-derived Growth Factors (PDGF-AA, AB, or BB)	Platelets, monocytes, activated macrophages, endothelial cells	Interactions unknown	Most cells of mesoderm origin	Activates a tyrosine kinase receptor

* TGF-β = transforming growth factor β; BMP = bone morphogenetic protein; aFGF = acidic FGF; bFGF = basic FGF.

** HSPG = heparan sulfate proteoglycan

ing. Experimentally, growth factors are localized to cells and regions within the callus by immunostaining the fracture callus with monospecific antibodies. Gene expression for different growth factors is detected by Northern analysis, if expression occurs at high levels, or by amplification techniques (polymerase chain reaction, PCR), if the growth factor gene is expressed at low levels or by a small number of cells.[1]

Growth Factor Gene Expression During Fracture Healing

To determine whether growth factors are expressed by cells within the fracture callus, and, if so, at which stages of the fracture healing process, total cellular RNA extracted from the callus was evaluated by Northern hybridization for TGF-β1, bone morphogenetic protein-2 (BMP-2) and BMP-7, and PDGF gene expression[28] and by reverse transcription followed by PCR amplification for aFGF and bFGF (S Jingushi, L Hjelmeland, ME Bolander, unpublished data). These studies show that the levels of growth factor gene expression vary with the progression of fracture repair (Table 2). Expression of the TGF-β1 gene is high during chondrogenesis and endochondral ossification, but lower during membranous bone formation. Acidic FGF gene expression also varies with the stage of repair, and maximal expression is seen during chondrogenesis. Constant levels of bFGF and PDGF B chain expression are detected during all stages of fracture repair. Localization of these factors is limited to areas of immature cells during the early stages of chondrogenesis. Although several authors have speculated about the role of BMPs in the fracture repair process, no expression of BMP-2 and -7 was seen in the callus on Northern analysis (ME Bolander and S Jingushi, unpublished data).

These observations suggest that different growth factors are expressed in the callus during the progression of cartilage and bone formation. High levels of TGF-β1 and aFGF in chondrogenesis suggest that chondrocytes synthesize high levels of these growth factors. Lower levels of expression for other growth factors suggest that these growth factors are also synthesized by cells in the callus, but this analysis does not detect changes in the relative level of gene expression.

Growth Factor Immunolocalization During Fracture Healing

Growth factors in the fracture callus can be localized to specific cell types by immunostaining with monospecific antibodies (S Jingushi, L Hjelmeland, ME Bolander, unpublished data).[29] Using the histologic characterization of fracture

Table 2 Growth factor gene expression during fracture repair

Growth Factor*	Membranous Ossification	Chondrogenesis	Endochondral Ossification
TGF-β1	+ +	+ + + +	+ + +
BMP-2	0	0	0
BMP-7	0	0	0
aFGF	+	+ +	+
bFGF	+	+	+
PDGF-B	+ +	+ +	+ +

* TGF-β = transforming growth factor-β; BMP = bone morphogenetic protein; aFGF and bFGF = acidic and basic fibroblast growth factor; PDGF = platelet-derived growth factor.

healing as a reference, distinct immunostaining patterns are seen for TGF-β1, aFGF, bFGF, and the TGF-β-related factors BMP-2 and -7.

Extracellular TGF-β1 is localized to the hematoma as early as 24 hours after fracture, both at the fracture site and along the periosteum (Table 3). Immunostaining of the periosteum and hematoma persist after injury and precisely define the region of periosteal proliferation and membranous bone formation. During membranous bone formation, bone adjacent to the fracture site demonstrates intercellular staining of osteoblasts in the bone spicules for TGF-β1. During chondrogenesis, mesenchymal cells and immature chondrocytes stain intensely for intercellular TGF-β1, whereas surrounding hematoma and matrix demonstrate extracellular TGF-β1 staining. The cartilaginous matrix surrounding mature chondrocytes demonstrates little or no TGF-β1 staining, whereas the matrix surrounding hypertrophic chondrocytes stains strongly for TGF-β1.

Similar studies have evaluated bFGF in the fracture callus. Anti-basic FGF antibodies stain macrophages in the hematoma and granulation tissue. Immature chondrocytes stain for bFGF in the nucleus, whereas mature chondrocytes stain intensely in the peripheral regions of the cytoplasm. Osteoblasts and bone matrix stain for bFGF only during endochondral ossification.

In contrast to the intercellular and extracellular staining for both TGF-β and bFGF, immunologic staining with aFGF antibodies show exclusive intercellular staining of cells. Macrophages in the hematoma and the early callus stain intensely for aFGF, whereas preosteoblasts in the upper regions of the periosteum and during endochondral ossification also stain for aFGF. Immature chondrocytes stain intensely for aFGF, while little staining is seen in mature or hypertrophic chondrocytes.

Correlation of Growth Factor Expression With the Histologic Progression of Repair

Correlating the expression and localization of the growth factor with changes in the histology of the callus may suggest the source of a growth factor and its role in cell regulation. This analysis implies that TGF-β1 detected in the fibrous periosteum is not the result of synthesis by periosteal cells, because the level of

Table 3 Immunostaining for growth factors in the fracture callus

| Growth Factors* | Hematoma** | Periosteum** | Cartilage** | | | Bone |
			Proliferating/ Immature	Mature	Hypertrophic	
TGF-β	+ +	+ +	+ + +	+	+ + +	+
bFGF	+ Macrophages	0	+ Nuclear	+ + Cytoplasm	+ Cytoplasm	+ Endochondral ossification
aFGF	+ Macrophages	+	+ + + Cytoplasm	0	0	+ Immature osteoblasts
BMP-2	0	0	+	0	0	0
BMP-7	0	0	+ +	0	0	0

*TGF-β = transforming growth factor-β; aFGF and bFGF = acidic and basic fibroblast growth factors; BMP = bone morphogenetic protein.
**0 = no immunostaining; + = slight immunostaining; + + = intermediate immunostaining; + + + = strong staining.

TGF-β gene expression at that time is very low. Significant concentrations of TGF-β are released from platelets at the time of injury, suggesting that platelets are the source of TGF-β seen in the periosteum. The clear association between TGF-β1 staining of the periosteum and the extent of callus formation suggest that TGF-β1 may stimulate proliferation during initial callus formation. TGF-β in chondrocytes probably is synthesized by these cells, because high levels of TGF-β gene expression are detected in the cartilage. Accumulation of TGF-β in the cytoplasm of mature chondrocytes and the extracellular matrix around hypertrophic chondrocytes suggests that chondrocytes transport this growth factor from intracellular sources into the extracellular matrix during hypertrophy. TGF-β in this matrix may have a role in regulating cartilage matrix calcification and endochondral ossification.

Acidic FGF is expressed at lower levels than TGF-β, but increased expression during chondrogenesis suggests a role for this growth factor in regulating the development of chondrocytes from their precursors. Basic FGF and PDGF are expressed at relatively constant levels throughout the development of the callus; consequently, this analysis is not informative about the possible regulatory functions of these growth factors in the fracture callus.

Although an increase in growth factor gene expression preceding a histologic or cellular event suggests a role for growth factor regulation, the evidence is only correlative and does not provide direct data on the role of the growth factor. Direct evidence for growth factor regulation can be obtained by adding exogenous factors to specific stages of fracture healing in vivo and in vitro, or by testing growth factors in models of different aspects of the factor repair response.

Growth Factors in Fracture Repair Models

Identification of growth factor gene expression and immunolocalization is only suggestive evidence of growth factor function, and does not provide direct data on the regulatory roles of various growth factors found in the callus. The addition of exogenous growth factors to specific stages of fracture healing in vivo has been informative for growth factors with relatively limited effects, as demonstrated below for aFGF. For growth factors with a broader range of effects, such as TGF-β, it can be difficult to interpret the histologic results after the addition of exogenous growth factors to the callus in vivo. To solve this problem, growth factors have been studied in organ culture of the fracture callus and in in vivo models of fracture callus formation.

TGF-β Released From Platelets at the Time of Fracture Initiates Callus Formation

Platelets are the first source of growth factors at the region of injury after fracture. In addition to coagulation factors and other proteins, platelet alpha granules contain TGF-β1 and PDGF.[25] Degranulation of platelets at the time of fracture releases high concentrations of these factors into the immediate region of injury. Because there is no evidence for TGF-β gene expression on Northern analysis of early fracture callus RNA, the intense TGF-β immunostaining observed in the fibrous periosteum is likely the result of TGF-β release by platelets. The strong correlation between TGF-β immunostaining of the periosteum and the extent of the fracture callus suggested a role for TGF-β in the initiation of periosteal cell proliferation and callus formation. This view was tested by initiation of short-term injection of TGF-β into the early fracture callus. These experiments showed marked abnormalities in the callus structure, thereby suggesting that TGF-β has a profound effect on multiple cells in the callus, but the experiments were not otherwise informative. It then was hypothesized that if cells in the periosteum responded to TGF-β release from platelets after fracture, these cells might also respond to TGF-β stimulation in the absence of fracture. This hypothesis was tested by injecting TGF-β into the subperiosteal tissue of uninjured femurs.

Subperiosteal injection of TGF-β into the nonfractured femurs resulted in mesenchymal cell proliferation, the initiation of chondrogenesis, and membranous bone formation.[29] Mesenchymal cell proliferation in the inner cambial layer of the periosteum was seen after injection of 200 ng of TGF-β1 or 20 ng of TGF-β2. After 4 days, chondrocytes were identified above the cortex at the injection site. The size of the cartilage tissue mass increased several fold with continued TGF-β injection. As the cartilage mass enlarged, hypertrophic chondrocytes developed near the underlying cortex, and smaller, proliferating chondrocytes were seen near the fibrous periosteum. The cartilage mass was replaced with bone by endochondral ossification. New bone formed in the subperiosteal region, lateral to cartilage, by membranous ossification. Bone in both locations underwent active remodeling by osteoclasts, which finally resulted in the thickening of the cortical bone.

Histologic and molecular evaluation of this mass demonstrates all the cellular events known to occur during callus formation. Consequently, this observation is interpreted as demonstrating that TGF-β directly or indirectly initiates a cascade of cellular events resembling those seen in fracture repair.[29] The requirement for continued daily injections of TGF-β suggests this model differs from normal fractures with respect to the activation and release of TGF-β from the periosteum. The data that support the concept that TGF-β plays a critical role in the initiation of fracture repair are strong, but confirmation of this view requires further understanding of the activation of TGF-β in the early callus, the demonstration of TGF-β receptors on cells in the callus that undergo proliferation and differentiation, and elucidation of the regulatory cascade resulting in chondrogenesis, including additional growth factors synthesized after TGF-β release from platelets.

aFGF Expression Regulates the Proliferation and Differentiation of Chondrocyte Precursors

To evaluate the significance of increased expression of aFGF in the early stages of chondrogenesis, aFGF was injected into the soft callus in a standard model of rat femur fracture repair at times that corresponded to aFGF expression by macrophages in the callus.[30] Histologic analysis of the callus demonstrated increased cartilage, indicated by increased type II procollagen, and a delay in the initiation of endochondral ossification, indicated by delayed expression of alkaline phosphatase on Northern analysis. These observations were interpreted as consistent with aFGF stimulation of chondrocyte proliferation, and chondrocyte hypertrophy and endochondral ossification were assumed to be secondarily delayed. No effects of aFGF injection were seen in other cell types in the callus. Bone formation, as evidenced by endochondral ossification and the development of increased force to failure and stiffness in mechanical tests, was unaffected (unpublished data).[30]

Based on this observation, the periosteum or surrounding soft tissues were hypothesized to contain a population of chondrocyte precursors that are stimulated by aFGF to differentiate and/or proliferate. If true, this hypothesis implies that aFGF injection into the periosteum stimulates the differentiation and proliferation of these cells in the absence of fracture. To test this hypothesis, aFGF was injected into the subperiosteum of intact femurs and the cellular response was followed (S Jingushi, L Hjelmeland, ME Bolander, unpublished data). Histologic examination of injected femurs demonstrated proliferation of undifferentiated mesenchymal cells that appear to arise from the periosteum. As long as aFGF injection is continued, these cells proliferate and remain undifferentiated. When aFGF injection was withdrawn, however, cells began the process of chondrocyte differentiation and hypertrophy, and they subsequently underwent endochondral ossification. These observations were interpreted as consistent with the hypothesis that aFGF regulates proliferation in the early fracture callus. When aFGF expression decreased, proliferation also decreased, and cells differentiated into chondrocytes. Confirmation of this hypothesis also will require further experimentation, including blocking the action of aFGF in the callus and identifying of factors that initiate chondrogenesis by down-regulating aFGF expression.

TGF-β Regulates Chondrocyte Maturation and the Initiation of Endochondral Ossification

The histology of the fracture callus in the rat femur fracture model shows marked changes in chondrocytes as cells hypertrophy and initiate endochondral ossification. These changes progress rapidly between day 9, the beginning of vascular invasion into the cartilage, and day 13, when vascular invasion of the cartilage-bone interface is completed. During this period, TGF-β1 expression in the soft fracture callus increases, and antibodies against TGF-β stain the matrix around hypertrophic chondrocytes. These observations indicate increased expression of this growth factor and suggest that TGF-β may have a role in regulating these changes in the cartilage. TGF-β is known to modulate the expression of type II procollagen by cultured chondrocytes, and overexpression of TGF-β has been observed in cases of pathologic cartilage matrix calcification.

TGF-β was hypothesized to perform regulatory functions in the fracture callus related to the modulation of type II procollagen expression and matrix mineralization. This hypothesis was evaluated in an organ culture model of the fracture callus, in which the exogenous administration of TGF-β could be controlled and the effects on specific cells evaluated. In this model, fracture calluses were stabilized in organ culture and then treated with varying doses of the growth factor. TGF-β stimulated a dose-dependent decrease in expression of genes related to cartilage, type II procollagen, and aggrecan, and an increase in expression of genes related to matrix mineralization, type I procollagen, osteonectin, and alkaline phosphatase. These observations are thought to indicate that TGF-β has profound effects on chondrocyte gene expression, and these results are viewed as indicating that TGF-β, in conjunction with other growth factors in the cartilage, regulates the process of chondrocyte maturation and hypertrophy. This hypothesis also must be subjected to further experimentation. Significant experimental tests would identify and characterize TGF-β receptors in the cartilage and identify factors that stimulate or modulate TGF-β synthesis. Even in the absence of additional experimental data, however, current observations strongly support the view that TGF-β has a major regulatory role in fracture repair.

Summary

Fractured bones heal by a cascade of cellular events in which mesenchymal cells respond to regulatory factors by proliferating, differentiating, and synthesizing extracellular matrix. Current literature suggests that growth factors regulate different steps in this cascade. Recent studies indicate regulatory roles for PDGF, aFGF, bFGF, TGF-β and possibly BMP-2, BMP-5, and BMP-7 in the initiation and development of the fracture callus. Fracture healing begins immediately following injury when growth factors, including TGF-β1 and PDGF, are released into the fracture by platelets and inflammatory cells. TGF-β1, BMP-2, BMP-7, and FGF are synthesized by osteoblasts and chondrocytes throughout the healing process. TGF-β appears to influence the initiation of fracture repair and the formation of cartilage and membranous bone. Acidic FGF is synthesized by chondrocytes, chondrocyte precursor cells, and macrophages; it appears to stimulate the proliferation of immature chondrocytes or their precursors, and indirectly regulates chondrocyte maturation and the expression of the cartilage matrix. Presumably, growth factors in the callus at later times regulate additional steps in fracture repair.

These studies suggest that growth factors are central regulators of cellular proliferation, differentiation, and extracellular matrix synthesis during fracture repair. Abnormal growth factor expression has been implicated as causing impaired or abnormal healing in other tissues, suggesting that altered growth factor expression also may be responsible for abnormal or delayed fracture repair. As a complete understanding of fracture healing regulation evolves, new insights into the etiology of abnormal or delayed fracture healing will be gained, and possible new therapies for these difficult clinical problems will result.

References

1. Jingushi S, Joyce ME, Bolander ME: Genetic expression of extracellular matrix proteins correlates with histologic changes during fracture repair. *J Bone Miner Res* 1992;7:1045–1055.
2. Joyce ME, Jingushi S, Scully SP, et al: Role of growth factors in fracture healing, in Barbule A, Caldwell MD, Eaglstein WH (eds): *Clinical and Experimental Approaches to Dermal and Epidermal Repair: Normal and Chronic Wounds*. New York, NY, Wiley-Liss, 1991, pp 391–416.
3. Duhamel HL: Quatriéme mémoire sur les os. *Mém Acad R Sci* 1743;56:87.
4. Dupuytren G: On the injuries and diseases of bones: Being selections from the collected edition of the clinical lectures of Baron Dupuytren. Le Gros Clark F (ed and trans). London, Sydenham Society, 1847.
5. von Haller: Quoted from Howship, J (1818). *Med Chir Trans* 1770;9:165.
6. Hunter J, in JF Palmer (ed): *The Works of John Hunter, F.R.S. With Notes*. London, Longman, 1835.
7. Ham AW: A histological study of the early phases of bone repair. *J Bone Joint Surg* 1930;12:827–844.
8. Tonna EA, Cronkite EP: Periosteum: Autoradiographic studies on cellular proliferation and transformation utilizing tritiated thymidine. *Clin Orthop* 1963;30:218–232.
9. Macey LR, Kana SM, Jingushi S, et al: Defects of early fracture-healing in experimental diabetes. *J Bone Joint Surg* 1989;71A:722–733.
10. Stanisavljevic S, Babcock AL: Fractures in children treated with methotrexate for leukemia. *Clin Orthop* 1977;125:139–144.
11. Ham AW, Harris WR: Repair and transplantation of bone, in Bourne GH (ed): *The Biochemistry and Physiology of Bone*, ed 2. New York, NY, Academic Press, 1972, vol 3, pp 337–399.

12. Owen M: The origin of bone cells in the postnatal organism. *Arthritis Rheum* 1980; 23:1073–1080.
13. Pritchard JJ: Histology of fracture repair, in Clark JMP (ed): *Modern Trends in Orthopedics*. London, Butterworths, 1964, pp 69–90.
14. McLean FC, Urist MR: *Bone: An Introduction to the Physiology of Skeletal Tissue*, ed 2. Chicago, IL, University of Chicago Press, 1955.
15. McLean FC, Urist MR: *Bone: Fundamentals of the Physiology of Skeletal Tissue*, ed 3. Chicago, IL, University of Chicago Press, 1968, pp 5, 12, 18.
16. Trueta J: The role of the vessels in osteogenesis. *J Bone Joint Surg* 1963;45B:402–418.
17. Harada K, Oida S, Sasaki S: Chondrogenesis and osteogenesis of bone marrow-derived cells by bone-inductive factor. *Bone* 1988;9:177–183.
18. Huang S, Terstappen LW: Formation of haematopoietic microenvironment and haematopoietic stem cells from single human bone marrow stem cells. *Nature* 1992; 360:745–749.
19. Brighton CT: Principles of fracture healing: Part I. The biology of fracture repair, in Murray JA (ed): *The American Academy of Orthopaedic Surgeons Instructional Course Lectures XXXIII*. St Louis, MO, CV Mosby, 1984, pp 60–82.
20. Cruess RI, Dumont J: Fracture healing. *Can J Surg* 1975;18:403–413.
21. Henricson A, Hulth A, Johnell O: The cartilaginous fracture callus in rats. *Acta Orthop Scand* 1987;58:244–248.
22. Hulth A: Current concepts of fracture healing. *Clin Orthop* 1989;249:265–284.
23. Nemeth GG, Bolander ME, Martin GR: Growth factors and their role in wound and fracture healing, in Barbul A, Pines E, Caldwell M, et al (eds): *Growth Factors and Other Aspects of Wound Healing: Biological and Clinical Implications*. New York, NY, Wiley-Liss, 1988, pp 1–17.
24. Pan WT, Einhorn TA: Mini-symposium: Principles of fracture management: (i) The biochemistry of fracture healing. *Curr Orthop* 1992;6:207–213.
25. Assoian RK, Sporn MB: Type-β transforming growth factor in human platelets: Release during platelet degranulation and action on vascular smooth muscle cells. *J Cell Biol* 1986;102:1217–1223.
26. Hauschka PV, Mavrakos AE, Iafrati MD, et al: Growth factors in bone matrix: Isolation of multiple types by affinity chromatography on heparin-sepharose. *J Biol Chem* 1986;261:12665–12674.
27. Sporn MB, Todaro GJ: Autocrine secretion and malignant transformation of cells. *N Engl J Med* 1980;303:878–880.
28. Nemeth GG, Heydemann A, Bolander ME: Isolation and analysis of ribonucleic acids from skeletal tissues. *Anal Biochem* 1989;183:301–304.
29. Joyce ME, Roberts AB, Sporn MB, et al: Transforming growth factor-β and the initiation of chondrogenesis and osteogenesis in the rat femur. *J Cell Biol* 1990;10: 2195–2207.
30. Jingushi S, Heydemann A, Kana SK, et al: Acidic fibroblast growth factor (aFGF) injection stimulates cartilage enlargement and inhibits cartilage gene expression in rat fracture healing. *J Orthop Res* 1990;8:364–371.

Chapter 12

Circulation, Blood Flow, and Interstitial Fluid Flow in Fracture Healing

Patrick J. Kelly, MD
James T. Bronk

Introduction

This chapter relates blood flow and interstitial fluid flow to bone repair, in particular to the healing process of a fracture. Methodology is discussed first, followed by the effects of fixation devices on blood flow to the fracture. One major aim of fixation of fractures is to increase function, which, in turn, may stimulate the healing process. Fluid flow in bone is an important aspect of tissue nutrition. Flow of electrolytes in the pore system of bone, a part of the circulation, may be related to important electrokinetic phenomena that help control the healing process.

Fractures

Methods to Measure Blood Flow

It is difficult to measure blood flow in any tissue, but the difficulty is compounded in bone because it has three separate anatomic vascular supplies—nutrient medullary, epiphyseal-metaphyseal, and periosteal.

Most techniques used to measure bone blood flow in animal models are invasive and many require that the animal be killed. The methods used to measure bone blood flow in humans are bone imaging and laser Doppler flowmetry.

Clearance This method depends on the assumption that the amount of tracer accumulated in the tissue after its injection into the general circulation is the difference between inflow and outflow. By definition, clearance is the minimal volume of blood entering an organ per unit time that could supply the amount of tracer or indicator removed from the blood during its passage through the organ. While the method is useful, there are major disadvantages.

Determination of clearance is not a true measure of blood flow, even though the units of measurement are ml/g of tissue. Blood flow is equal to the clearance divided by the extraction, which is the fraction of tracer removed with each passage through the capillary bed. Because extraction is low with high flow and high with low flow, clearance does not necessarily equal blood flow. Also, there may be tracer loss via the lymphatic exits. Dynamic bone imaging is a clinical counterpart of the clearance technique and can be used to indicate circulation if the earliest part of the curve is used.[1] The technique can give useful information if properly interpreted.

Microspheres The theory for microsphere usage is that if an indicator is evenly mixed in the heart and totally trapped by tissue, its distribution will reflect the distribution of cardiac output to that organ or tissue. Put another way, the fractional amount of tracer in the tissue of interest will represent the fraction of cardiac output perfusing that tissue. Hence, the extraction problem associated with clearance is removed. The concept is relatively simple, but the technique requires careful preparation and adherence to the details of the method. Serial flows can be determined in the same animal. Cardiac output and regional and total organ flow can be determined simultaneously because a withdrawal pump is used as a reference organ.

The use of microspheres of the proper size is essential; if they are too small, there will be throughput of microspheres (ie, extraction less than 100%) and the value for tissue blood flow will be incorrect. Uniformity of mixing is also essential. There must be a sufficient number of spheres to calculate the flow in the sample studied. Disadvantages are the expense of the spheres and the problems involved in disposing of radioactive substances. The latter problem may be mitigated by the use of fluorescent-labeled microspheres.[2] Also, the method is invasive and requires sacrificing the subject. The methods and theory have been published.[3-6]

Laser Doppler Flowmetry This technique for evaluation of circulation has been used for soft tissues and now is being applied to bone. Its advantages are that it allows multiple measurements in the same animal at different time intervals and allows "real time" measurements. The technique is not a true measurement of blood flow in ml/min/g of bone. Because it measures a small volume, heterogeneity of flow creates a problem . The opacity of bone to light also causes problems in interpretation.[7] Nonetheless, if it is applicable to clinical use, this method may represent an important advance.

Positron Emission Tomography Water labeled with [15]O has been used to measure bone blood flow in human volunteers with closed unilateral tibial fractures. Increased tibial blood flow was observed at levels 14 times normal 2 weeks after fracture. Absolute values of flow have not been calculated because arterial cannulation was not done.[8,9]

Effects of Fixation on Blood Flow

Common Forms of Fixation Plate, intramedullary rods, and external fixation are used in clinical practice. Plate fixation is usual for forearm fractures and is also used for humeral fractures if nonoperative methods are not applicable. In the tibia, plates, external fixation, and intramedullary rods that are inserted after reaming have been used at various times. In many centers, casts still are used for tibial and humeral fractures. For the diaphyseal femoral fracture, the intramedullary rod is almost universally the favorite form of fixation.

Each method of fixation has advantages and disadvantages. Rods do not control rotation as well as plates, plates are thought to produce excessive porosity, and external fixation is not well accepted by the patient. Furthermore, pin site infection can be a problem in external fixation. The canine tibia provides a good model to test each form of fixation on an experimental fracture.[10] The use of microspheres provides an opportunity to measure blood flow serially (at different time intervals). Microradiography and tetracycline labeling make it possible to evaluate the degree of bone remodeling and cortical porosity that occurs following use of all these forms of fixation.

Changes in Blood Flow After Fixation Three specific areas of cortical bone were studied: the endosteal cortex, the periosteal cortex, and the area under the plate (the subplate cortex). Microspheres were used to measure blood flow before osteotomy (experimental fracture) and at 10 minutes and 4 hours after osteotomy without fixation. Blood flow also was measured at 4 hours, 48 hours, 14 days, and 90 days after fixation. At 90 days, a cross section was studied by combined tetracycline-microradiographic analysis for bone formation and porosity. Osteotomy without fixation decreases blood flow by one half at 10 minutes and by two thirds at 4 hours when compared to control values. At 4 hours, the fractures fixed with a rod had significantly less endosteal cortical flow than those fixed with plates or externally fixed. At 14 days, endosteal cortex blood flow was still less in rod-fixed than in externally fixed fractures. Only subplate cortical flow was decreased significantly at 4 hours in fractures fixed with a rod. At 90 days, blood flow to the subplate region was significantly higher in plate-fixed fractures than in rod-fixed fractures. It thus appears that intramedullary rods decrease blood flow the most and external fixators the least. Plate fixation did not decrease flow early in the experiments, and regional flow beneath the plate was actually higher at 90 days than in either the external fixator or rod-fixed fractures. In unfractured long bones, an increase in strontium clearance has been observed in the segment of bone beneath the plate at 7 days and at 1 to 2 months. This is interpreted as an increase in blood flow.[11]

Effects of Revascularization on Porosity of Bone Porosity of cortical bone was increased in all fractures,[10] but there was no significant difference between rods, plates, or external fixators at 90 days. Reports of many studies have mentioned the increased porosity after application of plates.[12–16] These morphologic studies did not compare plates to intramedullary rods or external fixators. It would appear, at least from our study,[10] that at 90 days, not only does stability of fixation play a role, but revascularization, particularly by collateralization and ingrowth of new vessels, may be the significant determinant of porosity (Fig. 1).

One curious aspect of plate fixation is the increased blood flow noted in bone beneath the plate at 90 days.[10] At 8 weeks, increased bone remodeling beneath the plate was observed by Gunst.[17] This observation has been attributed to disturbed blood supply and has been repeated by a host of investigators.[18–20] Studies with vital dyes, such as disulphine blue, have been made very soon after plate application. These studies suggest blockage of capillary filtration, perhaps caused by increased pressure within the interstitial fluid space. Blockage of exiting periosteal lymphatics is another possibility, because the molecular weight of this dye, 566.70, suggests it should behave similarly to sucrose. If bone behaves in accordance with Starling's phenomenon,[21] a new steady state of capillary and fluid space pressures may result. This new steady state may, at a later time, actually result in enhanced capillary filtration due to a chronic venous and lymphatic obstruction. This obstruction, in turn, may promote increased remodeling as has been observed by others.[22] Certainly, blockage or failure in uptake of a vital dye could be a function of impaired passage across the capillary, resulting from transient increase in the extracapillary pressure.

Effects of Function on Fracture Healing

Surgically Created Defects in Tibia For over 50 years, mechanical stimulation has been considered a factor in determining organ weights.[23] There are conflicting reports on the effects of weightbearing on bone healing. To test the hy-

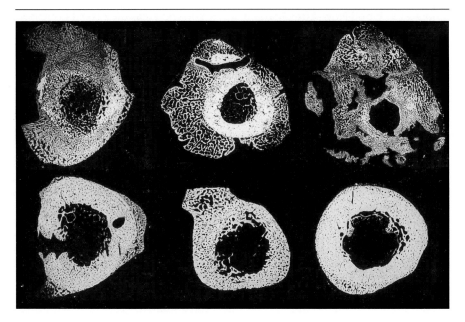

Fig. 1 Cross sections from tibias of dogs fixed with plates (PL), external fixators (EF), or intra-medullary rods (IM) from left to right. Top row compared to bottom row shows the great variability at 90 days. This suggests that revascularization may be as important or more important than stress protection from fixation during the first 90 days of the healing process.

pothesis that weightbearing affects bone formation, a small, surgically created defect was used to evaluate bone healing.[24] The period of study was 28 days, and adult dogs of uniform age were chosen. Evolution of the woven bone in the 11 × 4.5-mm defect was uniform in amount and rate. Significantly less bone was formed in the defect in a nonweightbearing tibia than in a weight-bearing tibia. The conclusion was that weightbearing is a permissive factor in the formation of woven bone; excessive or increased weightbearing did not increase woven bone formation.[25]

Capillary Filtration and Bone Repair (Tibial Defect) An 11 × 4.5-mm defect[26] was again studied for 28 days in dogs with one limb elevated, one weightbear-ing, and a control group with both limbs weightbearing. Again, less woven bone was seen in the defect of the elevated limb compared to the weightbearing one. The interstitial fluid space of the woven bone in the elevated tibial defect was significantly less at 7 and 14 days compared to that of the weightbearing defect. At 7 days, the interstitial fluid space, as measured using ^{14}C sucrose, was 0.72 ± 0.04 ml/ml bone in the elevated defect compared to 0.86 ± 0.05 ml/ml bone in the weightbearing defect. At 14 days, the interstitial space was 0.57 ± 0.04 ml/ml bone in the elevated tibial defect compared to 0.64 ± 0.04 ml/ml bone in the weightbearing defect. The interpretation was that fluid flow was decreased in the elevated defect due to a decrease in osseous venous resistance. This was supported by measurements of medullary pressures from day 0 to day 5, in which pressures were significantly less in the elevated tibia than in the weightbearing tibia.[26]

Effect of Weightbearing on Tibial Fracture Healing Tibial fractures in adult ca-nines were normally loaded, unloaded, or overloaded, and healing was studied at 6 and 12 weeks. Periosteal bone formation in the overloaded fractures was increased compared to that in the unloaded at 6 and 12 weeks and to that in the normally loaded tibial fractures at 6 weeks. Mechanical studies indicated significantly stronger fractures at both time intervals.[27] These results differ from those in the studies of a tibial defect. With movement at the fracture site, micromotion[28] as well as mechanoreceptors may play a role in repair of bone.[29]

Fluid Flow in Bone

Anatomy

Conduit Vessels The anatomy of the vascular network of bone is well known. However, the exchange mechanism for transport beyond the capillary has been poorly understood until recent years. Each new group of bone circulatory anatomists[30–32] has confirmed studies of the 19th century anatomists.[33] Injections of silicone rubber identified a parallel circulation to marrow and cortex. In the canine, the tibial nutrient artery supplies independent sets of arterioles that, in turn, supply terminal capillary beds of bone and marrow.[34] This system constitutes the only vascular supply to the bone. This conduit system also leads to the first barrier to exchange, the capillaries of bone. The fluid then passes through the capillaries to the lacunar-canalicular system. The interstitial fluid, which bathes the cells of bone, forms the fluid phase of bone.[35] The fluid then returns to the general circulation by the alymphatic system of bone.[36]

Capillaries The capillary is the first exchange barrier within bone for ions and molecules entering bone tissue. Knowledge about the structure of capillaries within bone rests on electron microscopic studies of the dog[37] and the rat.[38] Capillaries in cortical bone appear to be mostly closed, but some fenestrae are seen. Capillary structure in marrow-forming blood elements is discontinuous, but capillaries are continuous in the fatty marrow.

Interstitial Fluid Phase

Hydrophilic ions and molecules diffuse to the interstitial spaces from the capillary space via pores or clefts between the endothelial cells.[35] What is less certain is the presence of a defined lymphatic system. Evidence has been offered that hydrophilic ions, lipophilic substances, and large proteins pass through to the interstitial fluid space and later the lymphatic system.[35] Steady-state studies using volume of distribution methods have made it possible to estimate the various fluid spaces of canine cortical bone (Table 1). Total water of cortical bone has been estimated.[39] In addition, morphologic methods have been used in combination with tracer techniques to estimate fluid spaces in mature bone.[35,40] Changes in fluid space are observed with aging.[41] From these studies it is possible to conceptualize a scheme for an extracapillary fluid space that is in intimate contact with the cells of cortical bone (Fig. 2).

Exchange Mechanisms Across the Capillary

The skeleton is an enormous storehouse for ions, chiefly calcium ions, and this is especially true of fracture callus. Therefore, in a situation in which bone forms rapidly, such as a healing fracture, the concentrations of various ions, such as fluoride and strontium, and of molecules, such as diphosphonates, have been used in dynamic bone imaging, a common clinical tool. It has been possible to

Table 1 Fluid spaces of canine cortical bone

Space	Method	Fluid Spaces ml/ml bone ± S.D.	Obs
Haversian	morphology	0.015 ± 0.006	(6)
Lacunar	morphology	0.015 ± 0.004	(6)
Plasma	[111]In	0.008 ± 0.003	(5)
Red Blood Cells	^{99}Tc-Rbc	0.005 ± 0.002	(10)
Extracellular	[14C]inulin	0.042 ± 0.001	(4)
Extracellular	[14C]sucrose	0.043 ± 0.001	(9)
Total Water	[3]H$_2$O	0.245 ± 0.003	(4)

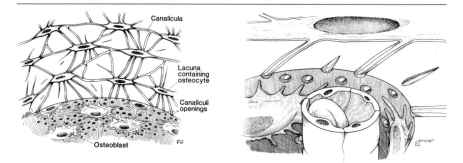

Fig. 2 Left, Representation of osteocytes, osteoblasts, and canaliculi of bone cells. **Right,** Diagrammatic scheme for the capillary containing a red cell and plasma. Fluid passes from the capillary to the fluid space outside the capillary that is in intimate contact with the cells of bone. (Reproduced with permission from Kelly PJ: Pathways for transport in bone, in Shephard JF, Abboud FM (eds): *Handbook of Physiology.* Baltimore, MD, Williams & Wilkins, 1983, pp 371–396.)

evaluate mechanisms of this process by determining the maximum extraction (E_{max}), of various-sized ions and molecules that tend to concentrate in bone. Results of many studies in which fractional extraction, E(t), of permeant tracers was used indicate early extraction of hydrophilic ions and molecules as determined by the diffusion coefficients of the ions or molecules (Fig. 3).[35] It was thought that there was a blood-bone barrier to antimicrobials. This is not true, for antibiotics and antibacterials do penetrate bone,[42,43] especially since many are weakly lipophilic.

A theory was proposed[44] that extracellular fluid space was compartmentalized by a cell layer that separates fluid beyond the capillary from fluid next to the crystal; ie, that a concentration gradient existed between interstitial fluid and fluid adjacent to bone mineral. Special indicator dilution and washout techniques adapted to bone for strontium ([85]Sr), a calcium tracer, and potassium ([42]K) revealed that this apparent compartmentalization probably could be explained by the rapid rate of uptake at extravascular binding sites on bone surfaces for Sr^{++}, or by absorption sites within the interstitium or on the bone surfaces. The apparent volume of distribution for strontium was much larger than for potassium, which, as in other tissues, is concentrated within the cells.[45]

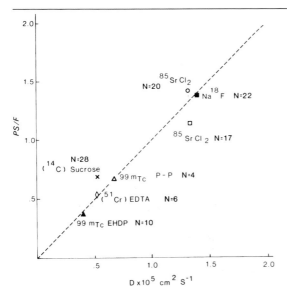

Fig. 3 Comparison of the ratio of permeability surface product (PS) to the flow of fluid (F) containing the tracer to the diffusion coefficients of the ion or molecules in dilute solutions at 25° C. The method used was an indicator-dilution method. (Reproduced with permission from Williams EA, Fitzgerald RH Jr, Kelly PJ: Microcirculation of bone, in Mortillaro NA (ed): *The Physiology and Pharmacology of the Microcirculation.* New York, NY, Academic Press, 1984, vol 2, pp 267–323.)

Further studies by the volume of distribution method were performed using dogs that were made hyper- or hypoparathyroid. Results of these studies implied a concentration-dependent binding mechanism for calcium in the extravascular fluid space of bone.[46] The binding capacity of canine bone is age dependent, and readily exchangeable calcium-binding capacity decreased from pup to adolescent to mature/old dogs by a factor of 34 times.[47]

Lymphatics of Bone

There is evidence of a fluid transport system in bone that is faster than simple diffusion. Markers such as thoratrast, horseradish peroxidase, and ferritin suggest transport within minutes through osteocyte lacunae and canalicular systems.[48–52] Injections of ferritin into the tibial nutrient artery of the mature dog as well as a dog with experimental tibial osteomyelitis allowed a more precise description of the fluid-phase movements through lymphatic channels. Movement appeared less impeded in infected bones.[36] Fluid that filters out of the capillary can be absorbed further down the pathway by capillaries in adjacent osteons. Perivascular prelymphatics may pick up interstitial fluid and then, via Volkmann's canals, drain to periosteal lymphatics or veins on the periosteal surface. Prelymphatic channels in the matrix, matrix prelymphatics, then join perivascular prelymphatics. Halos of ferritin form about the osteons, advance towards the periosteum, and coalesce into a ferritin front, which then permeates the appositional bone barrier to reach the periosteal surface (Fig. 4).

The appositional bone layer just adjacent to the periosteal surface limits fluid movement toward the periosteal exit. This is not the case in the immature dog as shown by in vitro observations in growing and adult dogs in which permeability of adult cortical bone is one sixth that seen in immature bone.[53] In adult canine bone with osteomyelitis, matrix prelymphatics could be seen penetrating the cortex periosteally. Timed injections allowed researchers to assess the movement of interstitial fluid in cortical bone. The pattern of movement of ferritin was consistent with bulk interstitial fluid flow influenced by hydrostatic pressure. The matrix prelymphatics and perivascular prelymphatics lack an endo-

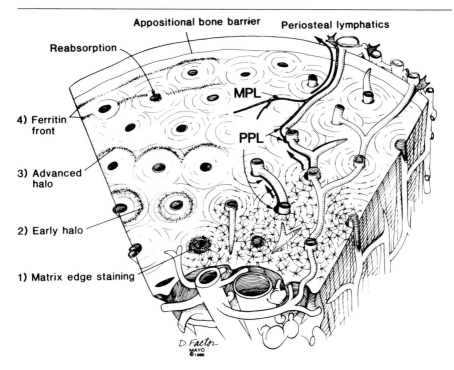

Fig. 4 Schematic diagram of lymphatic channels as described in text. MPL are matrix prelymphatics, PPL are perivascular prelymphatics. Fluid filtration is marked by movement of ferritin out of the capillary. An early halo of the marker ferritin may advance and form a front of ferritin that may penetrate through the appositional bone barrier to reach the periosteal surface and empty into the general circulation. Alternatively, the fluid may be reabsorbed by adjacent capillaries of osteons further down the pathway. Another route may be via MPL, which empty into PPL and then the fluid exits by Volkmann's canals.

thelium, and cortical bones are therefore termed an alymphatic system similar to the eye and brain.[54]

Relationships of Hydrostatic Pressure and Capillary Filtration

In all tissues, transport of substances, particularly those of large size, is by openings between the endothelial cells of capillaries. Intracellular clefts or pores in canine cortical bone capillaries are estimated to be about 175Å.[37] Other studies indicate these clefts between the endothelial cells of capillaries to be 90Å (Fig. 5).[55] Hydrophilic substances move through endothelial pores or clefts, and the lipid substances cross the endothelial cells by diffusion. However, ferritin studies indicate that larger molecules, such as albumin, ferritin, or growth hormone, move, not by diffusion, but by bulk fluid flow that depends on capillary hydrostatic pressure.[36] Bone (especially long bones) has a venous system that collects blood within the central medullary sinus. Detailed studies show that central medullary pressure is equivalent to osseous venous resistance in the canine tibia.[56] Therefore, if osseous venous resistance increases, bulk fluid movement should be from the capillary to the interstitium according to Starling's law.[21]

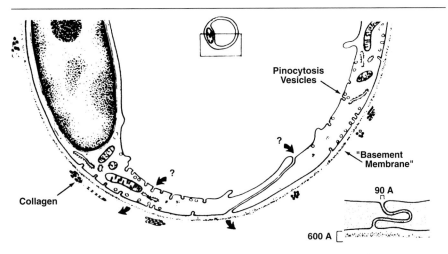

Fig. 5 Diagram of a capillary. The capillary is the end of the transport system to the cells. Fluid filters out of the pores or slits into the capillary. The capillary is a molecular sieve. Movement can be by diffusion but also by filtration which will be influenced by pressure within the capillary and pressure within the interstitium. (Reproduced with permission from Landis EM, Pappenheimer JR: Exchange of substances through the capillary walls, in Hamilton WF, Dow P (eds): *Handbook of Physiology*. Washington, DC, American Physiological Society, 1963, sect 2, vol II, pp 961–1034.)

Common examples of this are peripheral edema as well as pulmonary edema associated with congestive heart failure. Fluid flow in tissues other than bone, also called lymph flow, is an area of intense research activity with computer modeling used to validate theories.[57,58]

Stress-Related Potentials in Bone

The electromechanical characteristics of physiologically moist bone were first reported in 1968.[59] Since that time, the physical mechanism generating these endogenous electric signals has been determined to be the electrokinetic phenomenon known as streaming potentials.[59] Streaming potentials occur when electric charge is transported by fluid flow through the porous bone matrix.

The descriptions of fluid flow through a tube (Poiseuille's Law) and through a porous medium (Darcy's Law) both suggest a possible relationship between increased osseous resistance (resulting in a greater transcapillary pressure difference) and the bone formation seen distal to a venous tourniquet. Indeed, transcortical streaming potentials arise from circulatory pressures[60] and increase in magnitude in response to increases in venous pressures resulting from use of an inflatable cuff.[61]

Streaming potentials are also known to arise from fluid flow in response to mechanical loading of bone.[59,60] Thus, it has been hypothesized that streaming potentials may be an intermediary between mechanical loading and bone remodeling.

If fluid composition remains constant, the streaming potential, as defined mathematically,[62] is proportional to ΔP, the pressure difference driving the flow. A series of articles have emphasized the poroelastic structure of bone and coupled this to electrokinetic theory to explain the mechanism of change in bone formation in response to functional activity.[63,64]

In contrast, stretch[65] is emphasized in articles whose authors invoke known messengers to cells (ie, cyclic AMP [cAMP]), calcium, and prostaglandins that stimulate bone formation in response to their function.[66] Flow of extracapillary fluid would occur during mechanical loading. Nonetheless, shear stress would create a mechanical effect and, also, a streaming potential due to electrolyte solutions moving past a charged surface.[67] To view fluid movements in a larger context it is proposed that (1) fluid pressure would stimulate cells; (2) stress-induced fluid flow would aid in transport of substrates to cells, ie, have a nutritional effect; or (3) streaming potentials would be produced which would stimulate cells.[68]

In summary, it appears that fluid movement plays an important role in the response of bone to loading. Theories are complex. Electrokinetics appear important in this process. Changes in capillary filtration in response to stress indicate that changes in osseous venous resistance could play an important role, principally by increasing nutrition to cells.

Animal Models That Link Increased Fluid Movement and Bone Formation

A successful and consistent means of increasing bone formation in the canine model is the experimental arteriovenous fistula or venous tourniquet.[69–71] In growing canine tibias distal to an venous tourniquet, venous pressure and then tibial medullary canal pressure are elevated. Within 24 hours of tourniquet application, exchangeable water rose compared to the control tibia. This flux of fluid appeared to be at the expense of the vascular space. By 7 days, periosteal new bone formation increased significantly, and it continued to increase over a 42-day period.[70] The data support a view that increased venous pressure is followed by increased transcapillary fluid flow and then, in turn, by increased periosteal bone formation. The final mechanism may be simply a better delivery of substrate to the cells of bone resulting from increased bulk fluid flow. An alternative is that flow of fluid through pores or clefts in the capillary to the extracellular fluid space or even further into bone structure evokes streaming potentials. The electrical response could play a role in stimulating the cell or be an effect similar to the electric activity of functioning cardiac or skeletal muscle.

The production of increased bone remodeling is not confined to the tibia of growing dogs, but is also seen in the mature dog with an experimental ulnar fracture, a tibial defect, or an experimental tibial fracture.[72] Studies were conducted on a standardized tibial defect in weightbearing and nonweightbearing tibias. The interstitial fluid space decreased in the nonweightbearing tibial defect as did woven bone formation. Medullary canal pressures were significantly less in the nonweightbearing tibias. The conclusion was that decreased function decreased osseous venous resistance, fluid flow, and nutrition to the osteoblast within the experimental defect.[26] However, a pressurized brace that increases medullary pressure in the tibia does not increase bone formation[73] although increased venous pressure and streaming potentials are observed in acute experiments.[61] The explanation is that such a brace, while increasing fracture stability, probably reduces capillary filtration because of direct pressure on the exiting lymphatics of the tibia.[74]

Measurement of Fluid Flow in Bone

As previously stated, fluid moves from capillary to interstitium by bulk filtration for large molecules and diffusion for hydrophilic ions and smaller molecules. Measurements of glucose in stressed and unstressed canine femurs in vitro indicate a diffusion coefficient of 3×10^{-9} cm²/s.[75] This implies a 4-hour period for substances of this molecular weight to traverse the haversian canal to a cement line. Turnover rates of albumin in the interstitial fluid space of bone have been used in an attempt to obtain in vivo measurements of fluid flow in bone of canines from 9 to 54 months of age.[76] Fractional removal rates were calculated to be 1.843 h^{-1}. This compares to turnover of interstitial albumin in rat skeletal muscle of 0.02 h^{-1} in anesthetized rats and 0.08 h^{-1} in awake rats.[77] Similar turnover rates of albumin in rabbit bone have been observed by Owen and associates.[78] These studies suggest a considerable flow of interstitial fluid in cortical bone as suggested by timed microscopic studies using ferritin.[36] Direct measurement of fluid flow is not possible in bone, whereas it is feasible in the liver.[79] Hence, some tracer techniques, perhaps combined with computer modeling, will be the best method to unravel these complex questions.

Discussion

Increases of blood flow to bone clearly show that it is achieved by recruitment, that is to say, resting capillaries become perfused. This is a metabolically driven effect. The pattern of blood flow is therefore nonuniform.[80] For this reason, heterogeneity of flow becomes an overriding consideration in methods to measure blood flow. At this time, microspheres appear to be the benchmark for measurement of blood flow. Different isotopes can be used to label the spheres to allow for serial measurements. If environmental concerns arise and isotopes become less available, other methods may be necessary such as colored or fluoroscent spheres. Bone has a highly reactive vasomotor system as shown by perfusion studies.[81] Serial studies of regional blood flow will become more important as technology advances and whole bone or joint replacements of allograft origin are employed rather than artificial replacement with metal and plastic. Other methods such as laser Doppler flowmetry or positron cameras may be applicable to patients; however, both methods require careful validation.

The effects of fixative devices on regional blood flow is a practical consideration that cannot be ignored by the orthopaedic surgeon. Studies clearly show the adaptability of the circulatory system of bone to the damage of the fracture itself as well as fixation of the fracture. Intramedullary fixation of a long bone experimental fracture clearly shows rods to be the most damaging technique. On the other hand, intramedullary fixation is the treatment of choice for shaft fractures of the femur. It appears that some open fractures of the femur can be managed by intramedullary nailing but not by plate fixation.[82] Even enthusiasts for immediate fixation of open fractures favor external fixation for severe open fractures. Clearly, external fixation does the least harm to regional blood flow of an experimental fracture.[10]

Porosity from plate fixation continues to be investigated. The plate may be criticized unfairly as a cause of postfracture porosity. Every study has compared the plated experimental fracture to unfractured bone, not to a fracture treated by fixation other than a plate. At least at 90 days, in the dog, it has been shown that all forms of fixation cause porosity, because all fractures call out a revascularization process. After the fracture heals, the long bone behaves as an intact bone with plate fixation and is subject to stress protection from the plate. Nonetheless, efforts should be expended to better understand the effect on postfixation porosity of plates, intramedullary rods, and external fixators, each of which currently has a role in fracture treatment.

A better understanding of fluid flow in bone is essential to understanding regeneration of bone and the effects of strain on maintenance of bone mass. A number of mechanisms probably are involved in this process, sometimes referred to as bone response to function or Wolff's law. It is possible that fluid flow beyond the capillary and into the porous architecture of bone is more complex than is presently thought. Furthermore, theory based purely on mechanical factors probably will not explain bone's response to function. Efficient delivery of various growth factors may be the true effector of fracture healing. An interesting factor, endothelial cell stimulating factor, ESAF, is observed to be higher in patients with tibial fractures than in normal controls. Furthermore, less ESAF is released in fractures fixed with intramedullary rods, a form of fixation known to decrease blood flow in the early stages of fracture healing.[83]

Micromotion at the fracture site may play a role in periosteal bone formation.[28] This might be related to published experiments on mediators of mechanical effects on bone remodeling.[65] Logic suggests that any mechanical or stress mechanism ultimately invokes a biologic effect.[29,67,84] Increasingly, the science of fracture healing becomes reductionist in its outlook, an approach common to all of science that may be fruitful or philosophically bleak,[85] depending on one's outlook.

References

1. Nutton RW, Fitzgerald RH Jr, Kelly PJ: Early dynamic bone-imaging as an indicator of osseous blood flow and factors affecting the uptake of ^{99m}Tc hydroxymethylene diphosphonate in healing bone. *J Bone Joint Surg* 1985;67A:763–770.
2. Mori H, Haruyama S, Shinozaki Y, et al: New nonradioactive microspheres and more sensitive x-ray fluorescence to measure regional blood flow. *Am J Physiol* 1992;263:H1946–H1957.
3. Buckberg GD, Luck JC, Payne DB, et al: Some sources of error in measuring regional blood flow with radioactive microspheres. *J Appl Phys* 1971;31:598–604.
4. Hales JRS: Radioactive microsphere techniques for studies of the circulation. *Clin Exp Pharm Phys [Suppl]* 1974;1:31–46.
5. Li G, Bronk JT, Kelly PJ: Canine bone blood flow estimated with microspheres. *J Orthop Res* 1989;7:61–67.
6. Morris MA, Kelly PJ: Use of tracer microspheres to measure bone blood flow in conscious dogs. *Calcif Tissue Int* 1980;32:69–76.
7. Swiontkowski MF: Techniques for quantitating bone blood flow. Workshop given at the Orthopaedic Research Society, March 6, 1991.
8. Ashcroft GP, Evans NTS, Roeda D, et al: Measurement of blood flow in tibial fracture patients using positron emission tomography. *J Bone Joint Surg* 1992;74B:673–677.
9. VanDyke D, Anger HO, Yano Y, et al: Bone blood flow shown with F^{18} and the positron camera. *Am J Physiol* 1965;209:65–70.
10. Smith SR, Bronk JT, Kelly PJ: Effect of fracture fixation on cortical bone blood flow. *J Orthop Res* 1990;8:471–478.
11. Daum WJ, Simmons DJ, Calhoun JH, et al: Regional alterations in long bone produced by internal fixation devices: Part I. ^{85}Sr clearance. *J Orthop Trauma* 1988;2:241–244.
12. Akeson WH, Woo SL-Y, Rutherford L, et al: The effects of rigidity of internal fixation plates on long bone remodeling: A biomechanical and quantitative histological study. *Acta Orthop Scand* 1976;47:241–249.
13. Mathews RS, Cooper EM: Cortical bone atrophy secondary to compression plate fixation: A clinical and pathophysiologic study. *Surg Forum* 1976;27:523–524.
14. Slatis P, Karaharju E, Holstrom T, et al: Structural changes in intact tubular bone after application of rigid plates with and without compression. *J Bone Joint Surg* 1978;60A:516–522.

15. Uhthoff HK, Finnegan M: The effects of metal plates on post-traumatic remodelling and bone mass. *J Bone Joint Surg* 1983;65B:66–71.
16. Uhthoff HK, Foux A, Yeadon A, et al: Two processes of bone remodeling in plated intact femora: An experimental study in dogs. *J Orthop Res* 1993;11:78–91.
17. Gunst MA: Interference with blood supply through plating of intact bone, in Uhthoff HK (ed): *Current Concepts of Internal Fixation of Fractures: Symposium on Current Concepts of Internal Fixation*. Berlin, Springer-Verlag, 1980, pp 268–276.
18. Jacobs RR, Rahn BA, Perren SM: Effects of plates on cortical bone perfusion. *J Trauma* 1981;21:91–95.
19. Lippuner K, Vogel R, Tepic S, et al: Effect of animal species and age on plate-induced vascular damage in cortical bone. *Arch Orthop Trauma Surg* 1992;111: 78–84.
20. Xu XX, Zhao YH, Liu JG: Blood supply and structural changes of canine intact tibia following plate fixation with different rigidities. *Chinese Med J* 1991;104: 1018–1021.
21. Starling EH: On the absorption of fluids from the connective tissue spaces. *J Physiol* 1895;19:312–326.
22. Simmons DJ, Daum WJ, Calhoun JH: Regional alterations in long bone ^{85}Sr clearance produced by internal fixation devices: Part II. Histomorphometry. *J Orthop Trauma* 1988;2:245–249.
23. Steinhaus AH, Hoyt LA, Rice HA: Studies in physiology of exercise: Effects of running and swimming on organ weights of growing dogs. *Am J Physiol* 1932;99: 512–520.
24. McInnis JC, Robb RA, Kelly PJ: The relationship of bone blood flow, bone tracer deposition, and endosteal new bone formation. *J Lab Clin Med* 1980;96:511–522.
25. Meadows TH, Bronk JT, Chao EYS, et al: Effect of weight-bearing on healing of cortical defects in the canine tibia. *J Bone Joint Surg* 1990;72A:1074–1080.
26. Bronk JT, Meadows TH, Kelly PJ: The relationship of increased capillary filtration and bone formation. *Clin Orthop* 1993;293:338–345.
27. O'Sullivan M, Bronk JT, Chao EYS, et al: Experimental study of the effect of weight bearing on fracture healing in the canine tibia. *Clin Orthop* 1994;302:273–283.
28. Goodship AE, Kenwright J: The influence of induced micromovement upon the healing of experimental tibial fractures. *J Bone Joint Surg* 1985;67B:650–655.
29. Davidson RM, Tatakis DW, Auerbach AL: Multiple forms of mechanosensitive ion channels in osteoblast-like cells. *Pflugers Arch* 1990;416:646–651.
30. Brookes M: The vascular architecture of tubular bone in the rat. *Anat Rec* 1958; 132:25–47.
31. de Marneffe R: Recherches morphologiques et expérimentales sur la vascularisation osseuse. *Acta Chir Belgica*. 1951, pp 469–488; 568–599; 681–704.
32. Trueta J, Morgan JD: The vascular contribution to osteogenesis: I. Studies by the injection method. *J Bone Joint Surg* 1960;42B:97–109.
33. Langer K: Ueber das gefassystem der rohrenknocken mit beitragen zur kennt niss des baues und der entwicklund des knockenge webes, Denkschr. Akad wissu, mathemat-naturn-schaft. *Classe Wien* 1876;36:40.
34. Lopez-Curto JA, Bassingthwaighte JB, Kelly PJ: Anatomy of the microvasculature of the tibial diaphysis of the adult dog. *J Bone Joint Surg* 1980;62A:1362–1369.
35. Kelly PJ: Pathways for transport in bone, in Shephard JF, Abboud FM (eds): *Handbook of Physiology*. Baltimore, MD, Williams & Wilkins, 1983, pp 371–396.
36. Montgomery RJ, Sutker BD, Bronk JT, et al: Interstitial fluid flow in cortical bone. *Microvasc Res* 1988;35:295–307.
37. Cooper RR, Milgram JW, Robinson RA: Morphology of the osteon: An electron microscopic study. *J Bone Joint Surg* 1966;48A:1239–1271.
38. Hughes S, Blount M: The structure of capillaries in cortical bone (Abstract). *Ann Royal College Surg Engl* 1979;61:312.
39. Robinson RA, Elliott SR: The water content of bone: I. The mass of water, inorganic crystals, organic matrix, and "CO_2 space" components in a unit volume of dog bone. *J Bone Joint Surg* 1957;39A:167–188.

40. Morris MA, Lopez-Curto JA, Hughes SPF, et al: Fluid spaces in canine bone and marrow. *Microvasc Res* 1982;23:188–200.

41. Pinto MR, Kelly PJ: Age-related changes in bone in the dog: Fluid spaces and their potassium content. *J Orthop Res* 1984;2:2–7.

42. Bloom JD, Fitzgerald RH Jr, Washington JA II, et al: The transcapillary passage and interstitial fluid concentration of penicillin in canine bone. *J Bone Joint Surg* 1980;62A:1168–1175.

43. Williams EA, Fitzgerald RH Jr, Kelly PJ: Microcirculation of bone, in Mortillaro NA (ed): *The Physiology and Pharmacology of the Microcirculation.* New York, NY, Academic Press, 1984, vol 2, pp 267–323.

44. Talmage RV, Meyer RA Jr: Physiological role of parathyroid hormone, in Greep RO, Astwood EB (eds): *Handbook of Physiology.* Washington, DC, American Physiological Society, 1976, sect 7, vol VII, pp 343–351.

45. Maltby B, Lemon GJ, Bassingthwaighte JB, Kelly PJ: Exchange of potassium and strontium in adult bone. *Am J Physiol* 1982;242:H705–H712.

46. Brindley GW, Williams EA, Bronk JT, et al: Parathyroid hormone effects on skeletal exchangeable calcium and bone blood flow. *Am J Physiol* 1988;255:H94–H100.

47. Pinto MR, Gorski JP, Penniston JT, et al: Age-related changes in composition and Ca^{2+} binding capacity of canine cortical bone extracts. *Am J Physiol* 1988; 255:H101–H110.

48. Dillaman RM: Movement of ferritin in the 2-day-old chick femur. *Anat Rec* 1984; 209:445–453.

49. Dillaman RM, Roer RD, Gay DM: Fluid movement in bone: Theoretical and empirical. *J Biomech* 1991;24:163–177.

50. Doty SB, Schofield BH: Metabolic and structural changes within osteocytes of rat bone, in Talmage RV, Munson PL (eds): *Calcium, Parathyroid Hormone, and the Calcitonins; Proceedings of the Fourth Parathyroid Conference. Chapel Hill, NC, March 15–19, 1971.* Amsterdam, Excerpta Medica, 1972, pp 353–364.

51. Lorenz M, Plenk H Jr: A perfusion method of incubation to demonstrate horseradish peroxidase in bone. *Histochemistry* 1977;53:257–263.

52. Seliger WG: Tissue fluid movement in compact bone. *Anatomic Rec* 1970;166:247–255.

53. Li G, Bronk JT, An KN, Kelly PJ: Permeability of cortical bone of canine tibiae. *Microvasc Res* 1987;34:302–310.

54. Casley-Smith JR, Földi-Börcsök E, Földi M: The prelymphatic pathways of the brain as revealed by cervical lymphatic obstruction and the passage of particles. *Br J Exp Pathol* 1976;57:179–188.

55. Landis EM, Pappenheimer JR: Exchange of substances through the capillary walls, in Hamilton WF, Dow P (eds): *Handbook of Physiology.* Washington DC, American Physiological Society, 1963, sect 2, vol II, pp 961–1034.

56. Wilkes CH, Visscher MB: Some physiological aspects of bone marrow pressure. *J Bone Joint Surg* 1975;57A:49–57.

57. Bert JL, Pinder KL: Lymph flow characteristics and microvascular exchange: An analog computer simulation. *Lymphology* 1982;15:156–162.

58. Bert JL, Bowen BD, Reed RK: Microvascular exchange and interstitial volume regulation in the rat: Model validation. *Am J Physiol* 1988;254:H384–H399.

59. Cochran GVB, Pawluk RJ, Bassett CAL: Electromechanical characteristics of bone under physiologic moisture conditions. *Clin Orthop* 1968;58:249–270.

60. Otter MW, Palmieri VR, Cochran GVB: Transcortical streaming potentials are generated by circulatory pressure gradients in living canine tibia. *J Orthop Res* 1990;8:119–126.

61. Otter MW, Bronk JT, Wu DD, et al: Pulsatile pressurization of an inflatable cuff produces pulsatile streaming potentials in living canine tibiae. Presented at Annual BRAGS meeting, Scottsdale, AZ, September 1991.

62. Eriksson C: Streaming potentials and other water-dependent effects in mineralized tissues. *Ann NY Acad Sci* 1974;238:321–338.

63. Salzstein RA, Pollack SR: Electromechanical potentials in cortical bone: II. Experimental analysis. *J Biomech* 1987;20:271–280.

64. Salzstein RA, Pollack SR, Mak AFT, et al: Electromechanical potentials in cortical bone: I. A continuum approach. *J Biomech* 1987;20:261–270.
65. Rodan GA, Bourret LA, Harvey A, et al: Cyclic AMP and cyclic GMP: Mediators of mechanical effects on bone remodeling. *Science* 1975;189:467–469.
66. Harell A, Dekel S, Binderman I: Biochemical effect of mechanical stress on cultured bone cells. *Calcif Tissue Res* 1977;22:202–207.
67. Reich KM, Gay CV, Frangos JA: Fluid shear stress as a mediator of osteoblast cyclic adenosine monophosphate production. *J Cell Phys* 1990;143:100–104.
68. Johnson MW: Behavior of fluid in stressed bone and cellular stimulation. *Calcif Tissue Int* 1984;36:S72–S76.
69. Keck SW, Kelly PJ: The effect of venous stasis on intraosseous pressure and longitudinal bone growth in the dog. *J Bone Joint Surg* 1965;47A:539–544.
70. Kelly PJ, Bronk JT: Venous pressure and bone formation. *Microvasc Res* 1990;39:364–375.
71. Kelly PJ, Janes JM, Peterson LFA: The effect of arteriovenous fistulae on the vascular pattern of the femora of immature dogs: A microangiographic study. *J Bone Joint Surg* 1959;41A:1101–1108.
72. Kruse RL, Kelly PJ: Acceleration of fracture healing distal to a venous tourniquet. *J Bone Joint Surg* 1974;56A:730–739.
73. Kelly PJ, Bronk JT: Effect of a tourniquet or Aircast brace on immature bone fluid. Presented at Second Scientific Meeting of the International Society for Fracture Repair, September 6–8, 1990, Rochester, MN and Minneapolis, MN.
74. Dale PA, Bronk JT, O'Sullivan ME, et al: A new concept in fracture immobilization: The application of a pressurized brace. *Clin Orthop* 1993;295:264–269.
75. Lang SB, Stipanich N, Soremi EA: Diffusion of glucose in stressed and unstressed canine femur in vitro. *Ann NY Acad Sci* 1974;238:139–148.
76. McCarthy ID, Bronk JT, Kelly PJ: The measurement of interstitial fluid flow in cortical bone. *FASEB* 1990;4:A1262.
77. Reed RK, Johansen S, Noddeland H: Turnover rate of interstitial albumin in rat skin and skeletal muscle. Effects of limb movement and motor activity. *Acta Physiol Scand* 1985;125:711–718.
78. Owen M, Howlett CR, Triffitt JT: Movement of ^{125}I albumin and ^{125}I polyvinylpyrrolidone through bone tissue fluid. *Calcif Tiss Res* 1977;23:103–112.
79. Elk JR, Drake RE, Williams JP, et al: Lymphatic function in the liver after hepatic venous pressure elevation. *Am J Physiol* 1988;254:G748–G752.
80. Hughes SPF, Lemon GJ, Davies DR, et al: Extraction of minerals after experimental fractures of the tibia in dogs. *J Bone Joint Surg* 1979;61A:857–866.
81. Driessens M, Vanhoutte PM: Vascular reactivity of the isolated tibia of the dog. *Am J Physiol* 1979;236:H904-H908.
82. Brumback RJ, Ellison PS, Poka A, et al: Intramedullary nailing of open fractures of the femoral shaft. *J Bone Joint Surg* 1989;71A:1324–1331.
83. Wallace AL, McLaughlin B, Weiss JB, et al: Increased endothelial cell stimulating angiogenesis factor in patients with tibial fractures. *Injury* 1991;22:375–376.
84. Guggino SE, Lajeunesse D, Wagner JA, et al: Bone remodeling signaled by dihydropyridine- and phenylalkalymine-sensitive calcium channel. *Proc Natl Acad Sci USA* 1989;86:2957–2960.
85. Davies P: The holy grail of physics. New York Times Book Review, March 7, 1993, pp 11–12.

Chapter 13

Angiogenesis and Basic Fibroblast Growth Factor During Wound Healing

Harold Brem, MD
Judah Folkman, MD

Introduction

Angiogenic growth factors stimulate angiogenesis and potentiate normal wound healing. Specific growth factors can reverse wound healing deficiencies that occur in pathologic conditions, such as diabetes, as well as those that result from the use of pharmacologic agents, such as chemotherapeutic agents and steroids. Growth factors accelerate normal wound healing by stimulating matrix production, potentiating angiogenesis including granulation tissue formation, increasing tensile strength, accelerating epithelialization and increasing the rate of contraction. The use of growth factors for the treatment of human wounds, eg, wound pharmacology,[1] is now an accepted modality.[2-4] However, the most efficacious applications of growth factors to wounds remain to be elucidated.

Wound healing occurs in response to a disruption in either the epithelium or the basement membrane. The healing response depends on the type of wound. For example, in a full-thickness wound, epithelialization, contraction, and formation of granulation tissue become the predominant responses; whereas in a linear surgical wound, ie, healing by primary intention, contraction plays a minimal role. The physiology of the type of wound being evaluated must be addressed because each growth factor may be therapeutically beneficial for only specific types of wounds.

Once growth factors and cytokines have been released into a wound, multiple aspects of wound healing occur simultaneously. Furthermore, similarly to other important physiologic responses, eg, coagulation, many of the elicited processes in the wound are redundant. There are multiple stimuli for angiogenesis in the first few hours after a wound is created, but it is usually 3 to 4 days before actual vessel formation can be visualized. Angiogenesis maintains a critical role in the healing response.[5-12]

The cellular response to a wound (Fig. 1) merits review because many of the cells recruited into the wound synthesize molecules, such as chemoattractants and mitogens, that propagate the angiogenic cascade and help explain the redundancy of wound healing. Platelets activated by thrombin and exposed collagen begin to accumulate almost immediately after a wound is created, and they potentiate local coagulation. They also release multiple potent chemoattractants that help initiate the wound-healing cascade.[13] One of the growth factors that platelets synthesize is transforming growth factor-beta (TGF-β), which is a potent chemoattractant for macrophages at femtomolar concentra-

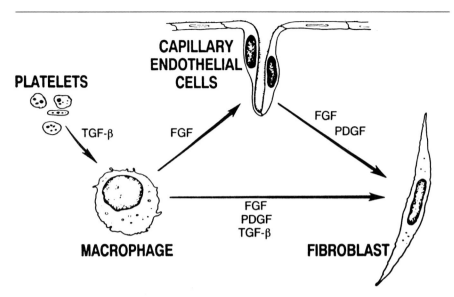

Fig. 1 Early events in wound healing. TGF-β = transforming growth factor-beta; FGF = fibroblast growth factor; and PDGF = platelet-derived growth factor.

tions.[14,15] Within 24 hours after wound creation, granulocytes replace platelets as the predominant cell type. Neutrophils and monocytes adhere to the endothelium adjacent to the site of injury. Lymphocytes emigrate from the postcapillary venule in an area termed the high-end venule.[16] Macrophages, which are in high concentration approximately 2 days after wounding, synthesize and release many important factors that stimulate angiogenesis and propagate the wound-healing response.[17,18]

The presence of macrophages in the wound appears to be an absolute requirement for normal healing to occur.[19] Macrophages have multiple effects in the wound, including (1) debridement;[20] (2) release of growth factors that are chemotactic, mitogenic,[10–12,17,18] and angiogenic;[21] and (3) stimulation of mesenchymal cells.[19] Macrophage depletion results in delays in wound debridement, deficient granulation-tissue formation, and reduced collagen accumulation.[19]

Angiogenesis is a major part of granulation-tissue formation. As early as day 3 after wound formation, blood vessels begin to form. Over the next several days, endothelial cells and fibroblasts enter the wound, followed by capillary formation and then collagen formation. During wound healing, angiogenesis occurs as part of the physiologic response to injury. In normal physiologic wound healing, angiogenesis is well-controlled; whereas, in many pathologic conditions, angiogenesis is not well regulated. Pathologic and, often, unregulated angiogenesis occur during many disease states,[21–26] eg, primary tumors, metastatic tumors, rheumatoid arthritis, retinopathy, and psoriasis. In many experimental studies[27–35] and in some clinical trials,[36–38] certain disease states are currently being treated successfully by angiogenesis inhibitors. Some of these angiogenesis inhibitors suppress wound healing.[6,39] Conversely, angiogenic growth factors significantly potentiate wound healing.[40–48] Further investigation into the contribution of the angiogenic response in wound healing is necessary.

Assays of Angiogenesis

In vitro assays are useful for the study of specific effects of a growth factor on endothelial cells. Capillary endothelial cells were first carried in long-term culture by Folkman.[49,50] The proliferative or inhibitory effect on endothelial cells of a specific growth factor (basic fibroblast growth factor [bFGF][51–56] or TGF-β,[56] respectively) can be studied using the capillary endothelial cell assay.[51–56] The angiogenic component of wound healing can be isolated and studied in a variety of in vivo models.

The rabbit[57–59] or rat cornea model,[60] provides a method for quantifying the rate of new vessel formation or inhibition. The cornea is normally avascular and, therefore, new vessel growth caused by a putative angiogenesis stimulator can be measured precisely. Similarly, a putative angiogenesis inhibitor can be assayed after cornea neovasularization is induced by a tumor,[58] endotoxin,[59] or bFGF.[60] The benefit of this model is that blood-vessel growth can be accurately quantitated. The disadvantage is the expense of rabbits and the necessity of ocular surgery.

The chick chorioallantoic membrane (CAM) assay to study angiogenesis inhibitors and stimulators is readily available, reproducible, inexpensive, and usable in large numbers.[61–65] This assay is more specific for inhibitors than stimulators because, in a background of growing vascular membrane, visualization of the absence of blood vessels is more reliable than quantification of new blood vessels. The usefulness of the CAM is based on the ability to visualize blood-vessel formation and inhibition directly.

Other animal models that have been used to study angiogenesis include the rabbit ear and the hamster cheek pouch. These are useful for studying a simple positive or negative response of a putative angiogenic modulator, but they are not quantitative. In another model, wound-healing angiogenesis is quantified by assaying the amount of radioactively labeled xenon that passes through a sponge implanted in rodents in a fixed time period.[66]

Quantitative confirmation of angiogenesis also can be obtained by intravascular injections (eg, india ink, latex, and microspheres) or specific stains such as factor VIII. Factor VIII is a highly specific marker for tumor angiogenesis in human tissue;[67,68] however, its use in wounds has not been well defined. It is our observation that the currently available animal antibodies to factor VIII are not as reliable as the human antibody to factor VIII. Laminin, fibronectin, and lectin are ubiquitous basement-membrane components that have been shown to be excellent markers for developing capillaries in normal tissue.[31] These immunohistochemical techniques can be effectively used to study angiogenesis in wound healing.

These models and assays are useful in screening for a putative angiogenic modulatory effect. If any or any combination of these studies demonstrate a significant effect, further evaluation should be performed in an in vivo wound-healing model.

Basic Fibroblast Growth Factor

When a wound is created, angiogenic molecules are released by many of the cells involved in wound healing, including macrophages,[69,70] platelets,[13] endothelial cells,[71,72] and keratinocytes.[73] We will review the biology of FGF and its role in wound healing.

FGFs consist of seven structurally homologous polypeptides found in many cell types and in most tissues.[74,75] Their similarity in structure is the primary component that places these polypeptides in one family.[8,10,74,75] Most of these proteins have different functions. Both acidic and basic FGF are very potent angiogenic proteins. We will limit this review to the applications of bFGF because it is currently the most widely available commercially and most studied of the FGF family. There is little doubt that other members of the FGF family, such as acidic FGF (aFGF, FGF-1) and keratinocyte growth factor (FGF-7), also have important roles in wound healing. FGF-6 may have exciting implications for wound healing because it has been derived from epithelial tissue and mediates epithelial cell proliferation.[76]

Basic FGF has a molecular weight of approximately 18,000 and binds heparin with a high affinity.[77,78] Basic FGF has been purified from a variety of tissues, including cartilage[42] and bone,[79] that often are involved in regeneration and wound healing. The predominant cells involved in wound healing that synthesize bFGF are macrophages[69] and endothelial cells.[80]

FGF is a potent mitogen for many of the constituent cells of a healing wound, eg, endothelial cells,[80] fibroblasts,[81] keratinocytes,[72] vascular smooth muscle cells,[82] and myoblasts.[83] On some cells, such as endothelial cells, bFGF functions as an autocrine growth factor, whereas on other cells it functions as a paracrine growth factor.[80,81]

In vitro, bFGF not only is a potent stimulator of capillary endothelial cells (in nanogram concentrations), but also stimulates capillary tubular networks.[84] These in vitro findings are consistent with investigations demonstrating the ability of bFGF in vivo, eg, in the cornea and in the chick chorioallantoic membrane models.[55,60] Davidson and associates[42] demonstrated that administration of bFGF to a wound results in a significant increase in the amount of angiogenesis in that wound. Furthermore, topical bFGF applied to a healing wound has been demonstrated to increase significantly the influx of capillary endothelial cells and formation of new blood vessels,[44,47] both of which have been associated with a significant acceleration of the healing response. Furthermore, exogenous bFGF is a more potent stimulator of angiogenesis than are most other growth factors assayed.[46] Thus, the role of FGF in wound healing is partially explained by its potent ability to stimulate mitogenesis and chemotaxis for fibroblasts and endothelial cells as well as directly stimulating angiogenesis.

In contrast to platelet-derived growth factor and TGF-β, FGF is not normally secreted.[85] However, bFGF is released into the subendothelial cell extracellular matrix.[86] FGF's mechanism of release during traumatic (eg, surgical) wound healing may be analogous to that in corneal wounding. When Descemet's membrane, the cornea's equivalent to the extracellular matrix, is injured, bFGF is released.[87] Data from those experiments and others suggest that bFGF may be released in response to injury of the basement membrane.[87] It is also possible that bFGF in a wound may acquire a unique form that allows it to be secreted. A secreted form of bFGF has been purified from a fibrosarcoma tumor,[51] but not from a healing wound.

In order to determine whether bFGF maintained a critical role in a healing wound, Broadley and associates[88] administered blocking antibodies to bFGF in a healing wound. They found that locally administered blocking antibodies to bFGF significantly decreased the wound healing response and decreased DNA proliferation, protein content, collagen content, and angiogenesis in these wounds.[88] These experiments demonstrated the importance of bFGF in wound healing, and this "causality" experiment demonstrated that a growth factor is necessary for normal wound healing to occur.

Role of bFGF in Accelerating Nonpathologic Wound Healing

Basic FGF accelerates normal wound healing by increasing the number of fibroblasts, endothelial cells, and monocytes released into the wound and by increasing angiogenic response. Basic FGF accelerates the healing response in many types of wounds, as can be seen in the following examples. The administration of topical bFGF to linear rat incisions on postwounding day 3 resulted in significant increases in tensile strength.[89] Basic FGF accelerated epithelialization of porcine partial-thickness wounds;[44] accelerated tympanic membrane closure;[90] resulted in significant neuronal regeneration after transection of the associated nerves;[91,92] and increased angiogenesis and accelerated epithelialization in a dermal ulcer model.[93]

In most types of wound healing in an unimpaired host, bFGF is not necessary to accelerate healing. However, when the wound results in significant morbidity, for example, in peptic ulcer disease, an angiogenic response is required for adequate healing. Oral bFGF has been shown to be more effective, on a molar basis, than any other agent, including cimetidine, in stimulating angiogenesis, accelerating healing, and preventing perforation of these ulcers in rats. It originally was shown that bFGF was inactivated by the acid milieu of the stomach and by proteolytic enzymes. However, bFGF becomes acid stable when its structure is modified by the replacement of two cysteines with serines; this form of bFGF is termed bFGF-CS23.[94] Alternatively, for duodenal ulcers bFGF may be administered with oral sucralfate, which binds bFGF and protects it from acid degradation. Taken together, these data suggest that peptic ulcer healing depends on the concentration of active bFGF and the amount of angiogenesis in the wound or ulcer.[9,47]

We have demonstrated that concentrations of bFGF reach a peak 12 to 14 days after full-thickness wounds are created.[95] In these wounds, the amount of bFGF does not begin to rise significantly until 8 days after wounding, suggesting that the bFGF was derived from cells that had been recruited into the wound, ie, from endothelium and/or fibroblasts. It is possible that the bFGF originally synthesized by macrophages in the wound stimulates endothelial cells to migrate and proliferate. Once these new blood vessels have grown in the wound, they may release additional bFGF, which serves to stimulate chemotaxis and proliferation of additional endothelial cells and fibroblasts. On approximately day 8, when the number of fibroblasts and endothelial cells in the wound is maximal, we found a rapid two- to fourfold increase in the amount of bFGF in the wound. On the twelfth day after wounding, even in a wound that is fully contracted, a high density of blood vessels occurs, which correlates with the peak occurrence of bFGF in the wound.

Role of bFGF in Accelerating Pathologic Wound Healing

The administration of exogenous bFGF in most types of wounds is not necessary because there already are multiple redundant steps of wound healing. However, in certain clinical conditions, impaired wound healing contributes to a significant amount of morbidity to patients. Some of these conditions can be correlated with an impaired angiogenic response in the healing wound. In experimental rodent models with impaired healing, topical application of bFGF accelerated healing in the following ways.

Topical bFGF dramatically accelerated wound healing contraction in mice treated with systemic steroids.[96] The rate of wound healing in diabetic rats with linear incisions was accelerated by topical bFGF.[97] The concentration of angiogenesis and healing was significantly increased in genetically diabetic mice.[43,96,98] The rate of contraction in full-thickness wounds, the healing of which was impaired by bacterial contamination, was accelerated significantly when topical bFGF was applied. This effect was not secondary to any bactericidal effect of bFGF; the bacteria counts did not change in any of the groups.[99] In genetically obese mice, full-thickness wounds that had not been treated remained 100% uncontracted with virtually no healing response 12 days after a wound was made. In comparison, the wound healing deficiency was completely reversed in topical bFGF-treated wounds in these obese mice, such that 90% of the wound had contracted 12 days after a wound was made.[96]

These experimental studies have been translated into clinical efficacy. It has now been shown, in a randomized, placebo-controlled, human trial, that recombinant bFGF applied topically to the wounds of patients with chronic pressure sores has the following effects: (1) there is a marked increase in fibroblasts and capillaries in the wounds and (2) a significantly higher percentage of patients achieve 70% volume reduction of their wounds.[4]

In the future it may be possible to deliver growth factors to wounds in higher concentration over prolonged periods by use of slow release polymers. The technology for these polymers has already been developed for treatment of some solid tumors.[100]

Acknowledgment

This work was supported in part by grants to Dr. Brem from the Association for Academic Surgery and the Leon Hirsch Fellowship.

References

1. Folkman J: Editorial: Is there a field of wound pharmacology? *Ann Surg* 1992;215:1–2.
2. Brown GL, Curtsinger L, Jurkiewicz MJ, et al: Stimulation of healing of chronic wounds by epidermal growth factor. *Plast Reconstr Surg* 1991;88:189–194.
3. Knighton DR, Ciresi K, Fiegel VD, et al: Stimulation of repair in chronic, non-healing, cutaneous ulcers using platelet-derived wound healing formula. *Surg Gynecol Obstet* 1990;170:56–60.
4. Robson MC, Phillips LG, Lawrence WT, et al: The safety and effect of topically applied recombinant basic fibroblast growth factor on the healing of chronic pressure sores. *Ann Surg* 1992;216:401–408.
5. Arnold F, West DC: Angiogenesis in wound healing. *Pharmacol Ther* 1991;52:407–422.
6. Brem H, Tsakayannis D, Folkman J: Time dependent suppression of wound healing with the angiogenesis inhibitor, AGM 1470. *J Cell Biol* 1991;115:403a.
7. D'Amore PA, Klagsbrun M: Angiogenesis: Factors and mechanisms, in Sirica AE (ed): *The Pathobiology of Neoplasia*. New York, NY, Plenum Press, 1989, pp 513–531.
8. Folkman J: The angiogenic activity of FGF and its possible clinical applications, in Sara VR, Hall K, Löw H (eds): *Growth Factors: From Genes to Clinical Application*. Karolinska Institute Nobel Conference Series. New York, NY, Raven Press, 1990, pp 201–216.
9. Folkman J, Szabo S, Stovroff M, et al: Duodenal ulcer: Discovery of a new mechanism and development of angiogenic therapy that accelerates healing. *Ann Surg* 1991;214:414–427.

10. Folkman J, Brem H: Angiogenesis and inflammation, in Gallin JI, Goldstein IM, Snyderman R (eds): *Inflammation: Basic Principles and Clinical Correlates*, ed 2. New York, NY, Raven Press, 1992, pp 821–839.
11. Hunt TK, Knighton DR, Thakral KK, et al: Studies on inflammation and wound-healing: Angiogenesis and collagen synthesis stimulated in vivo by resident and activated wound macrophages. *Surgery* 1984;96:48–54.
12. Whalen GF, Zetter BR: Angiogenesis, in Cohen IK, Diegelmann RF, Lindblad WJ (eds): *Wound Healing: Biochemical and Clinical Aspects*. Philadelphia, PA, WB Saunders, 1992, pp 77–95.
13. Heimark RL, Twardzik DR, Schwartz SM: Inhibition of endothelial regeneration by type-beta transforming growth factor from platelets. *Science* 1986;233:1078–1080.
14. Wahl SM, Hunt DA, Wakefield LM, et al: Transforming growth factor type beta induces monocyte chemotaxis and growth factor production. *Proc Natl Acad Sci USA* 1987;84:5788–5792.
15. Wahl LM, Wahl SM: Inflammation, in Cohen IK, Diegelmann RF, Lindblad WJ (eds): *Wound Healing: Biochemical and Clinical Aspects*. Philadelphia, PA, WB Saunders, 1992, pp 40–62.
16. Harlan JM: Leukocyte-endothelial interactions. *Blood* 1985;65:513–525.
17. Cai JP, Harris B, Falanga V, et al: Recruitment of mononuclear cells into wounded skin: Mechanism and modulation. *Prog Clin Biol Res* 1991;365:243–256.
18. Nathan CF: Secretory products of macrophages. *J Clin Invest* 1987;79:319–326.
19. Leibovich SJ, Ross R: The role of the macrophage in wound repair: A study with hydrocortisone and antimacrophage serum. *Am J Pathol* 1975;78:71–100.
20. Wornon II, Buchman SR: Bone and cartilaginous tissue, in Cohen IK, Diegelmann RF, Lindblad WJ (eds): *Wound Healing: Biochemical and Clinical Aspects*. Philadelphia, PA, WB Saunders, 1992, pp 356–383.
21. Knighton DR, Hunt TK, Scheuenstuhl H, et al: Oxygen tension regulates the expression of angiogenesis factor by macrophages. *Science* 1983;221:1283–1285.
22. Folkman J: The role of angiogenesis in tumor growth. *Semin Cancer Biol* 1992;3:65–71.
23. Brem H, Tamargo RJ, Guerin C, et al: Brain tumor angiogenesis, in Kornblith PL, Walker MD (eds): *Advances in Neuro-Oncology*. Mount Kisco, NY, Futura Publishing Co, 1988, pp 89–108.
24. Folkman J: Editorial: What is the evidence that tumors are angiogenesis dependent? *J Natl Cancer Inst* 1990;82:4-6.
25. Klagsbrun M, Folkman J: Angiogenesis, in Sporn MB, Roberts AB (eds): Series: Handbook of Experimental Pharmacology, in *Peptide Growth Factors and Their Receptors, Part II*. Berlin, Springer-Verlag, 1990, vol 95, pp 549–586.
26. Klagsbrun M, D'Amore PA: Regulators of angiogenesis. *Annu Rev Physiol* 1991;53:217–239.
27. Brem H, Folkman J: Analysis of experimental antiangiogenic therapy. *J Ped Surg* 1993;28:445–451.
28. Brem H, Gresser I, Grosfeld J, et al: The combination of antiangiogenic agents to inhibit primary tumor growth and metastasis. *J Ped Surg* 1993;28:1253–1257.
29. Brem SS, Zagzag D, Tsanaclis AM, et al: Inhibition of angiogenesis and tumor growth in the brain: Suppression of endothelial cell turnover by penicillamine and the depletion of copper, an angiogenic cofactor. *Am J Pathol* 1990;137:1121–1142.
30. Brem H, Ingber D, Blood CH, et al: Suppression of tumor metastasis by angiogenesis inhibition. *Surg Forum* 1991;42:439–441.
31. Folkman J: Editorial: Successful treatment of an angiogenic disease. *N Engl J Med* 1989;320:1211–1212.
32. Ingber D, Fujita T, Kishimoto S, et al: Synthetic analogues of fumagillin that inhibit angiogenesis and suppress tumour growth. *Nature* 1990;348:555–557.
33. Ingber D, Folkman J: Inhibition of angiogenesis through modulation of collagen metabolism. *Lab Invest* 1988;59:44–51.

34. Miller JW, Stinson WG, Folkman J: Regression of experimental iris neovascularization with systemic alpha-interferon. *Ophthal* 1993;100:9–14.
35. Moses MA, Langer R: A metalloproteinase inhibitor as an inhibitor of neovascularization. *J Cell Biochem* 1991;47:230–235.
36. Maragoudakis ME, Missirlis E, Sarmonika M, et al: Basement membrane biosynthesis as a target to tumor therapy. *J Pharmacol Exp Ther* 1990;252:753–757.
37. Tamargo RJ, Leong KW, Brem H: Growth inhibition of the 9L glioma using polymers to release heparin and cortisone acetate. *J Neurooncol* 1990;9:131–138.
38. Tamargo RJ, Bok RA, Brem H: Angiogenesis inhibition by minocycline. *Cancer Res* 1991;51:672–675.
39. Stout AJ, Gresser I, Thompson WD: Inhibition of wound healing in mice by local interferon alpha/beta injection. *Inter J Exp Pathol* 1993;74:79–85.
40. Broadley KN, Aquino AM, Hicks B, et al: Growth factors bFGF and TGF-beta accelerate the rate of wound repair in normal and in diabetic rats. *Int J Tiss Reac* 1988;10:345–353.
41. Connolly DT, Heuvelman DM, Nelson R, et al: Tumor vascular permeability factor stimulates endothelial cell growth and angiogenesis. *J Clin Invest* 1989;84:1470–1478.
42. Davidson JM, Klagsbrun M, Hill KE, et al: Accelerated wound repair, cell proliferation, and collagen accumulation are produced by a cartilage-derived growth factor. *J Cell Biol* 1985;100:1219–1227.
43. Greenhalgh DG, Sprugel KH, Murray MJ, et al: PDGF and FGF stimulate wound healing in the genetically diabetic mouse. *Am J Pathol* 1990;136:1235–1246.
44. Hebda PA, Klingbeil CK, Abraham JA, et al: Basic fibroblast growth factor stimulation of epidermal wound healing in pigs. *J Invest Dermatol* 1990;95:626–631.
45. Mustoe TA, Purdy J, Gramates P, et al: Reversal of impaired wound healing in irradiated rats by platelet-derived growth factor-BB. *Am J Surg* 1989;158:345–350.
46. Sprugel KH, McPherson JM, Clowes AW, et al: Effects of growth factors in vivo: I. Cell ingrowth into porous subcutaneous chambers. *Am J Pathol* 1987;129:601–613.
47. Szabo S, Vattay P, Scarbrough E, et al: Role of vascular factors, including angiogenesis, in the mechanisms of action of sucralfate. *Am J Med* 1991;91:158S–160S.
48. Folkman J, Klagsbrun M: Angiogenic factors. *Science* 1987;235:442–447.
49. Folkman J, Haudenschild CC, Zetter BR: Long-term culture of capillary endothelial cells. *Proc Natl Acad Sci USA* 1979;76:5217–5221.
50. Folkman J, Haudenschild C: Angiogenesis in vitro. *Nature* 1980;288:551–556.
51. Kandel J, Bossy-Wetzel E, Radvanyi F, et al: Neovascularization is associated with a switch to the export of bFGF in the multistep development of fibrosarcoma. *Cell* 1991;66:1095–1104.
52. Ingber DE, Folkman J: Mechanochemical switching between growth and differentiation during fibroblast growth factor-stimulated angiogenesis in vitro: Role of extracellular matrix. *J Cell Biol* 1989;109:317–330.
53. Sharpe RJ, Arndt KA, Bauer SI, et al: Cyclosporine inhibits basic fibroblast growth factor-driven proliferation of human endothelial cells and keratinocytes. *Arch Dermatol* 1989;125:1359–1362.
54. Shing Y, Folkman J, Sullivan R, et al: Heparin affinity: Purification of a tumor-derived capillary endothelial cell growth factor. *Science* 1984;223:1296–1299.
55. Shing Y, Folkman J, Haudenschild C, et al: Angiogenesis is stimulated by a tumor-derived endothelial cell growth factor. *J Cell Biochem* 1985;29:275–287.
56. Boes M, Dake BL, Bar RS: Interactions of cultured endothelial cells with TGF-beta, bFGF, PDGF and IGF-I. *Life Sci* 1991;48:811–821.
57. Gimbrone MA Jr, Cotran RS, Leapman SB, et al: Tumor growth and neovascularization: An experimental model using the rabbit cornea. *J Natl Cancer Inst* 1974;52:413–427.
58. Brem H, Folkman J: Inhibition of tumor angiogenesis mediated by cartilage. *J Exp Med* 1975;141:427–439.

59. Folkman J, Weisz PB, Joullie MM, et al: Control of angiogenesis with synthetic heparin substitutes. *Science* 1989;243:1490–1493.
60. Kusaka M, Sudo K, Fujita T, et al: Potent anti-angiogenic action of AGM-1470: Comparison to the fumagillin parent. *Biochem Biophys Res Commun* 1991;174:1070–1076.
61. Barnhill RL, Ryan TJ: Biochemical modulation of angiogenesis in the chorioallantoic membrane of the chick embryo. *J Invest Dermatol* 1983;81:485–488.
62. Dusseau JW, Hutchins PM, Malbasa DS: Stimulation of angiogenesis by adenosine on the chick chorioallantoic membrane. *Circ Res* 1986;59:163–170.
63. Okamoto T, Oikawa S, Toyota T, et al: Angiogenesis factors in ocular tissues of normal rabbits on chorioallantoic membrane assay. *Tohoku J Exp Med* 1988;154:63–70.
64. Splawinski J, Michna M, Palczak R, et al: Angiogenesis: Quantitative assessment by the chick chorioallantoic membrane assay. *Methods Find Exp Clin Pharmacol* 1988;10:221–226.
65. Flamme I, Schulze-Osthoff K, Jacob HJ: Mitogenic activity of chicken chorioallantoic fluid is temporally correlated to vascular growth in the chorioallantoic membrane and related to fibroblast growth factors. *Development* 1991;111:683–690.
66. Andrade SP, Fan TP, Lewis GP: Quantitative in-vivo studies on angiogenesis in a rat sponge model. *Br J Exp Path* 1987;68:755–766.
67. Weidner N, Semple JP, Welch WR, et al: Tumor angiogenesis and metastasis: Correlation in invasive breast carcinoma. *N Engl J Med* 1991;324:1–8.
68. Weidner N, Carroll PR, Flax J, et al: Tumor angiogenesis correlates with metastasis in invasive prostate carcinoma. *Am J Pathol* 1993;143:401–409.
69. Schulze-Osthoff K, Risau W, Vollmer E, et al: In situ detection of basic fibroblast growth factor by highly specific antibodies. *Am J Pathol* 1990;137:85–92.
70. Banda MJ, Knighton DR, Hunt TK, et al: Isolation of a nonmitogenic angiogenesis factor from wound fluid. *Proc Natl Acad Sci USA* 1982;79:7773–7777.
71. Schweigerer L, Neufeld G, Friedman J, et al: Capillary endothelial cells express basic fibroblast growth factor, a mitogen that promotes their own growth. *Nature* 1987;325:257–259
72. Barnhill RL, Parkinson EK, Ryan TJ: Supernatants from cultured human epidermal keratinocytes stimulate angiogenesis. *Br J Dermatol* 1984;110:273–281.
73. Vlodavsky I, Fuks Z, Ishai-Michaeli R, et al: Extracellular matrix-resident basic fibroblast growth factor: Implication for the control of angiogenesis. *J Cell Biochem* 1991;45:167–176.
74. Brem H, Klagsbrun M: The role of fibroblast growth factors and related oncogenes in tumor growth, in Benz CC, Liu ET (eds): *Oncogenes and Tumor Suppressor Genes in Human Malignancies.* Boston, MA, Kluwer Academic Publishers, 1993, pp 211–232.
75. Cordon-Cardo C, Vlodavsky I, Haimovitz-Friedman A, et al: Expression of basic fibroblast growth factor in normal human tissues. *Lab Invest* 1990;63:832–840.
76. Finch PW, Rubin JS, Miki T, et al: Human KGF is FGF-related with properties of a paracrine effector of epithelial cell growth. *Science* 1989;245:752–755.
77. Folkman J, Shing Y: Control of angiogenesis by heparin and other sulfated polysaccharides. *Adv Exp Med Biol* 1992;313:355–364.
78. Klagsbrun M: The affinity of fibroblast growth factors (FGFs) for heparin: FGF-heparin sulfate interactions in cells and extracellular matrix. *Curr Opin Cell Biol* 1990;2;857–863.
79. Hauschka PV, Mavrakos AE, Iafrati MD, et al: Growth factors in bone matrix: Isolation of multiple types by affinity chromatography on heparin-Sepharose. *J Biol Chem* 1986;261:12665–12674.
80. Connolly DT, Stoddard BL, Harakas NK, et al: Human fibroblast-derived growth factor is a mitogen and chemoattractant for endothelial cells. *Biochem Biophys Res Commun* 1987;144:705–712.
81. Gospodarowicz D, Moran JS: Mitogenic effect of fibroblast growth factor on early passage cultures of human and murine fibroblasts. *J Cell Biol* 1975;66:451–457.

82. Weich HA, Iberg N, Klagsbrun M, et al: Expression of acidic and basic fibroblast growth factors in human and bovine vascular smooth muscle cells. *Growth Factors* 1990;2:313–320.

83. Allen RE, Boxhorn LK: Regulation of skeletal muscle satellite cell proliferation and differentiation by transforming growth factor-beta, insulin like growth factor-I, and fibroblast growth factor. *J Cell Physiol* 1989;138:311–315.

84. Montesano R, Vassalli J-D, Baird A, et al: Basic fibroblast growth factor induces angiogenesis in vitro. *Proc Natl Acad Sci U S A* 1986;83:7297–7301.

85. Vlodavsky I, Fridman R, Sullivan R, et al: Aortic endothelial cells synthesize basic fibroblast growth factor which remains cell associated and platelet-derived growth factor-like protein which is secreted. *J Cell Physiol* 1987;131:402–408,

86. Vlodavsky I, Folkman J, Sullivan R, et al: Endothelial cell-derived basic fibroblast growth factor; synthesis and deposition into subendothelial extracellular matrix. *Proc Natl Acad Sci U S A* 1987;84:2292–2296.

87. Folkman J, Klagsbrun M, Sasse J, et al: A heparin-binding angiogenic protein—basic fibroblast growth factor—is stored within basement membrane. *Am J Pathol* 1988; 130:393–400.

88. Broadley KN, Aquino AM, Woodward SC, et al: Monospecific antibodies implicate basic fibroblast growth factor in normal wound repair. *Lab Invest* 1989;61:571–575.

89. McGee GS, Davidson JM, Buckley A, et al: Recombinant basic fibroblast growth factor accelerates wound healing. *J Surg Res* 1988;45:145–153.

90. Mondain M, Saffiedine S, Uziel A: Fibroblast growth factor improves the healing of experimental tympanic membrane perforations. *Acta Otolaryngol (Stockh)* 1991;111:337–341.

91. Eckenstein FP, Shipley GD, Nishi R: Acidic and basic fibroblast growth factors in the nervous system: Distribution and differential alteration of levels after injury of central versus peripheral nerve. *J Neurosci* 1991;11:412–419.

92. Otto D, Frotscher M, Unsicker K: Basic fibroblast growth factor and nerve growth factor administered in gel foam rescue medial septal neurons after fimbria fornix transection. *J Neurosci Res* 1989;22:83–91.

93. Mustoe TA, Pierce GF, Morishima C, et al: Growth factor-induced acceleration of tissue repair through direct and inductive activities in a rabbit dermal ulcer model. *J Clin Invest* 1991;87:694–703.

94. Sano K, Sasada R, Iwane K, et al: Stabilizing basic fibroblast growth factor using protein engineering. *Biochem Biophys Res Commun* 1988;151:701–708.

95. Brem H, Shing Y, Watanabe H, et al: Temporal expression of basic fibroblast growth factor during wound healing. *Surg Forum* 1992;43:664–667.

96. Klingbeil CK, Cesar LB, Fiddes JC: Basic fibroblast growth factor accelerates tissue repair in models of impaired wound healing, in Barbul A, Caldwell MD, Eaglstein WH, et al (eds): *Clinical and Experimental Approaches to Dermal and Epidermal Repair: Normal and Chronic Wounds.* New York, NY, Wiley-Liss, Inc, 1991, pp 443–458.

97. Phillips LG, Geldner P, Brou J, et al: Correction of diabetic incisional healing impairment with basic fibroblast growth factor. *Surg Forum* 1990;41:602–603.

98. Tsuboi R, Rifkin DB: Recombinant basic fibroblast growth factor stimulates wound healing in healing-impaired db/db mice. *J Exp Med* 1990;172:245–251.

99. Hayward P, Hokanson J, Heggers J, et al: Fibroblast growth factor reserves the bacterial retardation of wound contraction. *Am J Surg* 1992;163:288–293.

100. Brem H, Walter KA, Tamargo RJ, et al: Drug delivery to the brain, in Domb AJ (ed): *Polymeric Site Specific Pharmacology.* New York, NY, John Wiley & Sons, 1994, pp 117–139.

Chapter 14

Enhancement of Fracture Healing by Molecular or Physical Means: An Overview

Thomas A. Einhorn, MD

Introduction

The biochemical or molecular enhancement of fracture healing can be formulated into both local and systemic applications. From a drug development point of view, systemic enhancement would seem to be best because it would avoid the need for an operative procedure, make the treatment more widely available to the patient population at large, and avoid the need for an interaction with a physician each time the treatment is administered. Because a systemic agent that would target the fracture healing process requires a high degree of tissue specificity, the introduction of such an agent will certainly require much more extensive investigation. However, several local methods to enhance fracture healing have already been developed, and these can be categorized into osteogenic, osteoconductive, and osteoinductive approaches.

Osteogenic methods to enhance fracture healing include the use of naturally occurring materials, which have been known to induce or support bone formation, such as autologous bone marrow grafts,[1,2] autologous or allogeneic bone grafts,[3,4] or the use of demineralized allogeneic bone matrices.[5–8] Osteoconduction is a process that supports the ingrowth of sprouting capillaries, perivascular tissues, and osteoprogenitor cells from the recipient host bed into the three-dimensional (3-D) structure of the implant or graft.[9] Osteoconductive substances that have been studied to date include calcium-phosphate ceramics of a variety of types, as well as bioactive glasses and polymers.[10,11] None of these materials would result in bone formation if it were to be implanted at a nonosseous site. Osteoinduction is a process that supports the mitogenesis of undifferentiated perivascular mesenchymal cells leading to the formation of osteoprogenitor cells with the capacity to form new bone.[12] These substances do lead to bone formation at nonosseous extraskeletal sites. As will be discussed below, a variety of growth factors or peptide signaling molecules may fall within the category of osteoinductive substances. Although individually these substances may not actually support osteogenesis de novo, when used in conjunction with each other, they may lead to the formation of substantial amounts of new bone.

Local Stimulation of Fracture Healing

Osteogenic Stimulation

This category includes the use of several naturally occurring bone graft materials. Because autografts and allografts will be discussed in other chapters of this book, they will not be reviewed here. The use of autologous bone marrow to enhance fracture healing is relatively new, and research in this area impacts directly on the behavior of cells and their responses to some of the other materials, most notably growth factors and cytokines.

The ability of red marrow to form bone was first suggested by Goujon[2] as early as 1869. A number of subsequent investigations on animals have shown that autologous bone marrow contains osteogenic precursors that contribute to bone formation.[13,14] Several investigators have used autologous marrow clinically to augment the osteogenic response to implanted allografts or xenografts,[3,15,16] bone-inducing or bone-conducting substances such as bone morphogenetic protein, or Kiel (animal) bone.[17,18] Connolly and associates[1] have refined these techniques for potential clinical application by harvesting autologous bone marrow and then centrifuging and concentrating the osteogenic marrow elements prior to implantation.

Osteoconductive Stimulation

Investigations into the use of materials that support osteoblastic activity and bone formation have been ongoing for several decades. The musculoskeletal literature is replete with reports of a variety of calcium phosphate-based materials and their use as osteoconductive implants for the filling of bone defects and augmentation of bone healing.[10] The rationale for the use of these materials is that, independent of any direct stimulation of cellular activity, normal osteoblastic or osteoblast-like cells have the ability to form bone on the appropriate surface. That surface must have the proper chemical composition and be distributed in space in such a way as to support cell growth and development. Most studies to date have suggested that specific pore sizes of between 100 and 400 μm (most of these calcium phosphate materials are porous) are ideal.[10] The osteoconductive material serves as a scaffold for "creeping substitution" by osteoblasts.

Some of the questions currently being asked concerning the utility of these materials include: (1) Is the material resorbed, and if so at what rate? (2) If materials are not completely resorbed, what are the effects of residual calcium phosphate ceramic material on the ultimate modeling, remodeling, and mechanical properties of bone? (3) How well does the material support cell growth, and are the effects based on chemical composition or architectural distribution? (4) What are the mechanical properties of the material at the time of implantation, and to what extent can they support mechanical loads during the process of incorporation? Each material that has been studied has had to be examined with regard to these questions. Because each material behaves in a slightly different fashion from the others, the present discussion will be limited to two materials that are now available for clinical use in orthopaedic patients.

Interpore® hydroxyapatite[19] is formed by the replamineform process of replicating life forms from inorganic materials. This predominantly hydroxyapatite biomatrix is formed by the conversion of a specific marine coral calcium phosphate to crystalline hydroxyapatite using a patented technology. These structures become templates for host bone growth and sustain new living tissue based, presumably, on their chemical and architectural composition (Fig. 1). Multicenter clinical trials have recently been completed demonstrating the efficacy of the material in orthopaedic clinical applications of bone defects and fractures with bone loss. A preliminary study which tested the use of this material in metaphyseal defects associated with tibial plateau fractures in 40 pa-

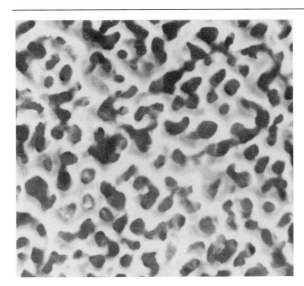

Fig. 1 Cross-section of Inter-pore® hydroxyapatite bone graft material demonstrating the porous nature of this calcium-phosphate ceramic. Note the similarity in appearance of this bone graft substitute to normal cancellous bone (original magnification × 3). (Reproduced with permission from Bucholz RW, Carlton A, Holmes R: Inter-porous hydroxyapatite as a bone graft substitute in tibial plateau fractures. *Clin Orthop* 1989;240:53–62.)

tients demonstrated equivalent efficacy to autogenous bone grafts at a minimum follow-up of 15.4 months.[19]

Another recently approved material, Collagraft®, is a mixture of hydroxyapatite, tricalcium phosphate porous ceramic beads, and fibrillar collagen.[20] When mixed with autogenous bone marrow, it serves as an effective bone graft substitute (Fig. 2). In 1986, 267 patients with fresh fractures were entered into a multicenter prospective randomized clinical trial in which Collagraft® was compared to autogenous iliac bone graft. Of these patients, 128 received cancellous autogenous bone grafts and 139 received Collagraft®. At 6- and 12-month follow-up periods, Collagraft® was shown to be as effective as autogenous bone graft in augmenting the healing of fresh fractures. As a graft material, Collagraft® is considered to be osteoconductive. However, when used in combination with an autogenous bone marrow aspirate, it is possible that certain osteoprogenitor cells may become incorporated into the final implanted material.[21]

Osteoinductive Materials

Over the past decade, considerable attention has been directed towards the development of recombinant proteins for use as growth factors in wound healing applications.[22] Although cell replication is maximal during the healing of most wounds, some wounds heal poorly, and enhancement of growth signals by exogenous factors would seem to be a logical therapy. This same logic can be applied to bone repair, a wound healing system in a mineralized tissue.

Before the enhancement of fracture healing can be approached, more information is required concerning the normal conditions that limit the rates of wound repair in general. Although several growth factors have been identified, their functions are unclear. In fact, the apparent activities of some of these factors appear to be redundant while others even seem antagonistic. As an example, interleukin-1 (IL-1) is found in wounds and accelerates the growth of fibroblasts in culture. It also stimulates the production of collagenase, and its

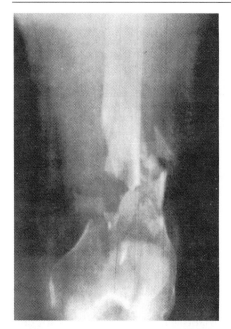

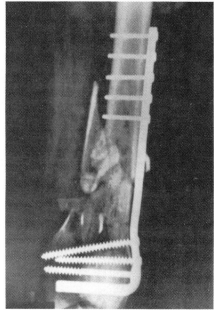

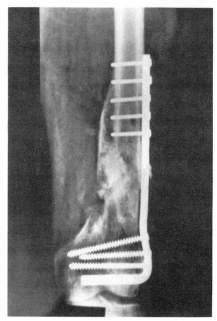

Fig. 2 Top left, Comminuted fracture of the left femur in a fifty-year-old patient. **Top right,** ORIF was performed using a blade plate and 31 ml of Collagraft.® **Bottom,** Follow-up at 7 months. Fracture judged to be healed with complete incorporation of the Collagraft® material. (Reproduced with permission from Cornell CN: Initial clinical experience with use of Collagraft® as a bone graft substitute. *Tech Orthop* 1992;7:55–63.)

use in wound healing has been associated with both positive and negative results.[22]

Although a plethora of papers have been published regarding the use of growth factors in the enhancement of soft-tissue wounds,[22] the study of growth factors in bone and cartilage systems has been limited to the use of certain peptide signaling molecules, such as transforming growth factor-beta

(TGF-β),[23-25] fibroblast growth factor (FGF),[26,27] platelet derived growth factor (PDGF),[28] and the bone morphogenetic proteins (BMP).[12,29-36]

Because it designates a family of molecules that may have repair-promoting properties for fractures, TGF-β will be discussed first. TGF-β is a homodimeric peptide with a molecular weight of 25 kd; its most abundant sources are platelets and bone. This multifunctional peptide has a broad range of cellular activities, including control of the proliferation and expression of the differentiated phenotype of several cell types specific to bone. Among these cell types are mesenchymal precursor cells, chondrocytes, osteoblasts, and osteoclasts.[23-25] Although TGF-β exists in several distinct forms, two of these, TGF-β1 and TGF-β2, have been isolated from bone in approximately a four to one ratio. In vivo studies based on both immunohistochemical staining and in situ hybridization have demonstrated the synthesis of TGF-β by both chondrocytes and osteoblasts, and the accumulation of TGF-β in models of endochondral ossification.[24,25] Studies on the potential role of TGF-β in soft-tissue wound healing have shown that this molecule initiates the healing process after it is released by degranulating platelets. In addition, exogenous application of TGF-β has been shown to stimulate healing of soft-tissue wounds.[37]

In a study in which TGF-β1 or 2 was introduced by daily injection into the subperiosteal region of newborn rat femurs, Joyce and associates[25] demonstrated that mesenchymal precursor cells in the periosteum were stimulated by TGF-β to proliferate and differentiate in much the same way as is observed in embryologic bone formation and early fracture healing. After the cessation of the injections, endochondral ossification also occurred, resulting in replacement of cartilage with bone. These investigators demonstrated the expression of type II collagen and the immunolocalization of types I and II collagen within the areas where TGF-β induced bone and cartilage. Moreover, injection of TGF-β2 stimulated the synthesis of TFG-β1 in chondrocytes and osteoblasts, suggesting positive autoregulation of TGF-β.[25]

The expression of TGF-β in fracture callus organ cultures was analyzed in subsequent studies.[26] It was shown that TGF-β's message is detected in the soft callus at approximately day 14 after fracture and in the hard callus on days 5 and 15. When fracture calluses were treated with TGF-β, inhibition of the expression of cartilage-specific genes was observed in day 7 fracture callus, but there was no effect on bone specific genes such as type I collagen or osteonectin. In later calluses on day 13, TGF-β stimulated a several-fold increase in type I collagen and osteonectin expression without affecting the cartilage specific gene, type II collagen. These studies suggest that TGF-β may have specific regulatory roles in the fracture healing process at different times.[26]

Several investigations on fracture healing have been conducted in which demineralized bone matrix, and its putative active component, BMP, were used. These investigations have included a series of studies in which demineralized bone matrix was applied to maxillocranial facial wounds in patients[7,8] and, subsequently, purified BMP was used in femoral and tibial nonunions in uncontrolled clinical trials.[30-32] In 1988, Wozney and associates[35] reported the sequencing and cloning of a BMP that could be produced by recombinant techniques. BMP refers to an activity derived from bone that induces the formation of cartilage and bone in vivo. The implantation of this protein (or proteins) leads to a series of developmental processes, including chemotaxis, proliferation, and differentiation, which result in the transient formation of cartilage and its replacement by living bone tissue complete with hematopoietic marrow.[12]

Several newly discovered factors, BMP-2, -3, -4, -5, -6, -7 and osteoinductive factor (OIF), have been implicated in the BMP process. BMP-3 is synonymous with the term osteogenin; BMP-4 is synonymous with BMP-2B; and BMP-7 is synonymous with the term OP-1. BMP-2 through BMP-7 are all members of the TGF-β superfamily of molecules and are closely related to two factors, Vg1 and DPP, which are involved in a variety of developmental processes during embryogenesis. BMP-2A and BMP-7 have been expressed as recombinant proteins, both of which have been shown to clearly induce the entire cartilage and bone formation process seen with bone-derived BMPs.[38] At the present time, two BMPs, BMP-2[33,35,36] and BMP-7[34] have been demonstrated to increase bone formation at extraosseous sites and to enhance fracture healing (Fig. 3).[33]

Other factors with wound-healing potential in the musculoskeletal system include acidic FGF (aFGF) and PDGF. Acidic FGF was tested in a fracture model in which 1 μg was injected into the fracture site either daily or on alternate days between the first and the ninth days postfracture.[26] The results

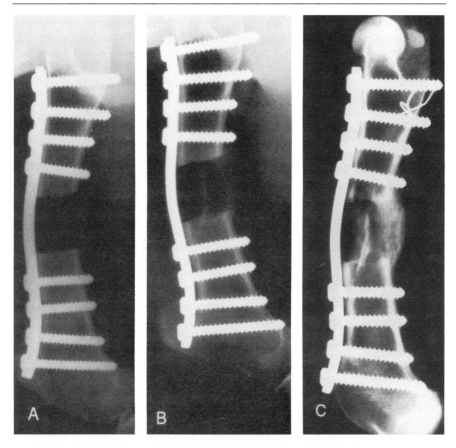

Fig. 3 Radiographs of the femoral defect site in a sheep that had been implanted with rhBMP-2. **Left,** Defect immediately after implantation. **Center,** Defect 6 weeks after implantation showing signs of new bone formation. **Right,** Defect at the time of euthanasia (12 weeks) demonstrating bridging of the fracture gap with new bone. (Reproduced with permission from Gerhart TN, Kirker-Head CA, Krig MJ, et al: Healing segmental femoral defects in sheep using recombinant human bone morphogenetic protein. *Clin Orthop* 1993;293:317–326.)

showed that aFGF-injected calluses were significantly larger than controls and that the total DNA and collagen contents were also greater (Fig. 4). The fracture calluses injected with aFGF remained larger than controls until the fourth

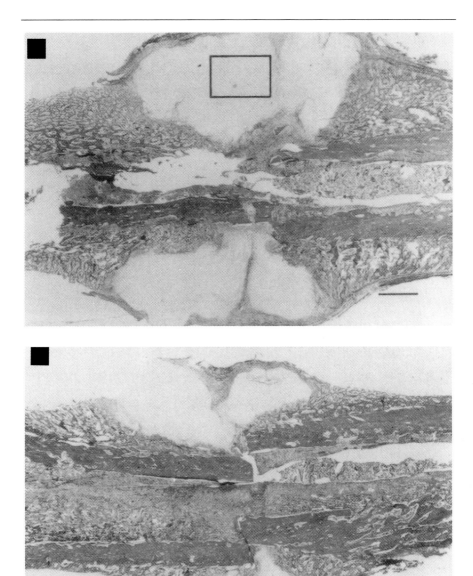

Fig. 4 Histology of an aFGF-injected callus that had been treated with 1 μg every other day postfracture. **Top,** aFGF-injected callus at 11 days postfracture. **Bottom,** Control callus that had not been injected. (Reproduced with permission from Jingushi S, Heydemann A, Kana SK, et al: Acidic fibroblast growth factor (aFGF) injection stimulates cartilage enlargement and inhibits cartilage gene expression in rat fracture healing. *J Orthop Res* 1990;8:364–371.)

week after fracture, at which time no difference was detected between aFGF-injected and control fractures. Northern analysis of total cellular RNA extracted from the cartilaginous soft callus and bony hard callus from the aFGF-injected fractures showed decreased expression of type II procollagen and proteoglycan core protein. Slight decreases in types I and II procollagen were also observed. The investigators concluded that aFGF injections in these experiments induced cartilage enlargement in the fracture calluses while decreasing expression of certain molecules potentially associated with cartilage development (Fig. 5).[26]

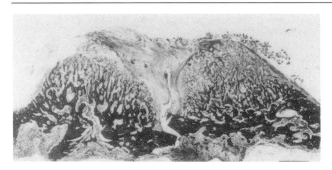

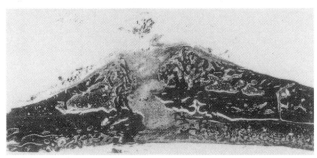

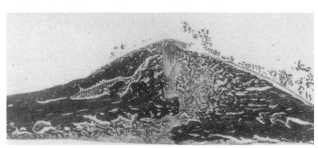

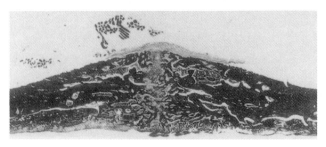

Fig. 5 Late effect of aFGF injections on callus histology. After making fractures, aFGF was injected every other day until day 9. The cartilaginous portion was substituted by trabecular bone at 3 and 4 weeks after fracture in both aFGF-injected and control calluses. **Top,** aFGF-injected at three weeks. **Center top,** Control at three weeks. **Center bottom,** aFGF-injected at four weeks. **Bottom,** Control at 4 weeks. (Reproduced with permission from Jingushi S, Heydemann A, Kana SK, et al: Acidic fibroblast growth factor (aFGF) injection stimulates cartilage enlargement and inhibits cartilage gene expression in rat fracture healing. *J Orthop Res* 1990; 8:364–371.)

The effect of exogenous PDGF on bone healing was studied in a pilot investigation of tibial osteotomies in rabbits. The results showed that, after 28 days of healing, there was radiographic, mechanical, and histologic evidence to suggest that a single application of PDGF at the time of fracture leads to enhanced healing.[28]

One of the most important issues currently limiting the potential use of these molecules in human applications is the development of an appropriate delivery system. The most critical feature of the delivery system is that it be biocompatible, meaning that it must be nonimmunogenic, nonreactive, and nontoxic either in its solid form or with respect to its degradation by-products. In addition, several other properties are desirable. It is considered optimal if a delivery system for a recombinant protein is bioabsorbable, ie, if it can be completely resorbed and replaced by bone. Porosity would facilitate the infiltration of the protein with fluids and, potentially, progenitor cells that express the receptors for the inductive molecules. Delivery systems could be liquid, viscous, semisolid, or solid, and each state has advantages and disadvantages that depend on the clinical application, eg, injection versus implantation. The delivery system must also be capable of being sterilized and must have a dose-flexibility, which allows titration depending on the desired response. In addition, certain optional properties may also be advantageous. For example, a delivery system with a timed-release capability would allow differing physiologic components of a biologic process, eg, fracture healing, to be enhanced at different times. Also, if a bone inductive protein is required in a weightbearing part of the skeleton, a delivery system with mechanical properties actually could support mechanical loads during the time that cartilage or bone is being formed.

Systemic Stimulation of Fracture Healing

The ability to enhance fracture healing through the use of a systemic agent, particularly one that would be administered orally, would have a substantial positive impact on the treatment of musculoskeletal injuries. The development of such an agent would depend on a number of conditions, but the most important would be specificity for only those cells and responses that participate in the healing.

Conditions are currently known in which enhancement of bone formation occurs systemically. The most obvious clinical examples of this may be the heterotopic ossification that occurs in conjunction with paralysis-producing injuries[39] or head trauma.[40–44] Bidner and associates[40] have shown that samples of sera from patients who had head injuries have a higher mitogenic activity against osteoblastic cells than sera from patients without head injuries. Moreover, when these experiments were conducted on nonosteogenic skin fibroblasts, the effect was not observed. These investigators concluded that there may be a humoral mechanism for the enhanced osteogenesis that accompanies head injury and that this effect may be dose-dependent.[40] Kurer and associates[39] noted similar results when sera from paraplegic patients with heterotopic ossification were studied in human osteoblast-like cultures.

Although the explanations for these findings are not clear, it is possible that a growth peptide could be released from injured neural tissue. Based on recent laboratory experiments on FGF[26] and in consideration of the fact that the largest source of FGF in the body is neural tissue,[45,46] it can be hypothesized that FGF or FGF-like peptides could be responsible for some of these observed effects.

An alternative explanation for the above clinical observations, which is consistent with other findings of systemic enhancement of osteogenesis, is the concept that these effects may be due to novel or unique circulating osteogenic growth peptides. Bab and associates[47–49] have shown, in a series of experiments, that direct or indirect injury to bone marrow is accompanied by a systemic osteogenic response. Einhorn and associates[50] have confirmed these findings and demonstrated that the effects result from bone marrow injury alone and not from an associated fracture of the cortex. Foldes and associates[51] demonstrated these effects in humans by showing increased levels of serum osteocalcin and bone-specific alkaline phosphatase in sera harvested from patients who had served as donors for bone marrow transplantation programs.

Another family of substances, which should be considered with respect to the systemic enhancement of fracture healing, are the prostaglandins. In recent years, it has become clear that prostaglandins have profound effects on the metabolism of bone and are among the most potent agents of resorption. It is also known that prostaglandin E_2 can stimulate bone formation[52] and inhibition of prostaglandins can impair fracture healing.[53] In studies in which prostaglandin E_1 was used to treat congenital cardiac defects in children, a side effect of increased periosteal reaction and cortical hyperostosis in long bones was observed.[54] Because much is already known about the use of this family of drugs in animal and human systems, the development of a prostaglandin-based substance that stimulates fracture healing may be worth investigating.

Physical Methods of Enhancing Fracture Healing

A fracture's mechanical environment greatly affects its healing. Consequently, it is reasonable to hypothesize that altering that mechanical environment in specific ways may enhance healing. This section will discuss the application of physical factors to fracture healing in terms of known physical/mechanical effects, such as the influences of stability, instability, and micromotion, as well as the effects of external biophysical phenomena, such as electrical stimulation, electromagnetic stimulation, and ultrasound. Although one of the most impressive and interesting mechanical phenomena to affect musculoskeletal medicine in the twentieth century is the distraction osteogenesis method of Ilizarov, those precepts and the results of those experiments will be discussed in a separate section of this book.

Mechanical Stimulation

The quantity and the quality of the callus tissue formed by a healing fracture are currently understood to be under the direct influence of the mechanical environment created by the orthopaedic treatment.[55] In general, if there is any degree of motion at the fracture site, callus will be formed.[56] Moreover, the more motion that occurs at a fracture site, the more callus that develops, and, if the motion becomes excessive, a hypertrophic nonunion may result. The converse is true with rigid internal fixation in which there is complete obliteration of motion. This is generally seen with the use of plates and screws in combination with compression devices. In these situations, fractures unite by primary healing in which no callus is formed, and the bone ends are bridged by direct cortical union.[56] Other forms of fixation, including casts, intramedullary devices (locked or unlocked), and external fixation frames, result in some degree of motion at the fracture site. To date, not one of these standard methods of treatment has been shown to be more effective than another in terms of the enhancement of fracture healing. Thus, the ability to enhance fracture healing through the use of direct mechanical means requires a more in-depth appreciation of the individual mechanical components of the fracture healing process.

Carter and associates[57,58] have modeled the influences of different mechanical loading conditions on tissue differentiation in a variety of musculoskeletal settings. They have presented a theory to relate mechanical loading history and tissue differentiation of preosseous mesenchymal tissue to the process of endochondral fracture healing. The theory identifies tissue vascularity and two key mechanical parameters, cyclic hydrostatic stress (pressure) and cyclic tensile strain, as important determinants of tissue differentiation. Using an osteotomized long bone as the experimental system for study, they performed a 3-D finite element analysis to model idealized fracture callus, including periosteal, endosteal, and interfragmentary callus regions. The investigators calculated stress and strain histories at each location within the callus. The results indicate that high levels of compressive hydrostatic stress are created within interfragmentary callus. At the mid-gap location, high levels of strain exist in the radial and circumferential directions. In periosteal and endosteal callus regions remote from the interfragmentary gap, low levels of hydrostatic stress and tensile strain exist. These findings suggest an association between: (1) intermittent compressive hydrostatic stress and chondrogenesis; (2) intermittent strain and fibrogenesis; and (3) low levels of mechanical stimulation and osteogenesis with good vascularity or chondrogenesis with poor vascularity. Finally, the investigators noted that once cartilage forms within the callus, moderate levels of cyclic tensile strain (or distortional strain) will accelerate endochondral ossification. Local cyclic hydrostatic compressive stress, however, will delay endochondral ossification, possibly due to an inhibitory influence on revascularization.[57,58]

To determine how mechanical perturbations may actually enhance the fracture healing process, Kenwright and associates[59,60] have examined the influence of axial movement and induced micromotion on the fracture-healing process. These investigators have shown, in both preclinical and clinical trials, that fracture healing can be enhanced by specific controlled degrees of induced micromotion. Figure 6 shows the experimental set-up in which these phenomena were studied in humans. As noted, direct strain measurements at the fracture site can be related to radiographic tissue quality and quantitated in terms of the induced mechanical input.[59,60]

The ability to produce similar or even advanced levels of healing as a result of distraction forces has also been studied extensively and will be discussed in a separate section of this book. Other mechanical effects on fractures or fracture callus can be produced by using intramedullary devices for internal fixation.[61,62] The effects of these constructs on fracture healing have been considered previously only in terms of the mechanical environments they create. However, recent evidence suggests that the use of an intramedullary device might also induce biochemical changes systemically,[61] and that these changes could enhance fracture healing. Moreover, the systemic osteogenic response observed as a result of bone marrow injury by the rod may also promote bone repair.[50]

Biophysical Stimulation

Several nonmechanical, physical methods, including bioelectricity, bioelectromagnetism, and ultrasound, have been tested with respect to their abilities to stimulate fracture healing. Most of the information on fracture repair using electric-based methods has come from studies of nonunion healing. Although

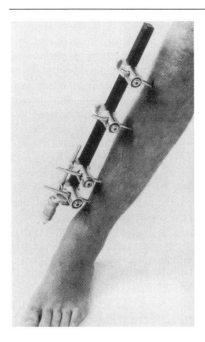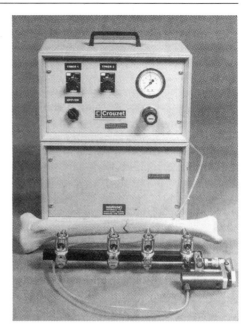

Fig. 6 Experimental set-up for the study of the effects of induced micromotion on fracture healing. **Left,** The unilateral frame is attached to the medial surface of the tibia by four Schantz screws. **Right,** Two sliding clamps are attached to the fixator column and to a spring assembly. They provide complete control of longitudinal displacement and load. A pneumatic pump is attached to the spring module and, hence, the sliding clamps so that small controlled increments of axial displacement can be applied. (Reproduced with permission from Kenwright J, Richardson JB, Cunningham JL, et al: Axial movement and tibial fractures. *J Bone Joint Surg* 1991;73B:654–659.)

much has been learned about electric stimulation, these results are not necessarily applicable to the augmentation or stimulation of fresh fracture healing. Therefore, this discussion will cover only what is known about fresh fracture stimulation. Most of the information on ultrasound stimulation that has come forth has been developed in studies on the healing of fresh fractures. To date, several investigations have been performed using animal models, and at least one large-scale multicenter clinical trial has been reported.[63] In studies of the enhancement of fracture healing by a biophysical signal, the investigator must distinguish between improvement in tissue quality and a stimulation of fracture callus quantity. Because most animal studies have used the acquisition of mechanical properties as the assay for fracture healing, it must be remembered that the geometric properties of the fracture callus can influence strength and stiffness significantly independent of any acceleration of biochemical or cellular pathways.

Several investigations have been attempted in which electrical stimulation was applied to fresh fractures. The data are conflicting; there is presently no agreement in the field that electrical stimulation or magnetic stimulation actually makes a meaningful difference to the healing of fresh fractures. However, Sharrard[64] has suggested that pulsed electromagnetic fields may enhance the healing of delayed fractures in humans. In a study of 45 conservatively treated tibial shaft fractures in which union was delayed for 16 but not less than 32 weeks, a double-blind multicenter analysis showed a statistically significant difference in the healing outcomes when pulsed electromagnetic fields were used. From these data it was concluded that pulsed electromagnetic fields significantly influence the healing of tibial fractures with delayed union.[64] These findings suggest that pulsed electromagnetic fields may enhance the fracture healing process when the healing phase is retarded or prolonged. In this sense, it would seem reasonable to conclude that pulsed electromagnetic fields have some stimulatory effect on the cells and tissues that contribute to early fracture healing.[65]

The effects of low-intensity pulsed ultrasound on the rate of fresh fracture healing in animals and patients have been reported.[63,66,67] In a study in which 139 mature New Zealand white rabbits underwent bilateral midshaft fibular osteotomies, and in which one limb was subjected to 20 minutes of ultrasonic stimulation per day, significant enhancement of fracture healing, as assessed by mechanical testing, was reported.[66] However, because the quality of the callus formed was not studied, it is unclear whether the ultrasonic input actually accelerated cellular and tissue level responses or simply produced more callus. Nevertheless, the early improvement in mechanical properties of the callus suggests a potential clinical role for this device. In a prospective, double-blind, randomized study evaluating the use of the same ultrasonic stimulator on the healing of 67 closed or grade I open tibial fractures in humans, there was both clinical and radiographic evidence of accelerated healing, and no serious complications were reported.[63]

Conclusions

The studies cited in this chapter provide several scientific leads that could result in the development of realistic methods to enhance fresh fracture healing. Although the notion that those biologic events that direct fracture healing are essentially optimized may be true, the ability to accelerate the process could greatly benefit patients and society. As investigations progress from the stages of preclinical to clinical trials, scientists must begin to use the tools of clinical outcomes research to assess the real value of these new therapies.

References

1. Connolly J, Guse R, Lippiello L, et al: Development of an osteogenic bone-marrow preparation. *J Bone Joint Surg* 1989;71A:684–691.
2. Goujon E: Recherches expérimentales sur les propriétés physiologiques de la moelle des os. *J Anat Physiol* 1869;6:399–412.
3. Burwell RG: Studies in the transplantation of bone: VII. The fresh composite homograft-autograft of cancellous bone: An analysis of factors leading to osteogenesis in marrow transplants and in marrow-containing bone grafts. *J Bone Joint Surg* 1964;46B:110–140.
4. Burchardt H: The biology of bone graft repair. *Clin Orthop* 1983;174:28–42.
5. Bolander ME, Balian G: The use of demineralized bone matrix in the repair of segmental defects: Augmentation with extracted matrix proteins and a comparison with autologous grafts. *J Bone Joint Surg* 1986;68A:1264–1274.
6. Einhorn TA, Lane JM, Burstein AH, et al: The healing of segmental bone defects induced by demineralized bone matrix: A radiographic and biomechanical study. *J Bone Joint Surg* 1984;66A:274–279.
7. Glowacki J, Kaban LB, Murray JE, et al: Application of the biological principle of induced osteogenesis for craniofacial defects. *Lancet* 1981;1:959–962.

8. Kaban LB, Mulliken JB, Glowacki J: Treatment of jaw defects with demineralized bone implants. *J Oral Maxillofac Surg* 1982;40:623–626.

9. Urist MR: Bone transplants and implants, in Urist MR (ed): *Fundamental and Clinical Bone Physiology.* Philadelphia, PA, JB Lippincott, 1980, pp 331–368.

10. Jarcho M: Calcium phosphate ceramics as hard tissue prosthetics. *Clin Orthop* 1981;157:259–278.

11. Elgendy HM, Norman ME, Keaton AR, et al: Osteoblast-like cell (MC3T3-E1) proliferation on bioerodible polymers: An approach towards the development of a bone-bioerodible polymer composite material. *Biomaterials* 1993;14:263–269.

12. Urist MR: Bone: Formation by autoinduction. *Science* 1965;150:893–899.

13. Owen M: Lineage of osteogenic cells and their relationship to the stromal system, in Peck WA (ed): *Bone and Mineral Research*, ed 3. Amsterdam, Elsevier, 1985, pp 1–25.

14. Friedenstein AJ, Chailakhyan RK, Gerasimov UV: Bone marrow osteogenic stem cells: In vitro cultivation and transplantation in diffusion chambers. *Cell Tissue Kinet* 1987;20:263–272.

15. Graham CE: Further experience with the bone grafting of fractures using xenografts mixed with autologous red marrow. *J Bone Joint Surg* 1982;64B:123.

16. Salama R, Weissman SL: The clinical use of combined xenografts of bone and autologous red marrow: A preliminary report. *J Bone Joint Surg* 1978;60B:111–115.

17. Takagi K, Urist MR: The role of bone marrow in bone morphogenetic protein-induced repair of femoral massive diaphyseal defects. *Clin Orthop* 1982;171:224–231.

18. Plenk H, Hollmann K, Wilfert K-H: Experimental bridging of osseous defects in rats by the implantation of Kiel bone containing fresh autologous marrow. *J Bone Joint Surg* 1972;54B:735–743.

19. Bucholz RW, Carlton A, Holmes R: Interporous hydroxyapatite as a bone graft substitute in tibial plateau fractures. *Clin Orthop* 1989;240:53–62.

20. Cornell CN: Initial clinical experience with use of Collagraft™ as a bone graft substitute. *Techniques Orthop* 1992;7:55–63.

21. Begley CT, Doherty MJ, Hankey DP, et al: The culture of human osteoblasts upon bone graft substitutes. *Bone* 1993;14:661–666.

22. Hunt TK, LaVan FB: Enhancement of wound healing by growth factors. *N Engl J Med* 1989;321:111–112.

23. Beck LS, Ammann AJ, Aufdemorte TB, et al: In vivo induction of bone by recombinant human transforming growth factor-β1. *J Bone Miner Res* 1991;6:961–968.

24. Joyce ME, Jingushi S, Bolander ME: Transforming growth factor-β in the regulation of fracture repair. *Orthop Clin North Am* 1990;21:199–209.

25. Joyce ME, Roberts AB, Sporn MB, et al: Transforming growth factor-β and the initiation of chondrogenesis and osteogenesis in the rat femur. *J Cell Biol* 1990;110:2195–2207.

26. Jingushi S, Heydemann A, Kana SK, et al: Acidic fibroblast growth factor (aFGF) injection stimulates cartilage enlargement and inhibits cartilage gene expression in rat fracture healing. *J Orthop Res* 1990;8:364–371.

27. Mohler DG, Cohen AM, Fehnel D, et al: Effect of basic fibroblast growth factor on angiogenesis and calcification of rat femoral defect. *Trans Orthop Res Soc* 1990;15:380.

28. Nash TJ, Howlett CR, Martin C, et al: Effects of platelet-derived growth factor on tibial osteotomies in rabbits. *Bone* 1994;15:203–208.

29. Lindholm TC, Lindholm TS, Alitalo I, et al: Bovine bone morphogenetic protein (bBMP) induced repair of skull trephine defects in sheep. *Clin Orthop* 1988;227:265–268.

30. Johnson EE, Urist MR, Finerman GAM: Bone morphogenetic protein augmentation grafting of resistant femoral nonunions. A preliminary report. *Clin Orthop* 1988;230:257–265.

31. Johnson EE, Urist MR, Finerman GAM: Repair of segmental defects of the tibia with cancellous bone grafts augmented with human bone morphogenetic protein: A preliminary report. *Clin Orthop* 1988;236:249–257.
32. Johnson EE, Urist MR, Finerman GAM: Distal metaphyseal tibial nonunion. Deformity and bone loss treated by open reduction, internal fixation, and human bone morphogenetic protein (hBMP). *Clin Orthop* 1990;250:234–240.
33. Gerhart TN, Kirker-Head CA, Kriz MJ, et al: Healing segmental femoral defects in sheep using recombinant human bone morphogenetic protein. *Clin Orthop* 1993;293:317–326.
34. Sampath TK, Maliakal JC, Hauschka PV, et al: Recombinant human osteogenic protein-1 (hOP-1) induces new bone formation in vivo with a specific activity comparable with natural bovine osteogenic protein and stimulates osteoblast proliferation and differentiation in vitro. *J Biol Chem* 1992;267:20352–20362.
35. Wozney JM, Rosen V, Celeste AJ, et al: Novel regulators of bone formation: Molecular clones and activities. *Science* 1988;242:1528–1534.
36. Yasko AW, Lane JM, Fellinger EJ, et al: The healing of segmental bone defects induced by recombinant human bone morphogenetic protein (rhBMP-2): A radiographic, histological, and biomechanical study in rats. *J Bone Joint Surg* 1992;74A:659–670.
37. Sporn MB, Roberts AB: Transforming growth factor-β: Multiple actions and potential clinical applications. *JAMA* 1989;262:938–941.
38. Wozney JM: Bone morphogenetic proteins. *Prog Growth Factor Res* 1989;1:267–280.
39. Kurer MH, Khoker MA, Dandona P: Human osteoblast stimulation by sera from paraplegic patients with heterotopic ossification. *Paraplegia* 1992;30:165–168.
40. Bidner SM, Rubins IM, Desjardins JV, et al: Evidence for a humoral mechanism for enhanced osteogenesis after head injury. *J Bone Joint Surg* 1990;72A:1144–1149.
41. Garland DE, Toder L: Fractures of the tibial diaphysis in adults with head injuries. *Clin Orthop* 1980;150:198–202.
42. Garland DE, Rothi B, Waters RL: Femoral fractures in head-injured adults. *Clin Orthop* 1982;166:219–225.
43. Smith R: Head injury, fracture healing and callus. *J Bone Joint Surg* 1987;69B:518–520.
44. Spencer RF: The effect of head injury on fracture healing. A quantitative assessment. *J Bone Joint Surg* 1987;69B:525–528.
45. Gospodarowicz D: Purification of a fibroblast growth factor from bovine pituitary. *J Biol Chem* 1975;250:2515–2520.
46. Gospodarowicz D, Bialecki H, Greenburg G: Purification of the fibroblast growth factor activity from bovine brain. *J Biol Chem* 1978;253:3736–3743.
47. Bab IA, Einhorn TA: Regulatory role of osteogenic growth polypeptides in bone formation and hemopoiesis. *Crit Rev Eukaryot Gene Exp* 1993;3:31–46.
48. Bab I, Gazit D, Massarawa A, et al: Removal of tibial marrow induces increased formation of bone and cartilage in rat mandibular condyle. *Calcif Tissue Int* 1985;37:551–555.
49. Bab I, Gazit D, Muhlrad A, et al: Regenerating bone marrow produces a potent growth-promoting activity to osteogenic cells. *Endocrinology* 1988;123:345–352.
50. Einhorn TA, Simon G, Devlin VJ, et al: The osteogenic response to distant skeletal injury. *J Bone Joint Surg* 1990;72A:1374–1378.
51. Foldes J, Naparstek E, Statter M, et al: Osteogenic response to marrow aspiration: Increased serum osteocalcin and alkaline phosphatase in human bone marrow donors. *J Bone Miner Res* 1989;4:643–646.
52. Voegeli TL, Chapman MW: Utilization of prostaglandins in fracture healing. *Trans Orthop Res Soc* 1985;10:134.
53. Allen HL, Wase A, Bear WT: Indomethocin and aspirin: Effect of non-steroidal and anti-inflammatory agents on the rate of fracture repair in the rat. *Acta Orthop Scand* 1980;51:595–600.

54. Olley PM, Coceani F: Prostaglandins and the ductus arteriosus. *Annu Rev Med* 1981;32:375–385.

55. McKibbin B: The biology of fracture healing in long bones. *J Bone Joint Surg* 1978; 60B:150–162.

56. Perren SM: Physical and biological aspects of fracture healing with special reference to internal fixation. *Clin Orthop* 1979;138:175–196.

57. Carter DR, Blenman PR, Beaupr GS: Correlations between mechanical stress history and tissue differentiation in initial fracture healing. *J Orthop Res* 1988;6:736–748.

58. Blenman PR, Carter DS, Beaupr GS: Role of mechanical loading in the progressive ossification of a fracture callus. *J Orthop Res* 1989;7:398–407.

59. Kenwright J, Richardson JB, Cunningham JL, et al: Axial movement and tibial fractures: A controlled randomised trial of treatment. *J Bone Joint Surg* 1991;73B:654–659.

60. Goodship AE, Kenwright J: The influence of induced micromovement upon the healing of experimental tibial fractures. *J Bone Joint Surg* 1985;67B:650–655.

61. Indrekvam K, Gjerdet NR, Engesaeter LB, et al: Effects of intramedullary reaming and nailing of rat femur. A mechanical and chemical study. *Acta Orthop Scand* 1991;62:582–586.

62. Reikeras O, Skjeldal S, Grogaard B: Mechanical effects of intramedullary reaming in pinned osteotomies in rats. *J Orthop Trauma* 1989;3:53–56.

63. Heckman JD, Ryaby JP, McCabe J, et al: Acceleration of tibial fracture-healing by non-invasive, low-intensity pulsed ultrasound. *J Bone Joint Surg* 1994;76A:26–34.

64. Sharrard WJW: A double-blind trial of pulsed electromagnetic fields for delayed union of tibial fractures. *J Bone Joint Surg* 1990;72B:347–355.

65. Pilla AA, Nasser PR, Kaufman JJ: On the sensitivity of cells and tissues to therapeutic and environmental electromagnetic fields. *Bioelectrochem Bioenerg* 1993; 30:161–169.

66. Pilla AA, Mont MA, Nasser PR, et al: Non-invasive low-intensity pulsed ultrasound accelerates bone healing in the rabbit. *J Orthop Trauma* 1990;4:246–253.

67. Pilla AA, Figueiredo M, Nasser P, et al: Acceleration of bone repair by pulsed sine wave ultrasound: Animal, clinical, and mechanistic studies, in Brighton CT, Pollack WR (eds): *Electromagnetics in Biology and Medicine.* San Francisco, CA, San Francisco Press, 1991, pp 331–341.

Section 2
Future Research Directions

Fracture Repair

Elucidate the cellular and molecular events that define injury to matrix, cells and molecules, and membranes in the bone at the time of fracture.

Little is known about the cellular events that occur at the time of injury. The stage of impact or injury may well dictate the rate of healing or whether or not the fracture heals at all. The rate, frequency, and amplitude of strain that cells experience at the time of injury need to be determined. Studies have demonstrated that a given cell may show a different response to stimuli, or behave in a different fashion, depending on its mechanical microenvironment. The mechanical microenvironment of a cell in fracture callus will depend on the stability of the fracture, the type of loading applied to that fracture, and the way by which those conditions are modulated by the matrix and through the cell's cytoskeleton. This will require correlation of anatomic studies with mathematical modeling. The cellular and molecular reactions that are set in motion at the time of injury, and the role that these play in the repair process, need to be elucidated.

Elucidate the cellular and molecular events that occur in the hematoma and the contribution of these events to the initiation and progression of the repair process.

At present, histologic analysis of fracture repair strongly suggests that events that occur during hematoma formation, such as the release of transforming growth factor β (TGF-β) and platelet-derived growth factor (PDGF) from platelets, initiate the formation of the callus. Current studies suggest that a cascade of cellular changes and regulatory processes, critical to normal repair, are initiated at this time. These processes have been incompletely evaluated so far in either normal or impaired fracture hematoma.

The role of the hematoma in initiating callus formation needs to be evaluated in both in vivo and in vitro models in which effects on cell proliferation and chemotaxis can be tested. Critical to these experiments is the development of appropriate controls.

Unlike mature bone or articular cartilage, fracture calluses include a heterogeneous population of cells whose distribution changes with time. Moreover, in the early stages of healing, discrete tissues, including periosteum, cortical bone, external soft tissues, and bone marrow, can be identified.

Methods to isolate the individual cell clones from loose mesenchymal, cartilaginous, or highly mineralized callus tissues are needed in order to investigate cellular mechanisms. In addition, the ability to correlate the findings of in vitro studies to the behavior of those same cell types in fractures in vivo must be established in experimental model systems.

Evaluate the role of inflammation in fracture healing.

Inflammation, including the influx of white blood cells and other inflammatory cells, and the concomitant release of cytokines, growth factors, and inflammatory mediators, occurs immediately after formation of the hematoma, and appears to be a critical step in the cascade of repair. Nevertheless, the specific contribution of these inflammatory events has not been defined.

As is true for studies of the hematoma, successful investigation of the role of inflammation will require carefully controlled studies comparing in vivo to in vitro experiments. Adequate models for these studies need to be developed. The in vivo bone chamber developed by Albrighton may be useful in this regard.

Identify the cells and regulatory signals that participate in intramembranous bone formation, including cell origins, local and systemic factors, and remodeling influences.

Despite the characterization of intramembranous bone formation at the histologic level, it has not been characterized at the cellular or molecular level. Although there are several cell culture models in which mineralization and bone nodule formation occur, there are no data to determine if the cell of origin, synthesis of matrix proteins, or regulation of bone formation is similar in these models to bone formation in the fracture callus. Also, the interplay of mechanical forces and the biologic events at this level have not been defined. Bone formation in cell cultures must be correlated with in vivo bone formation if reliable inferences are to be made about fracture repair in situ.

Identify the cells and regulatory signals that participate in chondrogenesis, including cell origins, local and systemic factors, and remodeling influences.

It appears that mechanical events dictate whether repair is by cartilage intermediates or by direct bone formation. In most clinical situations, repair occurs via cartilage intermediates. Despite many in vitro chondrogenesis models, correlation with in vivo chondrogenesis has not been made. This correlation must be made at the cellular and molecular levels in order to apply knowledge of regulatory mechanisms to clinical problems. Models of chondrogenesis should be validated by in vitro–in vivo comparisons.

Identify the cells and regulatory signals that participate in endochondral bone formation, including cell origins, local and systemic regulatory factors, and remodeling influences.

The process of endochondral ossification includes a complex sequence of histologic events, including cartilage maturation and hypertrophy, vascular invasion, and osteogenesis. Factors known to regulate endochondral ossification include mechanical and electrical factors, growth factors and their cognate receptors, general metabolic influences, and systemic and endocrine factors. These factors interact via complex and as yet undefined pathways.

A combined approach in which investigations of biologic and mechanical influences are correlated at both the cellular and molecular levels is required to study this complex problem in vivo. It is anticipated that this problem will require a team approach, fostering interaction between molecular biologists, engineers, and cell biologists.

Vascularization and Osteogenesis

Vascularization is intrinsically involved in osteogenesis; however, the specifics of the interactions between angiogenesis and osteogenesis remain to be elucidated. During bone formation multiple angiogenic modulators are expressed including basic fibroblast growth factor (bFGF). Furthermore, in experimental models, pathologic wound healing can be reversed when exogenous bFGF is administered. There is a need to better understand the vascular response during osteogenesis in the hope of providing therapy that will optimize the healing response.

Cellular infiltrate: Which cells regulate the angiogenic response during osteogenesis?

What is the role of the endothelial cell? Does it release growth factors that function as autocrine factors on endothelial cells and then as paracrine factors for the growth of other cells such as osteoblasts and myoblasts? What is the role of the pericyte? Does the pericyte regulate/inhibit or stimulate angiogenesis or osteogenesis? Does it serve as an osteogenic precursor cell?

What are the cell–cell interactions during angiogenesis and osteogenesis?

This is important because the study of each cell and its functions as isolated systems may not accurately depict the in vivo biology. For example, do endothelial cells and pericytes communicate with each other and then synthesize regulatory proteins, eg, TGF-β? Co-culture cell systems and the chick chorioallantoic membrane assay can be used to answer some of these questions. The role that selectins, gap junctions (connexins), matrix deposition (ie, collagen type IV), and the lamina obscurans play in the vascular response during osteogenesis requires study.

What is the role of endogenous angiogenesis stimulators and inhibitors during osteogenesis?

Growth factors and cytokines do not act in isolation but rather interact with each other. There may not be a simple initiation and termination of angiogenesis during osteogenesis, but rather a continuous balance between endogenous angiogenesis stimulators and inhibitors. Specific endogenous angiogenic proteins include acidic and basic fibroblast growth factors, vascular endothelial growth factor, TGF-β, TGF-α, tumor necrosis factor-α, platelet-derived growth factor-BB, and interleukin-8. Specific endogenous angiogenic inhibitors include α-interferon, cartilage derived inhibitor, and thrombospondin. TGF-β may represent the prototype bimodal angiogenic molecule. For example, in certain conditions it may function as a chemoattractant for macrophages and, therefore, elicit new angiogenic molecules, and in others, it acts as a potent endothelial cell inhibitor.

Determine the regulation and role of nutrients and oxygenation during the vascular response in osteogenesis.

Hypoxia is known to stimulate angiogenesis during wound healing. Hypoxia also exists in the early fracture callus, and the local Po_2 only returns to normal as healing occurs. Whether or not hypoxia is a stimulus to bone formation is not known. Future studies detailing the role of oxygenation during the vascular response and during osteogenesis may be of great therapeutic benefit.

Cell Lineages in Cartilage and Bone Formation

Determine the lineage of cells for cartilage during bone repair and regeneration.

The elucidation of the lineage pathways in the origin, commitment, and differentiation of cartilage cells is a prerequisite for optimal understanding of fracture repair. The precise origin of cells involved in cartilage formation is not known. The regulation of proliferation of stem cells for prechondrogenic lineage is a critical issue. The sequential differentiation of chondrogenic cells into cartilage is subject to modulation by multiple factors that need to be identified.

The identification and isolation of chondroprogenitor stem cells from the initial callus should receive high priority. The other sites from which progenitor cells should be isolated include the periosteum, endosteum, bone marrow stroma, and muscle. At the level of gene expression, is there a "master" control gene, such as the myo D, myogenin, and myf-5, which are involved in myoblast lineage? One potential approach for identifying such a gene may consist of subtraction hybridization of "naive" and committed cells. Another approach may consist of transferring bone morphogenic protein (BMP) and TGF-β genes into stromal precursor cells to induce cartilage phenotype. Finally, the use of transgenic and "gene knockout" approaches could be very rewarding. The major obstacle could be the rare occurrence of such master regulating genes.

Determine the origin and commitment of osteoblasts during bone repair and regeneration.

The delineation of the osteoblast lineage in the origin, commitment, and differentiation of osteoblasts during bone formation is a prerequisite for the full understanding and the optimal treatment of fracture repair. The origin of the osteoblast lineage in fracture repair is likely to be local. The initial commitment and clonal expansion of preosteoprogenitor cells are a central problem. It is necessary to examine the hypothesis that this step is induced by a member of the BMP family or by a novel helix-loop-helix (HLH) family member.

The influence of transfection of BMP genes into bone marrow stromal cells and skeletal muscle-derived mesenchymal cells should be investigated. The "transformation" of the phenotype could be monitored by bone-specific genes such as alkaline phosphatase and osteocalcin. Alternatively, an osteocalcin gene construct with the promoter could be used in a quantitative assay. The potential existence of a "master" gene for osteoblast lineage can be examined by "subtraction" hybridization methods. One approach will consist of determining differences between intramembranous and endochondral bone. The rarity of these genes may be a major obstacle. One additional difficulty may be that the isolated gene may not be the proximal one in the gene cascade.

Identify the signals and receptors governing commitment and differentiation.

The commitment and differentiation of chondrogenic and osteogenic cells are clearly dependent on and influenced by signals emanating from other cells (cell–cell interaction) from the matrix (matrix–cell interaction) and the general environment of the organism (systemic factors). Identification of these pathways of information transfer is important for recognizing deficiencies in disease and for controlling these processes therapeutically. The difficulties in embarking in these studies include the development of feasible models and proving their validity in vivo or in situ.

The current approaches include (1) identification of relevant osteogenic/chondrogenic activities, (2) isolation and characterization of the factors responsible for these activities, (3) identification and characterization of the "receptors" that sense these activities, and (4) elucidation of the signal transduction pathway. The signals can be divided into biologic (biochemical activities) and physical (mechanical/electrical); local and systemic; chondrogenic and osteogenic; morphogenic (induce commitment in predifferentiated cells) and osteogenic/chondrogenic (promote differentiation/maturation in committed cells). Furthermore, cells have only a few general signal transduction pathways, all of which affect the phosphorylation or dephosphorylation of specific proteins. The identity of these proteins determines the specificity of the cellular response, which in some cells includes gene transcription. Identification and characterization of the molecules involved in these pathways could help us understand and possibly control bone repair.

Section 3

Bone Remodeling

Section Editors:
Gary E. Friedlaender, MD
Lawrence G. Raisz, MD

Roland Baron, DDS, PhD
David R. Eyre, PhD
Gary E. Friedlaender, MD
Mark C. Horowitz, PhD
Mitsukazu Ishii, MD
Peter R. Jay, MD
Joan B. Levy, PhD

Richard R. Pelker, MD, PhD
He-Ying Qian, PhD
Lawrence G. Raisz, MD
Pamela Gehron Robey, PhD
Vicki Rosen, PhD
Nancy Troiano, MS

Chapter 15

The Cellular Basis of Bone Resorption: Cell Biology of the Osteoclast

Roland Baron, DDS, PhD

Introduction

The osteoclast is the cell responsible for the resorption of bone, a process that is required for the growth, remodeling, and repair of bone, and that is, under normal conditions, tightly coupled to the process of bone formation by osteoblasts. It is the balance between these two cellular activities, bone formation and resorption, that determines skeletal mass and shape at any point in time.

The osteoclast is a highly motile cell that attaches to and migrates along the surfaces of bone. The osteoclast is a multinucleated cell (although mononuclear osteoclasts are also encountered), which is formed by the asynchronous fusion of mononuclear precursors that are derived from the bone marrow and differentiate within the granulocyte-macrophage lineage. The cell attaches to the mineralized bone matrix that it is going to resorb by forming a tight ring-like zone of adhesion called the sealing zone. This attachment involves the specific interaction between adhesion molecules in the osteoclast's membrane (integrins) and some specific proteins found in the bone matrix or at the surface of bone. The space contained inside this ring of attachment and between the osteoclast and the bone matrix constitutes the bone resorbing compartment (Fig. 1). The attached osteoclast synthesizes several proteolytic enzymes that are then vectorially transported and secreted into this extracellular bone resorbing compartment. Simultaneously, the osteoclast lowers the pH of this compartment by extruding protons across its apical membrane (the membrane facing the bone matrix). The concerted action of the enzymes and the low pH in the bone-resorbing compartment leads to the extracellular digestion of the mineral and organic phases of the bone matrix. After resorbing the bone to a certain depth, which is determined by mechanisms that remain to be elucidated but may involve a calcium sensor, the osteoclast detaches and moves along the bone surface before reattaching and forming another resorption lacuna, usually in close proximity to the first one. In the process, a certain volume of bone matrix has been removed, only to be replaced a few days later, under normal circumstances, by newly formed matrix.

The osteoclast is, therefore, a cell that is morphologically and functionally polarized (Fig.1). One pole (the apical pole) faces the bone matrix at which attachment occurs and towards which most of the secretion is targeted. The other pole (the basolateral pole) faces the soft tissues in the local microenvironment (bone marrow or periosteum) and provides mostly, but not exclusively, regulatory functions.

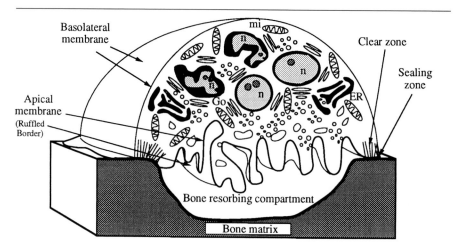

Fig. 1 Functional organization and polarity of the osteoclast; n = nuclei; Go = Golgi complexes; mi = mitochondria; ER = endoplasmic reticulum.

Osteoclast Secretions in the Bone Resorbing Compartment

The morphologic polarity of the osteoclast is paralleled by a functional polarity, with the osteoclasts synthesizing and vectorially secreting several classes of enzymes towards the apical ruffled border.[1,2] It is well established that these enzymes comprise acid phosphatases, aryl-sulfatases, β-glucuronidase, and β-glycerophosphatase as well as several cysteine-proteinases,[1-3] which are capable of fully digesting collagen at low pH. Recent evidence from several laboratories suggests that osteoclasts probably also secrete metalloproteinases (collagenase and stromelysin) and that these are important in the process of bone resorption.[4-7]

Thus, the cooperative action of a set of enzymes with acidic and neutral optimal pHs would lead to a complete degradation of the extracellular matrix at the resorbing site. During active resorption this action would allow matrix degradation over a broader range of pHs (ie, further away from the osteoclast membrane) and, after the osteoclast moves away, it would allow collagenase to complete the digestion of collagen at neutral pH.[4]

Hence, after attaching to the bone surface, the osteoclast secretes both lysosomal enzymes and metalloproteinases in the sealed-off bone-resorbing compartment, which, as discussed below, is acidified.

The Apical Membrane and the Process of Acidification

The apical membrane of the osteoclast, which is also called the ruffled border, is directly involved in the molecular mechanisms of bone resorption. It is the target for the specific delivery of the newly synthesized secretory enzymes,[1,2] and it is the site of proton extrusion for acidification of the bone-resorbing compartment.[1,8]

The protons are extruded by proton pumps, and the resulting osteoclast-mediated acidification is required for the dissolution of the mineral phase and the enzymatic degradation of the organic phase of the extracellular matrix.[1,3,8-11] The proton-transporting adenosine triphosphatases (H$^+$ ATPases) responsible for acidification in various cells and organelles are distinguished from each other on the basis of their structure and their sensitivity to various specific inhibitors.[12,13]

Based on pharmacologic and immunochemical data, it has been suggested that the H[+] ATPase present in osteoclast membranes is of the vacuolar-type, closely resembling the pumps present in kidney membranes.[8,14,15] There is, however, evidence in the literature that suggests the possibility that there are subtle differences in the properties and structure of mammalian vacuolar ATPases,[12,13,16] and recent results from my laboratory show that the osteoclast proton pumps, at least those in the chicken, differ from other known vacuolar ATPases.[11] Briefly, proton transport by osteoclast-derived vesicles is more sensitive to inhibition by vanadate and by nitrate than similar preparations derived from the kidney in the same animals. Furthermore, immunochemical data and purification of the enzyme have demonstrated that the osteoclast proton pump expresses isoforms of the common catalytic subunits of the vacuolar proton pump,[11] probably explaining the differences in pharmacology.

The osteoclast proton pump may, therefore, constitute a novel class of H[+] ATPase, which has a unique pharmacology and specific isoforms of two subunits in the catalytic portion of the enzyme. This H[+] ATPase is involved in the resorption of bone and, if expressed in a cell-specific manner, could open new possibilities for therapeutic intervention. Current efforts at cloning these various isoforms of the osteoclast proton pump's subunits found in chicken cells are under way in my laboratory and should allow the determination of the molecular basis for the unique pharmacology of this H[+] ATPase.

In parallel with proton pumping, the apical plasma membrane of the osteoclast also expresses chloride channels, measured as a chloride conductance. The extrusion of this anion (Cl^-) is absolutely required for the acidification process.[8,11]

Basolateral Ion Transport Systems and Apical Acidification

The apparently simple process of pumping protons across the ruffled border membrane to acidify the resorption lacuna imposes on the cell a complex and demanding set of ionic requirements. These requirements were designed essentially to maintain the electrochemical balance of the osteoclast during bone resorption. This ionic balancing act requires the coordinated activity of electrogenic ion pumps, ion channels, and electroneutral ion exchangers to maintain the cytoplasmic pH and the transmembrane electrical potential within narrow physiologic ranges.

Cytoplasmic pH is maintained near neutrality by the action of electroneutral ion exchangers in the basolateral membrane. There probably are a higher number of copies in the osteoclast than in other cell types, as a result of its very active proton transport. Both an acid extruder (the Na^+/H^+ exchanger) and an acid-loader (ie, base-extruder, the HCO_3^-/Cl^- exchanger) are present in the osteoclast.[17,18] The Na^+/H^+ exchanger is driven by a Na^+ gradient established across the basolateral membrane by the activity of the sodium pumps.[19]

The hyperpolarization, which results from the activities of the H[+] pump and the Na^+/K^+ ATPase, to which the activity of the Ca^{2+} ATPase also contributes,[20] is alleviated by the activity of voltage-sensitive ion channels that transport positively charged ions into the cell (K^+ channels) and/or negatively charged ions out of the cell (Cl^- channels), thus discharging the electrical potential.[21-26]

Regulation of H^+ transport at the apical surface of the osteoclast is, therefore, tightly linked to the regulation of intracellular pH and membrane potential, and it is accomplished mostly by exchangers, pumps, and channels present in the basolateral membrane of the cell. Evidence for this tight coupling is provided by the fact that inhibition of the sodium pump,[27] the HCO_3^-/Cl^- exchanger, or the Na^+/H^+ antiporter (Y Su and R Baron, unpublished results, 1992),[28] all lead to a profound inhibition of bone resorption. Furthermore, we found that calcitonin regulates, via G proteins and the activation of various protein kinases, both the Na^+/H^+ exchanger and the sodium pump in kidney cells,[29,30] thereby raising the possibility that the effects of this hormone on the osteoclast[31] are mediated via the same effectors.

Functional Role of the Proto-oncogene c-src

The discovery that deletion of the gene encoding c-src led to osteopetrosis, directly and unequivocally demonstrated that this protein tyrosine kinase plays a critical and unique role in bone resorption.[32] Follow-up studies have further shown that c-src is playing its critical role within the osteoclast itself, ie, that the osteopetrotic phenotype in these mutants is cell autonomous. First, pp60[c-src] is expressed at high levels in osteoclasts but not in other bone cells.[33] In osteoclasts, it is associated with both the plasma membrane and intracellular organelles. Second, mix and match experiments between mutant spleens or stromal cells and their wild type homologs showed the defect to be within the hematopoietic cells.[34]

While these initial studies did not attempt to identify specific function(s) of pp60[c-src] in osteoclastic bone resorption, some possibilities are suggested by considering the results of immunolocalization of c-src or some of its substrates as well as the known characteristics of these proteins in other cells.[33,35,36] The presence of c-src in the ruffled border and intracellular vesicles suggests that it may contribute to vesicle targeting or membrane fusion, a process required in the osteoclast for targeted delivery of intracellular vesicles to the apical surface in order to secrete enzymes into the resorption compartment and to insert the proton pump and other transporters involved in acid secretion at the apical ruffled border membrane.

The pp60[c-src] phenotype may also be involved in integrin-related attachment and signaling, another potential role that is of particular interest with regard to osteoclasts. Although confocal microscopic results fail to show a specific association of pp60[c-src] with adhesion structures,[33] integrin binding might nevertheless involve pp60[c-src] and provide a signal leading to the development of cell polarity and the formation of the ruffled border at the site of bone resorption. Consistent with this hypothesis, preliminary studies in my laboratory[37] show a rapid and transient wave of tyrosine phosphorylation in isolated osteoclasts exposed to arginine-glycine-aspartic acid (RGD)-peptides, and c-src has been suggested to form a complex with the vitronectin receptor in osteoclast-like cells.[38] Furthermore, src substrates are found in association with both the sealing zone and the ruffled border membrane. The c-src oncogene may, therefore, play several roles in osteoclast function, one or more of which cannot be compensated when the gene for c-src is deleted.[32]

Acknowledgments

This work was supported by grants #DE-04724, AR40185, and AR41339.

References

1. Baron R, Neff L, Louvard D, et al: Cell-mediated extracellular acidification and bone resorption: Evidence for a low pH in resorbing lacunae and localization of a 100-kD lysosomal membrane protein at the osteoclast ruffled border. *J Cell Biol* 1985;101:2210–2222.
2. Baron R, Neff L, Brown W, et al: Polarized secretion of lysosomal enzymes: G-distribution of cation-independent mannose-6-phosphate receptors and lysosomal enzymes along the osteoclast exocytic pathway. *J Cell Biol* 1988;106:1863–1872.
3. Vaes G: Cellular biology and biochemical mechanism of bone resorption: A review of recent developments on the formation, activation, and mode of action of osteoclasts. *Clin Orthop* 1988;231:239–271.
4. Delaissé JM, Neff L, Eeckhout Y, et al: Evidence for the presence of (pro)collagenase in osteoclasts, in Cohn DV, Gennari C, Tashjian AH Jr (eds): *Calcium Regulating Hormones and Bone Metabolism: Basic and Clinical Aspects*. Proceedings of the Eleventh International Conference on Calcium Regulating Hormones, Florence, April 24–29, 1992. Amsterdam, Excerpta Medica, 1992, vol 11, pp 161–164.
5. Everts V, Delaisse JM, Korper W, et al: Degradation of collagen in the bone-resorbing compartment underlying the osteoclast involves both cysteine-proteinases and matrix metalloproteinases. *J Cell Physiol* 1992;150:221–231.
6. Okamura T: Detection of collagenase in RNA in bovine root resorbing tissue by in situ hybridization. *Jpn J Oral Biol* 1992;34:95–111.
7. Case JP, Sano H, Lafyatis R, et al: Transin/stromelysin expression in the synovium of rats with experimental erosive arthritis: In situ localization and kinetics of expression of the transformation-associated metalloproteinase in euthymic and athymic Lewis rats. *J Clin Invest* 1989;84:1731–1740.
8. Blair HC, Teitelbaum SL, Ghiselli R, et al: Osteoclastic bone resorption by a polarized vacuolar proton pump. *Science* 1989;245:855–857.
9. Baron R: Molecular mechanisms of bone resorption by the osteoclast. *Anat Rec* 1989;224:317–324.
10. Blair HC, Kahn AJ, Crouch EC, et al: Isolated osteoclasts resorb the organic and inorganic components of bone. *J Cell Biol* 1986;102:1164–1172
11. Chatterjee D, Chakraborty M, Leit M, et al: Sensitivity to vanadate and isoforms of subunits A and B distinguish the osteoclast proton pump from other vacuolar H^+ ATPases. *Proc Natl Acad Sci USA* 1992;89:6257–6261.
12. Nelson N: Structure and pharmacology of the proton-ATPases. *Trends Pharmacol Sci* 1991;12:71–75
13. Forgac M: Structure and function of vacuolar class of ATP-driven proton pumps. *Physiol Rev* 1989;69:765–796.
14. Bekker PJ, Gay CV: Biochemical characterization of an electrogenic vacuolar proton pump in purified chicken osteoclast plasma membrane vesicles. *J Bone Miner Res* 1990;5:569–579.
15. Vaananen HK, Karhukorpi EK, Sundquist K, et al: Evidence for the presence of a proton pump of the vacuolar H^+-ATPase type in the ruffled borders of osteoclasts. *J Cell Biol* 1990;111:1305–1311.
16. Wang Z-Q, Gluck S: Isolation and properties of bovine kidney brush border vacuolar H^+-ATPase: A proton pump with enzymatic and structural differences from kidney microsomal H^+-ATPase. *J Biol Chem* 1990;265:21957–21965.
17. Teti A, Blair HC, Teitelbaum SL, et al: Cytoplasmic pH regulation and chloride/bicarbonate exchange in avian osteoclasts. *J Clin Invest* 1989;83:227–233.
18. Ravesloot JH, Boron WF, Baron R, et al: Proton extrusion in osteoclasts can occur via a basolateral-type Na^+/H^+ exchanger or via a Na^+-independent, amiloride-insensitive H^+ extruder. *J Bone Miner Res* 1992;7(suppl 1):S130.
19. Baron R, Neff L, Roy C, et al: Evidence for a high and specific concentration of (Na^+, K^+)ATPase in the plasma membrane of the osteoclast. *Cell* 1986;46:311–320.

20. Bekker PJ, Gay CV: Characterization of a Ca²⁺-ATPase in osteoclast plasma membrane. *J Bone Miner Res* 1990;5:557–567.

21. Ravesloot JH, Ypey DL, Vrijheid-Lammers T, et al: Voltage-activated K⁺ conductances in freshly isolated embryonic chicken osteoclasts. *Proc Natl Acad Sci USA* 1989;86:6821–6825.

22. Ravesloot JH, Ypey DL, Nijweide PJ, et al: Three voltage-activated K⁺ conductances and an ATP-activated conductance in freshly isolated embryonic chick osteoclasts. *Pflugers Arch* 1989;414:S166–S167.

23. Sims SM, Dixon SJ: Inwardly rectifying K⁺ current in osteoclasts. *Am J Physiol* 1989;256:C1277–C1282.

24. Sims SM, Kelly ME, Dixon SJ: K⁺ and Cl⁻ currents in freshly isolated rat osteoclasts. *Pflugers Arch* 1991;419:358–370.

25. Schoppa NE, Su Y, Baron R, et al: Identification of single ion channels in neonatal rat osteoclasts. *J Bone Miner Res* 1990;5(suppl 2):S204.

26. Blair HC, Teitelbaum SL, Tan HL, et al: Passive chloride permeability charge coupled to H(⁺)-ATPase of avian osteoclast ruffled membrane. *Am J Physiol* 1991; 260:C1315–C1324.

27. Baron R, Kellokumpu S, Neff L, et al: Sodium pumps and bone resorption: Presence of basolateral kidney type alpha subunits in osteoclasts, effects of ouabain on bone resorption and interactions with calcitonin in MDCK cells. *Calcif Tissue Int* 1988; 412:A14.

28. Hall TJ, Chambers TJ: Na⁺/H⁺ antiporter is the primary proton transport system used by osteoclasts during bone resorption. *J Cell Physiol* 1990;142:420–424.

29. Chakraborty M, Chatterjee D, Kellokumpu S, et al: Cell cycle-dependent coupling of the calcitonin receptor to different G proteins. *Science* 1991;251:1078–1082.

30. Chakraborty M, Su Y, Nathanson M, et al: The effects of calcitonin in rat osteoclasts and in a kidney cell line (LLC-PK1) are mediated via an inhibition of the Na⁺/H⁺ antiporter. *J Bone Miner Res* 1991;6(suppl 1):S134.

31. Su Y, Chakraborty M, Nathanson M, et al: Differential effects of the 3′,5′-cyclic adenosine monophosphate and protein kinase C pathways on the response of isolated rat osteoclasts to calcitonin. *Endocrinology* 1992;131:1497–1502.

32. Soriano P, Montgomery C, Geske R, et al: Targeted disruption of the c-src proto-oncogene leads to osteopetrosis in mice. *Cell* 1991;64:693–702.

33. Horne WC, Neff L, Chatterjee D, et al: Osteoclasts express high levels of pp60c-src in association with intracellular membranes. *J Cell Biol* 1992;119:1003–1013.

34. Lowe C, Yoneda T, Boyce B, et al: Osteopetrosis due to SRC-deficiency is caused by an osteoclast defect. *J Bone Miner Res* 1992;7(suppl 1):S98.

35. Boyce BF, Yoneda T, Lowe C, et al: Requirement of pp60c-src expression for osteoclasts to form ruffled borders and resorb bone in mice. *J Clin Invest* 1992;90: 1622–1627.

36. Boyce BF, Chen H, Bouton A, et al: A SRC tyrosine phosphoprotein substrate (P80/ 85) is localized to the ruffled border of osteoclasts. *J Bone Miner Res* 1992;7(suppl 1):S105.

37. Neff L, Horne WC, Male P, et al: A cyclic RGD peptide induces a wave of tyrosine phosphorylation and the translocation of a c-src substrate (p85) in isolated rat osteoclasts. *J Bone Miner Res* 1992;7(suppl 1):S106.

38. Rolnick F, Huskey M, Gupta A, et al: The signal generating complex of the occupied osteoclast α$_v$ β$_3$ integrin includes SRC, phosphatidyl inositol 3 kinase (PI 3 kinase) and phospholipase C$_\gamma$(PLC$_\gamma$). *J Bone Miner Res* 1992;7(suppl 1):S105.

Chapter 16

Bone Remodeling: Formation

Pamela Gehron Robey, PhD

Introduction

Bone is remarkable in that it is one of the few tissues of vertebrates that is capable of regeneration through a process of turnover. In bone turnover, small areas of the skeleton are destroyed by osteoclasts (bone resorption) and rebuilt by osteoblasts (bone formation).[1] Consequently, the ultrastructure and molecular composition of the adult skeleton at a particular site of remodeling are not static and depend on the stage of turnover. Unlike the developmental process, bone formation in the growing and mature skeleton occurs on a bony template, as opposed to de novo or by replacement of a cartilaginous structure, suggesting that the steps of the pathway and regulatory mechanisms may be different. This chapter contains a brief (and in some cases, speculative) discussion of the cell types involved, a description of their maturational pathway, and a discussion of the cellular mechanisms of mineralized matrix expression.

Bone-Forming Cells in Bone Remodeling

Although the cells that reform a packet of bone that has been excavated by an osteoclast are known to belong to the osteoblastic lineage, the members of this lineage have not yet been clearly identified. There have been many arguments that the differences in bone-forming cells observed both in vivo and in vitro are due to "different maturational stages;" however, it is still not clear whether complete bone formation is accomplished by one primordial stem cell type that, early in its pathway of development, gives rise to related but separate lines that cooperate, by more than one stem cell line, or by cells, which are at different stages of maturation, that must work together. This uncertainty is not clarified by examination of the situation during bone remodeling, because the origin of the cell(s) that rebuild is not unambiguous and there are several potential candidates within the area: osteocytes, lining cells, and marrow stromal fibroblasts.

Although often regarded as terminally differentiated cells, osteocytes should not be ruled out as potential candidates to repopulate the area. That osteocytes are not degenerating cells is evidenced by their normal-appearing nuclei. They maintain metabolic activity as evidenced by their continued synthesis and secretion of certain bone matrix proteins, and there may be some situations in which osteocytes may proliferate (as during fracture callus formation). Under normal circumstances, osteocytes are not able to proliferate because they are imprisoned by mineralized matrix, and it has been reported that osteoclasts will ultimately destroy osteocytes that they encounter during the resorptive process.[2]

Another candidate is the bone lining cell of the endosteal surface.[3] The origins of this cell are once again unclear. It has been suggested that, during the bone formation process, a single layer of osteoblasts that are tightly adherent to one another begins to reorganize as matrix apposition progresses. Under the influence of factors that have not yet been identified, a cell disengages from the osteoblastic layer, but maintains its tight associations (gap junctions) with its neighbors, thereby creating cell processes that are stretched between the two cells as the matrix mineralizes around them to form the osteocytic lacunae and canaliculae.[4] By depositing more matrix, the remaining osteoblasts continue to leave the new osteocyte behind, and the osteoblasts ultimately become a quiescent lining cell layer. The number of osteoblasts is higher than the total number of osteocytes and lining cells, suggesting that the remainder have an as yet unidentified fate (death?). In avian medullary bone, it is clear that lining cells can be metabolically activated very rapidly by estrogen, and begin bone formation,[5] but their activation in other animal species has not been well demonstrated. Lining cells also may actually be marrow stromal fibroblasts that are lying on the endosteal surface. The biochemical properties of lining cells have not been adequately delineated, but it has been reported that only a low percentage of them are alkaline phosphatase positive,[6] which may reflect different cellular pools from which they derive.

The last, and perhaps most likely candidates are the marrow stromal fibroblasts, which are at least in part osteogenic as demonstrated by the pioneering work of Friedenstein.[7] This population is highly pleiomorphic; it can give rise to fibroblasts that remain uncommitted, adipocytes, chondrocytes, osteoblasts, and perhaps even myoblasts, and certain fibroblasts that support hemopoiesis. It is possible that these cells are brought into the marrow environment by vascularization during development, because osteoprogenitor cells have been shown to be associated with invading capillaries.[8] Given the osteogenic capacity of a portion of this population, they are likely participants in the bone formation phase of bone turnover and, perhaps, in bone resorption as well.[9]

Information is somewhat incomplete concerning the biochemical nature of these three potential candidates before activation. Osteocytes and lining cells are amenable to biochemical characterization by in situ hybridization in that it is easy to identify them by their position within or on mineralized matrix. However, identification of resident marrow stromal fibroblasts is not routine until they become committed to a pathway and express a marker that gives their location away. While it remains to be determined how they compare to one another biochemically, it is clear that a common feature of all of these cells in vivo is that they are arrested in the G_o phase of the cell cycle, and are lying in wait for the moment when their bone-forming capacities are required.

Pathway of Maturation of Bone-Forming Cells

Chemotaxis

During the process of bone resorption, osteoclasts first demineralize and subsequently hydrolyze bone matrix, and the products of this process are liberated into the surrounding environment.[10] These products include the ions, Ca^{+2} and PO_4^{-2}, and fragments of mineralized matrix components, some of which maintain biologic activity. In response to the changing microenvironment (increasing ion concentration, calcitonin, and so forth), the osteoclast moves away from the resorption site, leaving behind an area of exposed bone. Within a certain time frame, which depends on the developmental age of the organism, this area is repopulated by one or a combination of osteoprogenitors. How did they get there? Although it is not a well described phenomenon in vivo, it is apparent that cells migrate into the area, perhaps as a chemotactic response to products of bone resorption that are diffusing away from the resorption site. The factors that cause the osteoprogenitor cells to "home" to a resorption lacuna have not been characterized, although it has been known for quite some time that type I collagen fragments have chemotactic activity.[11] This migration probably takes place before stimulation of proliferation; otherwise osteogenesis would occur wherever the osteoprogenitor is situated, causing islands of bone to form away from the trabecular surface. This latter process does not occur under normal circumstances.

A second implication of this observation is that stimulation of proliferation by factors released by resorption, such as transforming growth factor-betas (TGF-β), or bone morphogenetic proteins (BMPs), may not be effective unless the target cell is situated correctly; ie, in close proximity to or attached to mineralized matrix within an appropriate three-dimensional architecture. Bone matrix contains at least six putative cell attachment proteins,[12,13] and hydrolyzed fragments often have been found to maintain activity in some cases,[14] or exhibit new activities that were cryptic in the intact molecule.[15] These proteins or their fragments bind to integrins, cell surface receptors whose cytoplasmic extensions interact with intracellular signalling pathways.[16] Such cell-matrix interactions may play a critical role in initiation and subsequent maintenance of maturational events.

Although matrix synthesis and deposition in correlation to maturational stage have been well described during intramembranous and endochondral bone formation in development[13,17] and in vitro,[18] the bone matrix deposition phase in the adult skeleton has not been as well characterized. Results of recent studies in which marrow ablation was used in rat long bones indicate that the pattern of matrix protein expression is similar,[19] but because rat long bone contains few trabeculae and ablation is not the same as resorption, there may be differences in this process that have not yet been identified.

Proliferation of Osteoprogenitors

Osteoprogenitors proliferate, either in response to factors liberated by the resorption process or in response to other endogenous or exogenous factors. Interestingly, osteopontin has also been identified during the proliferative phase in rats[19] and in bovine bone cells,[20] and its expression in these circumstances may be analogous to its induction during transformation events in other cell types.[21] Because osteopontin contains an arginine-glycine-aspartic acid (RGD) sequence, it also may be mediating changes in cell matrix interactions. Following this burst, osteopontin expression decreases as the cell progresses toward becoming a preosteoblast.

Commitment of Preosteoblasts

Stimulation of proliferation is not enough to start the bone cell on its maturational pathway; other factors must come into play to cause commitment of the newly expanded population of cells to become preosteoblasts. This commitment is marked by the expression of alkaline phosphatase, the hallmark of the lineage. These cells synthesize a sparse extracellular matrix that is composed of type I collagen, but also contains significant amounts of type III collagen, the small proteoglycan decorin, fibronectin, and thrombospondin. Although decorin, fibronectin, and thrombospondin are often thought of solely as structural proteins, it is also apparent that they bind to and, therefore, may regulate activity of certain growth factors, in particular TGF-β.[22,23] Induction of these proteins may be a mechanism by which the potentially enormous amount of TGF-β in the area is held at bay. Although TGF-β stimulates proliferation of cells in the osteoblastic lineage, it decreases alkaline phosphatase expression. At the same time, fibronectin and thrombospondin may also be mediating cell-matrix interactions by binding to cell-surface integrins.[24] The identification of integrins on preosteoblastic cells is by no means complete, but it has been reported that they are moderately positive for α_v, and highly positive with an antibody that recognizes β_3 and β_5.[25] It is likely that the integrin expressed is $\alpha_v\beta_3$, because staining with antibodies against $\alpha_v\beta_5$ was almost undetectable. The expression of this integrin correlates with the appearance of its potential ligands, fibronectin and thrombospondin, whereas the ligand for $\alpha_v\beta_5$, vitronectin, is not associated with preosteoblasts. The nature of the intracellular pathways that may be stimulated by binding of the $\alpha_v\beta_3$ have not been characterized in osteoblastic cells.

Maturation of Osteoblasts

Subsequent to induction of alkaline phosphatase activity, preosteoblasts undergo several more mitoses (as can be determined by various different measures of mitotic activity)[26] before becoming nonproliferative. At this point, there is a major change in morphology from a spindle-shaped cell with relatively little rough endoplasmic reticulum (RER) to a somewhat cuboidal cell with enormously expanded biosynthetic apparati (RER, Golgi, secretory granules), the osteoblast. This expansion is required by the cell to carry out its primary mission, to secrete and deposit large amounts of osteoid. Concurrent with this morphologic change, there is also a switch in gene expression such that there is an increased amount of type I collagen, maintenance of decorin secretion, and induction of biglycan, the small proteoglycan, and osteonectin. Because decorin has been reported to regulate collagen fibril diameter, this change in the ratio of collagen to decorin may explain the relatively large size of collagen fibrils in osteoid.

The role of biglycan and osteonectin in the switch from preosteoblast to osteoblast is less clear. Biglycan has been localized to cell surface environments,[27] and its induction may indicate a change in cell-matrix interactions, or it may also be modulating TGF-β activity. Osteonectin has also been implicated in disrupting cell-matrix interactions and shape change (albeit in endothelial cells),[28] but as a result of its ability to bind collagen coupled with its affinity for calcium,[29] osteonectin may be a participant in subsequent matrix mineralization reactions. There is a marked increase in synthesis of fibronectin in the osteoblastic cell layer, and this coincides with an observed induction of the integrin subunit, α_4, which in combination with β_1, forms an integrin that is relatively specific for fibronectin.[24] However, β_1 has not yet been directly detected in the osteoblastic layer.

Following this initial phase of an osteoblast's life span, marked by secretion of a collagen-rich matrix, induction of another group of proteins that are associated more closely with matrix mineralization begins (a second phase of osteopontin, bone sialoprotein, and osteocalcin). Osteopontin and bone sialoprotein, by virtue of containing long stretches of acidic acid residues, have very high affinities for calcium.[30] It is not surprising that they are mineral associated, but the mechanisms by which they facilitate hydroxyapatite formation are unknown. Recent studies, which have immunolocalized the biosynthetic pathway of bone sialoprotein synthesis, secretion, and deposition, have revealed that bone sialoprotein is assembled in the intracellular environment in preformed packets of matrix that are secreted intact and immediately mineralize when exposed to the extracellular environment.[31] How or if the putative cell attachment activities of osteopontin and bone sialoprotein fit with a function in mediating matrix mineralization is not apparent. There is a case for speculating that binding of bone sialoprotein via its integrin (as yet, not identified in bone-forming cells) as it is trafficked through the cell may orient the bone sialoprotein in such a way that it binds appropriately to other proteins found in this preformed packet of material and may expose the acidic regions such that they are available as nucleation sites for hydroxyapatite deposition upon secretion.

Osteocalcin has a relatively weak affinity for calcium and hydroxyapatite compared to other bone matrix proteins. The precise point at which its synthesis is initiated is unclear and may differ from one animal species to another. In rats, mRNA for osteocalcin is clearly detectable in osteoblasts, but in spite of its appearance around the time of matrix mineralization, no abnormalities in hydroxyapatite formation are found when deposition of osteocalcin in matrix is inhibited.[32]

Formation of Osteocytes

As matrix deposition progresses, osteoblasts further elaborate a microenvironment that is conducive for mineralization by creating a secluded area (unmineralized osteoid sandwiched between the osteoblastic layer on one side and mineralized matrix on the other), with the appropriate concentration of ions and other factors that are required.[33] Certain cells dissociate from other cells in the osteoblastic layer, and the matrix surrounding them mineralizes, thereby forming the osteocytic lacunae and the cannaliculae. The biosynthetic capacity of these cells is decreased as evidenced by the reduction in the cytoplasmic volume, but they are not totally quiescent. Immunostaining and in situ hybridization indicate that synthesis and deposition of biglycan, thrombospondin, and fibronectin are maintained by osteocytes.[25,27] The pattern of integrin expression known to date indicates that osteocytes contain similar subunits to those identified on osteoblasts.[25] Other studies indicate that osteocalcin is also present at this stage of maturation, that osteocalcin may be synthesized after matrix mineralization, and that it may reflect the end point of the bone formation phase.[34]

Genetic Mechanisms of Cellular Maturation

A wealth of information specific for genes of bone matrix proteins has accompanied the vast expansion in the technology to isolate and characterize genes and the regulatory elements that control their activity. With the exception of decorin, the gene for which is larger than 40 kb,[35] virtually all of the structural matrix protein genes have been isolated in a number of animal species.[12,13] What is lacking at this point is an understanding of the sequence of events that causes genes to be up-regulated and down-regulated as the cells mature. Gene structure is highly complex. Genes are composed of exons, which contain the genetic information that is translated into protein; introns, which are spliced from the newly synthesized RNA prior to exclusion from the nucleus; and a promoter, which is responsible for regulation.

As in all genes, the promoter of bone matrix protein genes contains a number of regulatory elements (cis-acting) that facilitate binding of DNA polymerases and that serve as binding sites for nuclear factors (trans-acting elements).[36] DNA polymerases have been associated with "TATA" and "CAAT" boxes, and one or both of these transcriptional motifs have been found in the promoters of alkaline phosphatase, thrombospondin, collagen, fibronectin, matrix Gla protein, osteopontin, bone sialoprotein, and osteocalcin. Other unusual sequences have also been identified in the promoters of alkaline phosphatase (GC rich), osteonectin (GAGA), and biglycan (CA, CT repeats), which may confer unusual conformations or binding specificities to these promoters. Although the list of nuclear factors that bind to specific sequences in the promoters is by no means complete, consensus sequences have been identified that bind the nuclear factors NF1, SP1, AP1 and AP2. Many of these elements have been identified in the promoters in bone matrix genes to date, but there is no obvious pattern of elements that mark an "early" gene from a "middle" gene, from a "late" gene. For example, AP1 sites are found in the thrombospondin promoter, the production of which begins at early stages of maturation, and the osteopontin and osteocalcin promoters, both of which appear at late stages. This random distribution is not further clarified by the identification of hormone or factor response elements. Consensus sequences are now emerging for the binding of receptors with their ligands such as vitamin D (VDRE), glucocorticoids (GRE), retinoic acid (RAR, RXR), estrogen (ERE), and cAMP (CRE). Unfortunately, the identification of these response elements has not shed much light on the sequence of gene activation.[36]

However, certain features of gene activation are emerging, as can be seen by looking at the activation of the osteocalcin gene. It now appears the synthetic product of specific proto-oncogenes forms specific nuclear gene activating factors. For example, proto-oncogenes *fos* and *jun* are immediate response genes that become activated within moments of transduction events. Their products form homo- or hetero-dimers that cooperate with hormones and their receptors in binding to their response elements in the osteocalcin gene.[37] The presence or absence of these nuclear factors may either be stimulatory or inhibitory. Because the number of nuclear factors most likely is not limitless, gene activation probably is accomplished by a set of factors that cooperate and must come and go at the appropriate time during the biosynthetic lifetime of the cell.

Summary

Bone formation following resorption is a process that occurs as cells in the osteoblastic lineage pass through a series of maturational steps in a fashion similar, but not necessarily identical, to that during development. The composition of the extracellular matrix that these cells secrete changes such that at early stages of maturation, they synthesize a collagenous matrix with types I, III, and V collagens, decorin, thrombospondin, matrix Gla protein, and, sometimes, osteopontin; at intermediate stages, they switch to a type I collagen enriched matrix and also secrete fibronectin, biglycan, and osteonectin; and at late stages, osteopontin, bone sialoprotein, and osteocalcin. The pattern of integrin expression also changes with maturational stage, which may mediate changes in metabolism caused by extracellular matrix via intracellular signaling pathways yet to be defined. Further examination of the genomic events involved in the sequential expression of these bone matrix and related genes will be helpful in the development of strategies to manipulate bone cell activity therapeutically.

References

1. Raisz LG, Rodan GA: Cellular basis for bone turnover, in Avioli LV, Krane SM (eds): *Metabolic Bone Disease and Clinically Related Disorders*, ed 2. Philadelphia, PA, WB Saunders, 1990, pp 1–41.

2. Elmardi AS, Katchburian MV, Katchburian E: Electron microscopy of developing calvaria reveals images that suggest that osteoclasts engulf and destroy osteocytes during bone resorption. *Calcif Tissue Int* 1990;46:239–245.

3. Miller SC, Jee WSS: The bone lining cell: A distinct phenotype? *Calcif Tissue Int* 1987;41:1–5.

4. Palumbo C, Palazzini S, Marotti G: Morphological study of intercellular junctions during osteocyte differentiation. *Bone* 1990;11:401–406.

5. Wilson S, Duff SR: Morphology of medullary bone during the egg formation cycle. *Res Vet Sci* 1990;48:216–220.

6. Bianco P, Ballanti P, Mazzaferro S, et al: Combined use of tetracycline fluorescence and alkaline phosphatase cytochemistry in the evaluation of osteoblastic activity in bone biopsies. *Basic Appl Histochem* 1987;31(suppl):29.

7. Friedenstein AJ: Osteogenic stem cells in the bone marrow, in Heersche JNM, Kanes JA (eds): *Bone and Mineral Research: 7.* Amsterdam, Elsevier, 1990, pp 243–272.

8. Streeter GL: Developmental horizons in human embryos (fourth issue): Review of histogenesis of cartilage and bone. *Contrib Embryol Carnegie Inst* 1949;33:149–168.

9. Yamashita T, Asano K, Takahashi N, et al: Cloning of an osteoblastic cell line involved in the formation of osteoclast-like cells. *J Cell Physiol* 1990;145:587–595.

10. Zaidi M, Alam AS, Shankar VS, et al: Cellular biology of bone resorption. *Biol Rev Camb Philos Soc* 1993;68:197–264.

11. Gauss-Muller V, Kleinman HK, Martin GR, et al: Role of attachment factors and attractants in fibroblast chemotaxis. *J Lab Clin Med* 1980;96:1071–1080.

12. Gehron Robey P: The biochemistry of bone. *Endocrinol Metab Clin North Am* 1989;18:858–902.

13. Gehron Robey P, Bianco P, Termine JD: The cellular biology and molecular biochemistry of bone formation, in Favus MJ, Coe FL (eds): *Disorders of Bone and Mineral Metabolism.* New York, Raven Press, 1992, pp 241–263.

14. Nagai T, Yamakawa N, Aota S, et al: Monoclonal antibody characterization of two distant sites required for function of the central cell-binding domain of fibronectin in cell adhesion, cell migration, and matrix assembly. *J Cell Biol* 1991;114:1295–1305.

15. Mintz KP, Grzesik WJ, Midura RJ, et al: Purification and fragmentation of nondenatured bone sialoprotein: Evidence for a cryptic, RGD-resistant cell attachment domain. *J Bone Miner Res* 1993;8:985–995.

16. Ruoslahti E: Integrins. *J Clin Invest* 1991;87:1–5.

17. Strauss PG, Closs EI, Schmidt J, et al: Gene expression during osteogenic differentiation in mandibular condyles in vitro. *J Cell Biol* 1990;110:1369–1378.

18. Stein GS, Lian JB, Owen TA: Relationship of cell growth to the regulation of tissue-specific gene expression during osteoblast differentiation. *FASEB J* 1990;4:3111–3123.

19. Suva LJ, Seedor JG, Endo N, et al: Pattern of gene expression following rat tibial marrow ablation. *J Bone Miner Res* 1993;8:379–388.

20. Ibaraki K, Termine JD, Whitson SW, et al: Bone matrix mRNA expression in differentiating fetal bovine osteoblasts. *J Bone Miner Res* 1992;7:743–754.

21. Craig AM, Nemir M, Mukherjee BB, et al: Identification of the major phosphoprotein secreted by many rodent cell lines as 2ar/osteopontin: Enhanced expression in H-ras-transformed 3T3 cells. *Biochem Biophys Res Comm* 1988;157:166–173.

22. Ruoslahti E, Yamaguchi Y: Proteoglycans as modulators of growth factor activities. *Cell* 1991;64:867–869.

23. Murphy-Ullrich JE, Schultz-Cherry S, Hook M: Transforming growth factor-beta complexes with thrombospondin. *Mol Biol Cell* 1992;3:181–188.

24. Cheresh DA: Structural and biological properties of integrin-mediated cell adhesion. *Clin Lab Med* 1992;12:217–236.

25. Grzesik WJ, Gehron Robey P: Bone matrix RGD-glycoproteins: Immunolocalization and their interaction with human primary osteoblastic bone cells in vitro. *J Bone Miner Res,* in press.

26. Bianco P, Riminucci M, Bonucci E, et al: Bone sialoprotein (BSP) secretion and osteoblast differentiation: Relationship to bromodeoxyuridine incorporation, alkaline phosphatase, and matrix deposition. *J Histochem Cytochem* 1993;41:183–191.

27. Bianco P, Fisher LW, Young MF, et al: Expression and localization of the two small proteoglycans, biglycan and decorin, in developing human skeletal and non-skeletal tissues. *J Histochem Cytochem* 1990;38:1549–1563.

28. Sage EH, Vernon RB, Funk SE, et al: SPARC, a secreted protein associated with cellular proliferation, inhibits cell spreading in vitro and exhibits Ca^{+2}-dependent binding to the extracellular matrix. *J Cell Biol* 1989;109:341–356.

29. Termine JD, Kleinman HK, Whitson SW, et al: Osteonectin, a bone-specific protein linking mineral to collagen. *Cell* 1981;26:99–105.

30. Chen Y, Bal BS, Gorski JP: Calcium and collagen binding properties of osteopontin, bone sialoprotein, and bone acidic glycoprotein-75 from bone. *J Biol Chem* 1992;267:24871–24878.

31. Bianco P, Riminucci M, Silvestrini G, et al: Localization of bone sialoprotein (BSP) to Golgi and post-Golgi secretory structures in osteoblasts and to discrete sites in early bone matrix. *J Histochem Cytochem* 1993;41:193–203.

32. Price PA, Williamson MK: Effects of warfarin on bone: Studies on the vitamin K-dependent protein of rat bone. *J Biol Chem* 1981;256:12754–12759.

33. Gehron Robey P: Cell-mediated calcification in vitro, in Bonucci E (ed): *Calcification in Biological Systems.* Boca Raton, FL, CRC Press, 1992, pp 107–127.

34. Kasai R, Avioli LV, Noguchi A, et al: Distribution and regulation of an anti-proBGP cross-reacting protein in human serum, osteosarcoma and normal cells, and fetal bone. *J Bone Miner Res* 1989;4(suppl):S247.

35. Vetter U, Vogel W, Just W, et al: Human decorin gene: Intron-exon junctions and chromosomal localization. *Genomics* 1993;15:161–168.

36. Faisst S, Meyer S: Compilation of vertebrate-encoded transcription factors. *Nucl Acids Res* 1992;20:3–26.

37. Schule R, Umesono K, Mangelsdorf DJ, et al: Jun-Fos and receptors for vitamins A and D recognize a common response element in the human osteocalcin gene. *Cell* 1990;61:497–504.

38. Benayahu D, Gurevitch OA, Zipori S, et al: Bone formed by committed marrow osteogenic cells (MBA-15) does not support hemotopoietic microenvironment and osteoclastogenesis. *J Bone Miner Res* 1992;7(suppl):S104.

39. Ross FP, Chappel J, Alvarez JI, et al: Interactions between the bone matrix proteins osteopontin and bone sialoprotein and the osteoclast integrin $alpha_v beta_3$ potentiate bone resorption. *J Biol Chem* 1993;268:9901–9907.

40. Miyauchi A, Alvarez J, Greenfield EM, et al: Binding of osteopontin to the osteoclast integrin $alpha_v beta_3$. *Osteoporos Int* 1993;3(suppl 1):132–135.

41. Grzesik WJ, Gehron Robey P: The effect of extracellular-matrix glycoproteins on proteoglycan synthesis and secretion by human bone cells. *J Bone Miner Res* 1992;7(suppl):S221.

Chapter 17

Prostaglandins and Bone Metabolism

Lawrence G. Raisz, MD

Introduction

Prostaglandins (PGs), which are potent multifunctional regulators of bone metabolism, can both stimulate and inhibit bone formation and resorption.[1–4] Production of PGs by cells of the osteoblastic lineage is highly regulated.[5–8] Whereas exogenous PGs have been shown to stimulate bone resorption and formation, the specific roles of endogenous PGs are less well understood.[9–12] Nevertheless, based on indirect evidence obtained using nonsteroidal anti-inflammatory drugs (NSAIDs), it seems likely that PGs play an important role in mediating a number of physiologic and pathologic responses of the skeleton. Increased bone resorption in association with inflammation and change in mechanical forces, as well as that associated with heterotopic ossification, fracture healing, and impact loading, can be suppressed by NSAIDs.[13–20] This chapter will summarize the recent data concerning the effects of PGs on bone formation and resorption and the regulation of PG synthesis by bone cells.

PGs and Bone Resorption

In 1970, Chase and Aurbach[21] showed that not only parathyroid hormone (PTH) but also prostaglandin E_2 (PGE_2) could increase cyclic AMP (cAMP) concentration in bone. Subsequent studies showed that PGE_2 also shared with PTH the ability to stimulate bone resorption.[2] However, the resorptive response in fetal rat long bones is not as rapid for PGE_2 as it is for PTH. Moreover, while PTH has no direct effect on isolated osteoclasts, PGE_2 can produce a transient inhibition of osteoclast activity.[3,22,23] The structure-activity relations for stimulation of bone resorption have been studied extensively.[24–28] PGE_2 is probably the most potent, but other prostanoids, particularly prostacyclin (PGI_2) and $PGF_{2\alpha}$ are also quite effective, although PGD_2 does not stimulate resorption. Lipoxygenase products have been studied less extensively, but there is some evidence that they can also stimulate resorption.[29] The physiologic relevance of the transient inhibitory effect is not known. It has been difficult to demonstrate in organ culture or in vivo, but in animals given interleukin-1 (IL-1), there is a transient hypocalcemia which can be blocked by NSAIDs.[30] However, stimulation of bone resorption by PGE_2 has been implicated in the hypercalcemia of malignancy, although this is probably a relatively rare pathogenetic mechanism.[31,32] As noted above, there is also evidence that the increase in bone resorption in inflammation and immobilization can be mediated by PGs.

The precise mechanism by which PGs stimulate bone resorption is not fully understood, but in marrow culture systems PGs can increase osteoclast formation and can mediate or facilitate the effects of other agents that enhance osteoclast formation.[33–35] Whatever the mechanism, PGs mediate the resorptive response to many growth factors,[7,33,36] although some of these factors can also have direct PG-independent effects on bone resorption.[37] Moreover, PGs can produce synergistic enhancement of bone resorption in response to other agonists.[38]

PGs and Bone Formation

The effects of PGs on bone formation in vitro are clearly biphasic. High concentrations can inhibit collagen synthesis.[39] This effect has recently been shown to be due to selective inhibition of the transcription of the *COL1A1* gene in an immortalized rat osteoblastic cell line, Py1a.[40] The structure-activity relations for this inhibitory effect are quite different from those for bone resorption. $PGF_{2\alpha}$ is more potent than other prostanoids, and PGE_2 and PGD_2 are equally active.

Despite this direct inhibitory effect, the predominant effect of exogenous PGs in vivo, which can be duplicated in organ culture, is stimulation of bone formation.[4,10–12,41,42] In this regard, the action of PGs resembles that of PTH, which can also produce transcriptional inhibition of collagen synthesis, yet is anabolic in vivo, particularly when given intermittently.[43,44] In vitro, the best way to demonstrate the anabolic effect of PG is to add cortisol. Under these conditions, endogenous PG production is decreased, but the sensitivity to PGs may be increased. In the presence of physiologic concentrations of cortisol, PGE_2 can increase both cell replication and collagen synthesis in fetal rat calvariae.[4,41] PGE_2, like PTH, can increase insulin-like growth factor I (IGF-I) production in bone cell and organ cultures.[45–47] In addition, PGE_2 increases IGF binding proteins[48] and $PGF_{2\alpha}$ up-regulates IGF-I receptors.[49] However, changes in IGF response cannot entirely explain the anabolic effect, because it still occurs in the presence of inhibitory concentrations of IGF binding proteins.[46] Other growth factors may be important in the anabolic response.[50,51] The anabolic effect of PGE_2 is probably important in the response of the skeleton to impact loading.[52,53] When bones are subject to brief periods of impact, there is a subsequent increase in bone formation, which can be blocked by NSAIDs. PGI_2, as well as PGE_2, may mediate this response.[54] Heterotopic ossification may also be PG-dependent, because it can be blocked by NSAIDs.[15] The inhibitory effect of PGs on bone formation may be important in inflammation where the levels are extremely high.[55,56]

Regulation of PG Production in Bone

PGs are abundantly produced by bone cells, and many substances stimulate this production. These include all of the potent stimulators of bone resorption including PGs themselves, as well as cytokines, PTH, and 1,25-dihydroxyvitamin D.[57–61] However, these agents differ greatly in the magnitude of their effects on PG production. Many growth factors also stimulate PG production, and may interact synergistically with cytokines.[62,63] Cytokines and growth factors can have both PG-dependent and PG-independent mechanisms for stimulating bone resorption. In the case of IL-1, this may represent a sequential system. When IL-1 is injected over calvarial bone in rats, there is an initial stimulation of resorption which is largely PG-independent and a subsequent PG-dependent phase.[19]

Relatively few endogenous factors are known to inhibit PG production in bone. Glucocorticoids are probably the most effective.[59,64] Estrogens and androgens can inhibit PG production in bone, but in organ culture the effect is incomplete and the dose-response is biphasic.[65,66] Estrogens can also inhibit the cellular response to PGs.[67] The presence of a biphasic response in vivo is suggested by the observation that the anabolic effect of high doses of estrogen in rats is suppressed by indomethacin.[68] Interferon-gamma and vitamin K can inhibit PG production in bone cells.[69–71]

A number of studies have indicated that mechanical forces can stimulate PG production by bone cells. These include not only the indirect studies of the effect of NSAIDs in the response to impact loading in vivo but studies in which bone cell and organ cultures are subjected to stretch, compression, or fluid shear forces.[52,72,73] Under all of these conditions, there is an increase in PG production, but the responses are quite complex. Thus, immobilization may also increase PG production and excessive stretch decrease it.[74,75] In most experiments, PGE_2 has been the main product measured, but PGI_2 is also produced by bone in response to impact loading and may be the major product of osteocytes.[76,77]

The mechanisms by which prostaglandin production is controlled in skeletal tissues are just beginning to be elucidated. Activation of phospholipase A_2 and release of arachidonic acid could be important in the rapid responses to mechanical forces and kinins as well as hormones.[78] However, the production of large amounts of PGs probably depends on an increase in the prostaglandin endoperoxide synthase (PGHS) or cyclooxygenase enzymes. The recent discovery that there are two enzymes, the so-called "constitutive" PGHS-1 and "inducible" PGHS-2, which are differentially regulated, has provided new insights into the analysis of regulation of PG synthesis.[79] PGHS-1 and PGHS-2 are the products of different genes. Although there is 60% homology at both the nucleotide and amino acid levels, and the biochemical effects and cellular localization of the two enzymes are quite similar, the two enzymes clearly subserve different functions. PGHS-2 messenger RNA (mRNA) is larger and has a long, AUUA rich 3' end, which may be responsible for the fact that this message is usually expressed transiently.

Initial studies in which only PGHS-1 mRNA were examined showed relatively small changes that could not account for the large production of PGs in skeletal tissue. More recently, it has been shown that a number of the factors which increase PGE synthesis in bone, including PTH, IL-1, transforming growth factor-alpha (TGF-α), TGF-β, and serum, can produce a rapid increase in PGHS-2 mRNA, as measured by Northern blot analysis, and a subsequent increase in the protein, as measured by Western blot analysis.[64,80] PGHS-2 responses are also relatively transient with respect to mRNA levels, but the protein may persist. PGHS-1 also can respond to some of these stimuli, particularly serum, but the responses do not appear to be as large as for PGHS-2.[81]

One of the most interesting observations concerning PG synthesis is the recent evidence for autoamplification. PGs including $PGF_{2\alpha}$ and PGD_2, as well as PGE_2, can increase PGHS-2 mRNA and enzyme activity.[61] There is a smaller increase in PGHS-1 mRNA[58] so that the inducible enzyme probably accounts for most of the autoamplification response. This mechanism could be important in mediating the response to mechanical forces. Physiologic impact loading results in microstrain alterations in bone structure, which could produce small perturbations in the syncytium of osteocytes and osteoblasts in bone structural units. These small perturbations, either through altering fluid shear stress around the cell processes in the canaliculi connecting bone cells or through direct effects on the membrane of these cells, could result in a release of small amounts of arachidonate. PG formation by the constitutive enzyme could in turn induce PGHS-2 mRNA and amplify the larger signal.

PG Receptors and Signal Transduction

The specific receptors and signal transduction pathways for PGs in bone cells are poorly understood. Although the initial observation was that PGs stimulate cAMP production,[21] activation of phospholipase C and the phosphatidyl inositol pathway leading to activation of protein kinase C have also been implicated.[82–84] PGs can produce a rapid increase in intracellular calcium which also can activate protein kinase C. The specific receptors for PGs have not been studied in bone cells, and the structure-activity relations do not appear to fit any of the classic patterns that have been described for PG receptors in other tissues.[85] Nevertheless, the fact that different responses show different structure-activity relationships in bone cells holds promise for the development of more specific agents that could be therapeutically useful.

Conclusion

Although PGs are only one group among the many local factors that regulate bone cell function, they may play a central role in many skeletal responses. PGs appear to act as cofactors or amplifiers of the response to hormones, cytokines, and growth factors. There is evidence that PGs are involved in the response to mechanical forces and inflammation; however, their role in primary and secondary osteoporosis is less well established. PGs may be involved in the decrease in bone formation that occurs in glucocorticoid-treated patients as well as the increase in bone resorption that occurs in sex hormone deficiency. Because of the complexity of their actions and regulation, it may not be feasible to dissect the role of PGs simply by using NSAIDs. NSAIDs may have different effects on PGHS-1 and PGHS-2-mediated responses. Such a result has been obtained in preparations of cells transfected with the two enzymes,[86] but thus far we have not found differential NSAID effects on cells that express only one of the two enzymes (LG Raisz and PM Fall, unpublished observations). Moreover, although NSAIDs are potent inhibitors of PG production in bone, there is a paradoxical biphasic effect, that is, low concentrations of NSAIDs can increase PG production in bone.[87]

Acknowledgment

The author wishes to thank Ms. Lisa Godin for her careful preparation of this manuscript.

References

1. Raisz LG, Martin TJ: Prostaglandins in bone and mineral metabolism, in Peck WA (ed): *Bone and Mineral Research, Annual 2*. Amsterdam, Elsevier, 1984, pp 286–310.
2. Klein DC, Raisz LG: Role of adenosine-3′,5′-monophosphate in the hormonal regulation of bone resorption: Studies with cultured fetal bone. *Endocrinology* 1971; 89:818–826.
3. Fuller K, Chambers TJ: Effect of arachidonic acid metabolites on bone resorption by isolated rat osteoclasts. *J Bone Miner Res* 1989;4:209–215.
4. Raisz LG, Fall PM: Biphasic effects of prostaglandin E$_2$ on bone formation in cultured fetal rat calvariae: Interaction with cortisol. *Endocrinology* 1990;126:1654–1659.

5. Raisz LG, Vanderhoek JY, Simmons HA, et al: Prostaglandin synthesis by fetal rat bone in vitro: Evidence for a role of prostacyclin. *Prostaglandins* 1979;17:905–914.

6. Rodan SB, Rodan GA, Simmons HA, et al: Bone resorptive factor produced by osteosarcoma cells with osteoblastic features is PGE_2. *Biochem Biophys Res Commun* 1981;102:1358–1365.

7. Tashjian AH Jr, Voelkel EF, Lazzaro M, et al: α and β human transforming growth factors stimulate prostaglandin production and bone resorption in cultured mouse calvaria. *Proc Natl Acad Sci USA* 1985;82:4535–4538.

8. Raisz LG, Simmons HA: Effects of parathyroid hormone and cortisol on prostaglandin production by neonatal rat calvaria in vitro. *Endocr Res* 1985;11:59–74.

9. Norrdin RW, Jee WSS, High WB: The role of prostaglandins in bone in vivo. *Prostaglandins Leukot Essent Fatty Acids* 1990;41:139–149.

10. Jee WSS, Akamine T, Ke HZ, et al: Prostaglandin E_2 prevents disuse-induced cortical bone loss. *Bone* 1992;13:153–159.

11. Poznanski AK, Fernbach SK, Berry TE: Bone changes from prostaglandin therapy. *Skeletal Radiol* 1985;14:20–25.

12. Jee WSS, Ueno K, Deng YP, et al: The effects of prostaglandin E_2 in growing rats: Increased metaphyseal hard tissue and cortico-endosteal bone formation. *Calcif Tissue Int* 1985;37:148–157.

13. Saito S, Ngan P, Rosol T, et al: Involvement of PGE synthesis in the effect of intermittent pressure and interleukin-1 beta on bone resorption. *J Dental Res* 1991;70:27–33.

14. Plotquin D, Dekel S, Katz S, et al: Prostaglandin release by normal and osteomyelitic human bones. *Prostaglandins Leukot Essent Fatty Acids* 1991;43:13–15.

15. Wahlstrom O, Risto O, Djerf, K, et al: Heterotopic bone formation prevented by diclofenac: Prospective study of 100 hip arthroplasties. *Acta Orthop Scand* 1991;62:419–421.

16. Offenbacher S, Williams RC, Jeffcoat MK, et al: Effects of NSAIDs on beagle crevicular cyclooxygenase metabolites and periodontal bone loss. *J Periodon Res* 1992;27:207–213.

17. Engesaeter LB, Sudmann B, Sudmann E: Fracture healing in rats inhibited by locally administered indomethacin. *Acta Orthop Scand* 1992;63:330–333.

18. Solheim E, Pinholt EM, Bang G, et al: Inhibition of heterotopic osteogenesis in rats by a new bioerodible system for local delivery of indomethacin. *J Bone Joint Surg* 1992;74A:705–712.

19. Boyce BF, Aufdemorte TB, Garrett IR, et al: Effects of interleukin-1 on bone turnover in normal mice. *Endocrinology* 1989;125:1142–1150.

20. Hopps RM, Nuki K, Raisz LG: Demonstration and preliminary characterization of bone resorbing activity in freeze-dried gingiva of dogs. *Calcif Tissue Int* 1980;31:239–245.

21. Chase LR, Aurbach GD: The effect of parathyroid hormone on the concentration of adenosine $3',5'$-monophosphate in skeletal tissue in vitro. *J Biol Chem* 190;245:1520–1526.

22. Lerner UH, Ransjo M, Ljunggren O: Prostaglandin E_2 causes a transient inhibition of mineral mobilization, matrix degradation, and lysosomal enzyme release from mouse calvarial bones in vitro. *Calcif Tissue Int* 1987;40:323–331.

23. Conaway HH, Diez LF, Raisz LG: Effects of prostacyclin and prostaglandin E_1 (PGE_1) on bone resorption in the presence and absence of parathyroid hormone. *Calcif Tissue Int* 1986;38:130–134.

24. Dietrich JW, Goodson JM, Raisz LG: Stimulation of bone resorption by various prostaglandins in organ culture. *Prostaglandins* 1975;10:231–240.

25. Raisz LG, Dietrich JW, Simmons HA, et al: Effect of prostaglandin endoperoxides and metabolites on bone resorption in vitro. *Nature* 1977;267:532–534.

26. Collins DA, Chambers TJ: Effect of prostaglandin E_1, E_2 and $F_{2\alpha}$ on osteoclast formation in mouse bone marrow cultures. *J Bone Miner Res* 1991;6:157–164.

27. Raisz LG, Alander CB, Simmons HA: Effects of prostaglandin E_3 and eicosapentaenoic acid on rat bone in organ culture. *Prostaglandins* 1989;37:615–625.

28. Raisz LG, Woodiel FN: Effect of alterations in the cyclopentane ring on bone re-sorptive activity of prostaglandin. *Prostaglandins* 1989;37:229–235.

29. Meghji S, Sandy JR, Scutt AM, et al: Stimulation of bone resorption by lipoxygen-ase metabolites of arachidonic acid. *Prostaglandins* 1988;36:139–149.

30. Boyce BF, Yates AJP, Mundy GR: Bolus injections of recombinant human interleu-kin-1 cause transient hypocalcemia in normal mice. *Endocrinology* 1989;125:2780–2783.

31. Tashjian AH Jr: Editorial. Prostaglandins, hypercalcemia and cancer. *N Engl J Med* 1975;293:1317–1318.

32. Seyberth HW, Raisz LG, Oates JA: Prostaglandins and hypercalcemic states. *Annu Rev Med* 1978;29:23–29.

33. Shinar DM, Rodan GA: Biphasic effects of transforming growth factor-β on the production of osteoclast-like cells in mouse bone marrow cultures: The role of prostaglandins in the generation of these cells. *Endocrinology* 1990;126:3153–3158.

34. Collins DA, Chambers TJ: Prostaglandin E_2 promotes osteoclast formation in mu-rine hematopoietic cultures through an action on hematopoietic cells. *J Bone Miner Res* 1992;7:555–561.

35. Akatsu T, Takahashi N, Debari K, et al: Prostaglandins promote osteoclastlike cell formation by a mechanism involving cyclic adenosine 3',5'-monophosphate in mouse bone marrow cell cultures. *J Bone Miner Res* 1989;4:29–35.

36. Shibata Y, Ogura N, Moriya Y, et al: Platelet-activating factor stimulates produc-tion of prostaglandin E_2 in murine osteoblast-like cell line MC3T3-E_1. *Life Sci* 1991;49:1103–1109.

37. Lorenzo JA, Quinton J, Sousa S, et al: Effects of DNA and prostaglandin synthesis inhibitors on the stimulation of bone resorption by epidermal growth factor in fetal rat long-bone cultures. *J Clin Invest* 1986;77:1897–1902.

38. Raisz LG, Nuki K, Alander CB, et al: Interactions between bacterial endotoxin and other stimulators of bone resorption in organ culture. *J Periodon Res* 1981;16:1–7.

39. Raisz LG, Koolemans-Beynen AR: Inhibition of bone collagen synthesis by pros-taglandin E_2 in organ culture. *Prostaglandins* 1974;8:377–385.

40. Raisz LG, Fall PM, Petersen DN, et al: Prostaglandin E_2 inhibits α1(I) procollagen gene transcription and promoter activity in the immortalized rat osteoblastic clonal cell line Py1a. *Mol Endocrinol* 1993;7:17–22.

41. Chyun YS, Raisz LG: Stimulation of bone formation by prostaglandin E_2. *Prosta-glandins* 1984;27:97–103.

42. Mori S, Jee WSS, Li XJ: Production of new trabecular bone in osteopenic ovariec-tomized rats by prostaglandin E_2. *Calcif Tissue Int* 1992;50:80–87.

43. Kream BE, LaFrancis D, Petersen DN, et al: Parathyroid hormone represses α1(I) collagen promoter activity in cultured calvariae from neonatal transgenic mice. *Mol Endocrinol* 1993;7:399–408.

44. Gera I, Hock JM, Gunness-Hey M, et al: LG: Indomethacin does not inhibit the anabolic effect of parathyroid hormone on the long bones of rats. *Calcif Tissue Int* 1987;40:206–211.

45. McCarthy TL, Centrella M, Raisz LG, et al: Prostaglandin E_2 stimulates insulin-like growth factor-I synthesis in osteoblast-enriched cultures from fetal rat bone. *Endocrinology* 1991;128:2895–2900.

46. Raisz LG, Fall PM, Gabbitas BY, et al: Effects of prostaglandin E_2 on bone for-mation in cultured fetal rat calvariae: Role of insulin-like growth factor-I. *Endo-crinology* 1993;133:1504–1510.

47. Linkhart TA, MacCharles DC: Interleukin-1 stimulates release of insulin-like growth factor-I from neonatal mouse calvaria by a prostaglandin synthesis-de-pendent mechanism. *Endocrinology* 1992;131:2297–2305.

48. Schmid C, Schlapfer I, Waldvogel M, et al: Prostaglandin-E_2 stimulates synthesis of insulin-like growth factor binding protein-3 in rat bone cells in vitro. *J Bone Miner Res* 1992;7:1157–1163.

49. Hakeda Y, Harada S, Matsumoto T, et al: Prostaglandin $F_{2\alpha}$ stimulates proliferation of clonal osteoblastic MC3T3-E1 cells by up-regulation of insulin-like growth factor-I receptors. *J Biol Chem* 1991;266:21044–21050.

50. Pfeilschifter J, Bonewald L, Mundy GR: Characterization of the latent transforming growth factor β complex in bone. *J Bone Miner Res* 1990;5:49–58.

51. Harada S, Nagy JA, Endo N, et al: Induction of vascular endothelial growth factor expression by prostaglandin E_2 and E_1 in osteoblastic cells. *J Bone Miner Res* 1993; 8:S125.

52. Lanyon LE: Control of bone architecture by functional load bearing. *J Bone Miner Res* 1992;7:S369–S376.

53. Dallas SL, Zaman G, Pead MJ, et al: Early strain-related changes in cultured embryonic chick tibiotarsi parallel those associated with adaptive modeling in vivo. *J Bone Miner Res* 1993;8:251–259.

54. Zaman G, Suswillo RFL, Cheng MZ, et al: Effect of mechanical strain and exogenous prostaglandins on osteogenic responses in bone derived cells in culture. *J Bone Miner Res* 1993;8:S373.

55. Kream BE, Raisz LG, Sandberg AL: Activation of serum complement inhibits collagen synthesis in fetal rat bone in organ culture. *Calcif Tissue Int* 1982;34:370–375.

56. Sandberg AL, Raisz LG, Wahl LM, et al: Enhancement of complement-mediated prostaglandin synthesis and bone resorption by arachidonic acid and inhibition by cortisol. *Prostagland Leuk Med* 1982;8:419–427.

57. Pilbeam CC, Raisz LG: Effects of androgens on parathyroid hormone and interleukin-1-stimulated prostaglandin production in cultured neonatal mouse calvariae. *J Bone Miner Res* 1990;5:1183–1188.

58. Oshima T, Yoshimoto T, Yamamoto S, et al: cAMP-Dependent induction of fatty acid cyclooxygenase mRNA in mouse osteoblastic cells (MC3T3-E1). *J Biol Chem* 1991;266:13621–13626.

59. Klein-Nulend J, Pilbeam CC, Harrison JR, et al: Mechanism of regulation of prostaglandin production by parathyroid hormone, interleukin-1, and cortisol in cultured mouse parietal bones. *Endocrinology* 1991;128:2503–2510.

60. Klein-Nulend J, Pilbeam CC, Raisz LG: Effect of 1,25-dihydroxyvitamin D_3 on prostaglandin E_2 production in cultured mouse parietal bones. *J Bone Miner Res* 1991;6:1339–1344.

61. Raisz LG, Voznesensky OS, Alander CB, et al: Auto-amplification of inducible prostaglandin G/H synthase (cyclooxygenase) in osteoblastic MC3T3-E1 and Py1a cells. *J Bone Miner Res* 1993;8:S161.

62. Hurley MM, Fall P, Harrison JR, et al: Effects of transforming growth factor α and interleukin-1 on DNA synthesis, collagen synthesis, procollagen mRNA levels, and prostaglandin E_2 production in cultured fetal rat calvaria. *J Bone Miner Res* 1989; 4:731–736.

63. Lorenzo JA, Sousa S: Interleukin-1 synergistically enhances bone resorption stimulated by transforming growth factor alpha in fetal rat long bone cultures through prostaglandin synthesis. *J Bone Miner Res* 1987;2:Abstract 376.

64. Kawaguchi H, Pilbeam CC, Voznesensky OS, et al: Role of inducible prostaglandin G/H synthase (cyclooxygenase) in the regulation of prostaglandin production in cultured mouse calvariae. *J Bone Miner Res* 1993;8:S159.

65. Pilbeam CC, Klein-Nulend J, Raisz LG: Inhibition of 17β-estradiol of PTH stimulated resorption and prostaglandin production in cultured neonatal mouse calvariae. *Biochem Biophys Res Commun* 1989;163:1319–1324.

66. Feyen JHM, Raisz LG: Prostaglandin production by calvariae from sham operated and oophorectomized rats: Effect of 17β-estradiol in vivo. *Endocrinology* 1987; 121:819–821.

67. Tokuda H, Yoneda M, Oiso Y, et al: Inhibitory effect of 17β-estradiol on prostaglandin E_2-induced phosphoinositide hydrolysis in osteoblast-like cells. *Prostaglandins* 1992;43:271–280.

68. Chow JWM, Lean JM, Abe T, et al: The anabolic effect of 17β-oestradiol on the trabecular bone of adult rats is suppressed by indomethacin. *J Endocrinol* 1992; 133:189–195.

69. Hoffmann O, Klaushofer K, Gleispach H, et al: Gamma interferon inhibits basal and interleukin-1-induced prostaglandin production and bone resorption in neonatal mouse calvaria. *Biochem Biophys Res Commun* 1987;143:38–43.

70. Koshihara Y, Hoshi K, Shiraki M: Vitamin K2 (menatetrenone) inhibits prostaglandin synthesis in cultured human osteoblast-like periosteal cells by inhibiting prostaglandin synthethase. *J Bone Miner Res* 1993;8:S374.

71. Lacey DL, Shioi A, Tan HL, et al: IL-4 and PGEs 1,2 impact osteoclast-like cell formation by targeting bone marrow macrophages. *J Bone Miner Res* 1993:8:S397.

72. Reich KM, Frangos JA: Effect of flow on prostaglandin-E_2 and inositol triphosphate levels in osteoblasts. *Am J Physiol* 1991;261:C428-C432.

73. Reich KM, Frangos JA: Protein kinase-C mediates flow-induced prostaglandin-E_2 production in osteoblasts. *Calcif Tissue Int* 1993;52:62–66.

74. Thompson DD, Rodan GA: Indomethacin inhibition of tenotomy-induced bone resorption in rats. *J Bone Miner Res* 1988;3:409–414.

75. Nishioka S, Fukuda K, Tanaka S: Cyclic stretch increases alkaline phosphatase activity of osteoblast-like cells: A role for prostaglandin E_2. *Bone Miner* 1993;21: 141–150.

76. Okiji T, Morita I, Kawashima N, et al: Immunohistochemical detection of prostaglandin I_2 synthase in various calcified tissue-forming cells in rat. *Arch Oral Biol* 1993;38:31–36.

77. Cheng MZ, Zaman G, Lanyon LE: Estrogen enhances the osteogenic effects of mechanical loading and exogenous prostacyclin, but not prostaglandin E_2. *J Bone Miner Res* 1993;8:S151.

78. Schwartz Z, Dennis R, Bonewald L, et al: Differential regulation of prostaglandin-E_2 synthesis and phospholipase-A2 activity by 1,25-$(OH)_2$ D_3 in three osteoblast-like cell lines (MC3T3-E1, ROS 17/2.8, and MG-63). *Bone* 1992;13:51–58.

79. Xie W, Robertson DL, Simmons DL: Mitogen-inducible prostaglandin G/H synthase: A new target for nonsteroidal antiinflammatory drugs. *Drug Develop Res* 1992;25:249–265.

80. Pilbeam CC, Alander CB, Voznesensky OS, et al: Regulation of inducible prostaglandin G/H synthase (cyclooxygenase) by interleukin-1 and transforming growth factors-α and -β in osteoblastic cells. *J Bone Miner Res* 1993;8:S299.

81. Kawaguchi H, Yavari R, Stover ML, et al: Quantitation of constitutive prostaglandin G/H synthase (cyclooxygenase) mRNA expression in MC3T3-E1 cells using competitive polymerase chain reaction. *J Bone Miner Res* 1993;8:S299.

82. Hakeda Y, Hotta T, Kurihara N, et al: Prostaglandin E_1 and $F_{2\alpha}$ stimulate differentiation and proliferation, respectively, of clonal osteoblastic MC3T3-E1 cells by different second messengers in vitro. *Endocrinology* 1987;121:1966–1974.

83. Muallem S, Merritt BS, Green J, et al: Classification of prostaglandin receptors based on coupling to signal transduction systems. *Biochem J* 1989;263:769–774.

84. Toriyama K, Morita I, Murota S-I: The existence of distinct classes of prostaglandin E_2 receptors mediating adenylate cyclase and phospholipase C pathways in osteoblastic clone MC3T3-E1. *Prostaglandins Leukot Essent Fatty Acids* 1992;46:15–20.

85. Coleman RA, Kennedy I, Humphrey PPA, et al: Prostanoids and their receptors, in Hansch C, Sammes PG, Taylor JB (eds): *Comprehensive Medicinal Chemistry: The Rational Design, Mechanistic Study & Therapeutic Applications of Chemical Compounds.* Oxford, Pergamon Press, 1989, vol 3, pp 643–714.

86. Meade EA, Smith WL, DeWitt DL: Differential inhibition of prostaglandin endoperoxide synthase (cyclooxygenase) isozymes by aspirin and other nonsteroidal antiinflammatory drugs. *J Biol Chem* 1993;268:6610–6614.

87. Raisz LG, Simmons HA, Fall PM: Biphasic effects of nonsteroidal antiinflammatory drugs on prostaglandin production by cultured rat calvariae. *Prostaglandins* 1989; 37:559–565.

Chapter 18

Cytokine-Induced Signal Transduction Mediated by Nonreceptor Tyrosine Kinases in Bone Cells

Mark C. Horowitz, PhD
Peter R. Jay, MD
He-Ying Qian, PhD
Roland Baron, DDS, PhD
Joan B. Levy, PhD

Introduction

The formation and regeneration of bone involves a complex set of interactions between cells of the skeletal, hematopoietic, and, in some cases, immune systems. These interactions can be mediated by direct cell to cell contact, contact with matrix proteins, or binding of cytokines or growth factors to their cognate receptors. Cytokines appear to play an important role in the regulation of bone resorption and formation during pathologic bone remodeling and may also play a central role during normal remodeling. Osteoblasts respond to a specific set of cytokines restricted by the expression of cell surface receptors. Binding of cytokine (ligand) to its receptor generates a signal from the plasma membrane to the nucleus, which results in increases in the transcription of specific genes and, ultimately, the activation of different cellular processes. One result of activation is the secretion of a specific set of cytokines, which is dependent on the activation signal and limited to the repertoire of cytokines that osteoblasts are capable of secreting. The secretion and binding of cytokines and growth factors forms the autocrine and paracrine circuitry involved in the regulation of bone remodeling.

A new subfamily of cytokines has been identified in which the majority of the members are capable of modulating bone cell activity. These factors are related based on sequence homology, chromosome location, and the structure of their receptors.[1] This subfamily is composed of interleukin-6 (IL-6), IL-11, leukemia inhibitory factor (LIF), oncostatin-M (OSM), ciliary neurotrophic factor (CNTF), and granulocyte colony stimulating factor (G-CSF). The data known about these cytokines as they relate to bone are quite variable. Substantial information is known about LIF and IL-6,[2–9] while little is known about IL-11 and G-CSF[10–12] and almost nothing is available on OSM[13] and CNTF. Although some information is available about the receptors for these cytokines and the downstream events that occur following ligand binding in nonbone cell systems, the signal transduction cascade induced by these cytokines in bone cells remains to be elucidated.

It has been demonstrated in nonbone cell systems that signal transduction stimulated by this family of cytokines is mediated by tyrosine kinases. However, two major examples can be cited to demonstrate the importance of tyrosine phosphorylation in bone remodeling. Both examples involve altered bone remodeling as a result of genetic defects in some aspect of signal transduction that involves tyrosine phosphorylation. In the first, the op/op (osteopetrotic) mouse has a defect in the secretion of biologically active macrophage colony stimulating factor (M-CSF),[14] which can no longer signal through its receptor, c-*fms*, a receptor tyrosine kinase. The result of this defect is osteopetrosis. The second example involves c-*src*, a nonreceptor tyrosine kinase in which gene deletion by homologous recombination also results in overt osteopetrosis.[15] The importance of tyrosine phosphorylation in bone cells, mediated by the M-CSF receptor, c-*src*, and the cytokines mentioned above, requires further investigation.

Because many of the members of this subfamily of cytokines appear to play an important role in the regulation of bone formation and regeneration, a clearer understanding of the signal transduction pathways from the cell membrane to the nucleus is a critical element in understanding how these factors function in bone cell activation. In this chapter, we will present what is known about the signal transduction mechanism induced by these cytokines. These data are based, for the most part, on studies performed in nonbone cells. However, where possible we will relate our own experience using primary osteoblasts or osteosarcoma cells.

Receptor Assembly

The receptors used by these cytokines are composed of a set of proteins that are assembled in a defined order and that have specific functions. Figure 1 depicts a generic receptor applicable to this entire subfamily of cytokines.[16] However, because different members of the subfamily use some, but not all of the receptor components, the specificities of the receptor subunits for the relevant cytokines will be discussed.

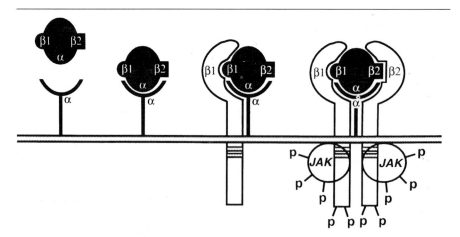

Fig. 1 Generic cytokine receptor with component assembly including: ligand; α component; β1 component; β2 component (gp130); JAK kinase; p signifies tyrosine phosphorylation sites; cross hatched portion in β components represents JAK kinase binding domains.

The ligand can possess at least three receptor binding sites. The first site binds the α component of the receptor, which, like the other components, is a cell surface expressed protein. The receptors for IL-6 and CNTF both have ligand binding α components, whereas the receptors for OSM and LIF lack this component, and it is not yet known whether the IL-11 receptor has an α component.[17-19] These proteins are often referred to as the IL-6 or CNTF binding proteins and lend specificity to the receptor. The CNTFα component is a glycosyl-phosphatidylinositol (GPI) anchored 41-kd protein.[17] This type of linkage is susceptible to enzymatic cleavage and may account for the presence of soluble α molecules (sCNTFα). Similarly, circulating levels of IL-6α chains (sIL-6α) can be detected. Although both CNTFα and IL-6α can be found in soluble form, the molecules have different characteristics. IL-6α is an 80-kd protein, which, unlike CNTFα, is not GPI anchored; it does traverse the plasma membrane and has a small intracytoplasmic tail, but cannot by itself mediate signal transduction.[18,20]

The other two binding sites on the ligand are required for interaction with the β1 and β2 components of the receptor. The β1 component is a transmembrane protein that forms a complex with the ligand and the α component, or with the ligand alone if the α component is absent. Whether a stable ligand-α-β1 or ligand-β1 intermediate exists for any appreciable time is unknown. Its presence, particularly in those receptors that lack an α component, lends specificity to the ligand-receptor interaction and confers high-affinity binding.[21,22] The β1 component has been found in the receptors of all subfamily members that have been examined. However, it is not necessarily the same molecule for every member. OSM and CNTF use the same β1 molecule that was originally identified for LIF, LIFRβ.[21-23] LIFRβ is the low affinity receptor for LIF.[22] IL-6 does not use LIFRβ, but instead uses gp130.[23] The β1 component for IL-11 is not characterized.[24]

The β2 component has been identified as gp130. Originally identified as a signal transducer for IL-6, gp130 is now known to be a common and obligatory component of the receptor for all of the cytokines in the subfamily (IL-6, IL-11, OSM, LIF, and CNTF) and is required for signal transduction.[19,20,25] The gp130 component has been referred to as a high-affinity converting subunit. An example of this is cell activation with LIF, which requires LIF, LIFRβ (the β1 component), and gp130. LIF can bind LIFRβ and transmit a signal suboptimally. However, the presence of gp130 allows for high-affinity binding, optimal signal transduction, and cell activation. With the exception of OSM, it appears that gp130 is the last member of the receptor components to bind the ligand and form the completed and functional receptor. As can be seen in Table 1, CNTF, LIF, and OSM use the LIFRβ subunit as the β1 component and gp130 as the β2 component for their receptor complexes, and IL-6 uses gp130 for

Table 1 Cytokine receptor composition

Cytokine (ligand)	Subunits		
	α	β1	β2
IL-6	IL-6Rα	gp130	gp130
CNTF	CNTFRα	LIFRβ	gp130
LIF	None	LIFRβ	gp130
OSM	None	LIFRβ	gp130
IL-11	Unknown	Unknown	gp130

both its β1 and β2 components. Like LIF, OSM uses gp130 as a high-affinity converting subunit. However, OSM presents a unique difference in that it preferentially binds gp130, and the resulting complex can suboptimally transduce a signal.[21,26,27] In addition, there is evidence indicating that OSM also binds a unique OSM receptor, which is not the LIFRβ component.[21,28] This alternate receptor complex also includes gp130.

Signal Transduction

A ligand's interaction with its receptor appears to occur in two settings, both of which can result in signal transduction. The first is the more conventional setting in which the ligand binds to its appropriate plasma-membrane-expressed receptor component (IL-6 or CNTF-α component; LIF-β1 component; OSM-β2 component; IL-11-unknown). This interaction initiates receptor component assembly, which culminates in a functional receptor capable of transmitting a signal to the interior of the cell. This form of ligand-receptor interaction can occur for all of the cytokine subfamily members.

The second setting is restricted to IL-6 (sIL-6Rα) and CNTF (sCNTFRα) by virtue of the ability of their receptors' α component to be cleaved from the membrane and function in soluble form. Soluble receptor can bind ligand, forming a complex that can interact with the appropriate β subunits to trigger signal transduction. This type of interaction could induce signal transduction in cells that would not normally be responsive to IL-6 or CNTF because they lack the appropriate α components. However, by expressing the correct β components, signal transduction can occur. This type of activation has been reported for sIL-6Rα and sCNTFRα in hematopoietic cells.[20,29] A similar interaction could explain some of the discrepancies observed for IL-6's activities on bone cells, and such a possibility is supported by the observation that gp130 does not directly bind IL-6, although this subunit does constitute both of IL-6's β chains.[6,7,19,20]

Ligand binding with concomitant receptor assembly results in signal transduction mediated by protein tyrosine phosphorylation (Fig. 1). Activation of the kinase(s) is assumed to result from dimerization of the receptor β chains following ligand binding. This dimerization can be between identical β chains (homodimers), as is the case for IL-6 (two gp130 molecules), or between two different β chains (heterodimers), as is the case for LIF and OSM (one gp130 and one LIFRβ). Phosphorylation resulting from this type of two-chain receptor dimerization is reminiscent of the mechanism known to be responsible for the activation of tyrosine kinase receptors (eg, c-*fms*, c-*kit*, or the receptors for platelet-derived growth factor and epidermal growth factor).[30,31] However, unlike receptor tyrosine kinases, none of the receptor components for these cytokines have intrinsic tyrosine kinase domains, suggesting that a nonreceptor tyrosine kinase is or becomes associated with the receptor and is required for signal transduction.

Recent evidence indicates that members of a new class of nonreceptor tyrosine kinases, known as the JAK family, are associated with the receptors for a variety of different cytokines, including interferon γ, erythropoietin (EPO), growth hormone, IL-3, granulocyte macrophage colony-stimulating factor (GM-CSF), and G-CSF.[32–34] The JAK family (also referred to as the Janus family or Just Another Kinase) presently includes three members, JAK 1, JAK 2, and Tyk 2, which range in size from 130 to 134 kd. These kinases can be distinguished from other nonreceptor tyrosine kinases in that they have no SH2 or SH3 (*src* homology) domains and contain two catalytic domains, one being the classical kinase domain and the second a kinase-related domain.[35-37] The JAK kinases bind to proline-rich regions of the β components found distal to the transmembrane domain.[38] This region of the EPO receptor displays homology to similar regions of gp130 and LIFRβ.[34,38] Different JAK kinases are activated depending on cell type and are ligand bound.[39]

Ligand binding to the receptor results in activation of the associated tyrosine kinase and phosphorylation of three groups of proteins (Fig. 2). The first group includes the β chains, β1 and β2, of the receptor itself. The second group includes the phosphorylated kinase itself, and the third group includes a series of cytoplasmic proteins. In other cell systems it appears that some of these cytoplasmic proteins may be transcription factors that, once phosphorylated, translocate to the nucleus and bind the appropriate DNA sequence, resulting in gene activation.[40-42] This is suggested by data, which show that IL-6, LIF, and OSM treatment of hematopoietic or immune cells leads to transcription of a characteristic set of immediate early response genes including junB, tis11, and EGR-1.[43-45]

Activation of Osteoblasts

We have started to analyze the response of bone cells to these cytokines by dissecting their signal transduction pathways and correlating each dissection to the resulting biologic consequences. To this end, primary murine calvarial osteoblasts were isolated by sequential collagenase digestion (population three to five), grown to confluence, and serum starved for 15 to 18 hours. The human osteosarcoma cell line U2OS was recovered from maintenance culture, grown to confluence, and also serum starved. The confluent monolayers were washed and stimulated with OSM for 5 minutes in medium with low serum content. Cell lysates were prepared, then the proteins were separated by SDS polyacrylamide gel electrophoresis and transferred to nitrocellulose membranes. Proteins phosphorylated on tyrosine residues were visualized by antiphosphotyrosine Western blot analysis. Figure 3 is a comparison of tyrosine-phosphorylated proteins derived from lysates of OSM-stimulated primary murine cal-

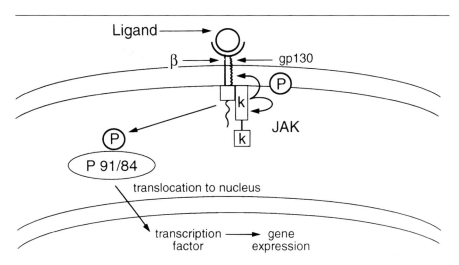

Fig. 2 Theoretical signal transduction pathway initiated by cytokine binding and ending in gene activation. P signifies tyrosine phosphorylation sites.

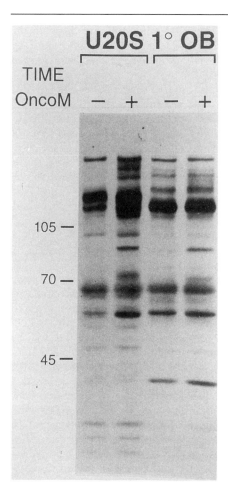

Fig. 3 Antiphosphotyrosine Western blot of lysates prepared from primary murine osteoblasts and the human osteosarcoma cell line U2OS. Osteoblasts were induced with 100 ng/ml of OSM for 5 minutes, washed, and lysates were prepared in the presence of protease inhibitors. Proteins phosphorylated on tyrosine were detected by protein immunoblotting with antibodies to phosphotyrosine.

varial osteoblasts and U2OS cells. In the primary osteoblasts, OSM specifically induced the tyrosine phosphorylation of proteins of 70, 90, and 130 kd; proteins with similar sizes were observed in the OSM-stimulated U2OS lysates. Additional proteins of 50, 60, 110, and 160 kd became phosphorylated in the U2OS cell lysates; these proteins were not observed in similarly treated primary osteoblast lysates. Thus, some similarities and clear differences apparently can be detected between stimulation of primary murine osteoblasts and of the human osteosarcoma cell line, at least with respect to tyrosine phosphorylation. Similarly, distinct differences exist between the pattern of phosphoproteins induced by OSM in osteoblasts as compared to endothelial cells.[46]

It is tempting to identify the proteins that are tyrosine phosphorylated by a simple comparison of the molecular weights of the bands to those of proteins already known to be associated with signal transduction. As an example, it would seem reasonable to assume that the band in the 130 to 150 kd range might be gp130 (glycosylation causes the protein to run at 150 kd). Confirmation of this identification will require immunoprecipitation using specific antibodies directed at gp130 followed by antiphosphotyrosine Western blotting to determine if gp130 is phosphorylated.

To investigate the biologic consequences of cytokine binding, primary murine osteoblasts were prepared as described above. OSM at 100 ng/ml was added for 48 hours, then the conditioned medium (CM) was collected and tested for the presence of IL-6 by proliferation of the IL-6 dependent cell line B9.[47] Production of IL-6 was determined because OSM is known to induce IL-6 secretion in nonbone cells.[48] As mentioned, IL-6 is produced by osteoblasts and affects bone cells.[5-10] Data in Figure 4 show that CM from primary osteoblasts stimulated with OSM induce B9 cell proliferation. Addition of neutralizing monoclonal anti-IL-6 antibodies blocks the B9 cell proliferation to background levels, confirming that the B9 cell proliferation was due to the presence of IL-6.

These data indicate that OSM receptors are present on both primary murine osteoblasts and the human osteosarcoma cell line U2OS; binding of OSM results in phosphorylation of specific proteins and leads to cell activation characterized by the secretion of biologically active factors such as IL-6. Although the data suggest that phosphorylation and IL-6 secretion are directly linked, this remains to be demonstrated conclusively.

Summary

It is becoming clear that cytokines play an important role in the regulation of both normal and pathologic bone remodeling. Regardless of the particular aspect of bone remodeling under investigation, when there is a cytokine-mediated pathway, there is a hierarchical order to the participation of the relevant cytokines. The subfamily of cytokines discussed in this chapter seem to have this attribute, with IL-6 and IL-11 on the more relevant end of the scale, LIF and OSM in the middle, and CNTF and G-CSF on the less relevant end. This hierarchy suggests that whereas certain cytokines are important to one set of cells, other members of the same family are equally important to cells of a different phenotype. Such is the case with CNTF, which appears to have a marginal effect on bone cells but is an important growth factor for certain types of neurons.[49] Similarly, OSM has distinct activity on osteoblasts, but also is a major growth factor for Kaposi's sarcoma.[50,51] The fact that different cytokines affect different cells, but are members of the same family by virtue of their receptors

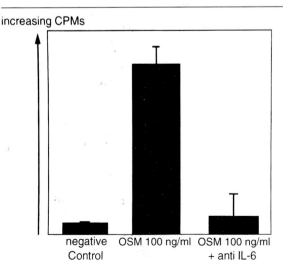

increasing CPMs

negative Control   OSM 100 ng/ml   OSM 100 ng/ml + anti IL-6

Fig. 4 IL-6 secretion by primary murine osteoblasts. Osteoblasts were stimulated with 100 ng/ml of OSM for 48 hours and the conditioned medium (CM) collected. B9 cells (10^4/well) were cultured in a total volume of 200 μl in the presence or absence of 10% added CM for 72 hours. B9 cell proliferation was measured by the incorporation of ^{3}H-thymidine (1 μCi/well S.A. 6–10 Ci/mmol) during the last 16 to 18 hours of culture. Monoclonal anti-IL-6 antibodies (4 μg/ml) were cultured with test CM for 30 to 45 minutes prior to addition of assay cells. OSM has no direct stimulating activity on B9 cells (data not shown).

and signal transduction pathway, suggests that they share common elements that are critical to cell activation. Potentially more important is the likelihood that elements of the pathway are unique to a specific cell phenotype; this uniqueness is how one cell responds differently from another when encountering the same cytokine.

If even some of the observations made in nonbone cells can be assumed to be applicable to bone cells, then important questions can be asked. As an example, the facts that all of the receptors are composed of multiple proteins and that bone cells almost certainly have their own unique elements in the signal transduction pathway provide a target-rich environment for therapeutic intervention. Therefore, it is important to identify the different components of the signal transduction cascade stimulated by cytokine activation of bone cells. Unfortunately, very little data exist on the signal transduction pathways used by bone cells when encountering this subfamily of cytokines.[13]

References

1. Rose TM, Bruce AG: Oncostatin M is a member of a cytokine family that includes leukemia-inhibitory factor, granulocyte colony-stimulating factor, and interleukin 6. *Proc Natl Acad Sci USA* 1991;88:8641–8645.
2. Abe E, Tanaka H, Ishimi Y, et al: Differentiation-inducing factor purified from conditioned medium of mitogen-treated spleen cell cultures stimulates bone resorption. *Proc Natl Acad Sci USA* 1986;83:5958–5962.
3. Metcalf D, Gearing DP: Fatal syndrome in mice engrafted with cells producing high levels of the leukemia inhibitory factor. *Proc Natl Acad Sci USA* 1989;86:5948–5952.
4. Lorenzo JA, Sousa SL, Leahy CL: Leukemia inhibitory factor (LIF) inhibits basal bone resorption in fetal rat long bone cultures. *Cytokine* 1990;2:266–271.
5. Feyen JH, Elford P, Di Padova FE, et al: Interleukin-6 is produced by bone and modulated by parathyroid hormone. *J Bone Miner Res* 1989;4:633–638.
6. Ishimi Y, Miyaura C, Jin CH, et al: IL-6 is produced by osteoblasts and induces bone resorption. *J Immunol* 1990;145:3297–3303.
7. al-Humidan A, Ralston SH, Hughes DE, et al: Interleukin-6 does not stimulate bone resorption in neonatal mouse calvariae. *J Bone Miner Res* 1991;6:3–8.
8. Horowitz M, Phillips J, Centrella M: TGFβ regulates interleukin-6 secretion by osteoblasts, in Cohn DV, Gennari C, Tashjian AH Jr (eds): *Calcium Regulating Hormones and Bone Metabolism: Basic and Clinical Aspects*. Amsterdam, Exerpta Medica, 1992, pp 275–280.
9. Jilka RL, Hangoc G, Girasole G, et al: Increased osteoclast development after estrogen loss: Mediation by interleukin-6. *Science* 1992;257:88–91.
10. Passeri G, Girasole G, Knutson S, et al: Interleukin 11 (IL-11): A new cytokine with osteoclastogenic and bone resorptive properties and a critical role in PTH- and 1,25(OH)$_2$ D$_3$-induced osteoclast development. *J Bone Miner Res* 1992;7:S110.
11. Horowitz M, Fields A, Zamparo J, et al: IL-11 secretion and its regulation in bone cells. *J Bone Miner Res* 1993;8:S143.
12. Felix R, Cecchini MG, Hofstetter W, et al: Production of granulocyte-macrophage (GM-CSF) and granulocyte colony-stimulating factor (G-CSF) by rat clonal osteoblastic cell population CRP 10/30 and the immortalized cell line IRC10/30-myc1 stimulated by tumor necrosis factor α. *Endocrinology* 1991;128:661–667.
13. Jay P, Lorenzo J, Centrella M, et al: Oncostatin M: A new cytokine with osteoblast activating activity. *J Bone Miner Res* 1993;8:S302.
14. Yoshida H, Hayashi S, Kunisada T, et al: The murine mutation osteopetrosis is in the coding region of the macrophage colony stimulating factor gene. *Nature* 1990;345:442–444.
15. Soriano P, Montgomery C, Geske R, et al: Targeted disruption of the c-src proto-oncogene leads to osteopetrosis in mice. *Cell* 1991;64:693–702.

16. Stahl N, Yancopoulos GD: The alphas, betas, and kinases of cytokine receptor complexes. *Cell* 1993;74:587–590.
17. Davis S, Aldrich TH, Valenzuela DM, et al: The receptor for ciliary neurotrophic factor. *Science* 1991;253:59–63.
18. Yamasaki K, Taga T, Hirata Y, et al: Cloning and expression of the human interleukin-6 (BSF-2/IFNβ2) receptor. *Science* 1988;241:825–828.
19. Hibi M, Murakami M, Saito M, et al: Molecular cloning and expression of an IL-6 signal transducer, gp130. *Cell* 1990;63:1149–1157.
20. Taga T, Hibi M, Hirata Y, et al: Interleukin-6 triggers the association of its receptor with a possible signal transducer, gp130. *Cell* 1989;58:573- 581.
21. Gearing DP, Comeau MR, Friend DJ, et al: The IL-6 signal transducer, gp130: An oncostatin M receptor and affinity converter for the LIF receptor. *Science* 1992; 255:1434–1437.
22. Gearing DP, Thut CJ, VandenBos T, et al: Leukemia inhibitory factor receptor is structurally related to the IL-6 signal transducer, gp130. *EMBO J* 1991;10:2839–2848.
23. Davis S, Aldrich TH, Stahl N, et al: LIFRβ and gp130 as heterodimerizing signal transducers of the tripartite CNTF receptor. *Science* 1993;260:1805–1808.
24. Yin T, Taga T, Tsang ML, et al: Involvement of IL-6 signal transducer gp130 in IL-11-mediated signal transduction. *J Immunol* 1993;151:2555–2561.
25. Ip NY, Nye SH, Boulton TG, et al: CNTF and LIF act on neuronal cells via shared signaling pathways that involve the IL-6 signal transducing receptor component gp130. *Cell* 1992;69:1121–1132.
26. Linsley PS, Bolton-Hanson M, Horn D, et al: Identification and characterization of cellular receptors for the growth regulator, oncostatin M. *J Biol Chem* 1989;264: 4282–4289.
27. Liu J, Modrell B, Aruffo A, et al: Interleukin-6 signal transducer gp130 mediates oncostatin M signaling. *J Biol Chem* 1992;267:16763–16766.
28. Gearing DP, Bruce AG: Oncostatin M binds the high-affinity leukemia inhibitory factor receptor. *New Biol* 1992;4:61–65.
29. Davis S, Aldrich TH, Ip NY, et al: Released form of CNTF receptor α component as a soluble mediator of CNTF responses. *Science* 1993;259:1736–1739.
30. Schlessinger J, Ullrich A: Growth factor signaling by receptor tyrosine kinases. *Neuron* 1992;9:383–391.
31. Ullrich A, Schlessinger J: Signal transduction by receptors with tyrosine kinase activity. *Cell* 1990;61:203–212.
32. Argetsinger LS, Campbell GS, Yang X, et al: Identification of JAK2 as a growth hormone receptor-associated tyrosine kinase. *Cell* 1993;74:237–244.
33. Silvennoinen O, Witthuhn BA, Quelle FW, et al: Structure of the murine JAK2 protein-tyrosine kinase and its role in IL-3 signal transduction. *Proc Natl Acad Sci USA* 1993;90:8429–8433.
34. Witthuhn BA, Quelle FW, Silvennoinen O, et al: JAK2 associates with the erythropoietin receptor and is tyrosine phosphorylated and activated following stimulation with erythropoietin. *Cell* 1993;74:227–236.
35. Firmbach-Kraft I, Byers M, Shows T, et al: Tyk2, prototype of a novel class of nonreceptor tyrosine kinase genes. *Oncogene* 1990;5:1329–1336.
36. Wilks AF, Harpur AG, Kurban RR, et al: Two novel protein-tyrosine kinases, each with a second phosphotransferase-related catalytic domain, define a new class of protein kinase. *Mol Cell Biol* 1991;11:2057–2065.
37. Harpur AG, Andres A-C, Ziemiecki A, et al: JAK2, a third member of the JAK family of protein tyrosine kinases. *Oncogene* 1992;7:1347–1353.
38. Murakami M, Narazaki M, Hibi M, et al: Critical cytoplasmic region of the interleukin 6 signal transducer gp130 is conserved in the cytokine receptor family. *Proc Natl Acad Sci USA* 1991;88:11349–11353.
39. Stahl N, Boulton TG, Farruggella T, et al: Association and activation of Jak-Tyk kinases by CNTF-LIF-OSM-IL-6 beta receptor components. *Science* 1994;263:92–95.

40. Sadowski HB, Shuai K, Darnell JE, et al: A common nuclear signal transduction pathway activated by growth factor and cytokine receptors. *Science* 1993;261: 1739–1744.

41. Larner AC, David M, Feldman GM, et al: Tyrosine phosphorylation of DNA binding proteins by multiple cytokines. *Science* 1993;261:1730–1733.

42. Shuai K, Stark GR, Kerr IM, et al: A single phosphotyrosine residue of Stat91 required for gene activation by interferon-γ. *Science* 1993;261:1744–1746.

43. Nakajima K, Wall R: Interleukin-6 signals activating junB and TIS11 gene transcription in a B-cell hybridoma. *Mol Cell Biol* 1991;11:1409–1418.

44. Lord KA, Abdollahi A, Thomas SM, et al: Leukemia inhibitory factor and interleukin-6 trigger the same immediate early response, including tyrosine phosphorylation, upon induction of myeloid leukemia differentiation. *Mol Cell Biol* 1991; 11:4371–4379.

45. Liu J, Clegg CH, Shoyab M: Regulation of EGR-1, c-jun, and c-myc gene expression by oncostatin M. *Cell Growth Differ* 1992;3:307–313.

46. Schieven GL, Kallestad JC, Brown TJ, et al: Oncostatin M induces tyrosine phosphorylation in endothelial cells and activation of p[62yes] tyrosine kinase. *J Immunol* 1992;149:1676–1682.

47. Aarden LA, DeGroot ER, Schaap OL, et al: Production of hybridoma growth factor by human monocytes. *Eur J Immunol* 1987;17:1411–1416.

48. Brown TJ, Rowe JM, Liu JW, et al: Regulation of IL-6 expression by oncostatin M. *J Immunol* 1991;147:2175–2180.

49. Stockli KA, Lottspeich F, Sendtner M, et al: Molecular cloning, expression and regional distribution of rat ciliary neurotrophic factor. *Nature* 1989;342:920–923.

50. Nair BC, DeVico AL, Nakamura S, et al: Identification of a major growth factor for AIDS-Kaposi's sarcoma cells as oncostatin M. *Science* 1992;255:1430–1432.

51. Miles SA, Martinez-Maza O, Rezai A, et al: Oncostatin M as a potent mitogen for AIDS-Kaposi's sarcoma-derived cells. *Science* 1992;255:1432–1434.

Chapter 19

Possible Roles for Growth Factors in Bone Remodeling

Vicki Rosen, PhD

Introduction

The adult skeleton is in a dynamic state of continuous turnover that occurs through the process of bone remodeling. Local regulation of the remodeling process is likely, because the resorption and formation events that constitute remodeling are themselves independent cellular activations and repressions occurring at multiple sites in the skeleton. Growth factors present in the microenvironment of bone have been identified as probable regulatory molecules during bone remodeling.

Investigations into the mechanisms controlling bone remodeling have taken two separate approaches. The first involves a highly detailed morphologic analysis of the cellular events observed during remodeling in vivo. Parfitt,[1] Frost,[2] and others[3] have created a precise histologic framework that can be used to evaluate the remodeling process as a physical event. The second approach is based on the molecular and biochemical characterization of the activities of growth factors and other locally acting regulators on the processes of bone formation and bone resorption in vitro. These in vitro studies have provided most of the currently available data on local regulation of remodeling. Although both of these approaches are useful, the correlation of in vivo morphologic data with in vitro biochemical information does little to establish a cause and effect relationship between the ability of individual growth factors to act during a specific phase of remodeling and the cellular events that are observed during that phase. At best, a postulated role for specific growth factors has been established, but the fundamental regulatory mechanisms that underlie the cellular processes of remodeling remain to be elucidated.

The aim of this chapter is to review the cellular events that make up the bone remodeling process and, in doing so, to identify possible steps in this sequence that could be under the control of locally acting factors. Candidate regulatory molecules normally present at the sites of bone formation and bone resorption and their known activities on the osteoblast and osteoclast cell lineages will be discussed.

Cellular Events in Bone Remodeling

Bone remodeling is a surface event, which occurs simultaneously at multiple sites along bone surfaces. Although the reason remodeling occurs at specific locations is unknown, initiation of the remodeling sequence has been shown to require the presence of mineralized bone matrix. However, once the remodeling process has begun, unmineralized matrix may also be removed. The remodeling process is executed by functionally differentiated osteoblasts and osteoclasts at discrete sites, and the amount of remodeling activity at a given site depends on the number of mature osteoblasts and osteoclasts at that site. Additionally, remodeling is influenced by the number of available precursor cells for these lineages that can mature and differentiate into active osteoblasts and osteoclasts.[1]

The majority of bone surfaces appear quiescent with regard to remodeling. An indication of this inactivity is the presence of lining cells on bone surfaces. The lining cell, a member of the osteoblast lineage, seems to provide a physical barrier to osteoclasts as they approach the mineralized surfaces. Lining cells that reside on these bone surfaces are no longer functionally able to synthesize or secrete matrix proteins and, thus, do not contribute to bone matrix accumulation. Whether lining cells were once active in matrix deposition at their present sites is unknown.[3]

Activation, the beginning of the resorption phase of remodeling, is the process by which osteoclasts gain access to the mineralized surfaces formerly occupied by bone lining cells. Although little is understood about the control of activation, it is hypothesized that osteoclasts gain access to the mineralized surfaces by a signaling interaction with lining cells. In any event, once they are able to interact with the mineralized bone surface, the osteoclasts begin the job of removing bone matrix. These resident osteoclasts, by themselves, are not sufficient to complete the resorption process, and additional osteoclasts, thought to come from progenitor cells at the site, are required to continue the bone removal process. Once the resorption cavity reaches a certain size or depth, the matrix removal process stops. Again, the control mechanisms for completion of resorption are unclear.[1-3]

The reversal phase, the time between the end of resorption and the beginning of formation at a specific site, is the time interval required by osteoblast progenitors at that site to differentiate into functionally mature osteoblasts, capable of laying down new bone matrix. This local differentiation of osteoblasts from progenitors, and perhaps mesenchymal stem cells, is a poorly understood process. Once enough osteoblasts are present at the resorption site and are aligned in the correct orientation to deposit bone matrix, they begin the formation phase of bone remodeling. Exactly how much new bone is formed appears to depend on the number of active osteoblasts that are present at the resorption site. After local bone replacement is complete, these osteoblasts become quiescent, and remodeling at that site is finished.[1,3] There are many obvious control points for these processes and many more unanswered questions as to how remodeling is controlled. Some of these are shown in Figure 1.

Growth Factors

Growth factors are an obvious choice for local factors involved in the regulation of the bone remodeling process. Although some growth factors may also be found in the systemic circulation, the focus of this discussion will be the local presence of these agents in the bone microenvironment. Bone matrix is a rich source of growth factors,[4] and in recent years, researchers have accumulated much data on both the increasing number of growth factors present in bone matrix and the importance of those factors in bone formation and repair.[5] There are multiple ways in which growth factors might be incorporated into bone matrix. Locally acting factors could be deposited after being produced by cells present in bone tissues and may accumulate in bone matrix by being

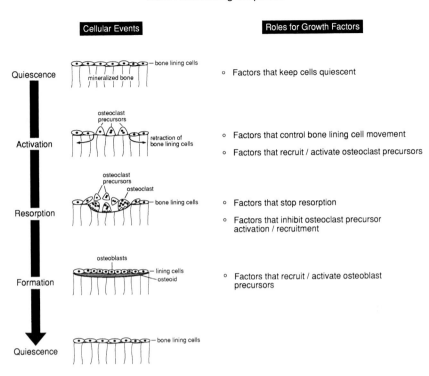

Fig. 1 Possible roles for growth factors during the bone remodeling sequence.

trapped and bound to matrix molecules. Alternatively, growth factors circulating in its blood supply could become trapped in the bone matrix. In either event, these factors would then be available to act as regulatory molecules at specific sites. In theory, growth factors could act at multiple stages in the remodeling process to control the recruitment, migration, proliferation, and differentiation of cells important to this process. The target cells for individual growth factors may change at each step of the remodeling sequence so that one growth factor might have multiple targets. Growth factors could also act together in their control of a particular step in remodeling and, in doing so, affect subsequent steps in the remodeling cascade. Although bone probably contains many yet to be discovered growth factors, the growth factors about which the most is known are discussed in this chapter. In the following sections, individual growth factors will be discussed on the basis of their availability in bone matrix and known biologic actions on bone formation and repair. Speculation on the roles of these growth factors in remodeling processes will be included in this section.

Insulin-Like Growth Factors (IGFs)

IGFs I and II are the products of two different genes, both of which are regulated by growth hormone. These proteins have significant amino acid homology to each other and overlapping biologic functions.[6] IGFs I and II are made by bone cells as well as by other tissues and are found in bone matrix, presumably having been secreted by bone cells.[7] In vitro, measurable amounts of secreted IGFs can be harvested from skeletal tissues in conditioned medium.[8] Signaling pathways for IGFs exist in bone; osteoblasts have receptors for both IGF-I and IGF-II.[9] Most of the biologic effects of IGFs are mediated through the IGF-I receptor, which is a transmembrane glycoprotein with homology to the insulin receptor. The IGF-II receptor has been shown to be the mannose-6-phosphate receptor; however, the role of the IGF-II receptor in mediating the effects of IGF-II in bone is unclear.

Effects of IGFs on target tissues are also regulated by binding proteins, and, to date, six known IGF binding proteins have been identified.[10] All of these IGF binding proteins are made by bone cells, as well as other tissues, and may greatly change the effects of IGFs on bone. Although little is known about the regulation of IGF binding proteins in bone, these binding proteins have been shown to both increase and decrease IGF activity in other tissues by sequestering IGF and, thereby, changing its availability to target cells. In addition, IGFs are known to interact with β2 microglobulin; this interaction results in an increase in IGF affinity for its receptor and thus increases the effects of IGFs in target tissues.[11]

In vitro, IGFs affect bone cells; they have been shown to increase bone collagen and matrix synthesis and also to increase osteoblast-precursor replication while decreasing bone collagen degradation.[12,13] These observed in vitro effects make IGF-I and IGF-II possible regulatory molecules in the formation stages of bone remodeling. IGFs, either made by bone cells in the area or released from matrix during resorption, might be used as a signal to increase osteoblastic activity, allowing for rapid replacement of bone lost during the resorption phase of remodeling. Although no direct effects of IGFs on osteoclast activity have been documented, a recent report on a novel IGF-like protein purified from deer antlers suggests that an IGF-like factor may have a role in the coupling of bone resorption and bone formation.[14]

Fibroblast Growth Factors (FGFs)

There are at least seven members of the FGF gene family,[15] but only two, acidic FGF (aFGF) and basic FGF (bFGF) are normally found in bone and are the products of bone cells.[16] Although FGFs are not secreted proteins, it is possible that FGFs made by bone cells may be released into the surrounding bone matrix at the time of cell death or they may be deposited in bone by cells not resident within bone matrix. Four genes encoding high affinity FGF receptors have been identified, and several low-affinity heparan sulfate proteoglycans also have been proposed to be involved in FGF-mediated signal transduction.[17] Bone tissue has been shown to have a high level of FGF receptors during embryonic development, but the level of receptor expression in adult bone is not well characterized.[18] In vitro, FGFs are mitogenic for bone cells, and the increase in osteoblastic cell replication results in a total increase in the number of osteoblasts synthesizing matrix proteins such as type I collagen.[19-21] A specific role for FGFs in normal bone physiology and remodeling is unclear, but these in vitro data suggest that FGFs may affect the osteoblast progenitor population, which is activated during the formation stage of bone remodeling, and, thus, increase the amount of new bone formed or its rate of formation.

Platelet-Derived Growth Factor (PDGF)

Platelet-derived growth factor, a polypeptide with a molecular weight of approximately 30,000, exists as a dimeric molecule composed of two A or two B subunits or as a heterodimer composed of an A subunit and a B subunit. Thus, there are three separate forms of PDGF. These subunits are the products of two separate genes. Although all three forms of the protein are found in bone matrix, only PDGF AA is made and secreted by bone cells in vitro. Little information on the regulation of PDGF production by bone cells exists.[22] However, a possible PDGF signaling pathway exists in bone. PDGF receptors have been identified on the surfaces of bone cells, and PDGF AA has been shown to bind primarily to the PDGF receptors found in bone with an approximate affinity constant (K_d) of 4 nM.[23] In contrast to IGFs and FGFs, PDGF has been shown to have bone resorbing activity, and a number of investigators have reported increased bone resorption in vitro in response to administration of physiologic doses of PDGF.[24] In addition, PDGF has been shown to increase osteoprogenitor cell replication.[25,26] These two activities allow us to predict that PDGF may be involved in both the resorption and formation phases of bone remodeling. There is no evidence to date that PDGF is able to couple bone resorption and bone formation, and PDGF is probably more likely to be involved in the local regulation of both processes, but is not an inducer of either one.

Transforming Growth Factor-β (TGF-β)

In recent years, available information about TGF-β and TGF-β receptors has made TGF-β a popular candidate for a signaling molecule in bone remodeling. Bone is the largest single source of TGF-β protein in the body, and bone matrix contains much TGF-β, which probably is deposited by osteoblasts during bone matrix formation.[27] At least five distinct isoforms of TGF-β are known, and of these, TGF-β1 and TGF-β2 are synthesized by bone cells. Most of the TGF-β present in bone is in latent form in vivo, and in vitro studies have shown that the majority of TGF-β synthesized and released during bone organ culture is also inactive.[28] There is some evidence for local activation of TGF-β in bone and other tissues, and these data suggest that some amount of the TGF-β found in bone may be available in active form and, thus, able to take part in the control of bone remodeling. Our knowledge of the TGF-β signaling pathway has advanced greatly in recent years, with the molecular cloning of three TGF-β receptor genes. The type III TGF-β receptor is a large (250 kd) glycoprotein that binds to TGF-β. However, this binding does not result in signal transduction, suggesting that the role of the type III receptor may be to modulate the amount of TGF-β available for binding to the other TGF-β receptors.[29] Both the type I and type II TGF-β receptors have been cloned recently and have been shown to contain a conserved serine/threonine kinase domain. Preliminary evidence suggests that a complex cooperative interaction between these two receptors exists.[30,31] The TGF–β type I receptor has been identified as being responsible for the regulation of cell matrix effects seen with TGF-β whereas the type II receptor is most probably involved in the potent antiproliferative activities of the molecule.

The reported effects of TGF-β on bone, in vivo and in vitro, are complicated and at times contradictory. This may be due to the large amounts TGF-β produced by the systems under study. Simply stated, TGF-β has been shown to affect both bone formation and bone resorption. Hormones that have the ability to stimulate bone resorption also increase the amount of active TGF-β released from bone.[32] TGF-β, once released, appears to decrease bone resorption by decreasing both the formation of osteoclasts and their activation. However, more recent evidence makes the direct action of TGF-β on bone resorption questionable. In an interesting set of experiments, Chen and Bates[33] found no direct effects of TGF-β addition on bone resorption in a bone organ culture system. Instead, TGF-β significantly increased the dry weight of the bone explants as a result of increased DNA synthesis and cell proliferation, which in turn resulted in increased collagen deposition.[33] Many other investigators have reported on the stimulatory and inhibitory effects of TGF-β on osteoblasts both in vivo and in vitro.[34,35] Centrella and associates[36] reported that TGF-β stimulated preosteoblastic cell replication and osteoblast cell collagen synthesis in the fetal rat calvaria system. In vivo studies have shown that injection or implantation of TGF-β onto bone surfaces increases bone formation in that local area.[37] These findings are interesting in light of the fact that bone contains abundant stores of TGF-β. At present, TGF-β is the lead candidate for a coupling factor that would not only affect the amount of bone resorption and subsequent new bone formation at a specific site, but would coordinate these activities as well. This hypothesis was recently reviewed by Mundy.[38]

Bone Morphogenetic Proteins (BMPs)

The discovery of BMPs as the osteoinductive components of bone matrix has added an additional group of growth factors to the list of locally acting bone regulatory molecules. The ability of BMPs to differentiate mesenchymal stem cells into cells of the osteoblast lineage suggests the BMPs may have a role in the formation phase of bone remodeling. BMPs were first identified by their property of osteoinduction and were shown by Urist[39] to be components of bone matrix. Based on the purification of BMPs from bone, the amount of BMPs present in bone matrix is small.

The BMPs constitute a large gene family within the TGF-β gene superfamily.[40,41] Unlike TGF-β, BMPs are secreted from the cell in active form. At present, there is no evidence to suggest that latent forms of BMPs are present in bone matrix, indicating that all of the BMP present in the bone microenvironment is biologically active. Multiple individual BMPs have been shown to be osteoinductive in vivo.[42–45] When implanted at ectopic or bony sites in rodents, each of these BMPs induces the endochondral bone formation sequence normally observed during embryonic skeletal formation and fracture healing.[46] BMP messenger RNAs are localized to sites of skeletal formation in the embryo; this observation is consistent with the osteoinductive activity seen in vivo.[47] Although BMP receptors have been described through binding studies, BMP receptor genes have only recently been cloned, and their localization during bone remodeling remains to be determined. Interestingly, the BMP-2 and -4 receptors also contain a serine/threonine domain that is homologous to the kinase domain in type I and II TGF-β receptors that was described above.[48]

The bone-forming effects of BMPs observed in vivo are also evident in vitro on cells of the osteoblast lineage. The primary effect of BMPs appears to be to induce progenitor cells to differentiate into mature osteoblasts. These effects have been observed on mesenchymal stem cells,[49] bone marrow stromal osteoprogenitor cells,[50] cells isolated from embryonic calvaria and limb bud,[51–54] and embryonic mesenchymal cells[55] from multiple species. A likely role for BMPs, based on these data, is control of the recruitment and differentiation of osteoprogenitor cells during the formation phase of bone remodeling. There is not enough information at present to suggest a role for BMPs in bone resorption.

Conclusions

Bone remodeling, the process by which skeletal homeostasis is maintained, is in actuality multiple locally regulated bone resorption and formation events that are tightly coupled in both a temporal and spatial manner. The importance of growth factors as regulators of both bone formation and resorption is well documented. Knowledge of possible candidate molecules for control of bone remodeling has increased dramatically in the last few years, based in part on the use of molecular techniques to identify and localize these molecules. Progress should continue with the use of transgenic technology in which overexpression or removal of specific factors may create animals in which remodeling is greatly affected, thus providing evidence for the importance of specific growth factors to bone remodeling in vivo.

References

1. Parfitt AM: The cellular basis of bone remodeling: The quantum concept reexamined in light of recent advances in the cell biology of bone. *Calcif Tissue Int* 1984; 36:S37–S45.
2. Frost HM: Dynamics of bone remodeling, in Frost HM (ed): *Bone Biodynamics*. Boston, MA, Little Brown, 1964, pp 315–333.
3. Eriksen EF, Vesterby A, Kassem M, et al: Bone remodeling and bone structure, in Mundy GR, Martin TJ (eds): *Physiology and Pharmacology of Bone*. Berlin, Springer-Verlag, 1993, pp 67–109.
4. Hauschka PV, Chen TL, Mavrakos AE: Polypeptide growth factors in bone matrix, in Evered D, Harnett S (eds): *Cell and Molecular Biology of Vertebrate Hard Tissues*. Chichester, Wiley, 1988, pp 207–225.
5. Canalis E, McCarthy T, Centrella M: The role of growth factors in skeletal remodeling. *Endocrinol Metab Clin North Am* 1989;18:903–918.
6. Czech MP: Signal transmission by the insulin-like growth factors. *Cell* 1989;59: 235–238.
7. Canalis E, McCarthy T, Centrella M: Isolation and characterization of insulin-like growth factor I (Somatomedin C) from cultures of fetal rat calvariae. *Endocrinology* 1988;122:22–27.
8. Frolik CA, Ellis LF, Williams DC: Isolation and characterization of insulin-like growth factor-II from human bone. *Biochem Biophys Res Commun* 1988;151: 1011–1018.
9. Centrella M, McCarthy TL, Canalis E: Receptors for insulin-like growth factors I and II in osteoblast-enriched cultures from fetal rat bone. *Endocrinology* 1990;126: 39–44.
10. Canalis E, McCarthy TL, Centrella M: Factors that regulate bone formation, in Mundy GR, Martin TJ (eds): *Physiology and Pharmacology of Bone*. Berlin, Springer-Verlag, 1993, pp 249–266.
11. Centrella M, McCarthy TL, Canalis E: β2-microglobulin enhances insulin-like growth factor I receptor levels and synthesis in bone cell cultures. *J Biol Chem* 1989;264:18268–18271.
12. Hock JM, Centrella M, Canalis E: Insulin-like growth factor I has independent effects on bone matrix formation and cell replication. *Endocrinology* 1988;122: 254–260.
13. McCarthy TL, Centrella M, Canalis E: Regulatory effects of insulin-like growth factors I and II on bone collagen synthesis in rat calvarial cultures. *Endocrinology* 1989;124:301–309.
14. Gutierrez G, Gallwitz W, Garrett IR, et al: Identification of a novel bone-derived growth regulatory factor which is expressed in osteoclasts. *J Bone Miner Res* 1993; 8(suppl 1):S146.
15. Klagsbrun M, Baird A: A dual receptor system is required for basic fibroblast growth factor activity. *Cell* 1991;67:229–231.
16. Globus RK, Plouet J, Gospodarowicz D: Cultured bovine bone cells synthesize basic fibroblast growth factor and store it in their extracellular matrix. *Endocrinology* 1989;124:1539–1547.

17. Johnson DE, Lee PL, Lu J, et al: Diverse forms of a receptor for acidic and basic fibroblast growth factors. *Mol Cell Biol* 1990;10:4728–4736.

18. Peters KG, Werner S, Chen G, et al: Two FGF receptor genes are differentially expressed in epithelial and mesenchymal tissues during limb formation and organogenesis in the mouse. *Development* 1992;114:233–243.

19. Canalis E, Centrella M, McCarthy T: Effects of basic fibroblast growth factor on bone formation in vitro. *J Clin Invest* 1988;81:1572–1577.

20. Rodan SB, Wesolowski G, Thomas K, et al: Growth stimulation of rat calvaria osteoblastic cells by acidic fibroblast growth factor. *Endocrinology* 1987;121:1917–1923.

21. McCarthy TL, Centrella M, Canalis E: Effects of fibroblast growth factors on deoxyribonucleic acid and collagen synthesis in rat parietal bone cells. *Endocrinology* 1989;125:2118–2126.

22. Centrella M, McCarthy TL, Canalis E: Relative effects of hetero- and homodimeric isoforms of platelet-derived growth factor in fetal rat bone cells, in Cohn DV, Glorieux FH, Martin TJ (eds): *Calcium Regulation And Bone Metabolism: Basic And Clinical Aspects*. Elsevier, Amsterdam, 1990, vol 10, pp 324–329.

23. Centrella M, McCarthy TL, Ladd C, et al: Expression of platelet-derived growth factor (PDGF) and regulation of PDGF binding are both isoform specific in osteoblast-enriched cultures from fetal rat bone. *J Bone Miner Res* 1990;5[suppl 2]:S86.

24. Tashjian AH Jr, Hohmann EL, Antoniades HN, et al: Platelet-derived growth factor stimulates bone resorption via a prostaglandin-mediated mechanism. *Endocrinology* 1982;111:118–124.

25. Centrella M, McCarthy TL, Canalis E: Platelet-derived growth factor enhances deoxyribonucleic acid and collagen synthesis in osteoblast-enriched cultures from fetal rat parietal bone. *Endocrinology* 1989;125:13–19.

26. Canalis E, McCarthy TL, Centrella M: Effects of platelet-derived growth factor on bone formation in vitro. *J Cell Physiol* 1989;140:530–537.

27. Centrella M, McCarthy TL, Canalis E: Transforming growth factor-beta and remodeling of bone. *J Bone Joint Surg* 1991;73A:1418–1428.

28. Bonewald LF, Mundy GR: Role of tranforming growth factor beta in bone remodeling: A review. *Connect Tissue Res* 1989;23:201–208.

29. Wang XF, Lin HY, Ng-Eaton E, et al: Expression cloning and characterization of the TGF-β type III receptor. *Cell* 1991;67:797- 805.

30. Lin HY, Wang XF, Ng-Eaton E, et al: Expression cloning of the TGF-β type II receptor, a functional transmembrane serine/threonine kinase. *Cell* 1992;68:775–785.

31. Ebner R, Chen R-H, Shum L, et al: Cloning of a type I TGF-β receptor and its effect on TGF-β binding to the type II receptor. *Science* 1993;260:1344–1348.

32. Shinar DM, Rodan GA: Biphasic effects of transforming growth factor-beta on the production of osteoclast-like cells in mouse bone marrow cultures: The role of prostaglandins in the generation of these cells. *Endocrinology* 1990;126:3153–3158.

33. Chen TL, Bates RL: Recombinant human transforming growth factor β1 modulates bone remodeling in a mineralizing bone organ culture. *J Bone Miner Res* 1993;8:423–434.

34. Noda M, Rodan GA: Type-β transforming growth factor inhibits proliferation and expression of alkaline phosphatase in murine osteoblast-like cells. *Biochem Biophys Res Commun* 1986;140:56–65.

35. Katagiri T, Lee T, Takeshima H, et al: Transforming growth factor-β modulates proliferation and differentiation of mouse clonal osteoblastic MC3T3-E1 cells depending on their maturation stages. *Bone Miner* 1990;11:285–293.

36. Centrella M, McCarthy TL, Canalis E: Transforming growth factor beta is a bifunctional regulator of replication and collagen synthesis in osteoblast-enriched cell cultures from fetal rat bone. *J Biol Chem* 1987;262:2869–2874.

37. Joyce ME, Jingushi S, Bolander ME: Transforming growth factor-β in the regulation of fracture repair. *Orthop Clin North Am* 1990;21:199–209.

38. Mundy GR: Cytokines of bone, in Mundy GR, Martin TJ (eds): *Physiology and Pharmacology of Bone*. Berlin, Springer Verlag, 1993, pp 185–214.
39. Urist MR: Bone: Formation by autoinduction. *Science* 1965;150:893–899.
40. Wozney JM, Rosen V, Celeste AJ, et al: Novel regulators of bone formation: Molecular clones and activities. *Science* 1988;242:1528–1534.
41. Celeste AJ, Iannazzi JA, Taylor RC, et al: Identification of transforming growth factor β family members present in bone-inductive protein purified from bovine bone. *Proc Natl Acad Sci USA* 1990;87:9843–9847.
42. Wang EA, Rosen V, D'Alessandro JS, et al: Recombinant human bone morphogenetic protein induces bone formation. *Proc Natl Acad Sci USA* 1990;87:2220–2224.
43. Sampath TK, Ozkaynak E, Jones WK, et al: Recombinant human osteogenic protein (hOP-1) induces new bone formation with a specific activity comparable to that of natural bovine osteogenic protein. *J Bone Miner Res* 1991;6(suppl 1):S155.
44. LaPan P, Bauduy M, Cox KA, et al: Purification, characterization and activities of recombinant human bone morphogenetic protein 4. *J Bone Miner Res* 1991;6(suppl 1):S153.
45. Wozney JM, Rosen V: Bone morphogenetic proteins, in Mundy GR, Martin TJ (eds): *Physiology and Pharmacology of Bone*. Berlin, Springer-Verlag, 1993, pp 725–748.
46. Reddi AH: Cell biology and biochemistry of endochondral bone development. *Collagen Relat Res* 1981;1:209–226.
47. Lyons KM, Pelton RW, Hogan BLM: Organogenesis and pattern formation in the mouse: RNA distribution patterns suggest a role for bone morphogenetic protein-2A (BMP-2A). *Development* 1990;109:833–844.
48. Yamaji N, Celeste AJ, Thies RS, et al: The molecular cloning of bone morphogenetic protein receptors. *J Bone Miner Res* 1993;8(suppl 1):S145.
49. Cox K, McQuaid DP, Rosen V: Use of cell capture chambers to study mesenchymal stem cells. Responses to recombinant human bone morphogenetic protein-2. *J Bone Miner Res* 1993;8(suppl 1):S179.
50. Thies RS, Bauduy M, Ashton BA, et al: Recombinant human bone morphogenetic protein-2 induces osteoblastic differentiation in W-20–17 stormal cells. *Endocrinology* 1992;130:1318–1324.
51. Takuwa Y, Ohse C, Wang EA, et al: Bone morphogenetic protein-2 stimulates alkaline phosphatase activity and collagen synthesis in cultured osteoblastic cells, MC3T3-E1. *Biochem Biophys Res Commun* 1991;174:96–101.
52. Yamaguchi A, Katagiri T, Ikeda T, et al: Recombinant human bone morphogenetic protein-2 stimulates osteoblastic maturation and inhibits myogenic differentiation in vitro. *J Cell Biol* 1991;113:681–687.
53. Rosen V, Capparella J, McQuaid D, et al: Development of immortalized cells derived from 13DPC mouse limb buds as a system to study the effects of rhBMP-2 on limb bud cell differentiation, in Fallon JF, Goetinck PF, Kelley RD, et al (eds): *Limb Development and Regeneration, Part A: Proceedings of the 4th International Conference on Limb Development and Regeneration, Asilomar, CA, July 1992*. Wiley-Liss, 1993, pp 305–315.
54. Carrington JL, Chen P, Yanagishita M, et al: Osteogenin (bone morphogenetic protein-3) stimulates cartilage formation by chick limb bud cells in vitro. *Dev Biol* 1991;146:406–415.
55. Katagiri T, Yamaguchi A, Ikeda T, et al: The non-osteogenic mouse pluripotent cell line, C3H10T1/2, is induced to differentiate into osteoblastic cells by recombinant human bone morphogenetic protein-2. *Biochem Biophys Res Commun* 1990;172:295–299.

Chapter 20

Abnormal Bone Remodeling: The Consequences of Therapeutic Drugs and Physical Modalities

Gary E. Friedlaender, MD
Nancy Troiano, MS
Mitsukazu Ishii, MD
Richard R. Pelker, MD, PhD
Roland Baron, DDS, PhD

Introduction

In the course of clinical practice, patients come in contact with a variety of therapeutic modalities that may also influence the skeleton.[1] These drugs and physical forces include systemic treatment, such as chemotherapy, nonsteroidal anti-inflammatory medication, immunosuppressive agents, and steroids, as well as focally delivered approaches, including irradiation and electric stimulation. In each case, these therapies exert their influence at the cellular and molecular levels, and may lead, in turn, to significant alterations in bone physiology and, therefore, biomechanical properties of bone. Such changes in the bone remodeling cycle may become apparent in the nature of bone homeostasis, fracture repair, or bone graft incorporation. These circumstances share common reparative and regenerative mechanisms that lead to bone remodeling.

The bone remodeling cycle, most simply stated, involves resorption activity by osteoclasts, new-bone formation mediated by osteoblasts, and a variety of molecular signals or factors that regulate these two opposing activities.[2-4] When resorption and formation are coupled and synchronous, which is the usual state during homeostasis, the mass of bone remains constant. Consequently, bone mass remains "normal" when resorption and formation are synchronously increased, regardless of how much, or synchronously reduced, even to the point of total cell death. That is not to suggest that the biologic and mechanical properties of bone tissue are divorced from cellular health. Although the material properties of dead bone are, in many ways, similar to those of live tissue, the fatigue characteristics of an inert bone are substantially less than those of a bone with synchronously coupled metabolic activity. This difference reflects the inability of bone with reduced cellular activity to remodel microfractures or to keep pace with the reparative activity required of bone subjected to repetitive loads.

A clinically significant alternate scenario to circumstances in which osteoclastic and osteoblastic activities are balanced is the uncoupling of resorption and formation with a subsequent change in bone mass (usually a reduction).

Uncoupling can occur for a variety of reasons including: (1) when an insult to cellular activity has a more profound influence on the metabolic activity of osteoclasts compared with osteoblasts (or the reverse); (2) when the recovery of these cell populations from sublethal injury occurs at differing rates; (3) when the local "restocking" of osteoclasts or osteoblasts from available progenitors or systemic pools happens at different speeds; or (4) when there is selective alteration of the cells from which are derived the molecules that regulate the bone remodeling system. In each of these cases, resorption and formation activity are no longer balanced, and bone mass changes from normal.

There are times when events that influence bone cell biology are inadvertent side effects of required treatment, often for nonskeletal disease. An example of such a circumstance is the use of chemotherapy for treatment of a soft-tissue sarcoma. At the other extreme, these same or similar therapies may prove purposefully useful to correct deficiencies in skeletal growth, homeostasis, or repair. For example, indomethacin and irradiation have been used to reduce heterotopic bone formation.[5,6]

Drugs Causing Abnormal Remodeling

Chemotherapy

Among the most blatant toxins directed against cell function are chemotherapeutic agents used deliberately for their antimetabolic activity in the treatment of malignant disease. Because the chemotherapeutic agents are systemic drugs, injury is not confined to specific or geographically localized cell populations, although more highly active cells are usually most susceptible to chemotherapy. In addition, different classes of chemotherapeutic agents differ in the mechanism by which they cause a metabolic dysfunction. Methotrexate, for example, is a competitive inhibitor of folic acid metabolism and, thereby, influences the entire spectrum of cellular activity from DNA synthesis to protein synthesis.[7] In addition to its applications in oncology, methotrexate is used in lower but more chronic doses to treat inflammatory arthropathies associated with connective tissue diseases, most notably rheumatoid arthritis.[8] Doxorubicin (Adriamycin) interferes with DNA replication by intercalation between adjacent base pairs.[9] By disrupting cell division, doxorubicin exerts a secondary influence on protein synthesis. This antracycline has been particularly efficacious in treating bone and soft-tissue sarcomas.[10]

The effect of these and other drugs or treatment modalities on bone has been explored in a rat model, in which tail vertebrae were either subjected to a systemic drug or became the direct target of a physical modality, such as irradiation. This treatment was followed by assessment using histomorphometry.[11] In the same animal, a midshaft fracture of the femur afforded the opportunity to evaluate fracture repair using histologic and biomechanical approaches.

Rats were evaluated 14 days after initiation of short-term administration of methotrexate, 0.75 mg/kg/d intraperitoneally for 5 days, or doxorubicin, 1.0 mg/kg/d intraperitoneally for 5 days. Methotrexate treatment resulted in a 27% decrease in net trabecular bone volume and doxorubicin in an 11.5% decrease (Table 1). Both drugs were associated with a 60% decrease in bone formation rates as well as profound reductions in a variety of static histomorphometric parameters of osteoblastic activity.[12]

Long-term administration of these same drugs (16 weeks) produced a different pattern. Doxorubicin-treated animals had no net change in bone volume after 4 months,[13] but bone formation rates continued to be reduced by at least

50%. This circumstance of unchanged bone volume with decreased bone formation rates requires synchronously reduced resorption activity. Both osteoclasts and osteoblasts appear similarly influenced (in net terms) by long-term exposure to doxorubicin. In contrast, long-term methotrexate treatment was associated with a 26% reduction in bone volume. This decrease could be appreciated as early as 2 weeks and remained constant thereafter, suggesting that osteoclasts initially were influenced less by methotrexate than osteoblasts but subsequently osteoclasts and osteoblasts were synchronously suppressed. Bone formation rates in this model were reduced approximately 40% (Table 2).

Other investigators have observed changes in skeletal repair associated with chemotherapy. Burchardt and associates[14] observed an increasing rate of segmental fibular autograft nonunions in dogs receiving 40 or 50 mg/m[2] of doxorubicin. They also demonstrated a reduction in new bone formation in dogs receiving methotrexate, and they noted that osteoclastic activity within autografts was less affected than osteoblastic function. Nilsson and associates[15] reported a 30% to 40% decrease in bone formation within heterotopically placed demineralized bone matrix in rats receiving methotrexate or doxorubicin.

Histologically, fracture repair (in the absence of rigid fixation without a gap) proceeds through a sequence of events characterized initially by injury, necrosis, inflammation, and a fibrovascular response. Activity then progresses through a cartilaginous phase followed by conversion of the callus to bone, which, in turn, is remodeled. Femoral fracture repair was assessed in the rat model, and the callus was found to be histologically mature by 12 weeks in untreated animals. In rats receiving methotrexate, fracture repair occurred at a slower and less reliable rate, with less than half demonstrating significant amounts of new bone in the callus during the 3-month period of observation (Table 3).[16]

Table 1 Effect of short-term administration of chemotherapeutic agent on cancellous bone of rat tail vertebrae

	Control N = 13	Doxorubicin* N = 12	Methotrexate** N = 10
Bone volume (%)†	18.2 ± 1.6	16.1 ± 3.1	13.3 ± 1.6
Bone formation rate (10^{-2} mm^3/mm^2/yr)†	25.2 ± 3.2	10.4 ± 5.1	10.6 ± 6.0

* 1.0 mg/kg/d for 5 days
** 0.75 mg/kg/d for 5 days
† one-way analysis of variance, $p < 0.01$

Table 2 Effect of chemotherapeutic agent administration (16 weeks) on cancellous bone of rat tail vertebrae

	Control N = 11	Doxorubicin* N = 8	Control N = 8	Methotrexate** N = 8
Bone volume (%)	22.6 ± 3.2	24.3 ± 9.5	21.0 ± 0.09	15.6 ± 2.9†
Bone formation rate (10^{-2} mm^3/mm^2/yr)	34.7 ± 6.8	14.1 ± 17.1†	33.9 ± 7.0	20.7 ± 15.1†

* 1.0 mg/kg/d, once each week until sacrifice
** 0.1 mg/kg/d, 5 of every 7 days until sacrifice
† $p < 0.05$

Biomechanical studies represent another method of assessing the biologic integrity of the skeleton. Fractures gradually regain strength during the repair process, and the progression or maturation of callus can be quantitated, for example, by subjecting healing fractures to torsional forces and measuring the energy and angle to failure and the stiffness. In addition, the pattern of failure (relationship of the "refracture" line to the original injury) also changes in a characteristic fashion as normal repair occurs.[17]

Using these biomechanical tools, substantial and persistent decreases in both strength and maturity of fracture callus have been demonstrated during treatment of animals with either methotrexate or doxorubicin (Table 4).[18] This finding is hardly a surprise, given the histomorphometric changes associated with these drugs. Khoo[19] demonstrated delayed fracture repair in rabbits receiving doxorubicin, and Haji and associates[20] also noted profound reduction in the mechanical strength of fractures in rats treated with weekly methotrexate. Both chemotherapeutic agents caused reduced strength in fibular autografts in a canine model evaluated by Burchardt and associates.[14]

Similar studies of humans have not been carried out; however, it is noteworthy that children receiving methotrexate for leukemia have been reported to develop osteoporosis and sustain spontaneous fractures.[21,22] It is also our impression that the osteosynthesis sites of osteochondral allografts used in limb-sparing tumor resections repair less reliably during long-term chemother-

Table 3 Effects of methotrexate and radiation therapy on histologic aspects of repair

	Score*		
Weeks	Control	Methotrexate**	Irradiation[†]
1	2.2 ± 0.20	2.6 ± 0.40	2.0 ± 0
2	4.6 ± 0.92	4.8 ± 0.48	2.2 ± 0.37
4	5.3 ± 0.25	5.0 ± 0	2.6 ± 0.60
8	5.8 ± 0.58	6.2 ± 0.80	3.4 ± 0.67
12	8.7 ± 0.33	5.8 ± 0.96	4.0 ± 0.63

* Effect measured using a point scoring scale in which 1 is least mature callus and 9 reflects advanced bone remodeling at the fracture site: 1 to 3 points for a fibrovascular callus; 4 to 6 points for a cartilaginous callus; and 7 to 9 points for a bony callus. N = 5 for each group
** 0.1 mg/kg/d for 5 of every 7 days until sacrifice
† 250 rad/d for 10 days

Table 4 Biomechanical changes in fracture repair in rats associated with 26 weeks of methotrexate and doxorubicin

	Control N = 35	Methotrexate* N = 11	Doxorubicin** N = 9
Torque to failure (Nm)	1.05 ± 0.51	0.85 ± 0.70†	0.45 ± 0.20‡
Stiffness	1.01 ± 0.76	0.85 ± 0.92	0.27 ± 0.21‡

* 0.1 mg/kg/d 5 of every 7 days until sacrifice
** 1.0 mg/kg/d once each week until sacrifice
† $p < 0.05$
‡ $p < 0.001$

apy, but can be salvaged by additional bone grafting after cessation of this drug treatment. These observations underscore the significance of the toxicity of some drugs to the skeleton in terms of clinical care and management.

Immunosuppressant Drugs

Cyclosporin-A has been evaluated in the rat model described above, and when the drug was administered at a dose of 7 mg/kg/d for 14 days, substantial changes from normal were found in the rates of both resorption and formation, with each reduced dramatically and in a synchronous fashion.[23] This profound reduction in remodeling, by approximately 90%, suggests absence of message(s) for remodeling rather than widespread cell necrosis (Table 5). Despite observed decreases in bone turnover, fracture repair, judged biomechanically, proceeded in a normal fashion in this model.[24] Much more needs to be assessed with respect to immunosuppressive agents and their interaction with the skeleton, particularly because there is evidence that many of the regulatory molecules involved in bone remodeling have their origin in cells associated with the immune system.[25]

Nonsteroidal Anti-inflammatory Drugs

There is limited information available concerning the influence of nonsteroidal anti-inflammatory drugs on bone metabolism. Evidence suggests that indomethacin reduces heterotopic bone in humans[6] and slows fracture repair in laboratory animals.[26,27] It is now important to determine if this or other commonly used nonsteroidal anti-inflammatory drugs also interfere with the biology of porous ingrowth, a crucial aspect of noncemented joint arthroplasties. Preliminary evidence suggests that ibuprofen, and presumably other nonsteroidals, does not significantly alter histomorphometric parameters of intact cancellous bone or biomechanical aspects of fracture repair in rats.[28]

Physical Modalities Causing Abnormal Bone Remodeling

Irradiation

Unlike that of chemotherapy, the influence of irradiation is localized. Only those cells directly in the path of the radiation source are affected. Irradiation is commonly used as a palliative approach to metastatic bone disease, including

Table 5 Influence of 14 consecutive days of cyclosporin-A (7 mg/kg/d) on bone of rat tail vertebrae

	% Change from Control		
	2 weeks*	4 weeks*	16 weeks*
Bone volume	0%	0%	0%
BFR**	− 83	− 93	− 75
BRR†	− 83	− 93	− 75

* Weeks after initiation of treatment
** BFR, bone formation rate as measured using pulse labeling with calcein
† BRR, bone resorption rate (derived)

pathological fractures, with total doses in the 2,500 rad range. Primary malignancies of bone and some soft-tissue sarcomas are treated with doses twice this level or higher, and adjacent bone may lie in the path of these treatment approaches.[29]

The rat model previously described has been used to assess the influence of palliative doses of irradiation (250 rad/d for 10 days) delivered to both intact tail vertebrae and a closed intact femoral fracture.[30] Three weeks following the onset of treatment, bone volume remained normal (Table 6). This lack of apparent change in the skeleton was the net result of substantial but synchronous reductions in resorption and formation activity. Some cells presumably sustained sublethal injuries, while other changes were permanent. By 7 weeks following irradiation, trabecular bone volume was decreased approximately 14% in this model, and it was reduced further by 11 weeks to nearly 70% of control values (a 30% loss of bone mass). The delayed drop in bone volume reflects disproportionately higher resorption than formation activity over time. This activity is apparently the result of earlier recovery from sublethal injury of osteoclasts compared with osteoblasts, and perhaps, of the more rapid recruitment, differentiation, or maturation of new osteoclasts from distant "reserves."

Again, histologic evidence of fracture repair following irradiation demonstrates not only incomplete repair, but a delay in progression through various stages of fracture healing. In the rat model, open fractures exposed to 2,500 rads failed to progress past the cartilaginous phase of callus maturation (Table 3).[16] Mechanically, irradiated fractures lagged temporally behind nonirradiated controls. Open fractures did not approach control values in 24 weeks, while closed fractures returned towards normal by 16 weeks.[31] Given the high level of clinical significance, much more information is required concerning the influence of irradiation on skeletal repair, with emphasis on exploring different times of delivery following injury and various dose fractionation schedules.

Electrical Stimulation

There is considerable evidence that bone subjected to electromagnetic forces or direct current stimulation responds with new bone formation.[32-34] Similarly, mechanical forces promote osteogenesis as well as cause measurable changes in the electric properties of bone.[35] It is apparent that a variety of physical and chemical activities can be translated at the cellular level, causing modulation of molecular events in cells responsible for either bone resorption or bone for-

Table 6 Influence of palliative doses of irradiation (2500 rads in 10 equally-divided daily doses) on bone of rat tail vertebrae

	% Change From Control		
	3 weeks*	7 weeks	11 weeks
Bone volume	0%	−14%	−29%
BFR**	−67	−50	+40
BRR†	−82	−77	+160

* weeks following initiation of irradiation
** BFR, bone formation rate as measured using pulse labeling with calcein
† BRR, bone resorption rate (derived)

mation. These modalities may produce enhanced or diminished osteogenesis, with either synchronous coupling of formation and resorption maintained and no net change in bone volume, or alteration of bone mass when the cellular events of the remodeling cycle are uncoupled. In each case, the nature of the resulting tissue varies from normal, and the significance of these changes is of clinical importance.

Conclusions

Bone is a remarkable tissue, characterized by the uncommon capacity to regenerate. This phenomenon is achieved through a series of events collectively referred to as the remodeling cycle, and these activities are central to homeostasis of intact bone, fracture repair, and bone graft incorporation. Remodeling is accomplished through a balance between resorption and formation activity, usually coupled and synchronous, and under the control of a cascading sequence of molecules responsible for the recruitment, differentiation, maturation, and regulation of osteoclasts and osteoblasts and their functions.

Under certain circumstances, resorption and formation activity are uncoupled, and then the biologic and biomechanical nature of the resultant skeletal tissue is affected. A variety of drugs are known to influence cellular metabolism on a systemic basis and have also been shown to specifically alter bone resorption or formation activity or both. Various chemotherapeutic agents (methotrexate, doxorubicin), nonsteroidal anti-inflammatory drugs (indomethacin), and immunosuppressants (cyclosporin-A) have demonstrated the ability to influence skeletal repair. This ability usually is observed as the inadvertent side effect of treatment modalities required for other important therapeutic purposes (the treatment of tumors, arthritis, or graft rejection). Irradiation and the application of electrical fields are examples of locally delivered modulators of cell function that also have impact on cells of the bone remodeling cycle.

References

1. Friedlaender GE: The influence of various physical modalities and drugs on bone regeneration and ingrowth, in Fitzgerald RH Jr (ed): *Noncemented Total Hip Arthroplasty.* New York, NY, Raven Press, 1988, pp 135–141.
2. Canalis E, McCarthy T, Centrella M: Growth factors and the regulation of bone remodeling. *J Clin Invest* 1988;81:277–281.
3. Frost HM: Skeletal physiology and bone remodeling: An overview, in Urist MR (ed): *Fundamental and Clinical Bone Physiology.* Philadelphia, PA, JB Lippincott, 1980, pp 208–241.
4. Raisz LG, Rodan GA: Cellular basis for bone turnover, in Avioli LV, Krane SM (eds): *Metabolic Bone Disease and Clinically Related Disorders.* Philadelphia, PA, WB Saunders, 1990, pp 1–41.
5. Coventry MB, Scanlon PW: The use of radiation to discourage ectopic bone: A nine-year study in surgery about the hip. *J Bone Joint Surg* 1981;63A:201–208.
6. Ritter MA, Gioe TJ: The effect of indomethacin on para-articular ectopic ossification following total hip arthroplasty. *Clin Orthop* 1982;167:113–117.
7. Bertino JR, Booth BA, Bieber AL, et al: Studies on the inhibition of dihydrofolate reductase by the folate antagonists. *J Biol Chem* 1964;239:479–485.
8. Weinblatt ME, Weissman BN, Holdsworth DE, et al: Long-term prospective study of methotrexate in the treatment of rheumatoid arthritis: 84-month update. *Arthritis Rheum* 1992;35:129–137.
9. DiMarco A: Adriamycin (NCS-123127): Mode and mechanism of action. *Cancer Chemother Rep* 1975;6:91–106.

10. Smith MA, Ungerleider RS, Horowitz ME, et al: Influence of doxorubicin dose intensity on response and outcome for patients with osteogenic sarcoma and Ewing's sarcoma. *J Natl Cancer Inst* 1991;83:1460–1470.

11. Baron R, Vignery A, Neff L, et al: Processing of undecalcified bone specimens for bone histomorphometry, in Recker RR (ed): *Bone Histomorphometry: Techniques and Interpretation.* Boca Raton, FL, CRC Press, 1983, pp 13–35.

12. Friedlaender GE, Tross RB, Doganis AC, et al: Effects of chemotherapeutic agents on bone: I. Short-term methotrexate and doxorubicin (Adriamycin) treatment in a rat model. *J Bone Joint Surg* 1984;66A:602–607.

13. Friedlaender GE, Baron R, Doganis AC, et al: Chronic effects of Adriamycin on bone volume in rats. *Trans Orthop Res Soc* 1983;8:297.

14. Burchardt H, Glowczewskie FP Jr, Enneking WF: The effect of Adriamycin and methotrexate on the repair of segmental cortical autografts in dogs. *J Bone Joint Surg* 1983;65A:103–108.

15. Nilsson OS, Bauer HCF, Brostrom LA: Comparison of the effects of Adriamycin and methotrexate on orthotopic and induced heterotopic bone in rats. *J Orthop Res* 1990;8:199–204.

16. Friedlaender GE, Goodman A, Hausman M, et al: The effects of methotrexate and radiation therapy on histologic aspects of fracture healing. *Trans Orthop Res Soc* 1983;8:224.

17. White AA III, Panjabi MM, Southwick WO: The four biomechanical stages of fracture repair. *J Bone Joint Surg* 1977;59A:188–192.

18. Pelker RR, Friedlaender GE, Panjabi MM, et al: Chemotherapy induced alterations in the biomechanics of rat bone. *J Orthop Res* 1985;3:91–95.

19. Khoo DBA: The effect of chemotherapy on soft tissue and bone healing in the rabbit model. *Ann Acad Med Singapore* 1992;21:217–221.

20. Haji A, Mnaymneh W, Ghandur-Mnaymneh L, et al: The effects of methotrexate on the healing of rats femora. *Trans Orthop Res Soc* 1981;6:79.

21. Ragab AH, Frech RS, Vietti TJ: Osteoporotic fractures secondary to methotrexate therapy of acute leukemia in remission. *Cancer* 1970;25:580–585.

22. Stanisavljevic S, Babcock AL: Fractures in children treated with methotrexate for leukemia. *Clin Orthop* 1977;125:139–144.

23. Friedlaender GE, Troiano N, McKay J Jr, et al: Cyclosporin-A induced changes in bone turnover. *Trans Orthop Res Soc* 1985;10:66.

24. Warren SB, Pelker RR, Friedlaender GE: Effects of short-term Cyclosporin-A on biomechanical properties of intact and fractured bone in the rat. *J Orthop Res* 1985;3:96–100.

25. Horowitz MC, Friedlaender GE: Immunologic aspects of bone transplantation: A rationale for future studies. *Orthop Clin North Am* 1987;18:227–233.

26. Allen HL, Wase A, Bear WT: Indomethacin and aspirin: Effect of non-steroidal anti-inflammatory agents on the rate of fracture repair in the rat. *Acta Orthop Scand* 1980;51:595–600.

27. Tornkvist H, Bauer FCH, Nilsson OS: Influence of indomethacin on experimental bone metabolism in rats. *Clin Orthop* 1985;193:264–270.

28. Huo MH, Troiano NW, Pelker RR, et al: The influence of ibuprofen on fracture repair: Biomechanical, biochemical, histologic and histomorphometric parameters in rats. *Trans Orthop Res Soc* 1990;15:168.

29. Suit HD: Role of therapeutic radiology in cancer of bone. *Cancer* 1975;35:930–935.

30. Friedlaender GE, Troiano N, McKay J Jr, et al: Irradiation induced changes in formation and resorption activity of bone. *Trans Orthop Res Soc* 1985;10:351.

31. Markbreiter LA, Pelker RR, Friedlaender GE, et al: The effect of radiation on the fracture repair process: A biomechanical evaluation of a closed fracture in a rat model. *J Orthop Res* 1989;7:178–183.

32. Bassett CAL, Pawluk RJ, Becker RO: Effects of electric currents on bone in vivo. *Nature* 1964;204:652–654.

33. Brighton CT: The treatment of nonunions with electricity. *J Bone Joint Surg* 1981; 63A:847–851.
34. Yasuda I, Noguchi K, Sata T: Dynamic callus and electric callus. *J Bone Joint Surg* 1955;37A:1292–1293.
35. Rubin CT, Lanyon LE: Regulation of bone formation by applied dynamic loads. *J Bone Joint Surg* 1984;66A:397–402.

Chapter 21

Biochemical Markers of Bone Remodeling: Emerging Technology

David R. Eyre, PhD

This chapter will review recent developments in the search for more specific and convenient biochemical assays for monitoring bone turnover that have clinical potential. Available assays for monitoring bone metabolism all rely on the measurement of (1) enzymes produced by osteoblasts or osteoclasts that escape into body fluids or (2) structural macromolecules of bone matrix synthesized by osteoblasts. The latter macromolecules can be measured in serum either as a spillover of osteoblast synthetic activity or as breakdown products of osteoclastic resorption. Table 1 lists the more commonly explored biochemical markers of bone formation and resorption.

Bone Formation Markers

Serum osteocalcin, alkaline phosphatase, and bone-specific alkaline phosphatase are the three markers of bone formation now in use. Osteocalcin or bone Gla protein (BGP), which can be measured in serum, is a component of bone matrix produced by osteoblasts.[1] Although serum osteocalcin might be expected to reflect a combination of bone resorption and formation, the intact molecule is primarily an index of bone formation activity.[2] The carboxypropeptide of type I collagen has proven to have some value as a serum marker of bone formation,[3] but it is presumed to reflect a summation of all synthetic

Table 1 Biochemical markers of bone metabolism

Formation	Resorption
Serum or Plasma	
• Alkaline phosphatase	• Tartrate-resistant acid phosphatase
• Bone specific alkaline phosphatase	• Collagen cross-links
• Osteocalcin (BGP)	
• Type I collagen carboxypropeptides	
Urine	
• Nondialyzable hydroxyproline	• Hydroxyproline
	• Hydroxylysine glycosides
	• Collagen cross-links
	• Total and free pyridinolines
	• Cross-linked type I collagen peptides

activity of type I collagen throughout the body and, therefore, is unlikely to be a bone-specific marker. An assay for serum N-propeptide of type I collagen[4] has the same theoretical disadvantage, with the added problem that collagen N-propeptides may be retained in the matrix, particularly of bone.[2]

Although serum osteocalcin (intact molecule) and skeletal alkaline phosphatase immunoassays are emerging as the best indicators of bone formation activity, they do not always show parallel responses. For example, serum osteocalcin correlates poorly with either total serum alkaline phosphatase activity or levels of the bone-specific enzyme molecule in Paget disease of bone.[5–7] The relative lack of correlation between osteocalcin and serum alkaline phosphatase probably reflects the expression of these proteins at different stages in preosteoblast and osteoblast development.[7] It should also be noted that platelets have recently been shown to contain osteocalcin messenger RNA (mRNA) and to synthesize osteocalcin. The significance of this phenomenon in understanding how serum levels of osteocalcin are related to osteoblast activity needs further study.[8]

The development of an immunoassay for the skeletal alkaline phosphatase molecule is clearly an improvement in convenience and specificity in comparison to total enzyme activity measurements.[9] Although some cross-reactivity is noted with the liver isoenzyme of alkaline phosphatase (at about 15% of the level of skeletal alkaline phosphatase[10]), the narrow normal range and marked elevation in Paget disease hold promise of clinical usefulness.

Bone Resorption Markers

Most of the biochemical tests for monitoring resorption are based on urinary measurements of collagen degradation products (Table 1). Total urinary hydroxyproline is the traditional index, but its usefulness is affected by dietary contributions, lack of specificity to bone collagen, degradation in the liver, and relatively tedious chemical assays. More precise chemical assays for hydroxyproline by high-performance liquid chromatography (HPLC) appear to offer greater specificity for bone metabolism than the traditional colorimetric assay.[11]

Plasma levels of tartrate-resistant acid phosphatase (TRAP), which is a prominent enzyme of osteoclasts, are elevated in clinical conditions that cause increased bone turnover, but the degree of specificity to osteoclasts is not well-defined.[12] The development of immunoassays for the enzyme molecule could prove more useful than enzyme activity measurements.[2]

In recent years, the bone resorption markers that have been considered to have the most promise are the pyridinoline cross-linking residues of collagen measured in urine.[13–23] These compounds appear not to be metabolized when tissue collagen is degraded and are excreted in urine primarily as small peptides with about 30% as the free amino acids.[13] Two forms exist: hydroxylysyl pyridinoline (HP; or simply pyridinoline, Pyr) and lysyl pyridinoline (LP; or deoxypyridinoline, Dpy). These forms are posttranslational chemical variants that reflect heterogeneity in the degree of hydroxylation of specific lysine residues at the triple-helical cross-linking sites in types I, II, III, and IX collagens.[24] Pyridinolines serve as mature cross-links in the collagens of most connective tissues other than skin. Because bone accounts for such a large proportion of total collagen in the body and turns over faster than most other connective tissues, urinary pyridinolines are derived primarily from bone resorption. This conclusion is supported by the similar ratios of HP to LP in adult human bone (3.5:1) and urine (2:1 to 7:1), in contrast with other connective tissues in which LP is usually present at less than 10% of the content of HP.[20,24,25]

Because bone is the primary store of LP in the body, this molecule presents a theoretically attractive, more specific marker of bone resorption than total pyridinoline, and, indeed, the clinical data from urinary measurements of HP and LP by HPLC support this concept.[14–23] The lower concentration of LP, and consequent larger analytical errors, tend to offset this advantage, however. It should also be clearly understood that even though the ratio of HP to LP is much higher in all other tissues than in bone, LP may actually be present in significant amounts, possibly as high as or even higher than concentrations in bone collagen, in certain tissues such as the vasculature.[20,26] This is because the total concentration of pyridinolines is actually quite low in bone collagen (about 0.3 moles per mole of collagen) compared with other tissue collagens (1.5 moles/mole in cartilage; 0.5 to 1.0 moles/mole in vascular tissue, tendon, ligament, fascia, lung, intestine, liver, muscle, etc.). Therefore, because not much is known about the collective turnover rates of collagen in these tissues relative to bone, it is questionable to what degree pyridinolines in total or LP in particular can be relied on as specific markers of bone resorption.

Because of reservations about the specificity of pyridinolines as bone resorption markers, including potential destructive losses of the 3-hydroxypyridinium ring in urine,[23] immunoassays for a collagen type-specific cross-linked peptide seem more attractive. We[27] isolated from urine a prominent cross-linked peptide that was derived from the N-telopeptide cross-linking domain of type I collagen (Fig. 1) and showed by its HP to LP ratio that it was derived exclusively from bone type I collagen. A monoclonal antibody, 1H11, was made that recognized the peptide conformations about this cross-linked fragment, but not the pyridinoline residue itself or the individual peptide sequences. A microtiter-plate immunoassay (ELISA) was developed with this antibody for application to urine. The results proved that this assay was significantly more specific than determination of pyridinolines (total or deoxypyridinoline) as a monitor of bone resorption.[28] The assay is applied directly to urine with no pretreatment,[27] and the latest commercial version is completed in 90 minutes. (Osteomark™, Ostex International, Inc.). Another immunoassay for a cross-linked collagen domain has been described that uses a polyclonal antiserum raised against an enriched peptide fraction that was derived from the C-telopeptide cross-linking

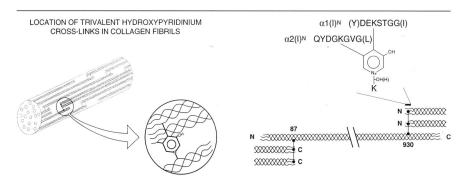

Fig. 1 Conceptual illustrations showing: **left,** the location of pyridinoline residues as intermolecular cross-links between three collagen molecules (two telopeptides to a triple-helical site) within a collagen fibril, and **right,** the structure and origin of the cross-linked N-telopeptide epitope recognized by mAb1H11 in human bone type I collagen (Reproduced with permission from Eyre DR: New molecular markers of bone metabolism. *Ther Ref* 1994;15:100–111.).

domain of human bone type I collagen.[29] This assay is applied to serum. Clinical evidence in support of this analyte as a specific indicator of bone resorbing activity has been disappointing.[30]

In another approach, the free pyridinoline pool in urine has been targeted for immunoassay.[31–33] Again, the advantage is that urine samples can be analyzed directly without hydrolysis or other pretreatment steps. A polyclonal antibody-based ELISA that recognizes pyridinoline was described.[31] The approach was developed into a urinary assay for free total pyridinolines[32] and, more recently, a monoclonal antibody-based ELISA that is specific for LP (deoxy-pyridinoline).[33] Available clinical data indicate that these assays correlate well with HPLC-based pyridinoline measurements. It remains to be seen, however, whether they represent an improvement in analyte specificity for bone resorption or will be limited by constraints that are now becoming apparent for total pyridinoline and deoxypyridinoline as analytes of bone resorption. With all these assays, no matter how compelling the theoretical arguments, the acid test of utility is the result of application to clinical samples.

Clinical Results

For any biochemical marker to be useful in the clinic, it eventually has to be able to provide meaningful results on an individual patient. To date, most studies of bone markers have presented cross-sectional data on subject groups that show statistically significant differences in formation or resorption rates, but no performance characteristics in longitudinal studies of individuals. Reported data monitoring individual subjects are few. Some of the newer immunoassays have the convenience and specificity to do this. For example, the short-term (2 weeks) and long-term (9 months) longitudinal coefficient of variance for the cross-linked N-telopeptide (NTx) urinary assay of bone resorption was 20% in early postmenopausal women (the placebo group in a bisphosphonate trial), compared with 60% for total pyridinolines by HPLC.[28] This NTx assay, therefore, has the potential to draw conclusions on the responsiveness of individual subjects to antiresorption therapies. Figure 2 shows an example of assay results from this study on an individual woman monitored for 9 months. The baseline value is the mean of samples taken 2 weeks apart just before a 6-week treatment with oral alendronate. Several recent studies[34–37]

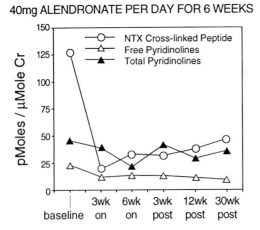

40mg ALENDRONATE PER DAY FOR 6 WEEKS

— NTX Cross-linked Peptide
— Free Pyridinolines
— Total Pyridinolines

y-axis: pMoles / μMole Cr

x-axis: baseline | 3wk on | 6wk on | 3wk post | 12wk post | 30wk post

Fig. 2 Comparative results of monitoring urinary total and free pyridinolines and cross-linked N-telopeptides (NTx) as measures of bone resorption in an individual early post-menopausal woman receiving a high dose of bisphosphonate (alendronate) for 6 weeks.

using the urinary NTx immunoassay support its specificity and responsiveness in monitoring bone resorption. For example, in a study of the short-term sequential effects of the bisphosphonate, pamidronate (to block resorption), and triiodothyronine (T3, to induce mild hyperthyroidism), NTx results showed an 83% fall in pamidronate compared with a 19% fall in free pyridinoline by day 8. Pamidronate pretreatment also blocked the subsequent T3-induced increase in NTx at day 16 more markedly than it blocked the increase in free pyridinoline, consistent with NTx providing a more selective index of bone resorption.[38]

Bone formation markers (intact osteocalcin and alkaline phosphatase) generally give tighter overall analytic and biologic coefficients of variance than urinary assays. This no doubt reflects in part the increased variance in having to normalize urinary values to a second analyte, creatinine. Serum formation markers, however, appear to respond more slowly to changes in bone turnover that occur naturally (eg, at menopause),[39] after surgical oophorectomy,[40] or on intervention with the antiresorptive agents, estrogen[41] or bisphosphonate.[42] In most clinical situations, coupling between resorption and formation appears to be tight, but there is usually a temporal lag in formation rate of several months behind resorption, whether the initial direction in resorption is up or down.

Circadian rhythms in bone biomarkers have been noted, with a peak in formation and resorption indices during the early morning hours and a nadir in late afternoon.[43,44] A nocturnal increase in bone resorption seen in the cross-linked N-telopeptide urine assay was most pronounced in young adults[45] and children (unpublished observations) in whom bone modeling was presumably still active, and less marked and not always evident on monitoring individual adult subjects.[45]

In summary, therefore, there is considerable promise that biochemical tests will find a place in the clinic in the diagnosis and therapeutic monitoring of patients with disorders of bone metabolism.

Conclusions

The prospects for applying specific biomarkers of bone metabolism in the clinical management of osteoporosis and other bone disorders are excellent. However, before any one marker gains acceptance, rigorous clinical evaluations are necessary to establish normal ranges and to confirm expected behavior in known clinical conditions of altered bone turnover. Longitudinal studies are necessary to establish the quantitative responsiveness of individual subjects and patients to antiresorptive and other therapeutic interventions. The great strides made in recent years in understanding basic bone biology and the growing focus of interest in osteoporosis ensure that biochemical tests for specifically probing bone turnover and cellular activity will continue to advance.

Acknowledgments

Research in the author's laboratory is supported in part by grants from the National Institutes of Health (AR37318 and AR36794) and Ostex International, Inc.

References

1. Price PA, Parthemore JG, Deftos LJ: New biochemical marker for bone metabolism: Measurement by radioimmunoassay of bone GLA protein in the plasma of normal subjects and patients with bone disease. *J Clin Invest* 1980;66:878–883.

2. Delmas PD: Biochemical markers of bone turnover for the clinical assessment of metabolic bone diseases. *Endocrinol Metab Clin North Am* 1990;19:1–18.

3. Parfitt AM, Simon LS, Villanueva AR, et al: Procollagen type I carboxy-terminal extension peptide in serum as a marker of collagen biosynthesis in bone: Correlation with iliac bone formation rates and comparison with total alkaline phosphatase. *J Bone Miner Res* 1987;2:427–436.

4. Kraenzlin ME, Mohan S, Singer F, et al: Development of a radioimmunoassay for the N-terminal type I procollagen: Potential use to assess bone formation. *Eur J Clin Invest* 1989;19:A86.

5. Delmas PD, Demiaux B, Malaval L, et al: Serum bone GLA-protein is not a sensitive marker of bone turnover in Paget's disease of bone. *Calcif Tissue Int* 1986;38:60–61.

6. Deftos LJ, Wolfert RL, Hill CS: Bone alkaline phosphatase in Paget's disease. *Horm Metab Res* 1991;23:559–561.

7. Parthemore JG, Burton DW, Deftos LJ: Associations and dissociations between serum bone GLA protein and alkaline phosphatase in skeletal metabolism. *J Orthop Res* 1993;11:671–676.

8. Thiede MA, Smock SL, Petersen DN, et al: Production of osteocalcin by platelets: A potentially important link of platelet action in bone turnover. *J Bone Miner Res* 1993;8(suppl 1):S147.

9. Hill CS, Wolfert RL: The preparation of monoclonal antibodies which react preferentially with human bone alkaline phosphatase and not liver alkaline phosphatase. *Clin Chim Acta* 1990;186:315–320.

10. Kress BC, Mizrahi I, Payne G: Skeletal alkaline phosphatase quantitation in serum using the immunoradiometric assay Tandem®-R Ostase™. *J Bone Miner Res* 1993;8(suppl 1):S257.

11. Dawson CD, Jewell S, Driskell WJ: Liquid-chromatographic determination of total hydroxyproline in urine. *Clin Chem* 1988;34:1572–1574.

12. Stepán JJ, Pospíchal J, Presl J, et al: Bone loss and biochemical indices of bone remodeling in surgically induced postmenopausal women. *Bone* 1987;8:279–284.

13. Gunja-Smith Z, Boucek RJ: Collagen cross-linking compounds in human urine. *Biochem J* 1981;197:759–762.

14. Robins SP, Stewart P, Astbury C, et al: Measurement of the cross-linking compound, pyridinoline, in urine as an index of collagen degradation in joint disease. *Ann Rheum Dis* 1986;45:969–973.

15. Black D, Marabani M, Sturrock RD, et al: Urinary excretion of the hydroxypyridinium cross-links of collagen in patients with rheumatoid arthritis. *Ann Rheum Dis* 1989;48:641–644.

16. Seibel MJ, Duncan A, Robins SP: Urinary hydroxypyridinium cross-links provide indices of cartilage and bone involvement in arthritic diseases. *J Rheumatol* 1989;16:964–970.

17. Uebelhart D, Gineyts E, Chapuy M, et al: Urinary excretion of pyridinium cross-links: A new marker of bone resorption in metabolic bone disease. *Bone Miner* 1990;8:87–96.

18. Beardsworth LJ, Eyre DR, Dickson IR: Changes with age in the urinary excretion of lysyl- and hydroxylysyl-pyridinoline: Two new markers of bone collagen turnover. *J Bone Miner Res* 1990;5:671–676.

19. Robins SP, Black D, Paterson CR, et al: Evaluation of urinary hydroxypyridinium crosslink measurements as resorption markers in metabolic bone diseases. *Eur J Clin Invest* 1991;21:310–315.

20. Seibel MJ, Robins SP, Bilezikian JP: Urinary pyridinium crosslinks of collagen: Specific markers of bone resorption in metabolic bone disease. *Trends Endocrinol Metab* 1992;3:263–270.

21. Body JJ, Delmas PD: Urinary pyridinium cross-links as markers of bone resorption in tumor-associated hypercalcemia. *J Clin Endocrinol Metab* 1992;74:471–475.

22. Thompson PW, Spector TD, James IT, et al: Urinary collagen cross-links reflect the radiographic severity of knee osteoarthritis. *Br J Rheumatol* 1992;31:759–761.

23. Eyre DR: Editorial: New biomarkers of bone resorption. *J Clin Endocrinol Metab* 1992;74:470A-470C.
24. Eyre DR: Collagen cross-linking amino acids, in Cunningham LW (ed): *Methods in Enzymology: Structural and Contractile Proteins*, Part D. Orlando, FL, Academic Press, 1987, vol 144, pp 115–139.
25. Eyre DR, Paz MA, Gallop PM: Crosslinking in collagen and elastin. *Annu Rev Biochem* 1984;53:717–748.
26. Eyre DR, Koob TJ, Van Ness KP: Quantitation of hydroxypyridinium crosslinks in collagen by high-performance liquid chromatography. *Anal Biochem* 1984;137: 380–388.
27. Hanson DA, Weis M-A E, Bollen A-M, et al: A specific immunoassay for monitoring human bone resorption: Quantitation of type I collagen cross-linked N-telopeptides in urine. *J Bone Miner Res* 1992;7:1251–1258.
28. Gertz BJ, Shao P, Hanson DA, et al: Monitoring bone resorption in early postmenopausal women by an immunoassay for cross-linked collagen peptides in urine. *J Bone Miner Res* 1994;9:135–142.
29. Risteli J, Elomaa I, Niemi S, et al: Radioimmunoassay for the pyridinoline cross-linked carboxy-terminal telopeptide of type I collagen: A new serum marker of bone collagen degradation. *Clin Chem* 1993;39:635–640.
30. Hassager C, Jensen LT, Pødenphant J, et al: The carboxy-terminal pyridinoline cross-linked telopeptide of type I collagen in serum as a marker of bone resorption: The effect of nandrolone decanoate and hormone replacement therapy. *Calcif Tissue Int* 1994;54:30–33.
31. Robins SP: An enzyme-linked immunoassay for the collagen cross-link pyridinoline. *Biochem J* 1982;207:617–620.
32. Seyedin SM, Kung VT, Daniloff YN, et al: Immunoassay for urinary pyridinoline: The new marker of bone resorption. *J Bone Miner Res* 1993;8:635–641.
33. Daniloff GY, Hesley RP, Ju J, et al: An immunoassay for deoxypyridinoline: A highly specific marker of bone resorption. *J Bone Miner Res* 1993;8(suppl 1):S357.
34. Rodriguez RR, Ries WL, Eyre DR, et al: Type I collagen cross-linked N-telopeptide excretion by osteopetrotic patients during interferon gamma therapy: A correlation with bone biochemical and densitometric markers. *J Bone Miner Res* 1993;8(suppl 1):S291.
35. Dickson IR, Arora MK, Coombes RC, et al: Pyridinolines and cross-linked type I collagen N-telopeptides as markers of bone metastases in breast cancer. *J Bone Miner Res* 1993;8(suppl 1):S288.
36. Blumsohn A, Al-Dehaimi AW, Herrington K, et al: Effect of timing of calcium supplementation on the circadian rhythm of bone collagen degradation. *J Bone Miner Res* 1993;8(suppl 1):S158.
37. Bell NH, Hollis BW, Shary J, et al: Diclofenac sodium is as effective as premarin in inhibiting bone resorption in postmenopausal women. *Am J Med*, in press.
38. Rosen HN, Dresner-Pollak R, Moses AC, et al: Specificity of urinary excretion of cross-linked N-telopeptides of type I collagen as a marker of bone turnover. *Calcif Tissue Int* 1994;54:26–29.
39. Ebeling PR, Atley LM, Eyre DR, et al: Sensitivity of type I collagen N-telopeptide cross-links in detecting early menopausal changes in bone turnover. *Proc ANZ Bone Miner Soc* 1993;A2.
40. Prior JC, Vigna YM, Schechter MT, et al: Spinal bone loss and ovulatory disturbances. *N Engl J Med* 1990;323:1221–1227.
41. Fledelius C, Eyre DR, Christiansen C: Urinary type I collagen cross-linked N-telopeptides: A new marker for bone resorption. Presented at the 4th International Symposium on Osteoporosis, Hong Kong, March 1993.
42. Harris ST, Gertz BJ, Genant HK, et al: The effect of short-term treatment with alendronate upon vertebral density and biochemical markers of bone remodeling in early menopausal women. *J Clin Endocrinol Metab* 1993;76:1399–1406.
43. Schlemmer A, Hassager C, Jensen SB, et al: Marked diurnal variation in urinary excretion of pyridinium cross-links in premenopausal women. *J Clin Endocrinol Metab* 1992;74:476–480.

44. Eastell R, Calvo MF, Burritt MP, et al: Abnormalities in circadian patterns of bone resorption and renal calcium conservation in type I osteoporosis. *J Clin Endocrinol Metab* 1992;74:487–494.
45. Blumsohn A, Al-Dehaimi AW, Herrington K, et al: Effect of timing of calcium supplementation on the circadian rhythm of bone collagen degradation. *J Bone Miner Res* 1993;8(suppl 1):S158.

Section 3

Future Research Directions

The explosion of information on bone cell biology has generated many questions concerning the functions of known regulatory factors and cell constituents in bone remodeling. We can ask a generic question for all of these activities: How are they controlled? We have listed below more detailed questions that the participants think are particularly important.

We recognize that the known factors and constituents probably represent only a small portion of those that will ultimately be found to be important in bone. For example, the factors responsible for the activation phase of bone remodeling have not been identified. Thus, some questions about bone remodeling may only be answered by identifying new cellular signals and pathways.

Finally, we need a better understanding of signal transduction by factors that influence bone metabolism. This knowledge will not only contribute to the understanding of bone physiology and pathology, but also enable the development of useful pharmacologic manipulation of bone remodeling.

In bone remodeling, what are the cellular and molecular events related to the initiation, arrest, and coupling of bone resorption and bone formation?

Control or mimicry of each event in the bone remodeling cycle would provide potential approaches to therapeutic intervention designed to restore bone mass. In the now well-established series of cellular events that constitute the process of bone remodeling (ie, activities that occur after the initial histogenesis of the tissue), (1) an area of the bone surface is recognized by osteoclasts and/or their precursors; (2) a discrete (limited) amount of preexisting matrix is resorbed by osteoclasts, following which this activity stops; (3) a reversed phase occurs in which mononuclear cells, possibly monophasic, are deposited; (4) osteoblasts and/or their precursors appear in the same area; and (5) limited amounts of new bone are formed, following which this activity stops.

Each of these steps must be initiated and stopped by specific molecular interactions between extracellular ligands (eg, soluble hormones or cytokines, or insoluble matrix proteins and/or soluble molecules absorbed on matrix proteins) and molecules at the surface of bone cells (ie, receptors). Molecules that would either mimic or compete with the ligands and/or the receptors for any of these interactions would allow shifting of the remodeling balance.

Approaches to the evaluation of the events of bone remodeling may include attention to a variety of working hypotheses. These hypotheses may be tested by the in vitro reconstitution of each of these events or as many as possible, one at a time, with isolated osteoblasts, isolated osteoclasts, bone substrate (slices) and enzymes, cytokines, and other molecules presumed important to remodeling activities.

307

Initiation of bone resorption could be investigated in the following ways: (1) physical exposure of the bone surface after trauma or microtrauma and retraction of the bone lining cells under hormonal, local, or mechanical influences; (2) binding of osteoclasts and/or their precursors to the matrix via integrin receptors and arginine-glycine-aspartic acid (RGD) containing matrix molecules; and (3) signal from osteocytes or lining cells to activate and/or recruit osteoclasts. Arrest of bone resorption could be investigated by determining (1) the inherent life span of the active osteoclast, (2) the role of the calcium receptor when high calcium occurs under osteoclasts, and (3) mechanical loads on trabecula thinned by resorption.

Coupling (ie, initiation) of bone formation should be elucidated by determining the following: (1) specific factors secreted by the osteoclast; (2) the role of the cement line, secretory products of the osteoclast (enzymes, osteopontin, BP II, etc) that may be the signal for osteoblast precursors; (3) the role of mononuclear cells in the reversal phase; and (4) the role of factors, such as growth factors and proteolytic fragments, released by the osteoclast from the bone matrix. Arrest of bone formation should be elucidated by determining the inherent life span of the active osteoblast and quantitating the mechanical load on the restored trabecula.

What are the receptors and signal transduction mechanisms (downstream elements) that activate and modulate osteoblast and osteoclast activity?

Signals that activate or regulate osteoblasts and osteoclasts require the presence of specific receptors. These receptors function to discriminate effectively what these cells see from the extracellular world. Once these receptors bind their ligand (eg, cytokines), a signal is transmitted to the interior of the cell that results in specific gene transcription and subsequent cellular activation. However, few of these receptors have been identified on either osteoblasts or osteoclasts. Even less is known about the specific intracellular proteins that constitute the downstream elements of the signal transduction pathways that follow ligand binding. Understanding these receptors and signal transduction pathways is seminal to understanding cell function and, therefore, to understanding bone remodeling. This information can also provide clues for developing therapeutic agents that can modify these pathways.

A variety of signals are known to activate osteoblasts and osteoclasts, including cytokines, growth factors, prostaglandins, hormones, and mechanical forces. Specific receptors for these signals can be identified using a number of approaches including measuring responses to specific ligands and analogs, binding of radiolabeled ligands, immunoprecipitation with antireceptor antibodies, and expression cloning.

Multiple signal transduction pathways are known to be involved in cell activation. These include phosphorylation of proteins on tyrosine or serine/threonine, stimulation of cyclic AMP, changes in Ca^{++} fluxes, activation of inositol phosphate, activation of protein kinase C, changes in intracellular pH, and formation of cyclic nucleotides. Standard methods exist to determine which of these pathways are involved for the different ligands.

What is the nature of interaction between osteoclastic precursors and stromal cells? Which type of stromal cell is involved?

Recent data indicate that a stromal cell population can induce formation of osteoclasts and that there is intimate association between osteoclastic precursors and stromal cells. The factors involved in this induction have not been definitively characterized, and this information is needed to be able to manipulate osteoclastogenesis, both in vivo and in vitro, in health and in disease. Given the heterogeneous nature of marrow stromal cells, identification of the particular population(s) that participate in this process will enable a search for the involved cell-signaling factors.

Further development of in vitro culture systems using either mixed populations of marrow stromal stem cells or cloned cells can be used to study osteoclast formation. Use of blocking antibodies against known factors in the cocultures with or without direct cell contact will help delineate which specific, known molecules are involved. If the factor(s) appear to be novel, conditioned medium from the stromal population can be used for purification by standard chromatographic procedures. In vivo, animal models or human diseased tissue in which a defect in osteoclastogenesis is present could be examined for any apparent disorganization in the marrow stroma. Stromal populations from gene knockout animals that exhibit abnormalities in bone resorption marrow could be examined for their ability to mediate osteoclast formation.

Are there hormonally-induced cytokines (activation factors) that directly stimulate mature osteoclasts?

Available evidence suggests that most systemic and locally acting hormones that stimulate bone resorption do not directly influence osteoclast activity. By contrast, osteoblasts and osteoblast-like cells express receptors for most of these hormones. Thus, many hormones presumably mediate osteoclast activity by inducing release of osteoblast-derived cytokines that in turn influence osteoclast activity or formation.

Although there are several osteoblast-derived factors that potentially increase osteoclast recruitment, little is known about molecules that can increase osteoclast activity. Indeed, whether osteoclast activity can be enhanced is controversial, because some evidence exists that osteoclasts are always fully activated. Nevertheless, in vivo evidence suggests that the rapid response of mature osteoclasts to such hormones as parathyroid hormone (PTH) reflects the presence of activating factors.

To identify hormonal factors that stimulate mature osteoclasts, candidate molecules must be defined and a detection system for osteoclast activation must be available. Continuous and primary osteoblast-like cells and stromal cell lines should be examined as a source for this activity. Decisions regarding the most appropriate detection systems for this activity are problematic. "Isolated" osteoclast culture systems are obviously contaminated by other cell types, and organ cultures, by their nature, contain a complex mixture of many cell types. Therefore, although initial screening can be accomplished in either of these systems, ultimately acute real-time effects must be demonstrated in living osteoclasts. Candidate molecules must be able to induce rapid changes in such osteoclast activities as mobility, shape change, cellular pH, and signaling molecules. Direct binding of such candidate molecules by osteoclasts will be critical evidence of their role as an activating molecule.

How are multiple growth factor signals coordinated by bone cells during bone remodeling?

Many growth factors are present in bone matrix and available to bone-forming and bone-resorbing cells during bone remodeling. In vitro, cells from both osteoblast and osteoclast lineages have receptors for and respond to some or all of these growth factors. However, the relevant importance of a specific growth factor or combination of growth factors in the regulation of specific steps in bone remodeling is difficult to assess in the context of the cellular microenvironment.

The use of transgenic animal models in which overexpression or loss of expression of individual growth factors has been accomplished may be an important tool in assigning specific roles for factors, individually or collectively, in bone remodeling. In addition, use of reverse transcriptase-polymerase chain reaction (RT-PCR), in situ hybridization, and other emerging techniques will provide access to and better control of the in vivo cellular microenvironment.

What are the factors that regulate activation, migration, proliferation, and differentiation of the osteogenic precursors that bring about bone formation following bone resorption?

Independent of where the osteoprogenitor cell resides, it is in a "quiescent" state, ie, not proliferating. Following bone resorption, that cell must become activated to leave its local environment and migrate into the area excavated by the osteoclast. Once it is located in the appropriate environment, the osteoprogenitor proliferates and passes through a maturation pathway that is similar, but not necessarily identical, to what has been described during development. However, the factors that regulate osteoprogenitor cell activation have not been determined, and the complex pathway of proliferation and maturation of the bone forming cell during the remodeling cycle is not well defined. Moreover, the sources of activation factors have not been identified. These agents could be released from bone matrix or secreted by osteoclasts or by the mononuclear cells (macrophages) seen near bone surfaces during the reversal phase.

Because the activation and migration of marrow stromal stem cells could be brought about by the products released from bone matrix during resorption, studies using partially degraded bone matrix, conditioned medium from resorbing organ cultures, or purified bone matrix proteins (or their fragments) would be most useful. Assessment of the potential factors involved in proliferation and differentiation could be carried out in in vitro studies using single factors or combinations of factors or in vivo models using transgenic animals (with either deletions or overexpression of specific factors).

What determines the pathways of differentiation of marrow stromal stem cells, and what are the markers that distinguish them from each other?

By analogy to the hematopoietic lineage, it is apparent that marrow stroma contains mesenchymal stem cells. This population is pluripotent and can give rise to a number of cell types including bone, cartilage, fat, and muscle. Currently, there are a limited number of markers that can distinguish one cell type from another, and their interrelationships are not well established. The ability to sort these stem cells would provide a unique opportunity to obtain an appropriate stem cell population to effect tissue repair.

In order to identify lineages of marrow stromal stem cells, identification of distinguishing markers through further development of monoclonal antibodies is needed. New molecular techniques such as subtraction libraries and differential displays could be applied to these cells to further characterize their similarities and differences. Incorporation of a marker into a stem cell during development and following the fate of its progeny could provide information on lineages and cellular interactions.

What factors initiate and direct the oriented deposition and determine the architecture of new bone matrix formed by osteoblasts?

Bone turnover involves the resorption of preexisting matrix characterized by spatially-oriented collagen and noncollagenous proteins as well as other molecules. This morphology provides site-specific structural and metabolic advantages. As new bone is laid down, these structural considerations must again be addressed. Combinations of physical and chemical signals must play a role in initiating, modulating, organizing, and terminating the deposition of matrix that reflects the special needs of this bone environment. This poorly understood control system requires better definition. Such knowledge may improve our understanding of how matrix is formed in pathologic states, including high turnover disease (Paget's disease), bone formed by sarcomatous stroma, and bone formed in response to injury. This information may suggest treatment strategies not only for those disorders but for other disorders of bone formation including "low turnover" osteoporosis.

What are the signaling pathways for PTH and prostaglandin[2] (PGE[2]) that are responsible for their peculiar ability to stimulate both formation and resorption in different experimental settings?

PTH and PGE_2 are both potent stimulators of bone resorption in a variety of experimental systems. Paradoxically, both agents are capable of stimulating bone formation in vivo and in vitro, although they also can inhibit bone collagen synthesis by direct transcriptional mechanisms. Understanding the signaling differences that underly these varied effects will lead to an improved ability to understand normal bone remodeling as well as enhance the potential therapeutic value of these molecules, or related pharmacologic agents.

PTH is largely catabolic in vitro when administered continuously, but intermittent treatment allows the hormone's anabolic properties to be expressed. PTH, when given intermittently, causes enhanced bone formation in both experimental animals and patients with osteopenia. Similarly, when injected systemically, PGE_2 causes a marked increase in bone turnover with formation greatly favored. Furthermore, the increase in bone formation noted in response to certain mechanical stimuli appears to be PGE_2 dependent. In vitro, PGE_2 is anabolic when coadministered with glucocorticoids.

Three levels of investigation may prove fruitful in studying the mechanisms of action of these molecules. The first level relates to the route and frequency of delivery. Thus, intermittent administration of PTH may more closely mimic the pulsatile nature of PTH's secretory pattern in vivo. Clinical trials are needed to investigate the optimum dosing intervals. The next level of investigation will be to determine which cytokines and growth factors are produced or released locally in bone in response to PTH and PGE_2 treatment. Differences in the pattern of secreted cytokines may provide clues as to how anabolic and catabolic effects are mediated. These studies can be carried out in vivo and in cell and organ culture. Finally, studies directed at understanding signal transduction will be central to understanding the effects of PTH and PGE_2 in bone. The recent cloning of the PTH receptor and several prostaglandin receptors should greatly advance these studies.

What is the role of the osteocyte in bone remodeling?

The network of osteocytes with their cell processes connected both to each other and to surface osteoblasts and lining cells provides a system for sensing small perturbations (strains) in skeletal structure and initiating remodeling. Osteocytes have been shown to have the capacity to synthesize specific bone proteins such as osteocalcin and regulatory molecules including prostaglandins. Surface markers that are relatively specific for osteocytes have been identified. Osteocyte isolation and culture systems have been developed.

These tools will assist in demonstrating the function of osteocytes in cell culture and in vivo; receptors, cell constituents, and secretory products of osteocytes need to be identified. Osteocyte-osteoblast model systems also should be examined for their intercellular signaling pathways.

Evaluate the influence on bone biology and bone function of various drugs and physical modalities used in the treatment of primarily nonskeletal diseases and disorders in order to: (1) understand, quantitate, and address clinically relevant changes in the structure and function of bone so treated; (2) serve as models for understanding mechanisms of bone remodeling and repair; and (3) develop potential treatment strategies for disorders of skeletal metabolism.

A wide variety of systemically administered drugs and physical modalities have already been shown to alter skeletal homeostasis as an indirect consequence of intended therapeutic applications. These include chemotherapeutic drugs (methotrexate, doxorubicin), nonsteroidal anti-inflammatory drugs (indomethacin), and immunosuppressant agents (cyclosporin-A), as well as irradiation and exposure to electromagnetic fields or direct current. The magnitude of these changes needs to be explored, including effects on histologic, histomorphometric, and biomechanical parameters of bone physiology and structure. Reversal or minimization of these untoward responses should be sought through changes in dosage and timing of these therapies.

Futhermore, the biochemical mechanisms by which these modalities alter the cellular and molecular biology of bone remodeling should be clarified. This will assist in a better understanding of normal physiologic events and, potentially, identify drugs or approaches that can be used to manipulate abnormally remodeled bone back toward normalcy. Animal models have been useful in preliminary approaches to these problems.

What are the important age-related changes in bone cell formation and regulation, and how do these influence remodeling?

Results of experiments on changes in function of bone cells with age are inconsistent. This apparent validity problem reflects differences in the models used for evaluation. Nevertheless, age-related changes in the numbers of progenitor cells, the production of systemic and local regulators, and the responsiveness of cells to these factors have been reported.

Systemic analysis of age-related changes in bone cells will require selection of suitable models and development of parallel methods for studying cell function in vivo and in vitro. Methods for quantitating local regulatory factors in vivo, which can be applied to tissues from older animals and humans, need to be developed.

What are the differences in bone remodeling at cortical and cancellous sites and between lamellar and woven bone? How do these differences affect bone quality?

Although a number of suggestions have been put forward, the physiologic functions of bone remodeling are not fully understood. The structure of remodeling units is quite different in cortical and cancellous bone. It is not clear how or when woven bone undergoes remodeling. There are probably site-specific differences as well, for example, between alveolar bone and the axial and appendicular skeleton. An understanding of these differences should provide clues to the nature and influence of bone remodeling on the structural integrity of skeletal tissues and their response to mechanical forces.

Systems for altering remodeling in vivo need to be developed which can be analyzed at the level of microarchitecture, not only by histomorphometric techniques, but also by mechanical testing at a microscopic level. The changes in local regulatory factors during remodeling are likely to be different in cancellous and cortical bone, and these changes need to be evaluated as well.

Can biochemical markers of formation and resorption be identified and validated that specifically quantify bone remodeling in patients and experimental systems?

More specific biomarkers of bone metabolism are needed for both clinical studies and experimental investigations in vivo and in vitro. The more traditional assays (eg, urinary hydroxyproline for resorption and total serum alkaline phosphatase activity for formation) lack the specificity to provide definitive information on bone turnover rates. The goal is to develop accurate, specific, and convenient assays (eg, immunoassays) that can be applied directly to body fluids or tissue culture media. Potentially useful assays that fulfill these criteria and selectively measure either resorption or formation are currently under study. The development and verification of such assays will provide the basis for investigating (1) normal and pathologic states of bone remodeling in clinical studies, (2) the effect of pharmacologic agents on bone remodeling, and (3) bone metabolism in vitro.

As more advanced assays for bone biomarkers are identified, they will need rigorous verification in carefully designed prospective clinical studies. One major difficulty in validation is the lack of "gold standards" for formation and resorption against which new markers can be tested. Therefore, the degree of sensitivity and selectivity in clinical and experimental situations in which bone formation or resorption is known to be selectively blocked or stimulated will remain the best evidence of validity of the underlying biochemical principle and of the potential clinical utility of the marker molecule.

What are the mechanisms of bone remodeling in pathologic conditions? Can these mechanisms be used to elucidate mechanisms of physiologic remodeling?

Past studies of bone remodeling in pathologic conditions have shed light on the factors and mechanisms that modulate bone remodeling (ie, studies of multiple myeloma leading to the identification of an osteoclast activating factor). The recent discovery that synthesis of a metalloprotein is stimulated by tumor cells demonstrates a novel mechanism of tumor-stimulated matrix resorption. These observations could be relevant to modulation of resorption by cell-cell interactions during normal remodeling. Extensive and rapid bone loss in infection without the presence of osteoclasts suggests the existence of additional mechanisms for matrix demineralization and resorption. Thus, pathologic conditions in which bone is resorbed or remodeled should be studied for the additional information that these conditions can provide on remodeling factors and mechanisms.

Elucidation of mechanisms and identification of factors in pathologic conditions will require the development of model systems that appropriately parallel these conditions in humans. Suitable animal and in vitro models can be adapted from current models of tumor metastasis to bone, infection, and prosthetic implant loosening.

Section 4

Biosynthetic Bone Grafting

Section Editors:
Carl T. Brighton, MD, PhD
A. Hari Reddi, PhD

Arnold I. Caplan, PhD
Dwight T. Davy, PhD
Victor M. Goldberg, MD
Jeffrey O. Hollinger, DDS, PhD
Ralph E. Holmes, MD
Sudha Kadiyala
Joseph M. Lane, MD

Cato T. Laurencin, MD, PhD
Kam W. Leong, PhD
Hungnan Lo
Meir Liebergall, MD
Naoto Ozawa, MD
James H. Reese, PhD
Randell G. Young, DVM

Chapter 22

Biodegradable Polymers as Synthetic Bone Grafts

Sudha Kadiyala
Hungnan Lo
Kam W. Leong, PhD

Introduction

Reconstruction of defective tissues by means of a graft material is a widely used procedure. The bone graft material that provides the best results is an autograft, most often obtained from the iliac crest. However, the supply of autografts is limited and the harvesting procedure can lead to postoperative complications. Allografts can also be used in some cases, but the problems of donor matching and tissue storage, coupled with the potential complications associated with blood-borne products, make the use of synthetic graft materials attractive.

Hydroxyapatite (HA) ceramics, which mimic the inorganic phase of bone, are an obvious choice and have been studied extensively.[1–13] In a study by Yamasaki and Sakai,[13] porous HA implanted under the skin of dogs was seen to elicit an osteogenic response at 3 months; dense HA, however, did not evoke such response. The osteoinductivity of the porous HA was attributed to the morphology of the implant in addition to the possibility of leaching of calcium phosphate from the ceramic. Even though the results are encouraging, several issues must be resolved before the use of HA becomes practical: a time course of 3 months for the nucleation of bone is too long; the high stiffness and low degradation rates of HA in the body are also undesirable.

A wide range of properties make biodegradable polymeric materials an attractive candidate for synthetic bone grafts. The polymeric materials can be used as osteoconductive material to encourage bone healing. The shape and morphology of the implants can be varied to achieve optimal bone growth, as is the case with the use of biodegradable foams, which provide pores in the range of several hundred micrometers for tissue ingrowth. Alternatively, the polymeric implant can be loaded with bone inductive factors, such as bone morphogenetic protein (BMP), for sustained release, to encourage bone growth. Another approach is to seed the implant with cells capable of providing differentiated function for bone healing.

Polymer Choice

Although there are a multitude of polymers available for use as osteosynthetic material, most of the studies and use have been limited to the α-hydroxy acid polymers, poly(lactic acid) (PLA) and poly(glycolic acid) (PGA), or a combination of the two (PLGA). These polymers were developed for use as sutures and have been used extensively in that role. The advantage of this polymeric system is that the breakdown products of the polymer are molecules that occur naturally in the body. Various studies have established the osteoconductive nature of these polymers.[13-30] They, however, are not osteoinductive and do not possess any unique advantage over other biodegradable polymeric systems when applied to the field of orthopaedics.

Because these polymers have been characterized extensively, they are the first biodegradable polymers to be widely used in clinical orthopaedics, especially in Europe. Several thousand clinical cases involving small-fragment fractures or osteotomies have been treated with these biodegradable polymers.[15-17] Efforts are continuously being made to improve their mechanical characteristics by fiber and particulate reinforcement.[11,26,31] In a large clinical study of PLA pins conducted by Bostman and associates,[15] about 8% of the patients developed an inflammatory response to the implant and had to be treated for related complications. The onset of the inflammation coincided with the degradation of the polymer. The inflammation is attributed to the autocatalytic breakdown of PLA, which results in a release of a copious amount of degradation products and the lowering of pH around the implant. It was recently reported that deep inguinal nodes of goats exhibited active sinus histiocytosis 2 years after implantation with PLA samples as femoral cortical plugs.[29]

All the other polymers are in the experimental stage. Polyanhydrides were initially designed to degrade heterogeneously and for drug delivery applications.[32] The anhydride bond is highly unstable hydrolytically. With a hydrophobic backbone to resist water penetration, polyanhydrides decompose from the surface. The biocompatibility of the copolymers of bis(p-carboxyphenoxy) propane and sebacid acid has been proven clinically in Phase III trials for use as a drug-carrier for chemotherapy of brain tumors. Having passed the formidable biocompatibility hurdle, polyanhydrides hold an advantage over other experimental biodegradable polymers in product development.

Poly(orthoesters) prepared from the condensation of 3,9-bis(ethylene 2,4,8,10-tetraoxaspiro[5,5] undecane) with either trans-1,4-cyclohexanedimethanol or 1,6-hexanediol have been studied for orthopaedic applications. Their mechanical properties are not as strong as that of high molecular weight PLA, but are comparable to those of PLAs with a molecular weight around 50,000. Reinforced with Ca-Na-metaphosphate fibers, they possess flexural strength approaching that of cortical bone.[33] Alzamer, the trade name for a poly(orthoester) with a different chemical structure, has also been used for the regeneration of calvarial defects in rats. The results show that the poly(orthoester) alone did not induce bony ingrowth, whereas the composite of the polymer and demineralized bone bridged the defect by bone.

In designing biomaterials for orthopaedic applications, we look for characteristics of versatility and osteoconductivity. We have developed a class of polymers that contain a phosphate group in the backbone of the polymer (Fig. 1).[34-37] In addition to making the polymer degradable, the phosphate group complexes with the calcium phosphate found in the bone tissue, thereby achieving a better interaction between the graft and the host bone. Also, be-

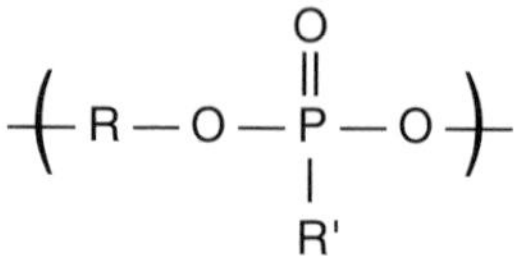

Fig. 1 Structure of poly(phosphoesters).

cause the phosphorus atom is pentavalent, a site is available for attachment of growth factors or drugs. The biocompatibility of the poly(phosphoesters) has been established in a variety of sites. In studies involving implantation of the poly(phosphoesters) in osseous sites, there was intimate contact between the polymer and the bone, without any interlacing fibrous tissue capsule.[35]

Growth Factor Delivery

Bone growth factors in various forms of purity, ranging from recombinant proteins to demineralized bone matrix, have been incorporated into polymer matrices for enhancement of bone growth. Hollinger and associates[20] successfully bridged a critical-size defect in the cranium of nonhuman primates using PLA to deliver bone morphogenetic protein (BMP) to the bone defect. Swoboda and associates[38] were able to elicit ectopic bone growth in rats by incorporating partially purified BMPs adsorbed onto PLA discs. Miyamoto and associates[39] also studied the efficacy of PLA polymers as a delivery vehicle for BMPs and found that among a range of molecular weights, only the 650 d polymer was able to induce ectopic bone growth. Lucas and associates[40] used a poly(anhydride) carrier to deliver water-soluble proteins extracted from bovine bone to a nonmuscular site in mice, and ectopic bone growth was observed in 50% of the cases.

The diverse responses observed by the different researchers are, in part, due to the different sites of implantation and different activities of the growth factor used. In many cases, the unknown nature of the growth factor also contributes to the unpredictability of the response. In almost all of the studies so far, the proteins have either been adsorbed onto the polymeric carrier or compression molded with the polymer. For the case of adsorption, unless the polymeric carrier is highly charged and can form an ionic complex with the protein, no sustained release can be expected. Even when the protein is physically dispersed in the polymeric matrix, the protein is almost completely released within the first week postimplantation.[41] This is expected because of the high driving force for the diffusional release of such hydrophilic compounds. This may be the reason that most of the studies carried out to date required a growth-factor concentration an order of magnitude higher than the physiologic levels. Polymers with lower degradation rates might retard protein release, but once the matrix is swollen or becomes porous as a result of degradation, diffusion becomes the dominant mode of release. Although studies have shown that bone growth activated by growth factors starts as early as 3 days postimplantation, vascularization of grafts, especially the larger ones, takes longer than a week. The sustained presence of the growth factor would lead to multinucleation of bone growth and earlier incorporation of the graft into the host tissue. To realize the potential of such growth factors, the protein might need to be covalently coupled to the polymeric carrier for a more sustained delivery.

Polymeric Foams

The use of polymeric foams as osteosynthetic materials is based on observations that devices with pore sizes in the range of 100 to 400 μm encourage bone growth. In addition, the foams can be used as carriers for cells, such as osteoblasts, that participate in the bone growth and healing process. Attempts to use foams as osteosynthetic graft materials have met with mixed success. Although researchers have been able to exhibit bone (or cartilage) growth in a variety of sites, the nature and time course of tissue formation are not optimal.[42-46] The results have shown that it is important to be able to control the pore size and distribution of the implant while ensuring that the structural rigidity is maintained in the early stages after implantation. There are a variety of foam fabrication techniques that produce foams with vastly different properties.

Mikos and associates[42] fabricated foams by solvent casting a mixture of poly(lactide-co-glycolide) (PLGA)-NaCl and followed by leaching the salt. The maximum level of porosity is limited because of the difficulty of suspending salt particulates in the solution as well as preventing the polymer from nucleating during the evaporation of the solvent. Furthermore, the crystalline structure of the sodium chloride salts gives sharp edges to the pores of the resulting foam. Some of the problems of this system can be overcome by laminating the porous thin films to form a three-dimensional structure. Nevertheless, complex implant shapes cannot be fabricated easily by compacting those films, and the process is time consuming.

Cima and associates[43] used a tassel of braided PLGA fibers 14 μm in diameter to fabricate a porous device. It may be difficult to control the pore size and pore size distribution in this process. Along the same line, Ito and associates[44] fabricated a scaffold for cell growth by overlapping and sewing two sheets of PLA and PGA nonwoven fabrics. The structural stability of the foam fabricated in this manner is limited. Another process that uses nonwoven PGA fibers was developed by Vacanti and associates.[45] They immersed the PGA mesh in a nonsolvent (methylene chloride) containing PLA or PLGA, to coat the fibers for improved structural stability. Mikos and associates[46] significantly improved the structural rigidity of the foam by using a fiber bonding technique. Briefly, a solution of a second polymer was poured into a mold containing the fiber mesh, and the solvent was allowed to evaporate, resulting in a polymeric composite. The second polymer was chosen to be nonmiscible with the polymer of interest in the melt state and to have a higher melting point. The composite was subjected to temperatures above the melting temperature of the mesh polymer, resulting in fiber bonding. The second polymer was subsequently dissolved, yielding a foam with a "bonded fiber structure." Porosity and pore distribution in this case are limited by that of the fiber mesh used in the fabrication.

None of the procedures described above are suitable for loading drugs or nutrients into the foams, because of either the high temperatures of fabrication or the need to leach out the porogens (materials added to induce pore formation). This limits the appeal of these porous scaffolds, because controlled drug delivery is a highly desirable feature.

We[47] have developed a fabrication technique that can yield foams with well-controlled porosity, pore-size distribution, and morphology, as shown in Figure 2. We have successfully cultured cells on these foams and are in the process of characterizing the functional activity of various cell types on foams fabricated by this process. Also, implants with complex shapes can be fabricated easily. A unique advantage of the foams fabricated by this procedure is that drugs or nutrients for sustained release can be incorporated into the foam during the fabrication procedure. Fluorescein isothiocyanate (FITC), a fluorescent dye, was used to demonstrate this principle. Distribution of dye in the polymer matrix was evaluated by confocal microscopy; incorporation of FITC inside the polymeric foam can be seen in Figure 3, *left*. To demonstrate the sustained release of incorporated nutrients or drugs, bromthymol blue was chosen as a model compound. Sustained release was observed in all cases (Fig. 3, *right*). The 10% loading foam leached out the marker at a faster rate than the 1% loading foam. There is, however, little difference between the release rates of the two foams with 95% and 99% porosity, indicating there is no mass transfer

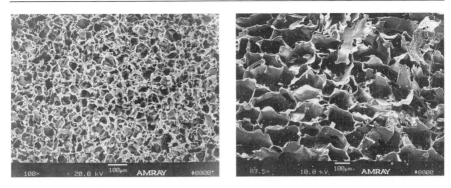

Fig. 2 Scanning electron micrographs of poly(L-lactic acid) foams with different porosities.

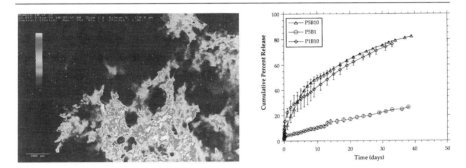

Fig. 3 Left, Confocal micrograph of a fluorescein isothiocyanate (FITC) containing poly(L-lactic acid) (PLLA) foam showing intimate dispersion of FITC inside the polymer matrix. **Right,** In vitro release curves of bromthymol blue from PLLA foams in 0.1M phosphate buffer (pH 7.4) at 37°C: 10 weight percent loading in 95% porous PLLA (P5B10); 1 weight percent loading in 95% porous PLLA (P5B1); and 10 weight percent loading in 99% porous PLLA (P1B10).

resistance to the interior of the foam. In loading alkaline phosphatase into these foams, about 30% of the enzymatic activity was lost during the process. This demonstrated the suitability of this fabrication technique in loading proteins or growth factors into the foam.

References

1. Damien CJ, Parsons JR, Benedict JJ, et al: Investigation of a hydroxyapatite and calcium sulfate composite supplemented with an osteoinductive factor. *J Biomed Mater Res* 1990;24:639–654.
2. Goshima J, Goldberg VM, Caplan AI: The origin of bone formed in composite grafts of porous calcium phosphate ceramic loaded with marrow cells. *Clin Orthop* 1991;269:274–283.
3. Gregoire M, Orly I, Menanteau J: The influence of calcium phosphate biomaterials on human bone cell activities: An in vitro approach. *J Biomed Mater Res* 1990;24:165–177.
4. Klein CP, Driessen AA, de Groot K, et al: Biodegradation behavior of various calcium phosphate materials in bone tissue. *J Biomed Mater Res* 1993;17:769–784.
5. Nelson JF, Stanford HG, Cutright DE: Evaluation and comparisons of biodegradable substances as osteogenic agents. *Oral Surg* 1977;43:836–843.

6. Ohgushi H, Okumura M, Yoshikawa T, et al: Bone formation process in porous calcium carbonate and hydroxyapatite. *J Biomed Mater Res* 1992;26:885–895.

7. Okazaki M: Fluoridated hydroxyapatites synthesized with organic phosphate ester. *Biomaterials* 1991;12:46–49.

8. Puleo DA, Holleran LA, Doremus RH, et al: Osteoblast responses to orthopedic implant materials in vitro. *J Biomed Mater Res* 1991;25:711–723.

9. Spivak JM, Ricci JL, Blumenthal NC, et al: A new canine model to evaluate the biological response of intramedullary bone to implant materials and surfaces. *J Biomed Mater Res* 1990;24:1121–1149.

10. Tencer AF, Woodard PL, Swenson J, et al: Bone ingrowth into polymer coated porous synthetic coralline hydroxyapatite. *J Orthop Res* 1987;5:275–282.

11. Verheyen CCPM, de Wijn JR, van Blitterswijk CA, et al: Hydroxylapatite/poly-(L-lactide) composites: An animal study on push-out strengths and interface histology. *J Biomed Mater Res* 1993;27:433–444.

12. Gomi K, Lowenberg B, Shapiro G, et al: Resorption of sintered synthetic hydroxyapatite by osteoclasts in vitro. *Biomaterials* 1993;14:91–96.

13. Yamasaki H, Sakai H: Osteogenic response to porous hydroxyapatite ceramics under the skin of dogs. *Biomaterials* 1992;13:308–312.

14. Bos RRM, Rozema FR, Boering G, et al: Degradation of and tissue reaction to biodegradable poly(L-lactide) for use as internal fixation of fractures: A study in rats. *Biomaterials* 1991;12:32–36.

15. Bostman O, Hirvensalo E, Makinen J, et al: Foreign-body reactions to fracture fixation implants of biodegradable synthetic polymers. *J Bone Joint Surg* 1990; 72B:592–596.

16. Bostman O, Makela EA, Tormala P, et al: Transphyseal fracture fixation using biodegradable pins. *J Bone Joint Surg* 1989;71B:706–707.

17. Bostman O, Vainionpaa S, Hirvensalo E, et al: Biodegradable internal fixation for malleolar fractures: A prospective randomised trial. *J Bone Joint Surg* 1987;69B: 615–619.

18. Casper RA, Dunn RL, Cowsar DR: Biodegradable fracture fixation plates for use in maxillofacial surgery, in Fraker AC, Griffin CD (eds): *Corrosion and Degradation of Implant Materials: Second Symposium, ASTM STP 859.* Philadelphia, PA, American Society for Testing and Materials, 1985, pp 340–348.

19. Eitenmueller J, Muhr G, Gerlach KL, et al: New semirigid and absorbable osteosynthesis devices with a high molecular weight polylactide (an experimental investigation). *J Bioactive Compat Polym* 1989;4:215–241.

20. Hollinger JO, Schmitz JP, Mark DE, et al: Osseous wound healing with xenogeneic bone implants with a biodegradable carrier. *Surgery* 1990;107:50–54.

21. Kumta SM, Spinner R, Leung PC: Absorbable intramedullary implants for hand fractures: Animal experiments and clinical trial. *J Bone Joint Surg* 1992;74B:563–566.

22. Majola A, Vainionpaa S, Vihtonen K, et al: Absorption, biocompatibility, and fixation properties of polylactic acid in bone tissue: An experimental study in rats. *Clin Orthop* 1991;268:260–269.

23. Makela EA, Vainionpaa S, Vihtonen K, et al: The effect of a penetrating biodegradable implant on the epiphyseal plate: An experimental study on growing rabbits with special regard to Polyglactin 910. *J Pediatr Orthop* 1987;7:415–420.

24. Schmitz JP, Hollinger JO: A preliminary study of the osteogenic potential of a biodegradable alloplastic-osteoinductive alloimplant. *Clin Orthop* 1988;237:245–255.

25. Wei G, Kotoura Y, Oka M, et al: A bioabsorbable delivery system for antibiotic treatment of osteomyelitis: The use of lactic acid oligomer as a carrier. *J Bone Joint Surg* 1991;73B:246–252.

26. Zimmerman M, Parsons JR, Alexander H: The design and analysis of a laminated partially degradable composite bone plate for fracture fixation. *J Biomed Mater Res* 1987;21:345–361.

27. Santavirta S, Konttinen YT, Saito T, et al: Immune response to polyglycolic acid implants. *J Bone Joint Surg* 1990;72B:597–600.

28. Winet H, Hollinger JO: Incorporation of polylactide-polyglycolide in a cortical defect: Neoosteogenesis in a bone chamber. *J Biomed Mater Res* 1993;27:667–676.

29. Verheyen CCPM, de Wijn JR, van Blitterswijk CA, et al: Examination of efferent lymph nodes after 2 years of transcortical implantation of poly(L-lactide) containing plugs: A case report. *J Biomed Mater Res* 1993;27:1115–1118.

30. Kinoshita Y, Kirigakubo M, Kobayashi M, et al: Study on the efficacy of biodegradable poly(L-lactide) mesh for supporting transplanted particulate cancellous bone and marrow: Experiment involving subcutaneous implantation in dogs. *Biomaterials* 1993;14:729–736.

31. Verheyen CCPM, de Wijn JR, van Blitterswijk CA, et al: Evaluation of hydroxylapatite/poly(L-lactide) composites: Mechanical behavior. *J Biomed Mater Res* 1992;26:1277–1296.

32. Leong KW, Domb A, Ron E, et al: Polyanhydrides, in Kroschwitz, JI (ed): *Encyclopedia of Polymer Science and Engineering*, New York, NY, Wiley, 1989, pp 648–665.

33. Andriano KP, Daniels AU, Heller J: Biocompatibility and mechanical properties of a totally absorbable composite material for orthopedic fixation devices. *J Appl Biom* 1992;3:197–206.

34. Richards M, Dahiyat BI, Arm DM, et al: Evaluation of polyphosphates and polyphosphonates as degradable biomaterials. *J Biomed Mater Res* 1991;25:1151–1167.

35. Kadiyala S, Richards M, Dahiyat B, et al: Poly(phosphoesters) as bioabsorbable osteosynthetic materials, in Cima LG, Ron ES (eds): *Tissue-Inducing Biomaterials*. Pittsburgh, PA, Materials Research Society, 1992, pp 311–320. Materials Research Society Symposium Proceedings, 252.

36. Lo H, Kadiyala S, Leong KW: Syntheses and evaluation of poly(phosphoro-amidates) and poly(phosphoesters) as biodegradable materials, in *Extended Abstracts*. New York, NY, American Institute of Chemical Engineers, 175a, 1992.

37. Kadiyala S, Guggino SE, Michelson JD, et al: Interactions of biodegradable poly(phospho-esters) with bone, in *Extended Abstracts*. New York, NY, American Institute of Chemical Engineers, 15f, 1991.

38. Swoboda HF, Wimmer FM, Pfeiffer K, et al: Ectopic bone induction by partially purified bone extract alone or attached to biomaterials. *Biomat Art Cells Art Organs* 1990;18:383–401.

39. Miyamoto S, Takaoka K, Okada T, et al: Evaluation of polylactic acid homopolymers as carriers for bone morphogenetic protein. *Clin Orthop* 1992;278:274–285.

40. Lucas PA, Laurencin C, Syftestad GT, et al: Ectopic induction of cartilage and bone by water soluble proteins from bovine bone using a polyanhydride delivery vehicle. *J Biomed Mater Res* 1990;24:901–911.

41. Meikle MC, Mak WY, Papaioannou S, et al: Bone-derived growth factor release from poly (alpha-hydroxy acid) implants in vitro. *Biomaterials* 1993;14:177–183.

42. Mikos AG, Wald HL, Sarakinos G, et al: Biodegradable cell transplantation devices for tissue regeneration, in Cima LG, Ron ES (eds): *Tissue-Inducing Biomaterials*. Pittsburgh, PA, Materials Research Society, 1992, pp 353–358. Materials Research Society Symposium Proceedings, 252.

43. Cima LG, Vacanti JP, Vacanti C, et al: Tissue engineering by cell transplantation using degradable polymer substrates. *J Biomech Eng* 1991;113:143–151.

44. Ito K, Fujisato T, Ikada Y: Implantation of cell-seeded biodegradable polymers for tissue reconstruction, in Cima LG, Ron ES (eds): *Tissue-Inducing Biomaterials*. Pittsburgh, PA, Materials Research Society, 1992, pp 359–365. Materials Research Society Symposium Proceedings, 252.

45. Vacanti CA, Cima LG, Ratkowski D, et al: Tissue engineered growth of new cartilage in the shape of a human ear using synthetic polymers seeded with chondrocytes, in Cima LG, Ron ES (eds): *Tissue-Inducing Biomaterials*. Pittsburgh, PA, Materials Research Society, 1992, pp 367–374. Materials Research Society Symposium Proceedings, 252.

46. Mikos AG, Bao Y, Cima LG, et al: Preparation of poly(glycolic acid) bonded fiber structures for cell attachment and transplantation. *J Biomed Mater Res* 1993;27: 183–189.

47. Lo H, Kadiyala S, Guggino SE, et al: Biodegradable microcellular foams for cell transplantation, in Mikos AG, Murphy RM, Bernstein H, et al (eds): *Biomaterials for Drug and Cell Delivery*. Pittsburgh, PA, Materials Research Society, 1994, pp 41–46. Materials Research Society Symposium Proceedings, 331.

Chapter 23

Poly(lactic acid) and Poly(glycolic acid): Orthopaedic Surgery Applications

Cato T. Laurencin, MD, PhD
Joseph M. Lane, MD

Introduction

Polymers are synthetic materials composed of small molecule repeating units. These materials have a wide range of properties and performance characteristics. Over the past three decades, interest has continued to grow in the development of degradable polymers for use in orthopaedic surgical applications. Materials required for use in this field ideally have tissue biocompatibility, mechanical integrity, and fabrication ease. The biodegradable polymers based on lactic acid and glycolic acid meet these requirements and have assumed a central place as degradable materials for orthopaedic applications. This chapter covers the development of degradable poly(lactide-co-glycolide) polymers from synthesis and fabrication, through in vitro characterization, to clinical application.

Synthesis and Fabrication

Poly(lactic acid)

Poly(lactic acid) (PLA) is a thermoplastic polyester formed from the homopolymerization of lactic acid (Fig. 1). A variety of polymers, including poly(L-lactic acid) (PLLA), poly(D-lactic acid) (PDLA), and poly(DL-lactic acid) (PDLLA), can be derived from D($-$) lactic acid, D($+$) lactic acid, L($-$) lactic acid, and L($+$) lactic acid. Lactic acid in its optically active form, L-lactic acid, or in its optically inactive racemic form, DL-lactic acid, can undergo acid catalyzed condensation to yield a lower molecular weight polymer ($<$ 3,000).[1] High-molecular-weight products can be formed by anionic ring opening polymerization of the cyclic diester of lactic acid, or lactide, catalyzed by zinc

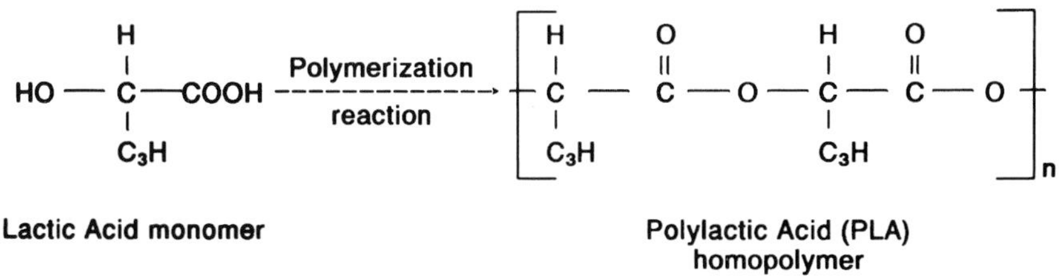

Fig. 1 Poly(lactic acid).

oxide.[1,2] Because only the L(+) form of lactic acid is metabolized in the body, PLLA is used much more commonly than PDLA.[3,4]

PLA homopolymer may be synthesized in various molecular weights depending on the applications sought. For example, molecular weights of 250,000 to 530,000 are suitable for solution-spun fibers, whereas molecular weights of 180,000 are sufficient for melt-spun fibers. For microparticle production for drug delivery systems, molecular weights from 2,000 to 120,000 can be used.[3,5] In addition, polymers with weights as low as 160 have been studied as carriers for bone morphogenetic protein (BMP).[6]

Poly(glycolic acid)

Poly(glycolic acid) (PGA) is a semicrystalline polymer that is formed most easily by the ring opening melt polymerization of glycolide. Glycolic acid can undergo thermal dehydration to form a low-molecular-weight polymer, which can then be pyrolized to form glycolide (Fig. 2).

PGA is insoluble in most common solvents and has a melting point of 224° to 226°C and a glass transition temperature of 36°C. PGA, with molecular weights ranging from 20,000 to 145,000, can be converted to fibers by melt extrusion.[7]

Copolymers and Self-reinforcing Materials

Lactic acid and glycolic acid molecules can be mixed together during polymer synthesis reactions to form copolymers called poly(lactide-co-glycolide) (PLAGA). The crystallinity of PLAGA polymers depends on the molar ratio of the two monomer components. PLAGA polymers containing less than 70% glycolide are almost entirely amorphous.[8] Although PLAGA is synthesized as a random copolymer, differences in monomer substitution along PLAGA polymers has resulted in copolymers with similar overall composition but dissimilar mechanical properties. This fact partly explains many of the experimental discrepancies found in reports of the characterization of these copolymers.

Recently, highly oriented polymer fibers have been bound together with a matrix polymer to achieve a self-reinforced material that is many times stronger than its constituents.[9-11] In one set of studies, investigators sintered PGA sutures together at high temperatures and pressures and then embedded them in a matrix of the same polymer. Self-reinforced rods constructed by these techniques have flexural strength near 370 MPa, making them some of the strongest reported totally biodegradable polymeric implants. These self-reinforced materials can then be fashioned into rods, plates, or screws. Experimental studies using these materials show that they degrade at a much slower rate and maintain their structural integrity for extended periods.[9]

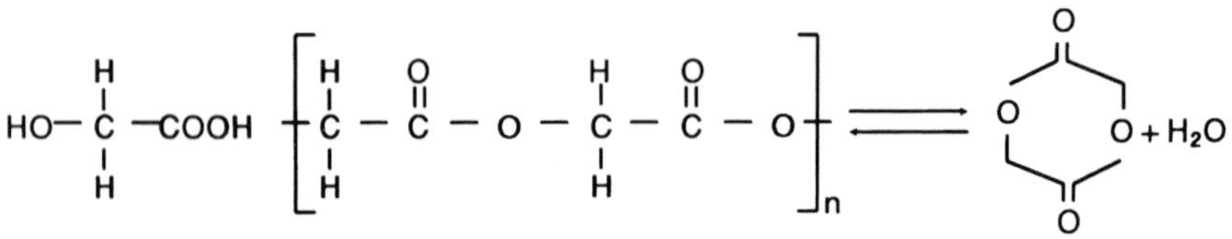

Glycolic Acid monomer   Polyglycolic Acid (PGA)   Glycolide

Fig. 2 Poly(glycolic acid).

Degradation

Pathways of Degradation and Metabolism

Polymers undergo degradation by various mechanisms, including heat, oxidation, hydrolysis, and enzymatic action. Like most degradable polymers for orthopaedic applications, the alpha-polyesters, such as PLA and PGA, degrade primarily through hydrolysis.[1,2] After nonspecific hydrolytic scission of PLA, lactic acid is formed. Lactic acid undergoes dehydrogenation to pyruvate and then to acetyl coenzyme A (CoA) for incorporation into the citric acid cycle (Fig. 3).[12,13] Resorption rate and route of elimination studies using ^{14}C-labeled polylactic acid have shown that 36.8% of the radioactivity is lost from polymer implants after 168 days with only 4.6% found in the urine, 2.8% found in the feces, and less than 0.3% found in the tissues. The authors have suggested that the elimination of radioactivity occurs mainly via respiration.[12]

PGA also undergoes hydrolysis to form its base monomer, glycolic acid, which can either be excreted in the urine or undergo further enzymatic alteration. Through reactions with glycolate oxidase and glycine transaminase, glycolic acid can be converted into serine, which can be transformed to pyruvate for use in the citric acid cycle (Fig. 4).[7,9,13]

Rate of Degradation

Several factors govern the degradation rate of polymers and copolymers composed of lactic acid and glycolic acid. The semicrystalline PLLA homopolymer degrades at a slower rate than the amorphous PDLLA homopolymer.[2] The degradation of copolymers of PLAGA has been found to depend to a large degree on the relative amounts of amorphous versus crystalline polymer domains, with increased degradation found in amorphous regions.[12,14,15]

Chu's[16] studies have characterized the mechanism of degradation of semicrystalline PLA. Homogeneous erosion of the polymer begins preferentially in amorphous regions of the polymer (where water penetrates better). Backbone ester linkages in tie-chain fragments, which make a path through the amorphous regions, are hydrolyzed. This reduces the degree of entanglement of the polymer and allows undegraded amorphous regions of polymer to rearrange into a crystalline structure.[16]

The molar ratio of the two monomers, lactic acid and glycolic acid, also governs the rate of degradation in these polymer systems. The degradation rate

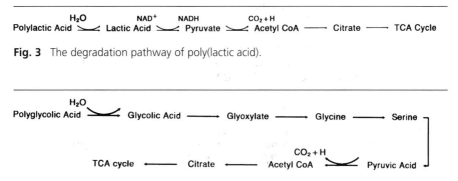

Fig. 3 The degradation pathway of poly(lactic acid).

Fig. 4 The degradation pathway of poly(glycolic acid).

of PLAGA polymers and copolymers can vary with half lives from 7 days to 6.5 months depending on composition and methods of synthesis/fabrication (Table 1).[12,14,15] It has been suggested that the methyl group on the lactic acid molecule offers steric hindrance, making hydrolysis of the lactic acid slower than that of glycolic acid. Therefore, generally, the greater the proportion of PLA the slower the rate of degradation of a copolymer. In addition to the molar ratios that compose a copolymer, the sequence of the monomers in the chain may influence the rate of degradation. For example, it is possible to have block polymers formed along a PLA:PGA copolymer. Block polymers would produce a degradation rate quite different from that of a sequence that has alternating lactic acid and glycolic acid units (Fig. 5). Block copolymers may be formed because of the higher reaction rate of glycolide as compared to the reaction rate of lactide during bulk polymerization.[17] However, situations where block co-polymer character predominates can be seen as an extreme. More often, co-monomer sequences are random. This variability is one reason why copolymers of the same molar ratios and levels of crystallinity may have different degra-dation rates.[5,18]

Environmental Effects

The local environment in which a polymer is placed will also affect its rate of degradation. If the material is placed in a highly vascular environment, its deg-radation rate may be more rapid than if it were placed in a more avascular environment. In 1992, Kumta and associates[19] used 1.5-mm polyglycolide rods (Biofix™) as intramedullary devices in rabbit femurs and implants in subcuta-neous tissue to study the rate of reduction in polymer strength. Two weeks after implantation there was a 73% reduction in strength of the intramedullary im-plants and a 64% reduction in strength of the subcutaneous implants.[19] The presence of cellular enzymes may also enhance degradation of the polymer and

Table 1 Polymer degradation

Ratio	Half-life
25PLA:75PGA	~ 14 days
50PLA:50PGA	~ 7 days
75PLA:25PGA	~ 14 days
100PLA	~ 6.5 months
100PGA	
Fast cure	~ 24 days
Slow cure	~ 5.0 months

Copolymers. Copolymers composed of the same monomers can possess different structural characteristics.

Random Copolymer	-ABBABABABBBAAABABAABAAB-
Block Copolymer	-AAAAAA-BBBBB-AAAAA-BBBBB-
Graft Copolymer	-AAAAAAAAAAAAAA-BBBBBBBBB-
	-BBBBBBBBBBBBB-AAAAAAAAA-

Fig. 5 Types of copolymers.

may help to explain the faster rate of degradation in a vascular environment that is rich in cellular elements.[20] The effects of pH on the degradation of polyglycolic sutures has also been studied in vitro. It was found that there was no significant difference in the degradation rate at pHs of 5.25 and 7.44. However, at 7 days, PGA sutures lost almost half of their original tensile strength at pH 10.09, while the same sutures retained more than 95% of their original breaking strength at the other two pHs.[21]

Tissue Response to Degradation

Use of experimental models to investigate the local tissue response to PLA and PGA and their copolymers has indicated that they are generally well tolerated by living tissue.[22] However, inflammatory reactions have been seen frequently around implants.[1,9,14,18,23–25] These reactions typically have been characterized as mild to moderate, and the accumulation of cells in most studies has been seen to be transient, decreasing to a process similar to a chronic resorption response. Local tissue response depends on the rate of degradation and the biologic compatibility of the materials as well as their breakdown products. It is hypothesized that the magnitude of the initial inflammatory response and the degree of chronic resorptive response are related to the rate of degradation and the length of time necessary to degrade the implant. Thus, if a material that is either large in size or slow in rate of degradation is implanted in the body, a minimal acute inflammatory reaction would be expected, followed by a well-developed, chronic resorption reaction. However, a small, rapidly absorbable material might elicit an acute response, while only eliciting a minimal chronic reaction.

The tissue reaction most commonly described in the literature can be summarized as follows.[1,23–25] In days, a reactive zone of inflammatory tissue is formed, which consists of polymorphonuclear leukocytes with occasional lymphocytes and a few eosinophils. Early signs of a connective tissue capsule formation can be observed. In weeks, a fibrous connective tissue capsule with parallel layers of fibroblasts and collagen is formed with minimal inflammatory cells penetrating the capsule. Occasional giant cells can be found attached to the polymer.

In weeks to months, the thickness of the fibrous connective tissue capsule decreases with formation of projections into the polymer. There is a decrease in the inflammatory reaction with minimal polymorphonuclear leukocytes, plasma cells, and lymphocytes noted. Multiple macrophages and small phagocytic cells forming occasional giant cells are evident surrounding the polymer. In months, the implant disappears. A few chronic inflammatory cells can continue to be observed in the tissue surrounding the implant.

Hollinger and Battistone[18] characterized the degradation of slowly biodegradable, biocompatible 50:50 PLAGA copolymer cylinders implanted in a rodent muscle pouch. They described a transient inflammatory response in the adjacent tissue. At 72 hours after implantation, a narrow zone of fibrinous exudate and edematous granulation tissue surrounded and penetrated the interstices of the implant, with a mixed infiltrate of polymorphonuclear and mononuclear leukocytes. By 7 to 14 days, the granulation tissue had matured into a thin, cellular fibrovascular capsule with lymphocytes and plasma cells. Inside the capsule, histiocytes and a few multinucleated giant cells lined the external surface of the implant. After 28 to 35 days, a thin rim of histiocytes and a large number of multinuclear giant cells lined the implant and interstices.[18]

The most consistent adverse tissue reaction to implanted biodegradable polymers of lactic acid and glycolic acid involves an inflammatory foreign-body reaction manifested as a sterile, discharging sinus. This adverse reaction has been described in nearly all published clinical studies on the use of absorbable fracture fixation implants made from PGA and PLAGA copolymers.[26] For example, Bostman and associates[27,28] reported the results of 516 patients with displaced malleolar fractures treated with either a rod made of PGA (Biofix™) or one made of lactide-glycolide copolymer (Polyglactin 910®). They reported a 1.2% materials failure necessitating reoperation, a 1.7% superficial bacterial wound infection rate, and a 7.9% rate of clinically manifested foreign-body reactions. This foreign-body reaction occurred after an average of 12 weeks, and produced a fluctuant swelling at the implantation site.[27,28]

Histologic examination of debris from the spontaneous sinus or from surgically drained radiolucent regions of malleolar bone revealed a nonspecific foreign-body reaction consisting of a sterile discharge with many macrophages and multinucleated giant cells along with polymorphonuclear leukocytes and small lymphocytes. A follow-up study was performed in which material aspirated from the effusion that occasionally forms around the implants was used to determine whether the PGA implants were immunologically inert.[29] The cells found in the effusion around the implants were mostly small lymphocytes, although some monocytes were also present. The investigators used gradient isolation of peripheral blood monocytes, and cultured them alone or with PGA in the experimental group or with phytohemagglutinin as a positive control. They used radiolabeled thymidine incorporation and immunostaining to detect activation and/or expression of markers. Cytologic results suggested that the predominance of lymphocytes may represent a lymphocyte-mediated immunologic reaction to the implant. The radiolabeled thymidine was not sensitive enough to detect activation of the lymphocyte in the PGA group, but did detect activation in the positive control group. However, using immunostaining, the PGA reportedly elicited expression of the interleukin-2 receptor and major histocompatibility complex-II (MHC-II) antigen. The authors[29] concluded that the PGA is immunologically inert; however, it may induce inflammatory mononuclear cell migration and adhesions, which may lead to nonspecific lymphocyte activation.

The implant's effect on the local environment must also be considered. If the rate of degradation exceeds the body's capacity to remove degradation products as well as debris, local changes can occur. The formation of osteolytic foci has been well documented and weakly associated with sinus tract formation. Bostman[26] analyzed the radiographs of 67 patients with displaced malleolar fractures treated using Biofix™ PGA rods. Of 17 patients who developed sinus tracts, 14 showed ovoid osteolytic foci occurring mostly in the deepest parts of the implant channels. Of the remaining 50 uneventful courses, only 20 showed evidence of osteolytic foci, mostly occurring at an intermediate depth along the implant channel. It was suggested that the lesions represented a sign of increased intraosseous pressure exerted by the liquid polymeric debris retained within the channel. This theory would support the observation that no osteolytic foci or manifest foreign body reactions were seen when the implant channel perforated the bone at both ends. All osteolytic foci resolved with restoration of normal bone structure.[26]

Alterations in the pH of the environment that contains the implant must also be considered, especially if the implant degrades at a rapid rate. As the production of the acidic by-products of the polymers supersedes the body's ability to eliminate these components, a local pH gradient can be potentially produced.

In the setting of a rapidly biodegradable implant placed in a poorly vascular environment, this situation potentially can be created. Vasenius and associates[30] studied possible lactic acidosis in rabbits after intramedullary SR-PDLLA and PLLA rods were implanted in both femurs of ten rabbits for 60 weeks. They found normal acid-base balances when measuring blood parameters.

Orthopaedic Applications of PLA, PGA, and Their Copolymers

Fracture Fixation

Early experimental studies using the class of biodegradable polymers known as polyesters for fracture fixation stemmed from the field of maxillofacial surgery. Devices made from PLA and PGA in the form of sutures, plates, screws, and rods were used for fixation of mandibular and orbital blowout fractures. Generally, investigators had excellent success with biodegradable polymer implants in these applications. The devices were well tolerated with minimal host inflammatory reaction. The fixation with these devices performed as well as, if not better than, fixation with their metal/alloy counterparts.

In 1971, Cutright and associates[23] used PLA sutures for internal fixation of midline symphysis fractures of the mandible in five rhesus monkeys. The sutures consisted of three 0.20-mm strands that were twisted together to form one 0.35-mm strand. Each 0.20-mm strand was constructed from 15 to 19 minor strands measuring 28 μm. The fractures healed without complications or deformity. The PLA sutures elicited only minimal inflammatory reaction.

In that same year, in a preliminary experiment, Kulkarni and associates[2] used extruded 1/8-in PDLLA rods to reduce mandibular fractures in dogs. They reported similar healing rates for the PDLLA rods and the stainless steel pin controls for their 8-month study. On examination of the implant, the 2-week pins were whitish in appearance, the 6-week pins appeared frayed, and the 3-month pins were progressively more so. After 8 months, the pins had disappeared.[2]

The following year, Cutright and Hunsuck[24] reported on the repair of orbital floor blowout fractures in 12 rhesus monkeys using 1.5-mm thick PLA sheets. They found normal healing of the fractures and normal globe movement. The PLA sheets were absorbed by phagocytes and giant cells with villous projections, and were still being absorbed at 38 weeks. Getter and associates[25] used nonreinforced, four-hole PLA plates and nonself-tapping threaded PLA screws to reduce six mandibular fractures in adult beagle dogs. The device was thermally fused intraoperatively to produce a one-piece system for stability and immobilization of the fragments. Throughout the study, only a slight inflammatory reaction was noted. At 24 weeks, the plates could not be seen or palpated. At 32 to 40 weeks, the fracture sites were indistinguishable from the adjacent bony area.[25]

In 1974, Roed-Peterson[31] used PGA sutures to treat two patients with severely dislocated fractures of the mandibular angle. These represented the first published studies on the use of degradable polyesters in humans for fracture fixation. Fixation using these polymers was continued for 6 weeks, during which healing was uneventful.

The preceding studies, as successful as they were, did not realistically approach a major problem involving the use of bioerodible polymers for fracture fixation: the maintenance of structural integrity under load. Studies in the

1970s in which bioerodible polyesters were used for long-bone fracture fixation (ie, fixation under load) met with quite poor results. It was not until a decade later that new work appeared in the literature on degradable materials for fracture fixation.

Vainionpaa and associates[32] studied diaphyseal fractures. Osteotomies were made in rabbit tibiae, and fracture fixation was accomplished by using a unique T-shaped implant. Two implants of this form were compared: one made of PGA/PLA and the other of poly-beta-hydroxy butyric acid (PHBA). Carbon reinforced $25 \times 5 \times 3$-mm sheets of the polymers were made by compression molding. Two pieces were united in a T-shape with cyanoacrylate glue. Group A adult rabbits were treated with the PGA/PLA implants and group B with PHBA implants. An oblong hole for the implant was made by a circular saw and drill on the medial side of the tibial diaphysis. The fibula was manually broken in the middle, and the implant was placed in the hole and secured with polyglycolic suture.

At 3 weeks, all of the rabbits of group A were walking compared to four out of five in group B. New bone was present in all group A rabbits and was found in three of five group B rabbits. Implant material was present at osteotomy in all animals. At 6 weeks, all rabbits used their legs normally. Implant material was observed in half the rabbits of both groups. In both groups, four rabbits had healed osteotomies. The most significant finding was at 12 weeks when only three of seven group A rabbits could bear weight on the limb compared to four of five in group B. Radiographs revealed that there were three cases of malalignment and three cases of nonunion in group A. There was only one case of nonunion in group B. At 24 weeks, half the group A rabbits could bear weight on the leg compared to four of five in group B. The polymer implants had disappeared in all rabbits.[32]

The investigators[32] concluded that both PHBA and PGA/PLA implants could be used for the fixation of rabbit osteotomies. PHBA was thought to provide better overall results in this study due to the fast degradation rate of PGA/PLA, which resulted in the PGA/PLA implant degrading before union of the fracture.

The same group[33] then used biodegradable rods for fixation of fractures involving cancellous bone. In the study, the rods were made of PGA. Dogs and cats with various fractures were studied. A channel was drilled crossing the fracture line, and a rod was interpositioned in the channel to provide equal support to both fragments.

All animals used their limbs during the first postoperative week. Within 6 weeks all animals except one could walk without lameness. The exception had a postoperative periosteal infection, and lameness ceased after antibiotic treatment. This study demonstrated successful fixation of cancellous bone in small animals. The investigators[33] concluded that PGA rods were successful in treating fractures that require 3 weeks to stabilize and 6 weeks to heal.

The first clinical study of fixation of physeal fractures of dogs and cats was accomplished by implantation of PGA rods in 1988.[34] Sizes of the rods were determined based on radiographs. After reduction of the fracture, a drill bit matching the size of the rod was used to make a hole on the epiphysis and the physeal plate into the metaphysis. The direction of the hole was perpendicular to the physeal plate.

All 14 animals used their limb in the first postoperative week. Twelve subjects walked without lameness in 3 weeks and the remaining two walked unhindered in 6 weeks. Radiographs revealed no angulation or dislocation had occurred in any of the patients. It was noted that the growing physeal plate was able to break a partially degraded PLA rod 3 to 4 weeks after fixation.

The ability to break a rod was a function of its diameter. Rod breakage was also a function of the size of the bone under fixation. Rods of 1 mm broke more easily than rods of 3.2 mm. The femur of a dog was able to break a rod of 3.2 mm in 3 postoperative weeks. The authors[34] believed that the ability of PLA rods to break made inhibition of growth less likely than with metallic implants.[34]

These investigators[35] also were the first to use polyglycolide rods across the growth plate to fix transphyseal fractures in humans. Three children with supracondylar fractures of the humerus were treated. Two channels of 1.5-mm diameter were drilled transphyseally crosswise through the fracture surfaces. One channel was through the lateral condyle into the proximal fragment and the other through the lateral column of the metaphysis distally into the medial part of the distal fragment. Polyglycolide pins of 1.5×50 mm or 1.5×60 mm were placed into the channels. A plaster cast with the elbow at 90° was worn for 4 weeks.

The three children successfully recovered with few complications. At 5 to 10 postoperative months, two of the patients had no significant change in the carrying angle and full movement of the elbow. Radiographs of the third patient showed a tilt of the distal fragment, and this resulted in a deformity of 10°.[35]

As early as 1985, Rokkanen and associates[36] reported on the use of poly-lactide-glycolide copolymer (Polyglactin 910®) for the treatment of displaced malleolar fractures. Their study involving 22 patients demonstrated no difference in healing between a group that was treated with conventional metallic implants and a group treated with the biodegradable implant. Later, Bostman and associates[37] used Polyglactin 910® cylinder-shaped rods, 3.2 or 4.5 mm in diameter and 50 to 70 mm in length, for fixation of malleolar fractures of the ankle in a prospective randomized trial in 56 humans. The immediate postoperative radiographs showed satisfactory initial reduction in 25 of 28 patients in the biodegradable fixation group and 26 of 28 patients in the control group. Subsequently, there was one failure of fixation and secondary displacement in each group. There were two disturbances in wound healing in both groups. Two patients with the biodegradable implants developed sterile wound sinus tracts 3 to 4 months after surgery, after an uneventful initial wound healing. Overall, the sinus tract formation was not found to affect final outcome.[37]

In another study, Bostman and associates[38] again used the malleolar fracture model. In this study of 102 patients, 39 were treated with the lactide-glycolide copolymer rod and 63 were treated with a self-reinforced polyglycolide rod. Ninety-three patients (91%) had exact initial reduction. Eight of the remaining nine had 1- to 2-mm displacement, and in one case of a comminuted osteoporotic bimalleolar fracture, a poor initial result was obtained. On follow-up, four of the 93 had secondary displacement. There were two superficial wound infections and six sinus-tract formations in a primarily uneventful healed wound 2 to 4 months postoperatively. These patients underwent surgical drainage of the tract. At 1 year follow-up, 84 patients showed no radiographic abnormalities. The 13 patients with incongruity of the joint were the same individuals who had either a primary or secondary displacement of the fracture. Because the few displacements that occurred after initial reduction occurred in the older population, and the only case of an unsatisfactory reduction was in osteoporotic bone, the authors[38] advise proper judgment when using biodegradable fixation methods in patients with decreased density of cancellous bone. In 1992, Kumta and associates[19] used 1.5-mm polyglycolide rods (Biofix™) as intramedullary devices to compare their ability to fix displaced, unstable fractures of the metacarpals and phalanges with that of Kirschner wires in a group of 30 patients. After a preliminary study in rabbit femurs showed at least a 73% reduction in strength of the intramedullary implants after 2 weeks, a loop wire was added to both groups for extra fixation. At 6 months, there was no significant difference between the two groups. All united by 16 weeks, with one loss of reduction in each group prior to uniting. There was no significant difference in deformity, stiffness, or return to normal activity between the groups. No inflammatory reactions were noted.[19]

Recently, Bucholz and associates[39] described the use of poly(lactide) screws for the management of closed displaced medial malleolar fractures in a prospective randomized study of the treatment of medial malleolar, bimalleolar, and trimalleolar ankle fractures. Eighty-three patients were treated with 4.0-mm "orientruded" poly(lactide) screws, while 72 control patients were treated using 4.0-mm stainless steel screws. Lateral malleolar fractures were stabilized with standard metallic implants. Functionally and radiographically, the results in the two groups were judged to be equivalent after an average follow-up of 37 months. The formation of sterile sinuses, seen in a number of other lower extremity fixation studies involving these polymers, did not occur with the "orientruded" poly(lactide) screws. While the study had the limitation of examining the fixation of fractures subject to low stress,[39] this work did demonstrate the ability of degradable poly(lactic) acid to act as a safe and effective alternative to stainless steel in a lower extremity fracture fixation setting. Overall, studies on the use of these polymers for fracture fixation offer exciting possibilities for novel ways to achieve osteosynthesis.

Drug-Delivery Systems

Delivery of Osteoinductive Proteins Since Urist and associates[40] reported the isolation of bone morphogenetic protein (BMP) in 1984, major advances have been made in fracture healing research using this osteoinductive isolate of bone matrix. In most studies reported, implantation of purified, water-soluble BMP alone typically fails to evoke an osteoinductive response, presumably because of the rapid diffusion of the protein from the implantation site. To solve problems of retention, biodegradable carrier systems based on PLA, PGA, and their copolymers have been used as controlled delivery vehicles. PLA homopolymers have been extensively investigated and successfully used for this purpose.[6,41,42] For example, Heckman and associates[41] established a nonunion model in the midpart of the radial diaphysis of dogs. The nonunion was treated with implantation of guanidine-extracted demineralized bone matrix (DBM), PLA alone, or a PLA/BMP delivery system. In this study, the PLA carrier was in the form of a friable block that could be transformed into the shape of the defect, whereas the guanidine-extracted matrix was carved to fit the defect. In the PLA implants, the BMP was polymerized with the PLA and the collagenous residue of the DBM was sandwiched around the BMP. The investigators[41] found that the guanidine-extracted DBM with or without BMP failed to induce any healing, whereas PLA alone showed a small amount of reparative new bone at 3 months. The PLA and BMP composite induced a significant increase in bone formation. The authors[41] felt that when implanted alone, the PLA acted as a crude osteoconductive scaffold, and in the presence of BMP, it provided osteoinductive potential in association with this scaffold.

Lovell and associates[42] reported the use of BMP in a canine segmental spinal fusion model. In this study, four individual spinal segments were isolated in each animal, and the following graft materials were tested in the decorticated spaces: control, corticocancellous bone strips, 50:50 plus BMP-impregnated

PLA strips, and bone strips plus PLA alone. The BMP/PLA strips resulted in fusion of five to seven of the segments tested and demonstrated two to three times more bone formation than the other groups. However, histologic examination of the BMP/PLA fusion levels revealed that the PLA strips were being separated from the host bone bed or autograft by a fibrous capsule. No bone was present inside the PLA or BMP/PLA strip in any animal, despite the fact that the strips were almost entirely surrounded by bone. In this study, it appeared that the BMP/PLA composite acted as an inductive material. However, it displayed minimal conductive ability and possibly created a barrier to the final stages of replacement by new bone because the strips were incompletely absorbed at the last time point.[42]

Miyamoto and associates[6] evaluated porous microspheres of differing molecular weights as carriers for BMP. Of the five molecular weights studied, only PLA 650/BMP composites were completely absorbed and replaced by new bone. The authors[6] suggested that this difference in ability to induce and conduct bone formation may be due to the varying tissue response elicited by the different spheres, as well as the morphologic differences in the final implant composite.

Most recently, studies on the use of recombinant BMP-2 for induction of bone formation have been performed by Yasko and associates[43] using a PLAGA matrix system. They found that 82% of segmental bone defects achieved clinical healing. Overall, the PLAGA/recombinant BMP-2 matrix achieved greater rates of healing than cancellous bone graft and a bone marrow/PLAGA matrix system.

Delivery of Anti-infective Agents The use of these polymers for drug release applications has proceeded beyond the delivery of BMP materials. For example, Wei and associates[44] have examined the use of lactic acid oligomers for the delivery of dideoxykanamycin B. In their rabbit implantation studies, polymer/drug rods placed in noninfected femurs were found to produce local drug levels exceeding the minimum inhibitory concentration for common infecting organisms of bone.[44] Sampath and associates[45] have reported on the preparation and characterization of degradable poly(lactic acid)-gentamicin delivery systems, whereas more recent studies by the same group[46] have demonstrated that these local delivery systems are capable of eradicating osteomyelitis in a dog hind tibia model. Although these studies did not demonstrate a statistically significant superiority of the biodegradable delivery system in eradicating infections over local nondegradable delivery systems based on polymethylmethacrylate or parenteral administration of gentamicin, the studies did demonstrate the overall efficacy of using degradable materials like PLAGA for local treatment of infections involving bone.[46]

Soft-Tissue Healing and Repair

Degradable polymers based on lactic acid and glycolic acid are currently being studied for use in soft-tissue repair, reconstruction, and regeneration. Speer and Warren[47] have reported on the development of degradable systems for the fixation of soft tissues to bone. Called the Suretac® (Fig. 6), the device is a cannulated tack made from a copolymer of glycolic acid and trimethylene carbonate. The bioabsorbable tack was specifically designed for use in intra-articular locations, such as the shoulder joint, in which the use of metallic implants has been fraught with problems of loosening, breakage, and migration. Warner and associates[48] reported on their first 20 patients treated with arthroscopic

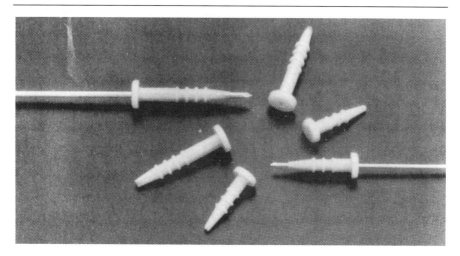

Fig. 6 The Suretac® degradable implant for soft-tissue fixation to bone.

Bankart repair for shoulder instability using the implant. At a minimum of 2 years follow-up, a recurrence rate of 10% (2 of 20) was found. Patients were able to achieve stable shoulders along with preserved range of motion.

Biodegradable PGA has been studied for use in reinforcing repairs of the anterior cruciate ligament after injury.[49] More recently, ligament augmentation devices made using PLA have been designed.[50] In in vitro and in vivo studies the materials were found to retain much of their tensile load-carrying capacity during the first 6 weeks after placement in an aqueous environment. Elongation to break was found to decrease with polymer degradation, probably as a result of relatively early loss of amorphous polymer regions with increased brittleness in vitro and in vivo. The authors[50] concluded that the absorbable braided PLA fibers showed promise in anterior cruciate ligament reconstruction.

A number of attempts at regenerating musculoskeletal soft tissue have been made, with some involving degradable polymers based on lactic acid and glycolic acid. For example, a filamentous PGA has been used for the induction of neotendon in the calcaneal tendon of sheep.[4] In this study, 2.5 to 4.0 cm of the calcaneal tendon was removed, then replaced with a polymer fiber matrix made from PGA. At follow-up, macroscopic examination revealed a thick, cylindrical, fibrous structure, with cross-sectional area two to three times greater than normal. Microscopically, the tissue was composed of multiple bundles of fibrous/collagenous tissue aligned in the long axis of the tendon.[4]

Regeneration of Bone and Cartilage

Laurencin and associates[51] have investigated the use of a number of degradable polymeric materials for the regeneration of bone tissue and have found osteoblast-polymer constructs based on copolymers of lactic acid and glycolic acid to be particularly well suited for osteoblast cell support. Using rat calvarial cells and cells from osteoblast cell clonal lines, they have demonstrated that this polymer environment supported the growth and phenotypic expression of osteoblast-like cells.[52] Most recent studies using three-dimensional polymer matrices made from degradable PLAGA have yielded lattice-works of osteoblasts in mineralized matrices (Fig. 7). Vacanti and associates[53] have engineered new

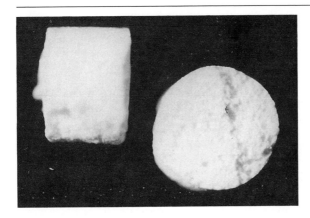

Fig. 7 Degradable 3-dimensional poly(lactide-co-glycolide) matrices for bone regeneration.

cartilage formation using PLAGA in a fiber network. After seeding chondrocytes and reimplanting the matrix, the regeneration of large cartilaginous structures was demonstrated.

In the areas of fracture fixation, drug delivery, promotion of healing, and tissue regeneration, degradable polymers based on lactic acid and glycolic acid have taken on important roles. The use of these and other degradable polymers in orthopaedic applications should increase in the future.

References

1. Kulkarni RK, Pani KC, Neuman C, et al: Polylactic acid for surgical implants. *Arch Surg* 1966;93:839–843.
2. Kulkarni RK, Moore EG, Hegyeli AF, et al: Biodegradable poly(lactic acid) polymers. *J Biomed Mater Res* 1971;5:169–181.
3. Conti B, Pavanetto F, Genta I: Use of polylactic acid for the preparation of microparticulate drug delivery systems. *J Microencapsul* 1992;9:153–166.
4. Howard CB, McKibbin B, Ralis ZA: The use of Dexon as a replacement for the calcaneal tendon in sheep. *J Bone Joint Surg* 1985;67B:313–316.
5. Jalil R, Nixon JR: Biodegradable poly(lactic acid) and poly(lactide-co-glycolide) microcapsules: Problems associated with preparative techniques and release properties. *J Microencapsul* 1990;7:297–325.
6. Miyamoto S, Takaoka K, Okada T, et al: Evaluation of polylactic acid homopolymers as carriers for bone morphogenetic protein. *Clin Orthop* 1992;278:274–285.
7. Frazza EJ, Schmitt EE: A new absorbable suture. *J Biomed Mater Res* 1971;5:43–58.
8. Gilding DK, Reed AM: Biodegradable polymers for use in surgery: Poly(glycolic)-poly(lactic acid) homopolymers and copolymers. *Polymer* 1979;20:1459–1464.
9. Majola A, Vainionpaa S, Vihtonen K, et al: Absorption, biocompatibility, and fixation properties of polylactic acid in bone tissue: An experimental study in rats. *Clin Orthop* 1991;268:260–269.
10. Tormala P, Rokkanen P, Laiho J, et al: Material for osteosynthesis devices. U.S. Patent, No. 4743257, 1988.
11. Tormala P, Vasenius J, Vainionpaa S, et al: Ultra-high strength absorbable self-reinforced polyglycolide (SR-PGA) composite rods for internal fixation of bone fractures: In vitro and in vivo study. *J Biomed Mater Res* 1991;25:1–22.
12. Brady JM, Cutright DE, Miller RA, et al: Resorption rate, route of elimination, and ultrastructure of the implant site of polylactic acid in the abdominal wall of the rat. *J Biomed Mater Res* 1973;7:155–166.

13. Hollinger JO: Preliminary report on the osteogenic potential of a biodegradable copolymer of polylactide (PLA) and polyglycolide (PGA). *J Biomed Mater Res* 1983;17:71–82.

14. Cutright DE, Perez B, Beasley JD III, et al: Degradation rates of polymers and copolymers of polylactic and polyglycolic acids. *Oral Surg Oral Med Oral Pathol* 1974;37:142–152.

15. Miller RA, Brady JM, Cutright DE: Degradation rates of oral resorbable implants (polylactates and polyglycolates): Rate modification with changes in PLA/PGA copolymer ratios. *J Biomed Mater Res* 1977;11:711–719.

16. Chu CC: Hydrolytic degradation of polyglycolic acid: Tensile-strength and crystallinity study. *J Appl Poly* 1981;26:1727–1734.

17. Gerlach KL, Krause HR, Eitenmuller J: Use of absorbable osteosynthesis material for mandibular fracture treatment of dog, in Pizzoferrato AMPG, Ravagliori A, Lee ACJ (eds): *Biomaterials and Clinical Applications: Advances in Biomaterials.* Amsterdam, Elsevier, 1987, vol 7, pp 459–464.

18. Hollinger JO, Battistone GC: Biodegradable bone repair materials: Synthetic polymers and ceramics. *Clin Orthop* 1986;207:290–305.

19. Kumta SM, Spinner S, Leung PC: Absorbable intramedullary implants for hand fractures: Animal experiments and clinical trial. *J Bone Joint Surg* 1992;74B:563–566.

20. Williams DF: Some observations on the role of cellular enzymes in the in vivo degradation of polymers, in Syrette BC, Acharya A (eds): *International Symposium on Corrosion and Degradation of Implant Materials.* Kansas City, MO, May 22–23, 1978. Philadelphia, PA, American Society for Testing and Materials, 1979, pp 61–75.

21. Chu CC: The in-vitro degradation of poly(glycolic acid) sutures: Effect of pH. *J Biomed Mater Res* 1981;15:795–804.

22. Iizuka T, Mikkonen P, Paukku P, et al: Reconstruction of orbital floor with polydioxanone plate. *Int J Oral Maxillofac Surg* 1991;20:83–87.

23. Cutright DE, Hunsuck EE, Beasley JD: Fracture reduction using a biodegradable material, polylactic acid. *J Oral Surg* 1971;29:393–397.

24. Cutright DE, Hunsuck EE: The repair of fractures of the orbital floor using biodegradable polylactic acid. *Oral Surg Oral Med Oral Pathol* 1972;33:28–34.

25. Getter L, Cutright DE, Bhaskar SN, et al: A biodegradable intraosseous appliance in the treatment of mandibular fractures. *J Oral Surg* 1972;30;344–348.

26. Bostman OM: Osteolytic changes accompanying degradation of absorbable fracture fixation implants. *J Bone Joint Surg* 1991;73B:679–682.

27. Bostman O, Hirvensalo E, Makinen J, et al: Foreign-body reactions to fracture fixation implants of biodegradable synthetic polymers. *J Bone Joint Surg* 1990;72B:592–596.

28. Bostman OM: Absorbable implants for the fixation of fractures. *J Bone Joint Surg* 1991;73A:148–153.

29. Santavirta S, Konttinen YT, Saito T, et al: Immune response to polyglycolic acid implants. *J Bone Joint Surg* 1990;72B:597–600.

30. Vasenius JM, Majola A, Miettinen EL, et al: Do intramedullary rods of self-reinforced poly-(L-lactide) or poly (DL/L-lactide) cause lactic acid acidosis in rabbits? *Clin Mater* 1992;10:213–218.

31. Roed-Peterson B: Absorbable synthetic suture material for internal fixation of fractures of the mandible. *Int J Oral Surg* 1974;3:133–136.

32. Vainionpaa S, Vihtonen K, Mero M, et al: Biodegradable fixation of rabbit osteotomies. *Acta Orthop Scand* 1986;57:237–239.

33. Axelson P, Raiha J, Sittnikow K, et al: The use of biodegradable implants in the fixation of small animal cancellous bone fractures. *Acta Vet Scand* 1988;29:469–476.

34. Rokkanen P, Bostman P, Hirvensalo E, et al: Three years' audit of biodegradable osteofixation in orthopedic surgery. *Acta Orthop Scand Suppl* 1988;59:18.

35. Bostman O, Makela EA, Tormala P, et al: Transphyseal fracture fixation using biodegradable pins. *J Bone Joint Surg* 1989;71B:706–707.

36. Rokkanen P, Bostman O, Vainionpaa S, et al: Biodegradable implants in fracture fixation: Early results of treatment of fractures of the ankle. *Lancet* 1985;1:1422–1424.

37. Bostman O, Vainionpaa S, Hirvensalo E, et al: Biodegradable internal fixation for malleolar fractures: A prospective randomised trial. *J Bone Joint Surg* 1987;69B:615–619.

38. Bostman O, Hirvensalo E, Vainionpaa S, et al: Ankle fractures treated using biodegradable internal fixation. *Clin Orthop* 1989;238:195–203.

39. Bucholz RW, Henry S, Henley MB: Fixation with bioabsorbable screws for the treatment of fractures of the ankle. *J Bone Joint Surg* 1994;76A:319–324.

40. Urist MR, Huo YK, Brownell AG, et al: Purification of bovine bone morphogenetic protein by hydroxyapatite chromatography. *Proc Natl Acad Sci USA* 1984;81:371–375.

41. Heckman JD, Boyan BD, Aufdemorte TB, et al: The use of bone morphogenetic protein in the treatment of non-union in a canine model. *J Bone Joint Surg* 1991;73A:750–764.

42. Lovell TP, Dawson EG, Nilsson OS, et al: Augmentation of spinal fusion with bone morphogenetic protein in dogs. *Clin Orthop* 1989;243:266–274.

43. Yasko AW, Cole BJ, Lane JM, et al: Comparison of recombinant human BMP-2 versus cancellous bone to heal segmental bone defects. *Trans Orthop Res Soc* 1993;18:100.

44. Wei G, Kotoura Y, Oka M, et al: A bioabsorbable delivery system for antibiotic treatment of osteomyelitis: The use of lactic acid oligomer as a carrier. *J Bone Joint Surg* 1991;73B:246–252.

45. Sampath SS, Garvin KL, Robinson DH: Preparation and characterization of biodegradable poly(L-lactic acid) gentamicin delivery systems. *Int J Pharm* 1992;78:165–174.

46. Garvin KL, Miyano JA, Giger DK, et al: The role of poly(lactide/glycolide) antibiotic implants in the treatment of osteomyelitis: An experimental canine model. *Trans Orthop Res Soc* 1993;18:463.

47. Speer KP, Warren RF: Arthroscopic shoulder stabilization: A role for biodegradable materials. *Clin Orthop* 1993;291:67–74.

48. Warner JJP, Pagnani M, Warren RF: Arthroscopic Bankart repair utilizing a cannulated absorbable fixation device. *Orthop Trans* 1991;15:761–762.

49. Cabaud HE, Feagin JA, Rodkey WG: Acute anterior cruciate ligament injury and repair reinforced with a biodegradable intraarticular ligament: Experimental studies. *Am J Sports Med* 1982;10:259–265.

50. Laitinen O, Tormala P, Taurio R, et al: Mechanical properties of biodegradable ligament augmentation device of poly(L-lactide) in vitro and in vivo. *Biomaterials* 1992;13:1012–1016.

51. Laurencin CT, Morris CD, Pierre-Jacques H, et al: Osteoblast culture on bioerodible polymers: Studies of initial cell adhesion and spread. *Polym Adv Tech* 1992;3:359–364.

52. Elgendy HM, Norman ME, Keaton AR, et al: Osteoblast-like cell (MC3T3-E1) proliferation on bioerodible polymers: An approach towards the development of a bone-bioerodible polymer composite material. *Biomaterials* 1993;14:263–269.

53. Vacanti CA, Langer R, Schloo B, et al: Synthetic polymers seeded with chondrocytes provide a template for new cartilage formation. *Plast Reconstr Surg* 1991;88:753–759.

Chapter 24

Animal Models for Assessing Bone Repair With Emphasis on Poly(α-hydroxy acid) Delivery Systems

Jeffrey O. Hollinger, DDS, PhD

Introduction

A class of polypeptides known as bone morphogenetic proteins (BMPs) is active in bone maintenance and pivotal to bone repair. To bring about responses similar to those caused by endogenous BMPs, synthetic BMPs must be administered using a delivery system that meets the following requirements: biocompatibility at implantation and during the biodegradation cycle; internal porous architecture that will promote osteoconduction; biophysical surface profile that will support cell-specific attachment; controlled mass loss to release BMP at the appropriate dose, duration, and time points; biodegradation in harmony with new bone formation; and physical properties consistent with those of the recipient bed.

Refinement of candidate delivery systems for BMP mandates assessment in characterized animal wound models. Fracture and gap models have been described for evaluating implantable materials. However, a liability of fracture wound models is the unpredictability of the resultant wound. A virtue of gap wound models is their reproducibility. A special type of gap wound is the intraosseous critical-size defect. The critical-size defect should be used to evaluate candidate delivery systems in species ranging from rodents through nonhuman primates. This chapter describes a number of reproducible osseous wound models and highlights candidate delivery systems for BMP.

Animal Wound Models

A virtue of reproducible, standard-sized animal wound models is the relative predictability of the wound bed response to trauma and implanted experimental material. Fracture and gap wound repair progresses through a time-dependent cascade of cellular, stromal, and biochemical events that result in regeneration of tissue. Recent research has focused on a special type of gap wound: the critical-size defect, which may be defined as the smallest intraosseous wound that will not regenerate completely with new bone. It is a unique type of nonunion in which less than 10% of the original osseous contour will be regained in the lifetime of the animal (Fig. 1). In contrast, a nonunion can be repaired by a combination of fibrous and osseous bridging (greater than 10% bone). It is unlikely that bony bridging and contour will be restored if

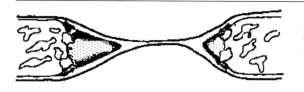

Fig. 1 Top, A critical-size defect. **Bottom,** An intraosseous wound that went on to bone repair.

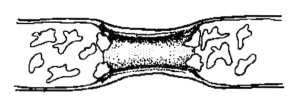

they are not achieved in approximately 6 months for rodents and rabbits and about 12 months for dogs and nonhuman primates.

The skeletal maturity of test animals must be validated radiographically; ie, through radiographic evidence of closure of the epiphyseal plates. An animal may be judged incorrectly to be skeletally mature if weight is the criterion of maturity. Skeletally mature animals should be used to study methods for bone repair because skeletally immature animals of most species heal more completely and rapidly than do adults. This is also true for humans. In children, the coronoid and articular surfaces of condyles will regenerate after hemimandibulectomies,[1] whereas adults may regenerate only about 5 to 8 mm of the mandible.[2] Rats are the exception to the rule; they grow continuously throughout their life. Although in most species a critical-size defect may decrease in size with advancing age, the size of the critical-size defect in rats remains relatively constant.

Consistency in observations between laboratories assessing experimental bone repair materials may be achieved through use of a characterized, standard, reproducible animal wound model. The critical-size defect can fulfill this extremely important role. Critical-size defects have been reviewed;[2] therefore, only a few examples will be presented as background for developing candidate delivery systems for osteoregenerative molecules such as the BMPs.

Rat Calvaria

Rats are preferable for general screening of experimental materials because they are relatively abundant, inexpensive, and hardy. In the rat calvaria, a critical-size defect is an 8-mm diameter defect in the parietal bones. In this wound model, experimental agents can be assessed over time, and dose-response studies can be executed.

The amount of rat skull that must be removed to develop a critical-size defect is extraordinary when compared to the amount of human skull that has the same effect. An 8-mm diameter critical-size defect in the rat is 80 times larger than a comparable defect in the human that will not heal by bone formation.

Takagi and Urist[3] described 8-mm diameter calvarial defects in 6-month-old Sprague-Dawley rats and noted fibrous unions at 12 weeks. Hollinger and associates[4] reported only fibrous tissue developed after 13 months' observation of 8-mm diameter calvarial defects that had been prepared in 28- to 35-day-old Long-Evans rats. Figure 2 reviews the sequence of a critical-size defect in a

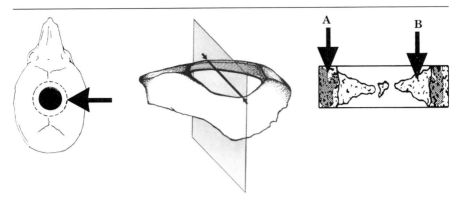

Fig. 2 Left, View of skull in which a critical-size defect has been prepared (black filled circle); the dotted line circle indicates host bone that would be removed with the critical-size defect at necropsy. **Center,** Calvarium with section through coronal plane of the critical-size defect. Arrows indicate coronal plane at 8-mm diameter. **Right,** Arrow A indicates bony margin; arrow B shows new bone formation; mid-coronal section.

rat treated with a bone regenerative material. Figure 3 depicts histologic responses of the critical-size defect to three types of treatments.

Bone repair systems have been tested using critical-size defects in a progression of species. The rat calvaria critical-size defect has become standard for screening. After successful dose-response and biocompatibility studies, testing continues with use of rabbit calvaria. A 15-mm diameter calvarial wound has been established as the critical-size defect for this species.[5,6]

Rabbit: Radius Ostectomy

A 15- to 20-mm piece of bone may be removed from the middle of the radial diaphysis. The proximal and distal segments of the radius are attached to the ulna by a combination of synchondroses and synostoses; therefore, the radius fragments remain stable. An external fixator or rigid internal fixation device is not required. However, absolute rigid fixation of the fragments cannot be assured in this wound model; only relatively rigid fixation can be assured. Figure 4 reveals the unremarkable progression of fibrous bridging that will occur in the nonrigidly fixed rabbit radius ostectomy wound model. Chai and Tang[7] evaluated 6-mm ostectomies in rabbit radii and reported that this size of wound healed by fibrous tissue formation.

Nonhuman Primate: Mandibular Critical-Size Defects

Mandibular defects have been described for several types of species.[2] Boyne[8] used a mandibular resection wound in rhesus monkeys; however, defects were treated with bone repair materials and it could not be determined from the report whether the mandibular wounds would have healed if left untreated.

A convenient mandibular defect model in skeletally mature Macaca mulatta (rhesus) has been refined by using anatomic osseous landmarks as defect delimiters, rather than absolute linear values. This strategy allows the use of animals with differently sized mandibles without requiring bone resection according to an artificially derived linear paradigm. Consequently, to obtain a common denominator of resection sizes, the canine eminence and the anterior border of

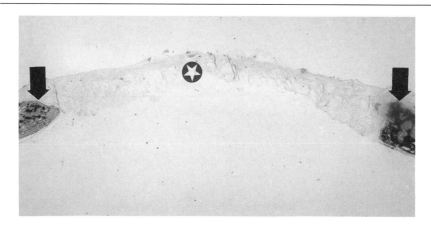

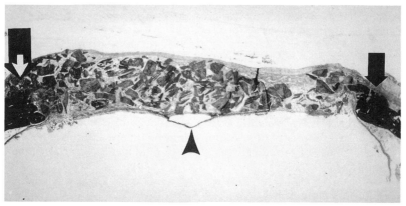

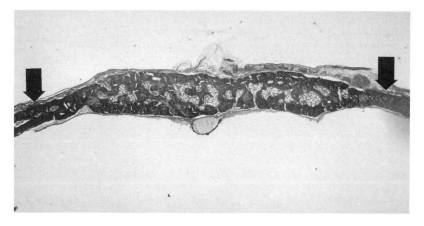

Fig. 3 Top, Coronal section through the 8-mm calvarial critical-size defect. Host bone (↓) and fibrous union (*). Left untreated, osseous union did not occur after 28 days. **Center,** An 8-mm critical-size defect in the rat (coronal plane) reveals new bone formation 28 days posttreatment. Host bone (↓) and new bone admixed with remnants of implanted demineralized bone matrix (between arrows). Mid-sagittal sinus (Δ). **Bottom,** A more robust bone response from another type of bone regenerative protein combination in the same model as above. Host bone (↓) and new bone (between arrows).

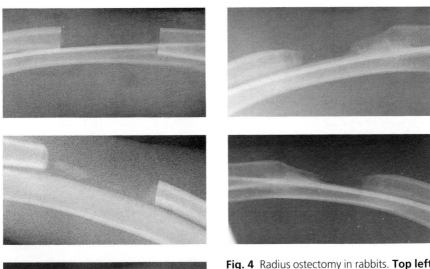

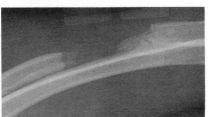

Fig. 4 Radius ostectomy in rabbits. **Top left,** time of resection; Two weeks (**top right**), 4 weeks (**center left**), 6 weeks (**center right**), and 8 weeks (**bottom left**) after surgery.

the ascending ramus were chosen as delimiters for the ostectomy gap. Removal is recommended of at least 25% of the mid body of the mandible from the canine eminence to the anterior border of the ascending ramus to achieve the criterion of a critical-size defect (unpublished data).

The sequence for this wound model involves extraction of the teeth distal to the canine, mild alveoloplasty, soft-tissue closure, and waiting 8 to 10 weeks for mucosal/gingival healing. A modified Risdon neck dissection then allows access to the mandibular mid body. The desired percent of the ostectomized mandible is visualized, and the proximal and distal fragments are fixed with a reconstruction plate using at least six cortices on each side of the resection. Figure 5 shows the surgical sequence. Histologic examination of the resected site after 6 months reveals fibrous union (Fig. 5, *bottom right*).

Dog: Preliminary Information

In the later stages of identifying candidate delivery systems and refining them to improve safety and efficacy, certain bone physiology parameters in the animal model must be homologous to those of humans. Jowsey[9] indicated that haversian systems in dogs are similar to those in humans, with an average size of approximately 223 µm. Haversian systems carry the vascular elements required for skeletal viability, the biochemical messengers needed for regulatory homeostasis, and the precursor elements capable of expressing bone cell phenotypes. Therefore, the natural engineering of the haversian canal space should be reproduced in a synthetic delivery system. Spaces (channels) should be en-

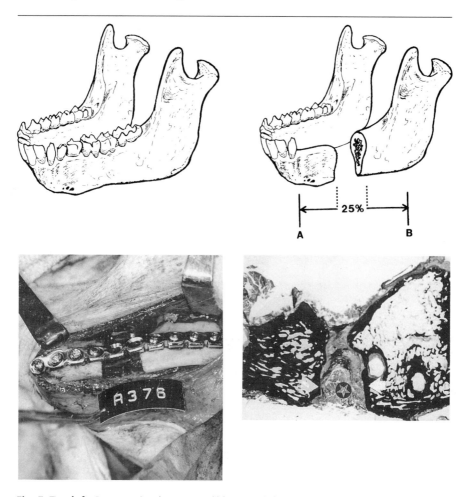

Fig. 5 Top left, Preoperative rhesus mandible. **Top right,** Resection of 25% of the mandible using landmarks of the canine eminence (A) and the anterior border of the ascending ramus (B). **Bottom left,** Clinical view of rhesus mandible at the time of surgical resection with fixation using a reconstruction plate (R376). **Bottom right,** Six months postoperatively, a fibrous bridge (*) formed across the osteotomized mid body of the mandible (⇒⇐).

gineered as potential vascular conduits to enable sprouting vessels to progress from host bone margins throughout the implant system. Therefore, the design for monolithic or block-type delivery system should include an average pore size (equivalent circular diameter) of approximately 200 to 400 μm with a pore density of about 75%.[10]

In dogs, osteoclast cutting cones erode approximately 40 μm per day longitudinally and 7 μm per day radially.[11] Data for nonhuman primates suggest that these values probably are related closely to osteoclastic resorption in humans.[12] In the remodeling process, resorption and formation are linked. Therefore, once the candidate delivery system has passed efficacy and safety assessments in lower-order species, fine tuning for the remodeling should include a resorption profile in concert with the remodeling of higher-order species, such as dogs and nonhuman primates, that have homology to humans.

Nasoalveolar Cleft

Osseous wound models in calvariae, mandibles, and long bones in dogs have been reviewed.[2, 13] With the exception of the calvaria, these locales require rigid fixation to ensure fragment stability proximal and distal to the ostectomy. Fixation devices are an additional variable within a wound bed; therefore, a virtue of the nasoalveolar cleft model is that fixation is not required.

A nasoalveolar cleft model modified from Marx and associates[14] was treated with an osteoregenerative composition. Briefly, the surgical sequence involves extraction of the maxillary incisors, alveoloplasty, and removal of sufficient bone in the premaxilla to achieve a through-and-through communication with the floor of the nose. The dry skull illustrations reveal the dentulated maxilla, palatal view (Fig. 6, *left*), and the partially edentulous premaxilla with nasal communication (Fig. 6, *center*). The radiograph of an experimental wound site treated with an osteoregenerative compound (Fig. 6, *right*) reveals regeneration of deficient bone, whereas bone formation did not develop in the contralateral, untreated cleft.

Osseous Wound Healing

The time-dependent biochemical and cellular events involved in osseous wound repair have been detailed.[10] Features of osteoinduction, callus development, fracture, and gap repair have been described in the literature,[15-19] and the biologic responses of host beds to autogenous grafts and allogeneic bone implants have been covered in several key works.[20-22] Development of bone repair materials that may replace autografts and allografts requires knowledge of both the biologic responses associated with these materials and the orderly progression of physiologic events in osseous wound healing. A laboratory-synthesized product must be engineered to have biologic features inherent to autografts and to have the biochemical, structural, and biomechanical properties needed to promote regeneration of osseous form and function to deficient skeletal tissue.

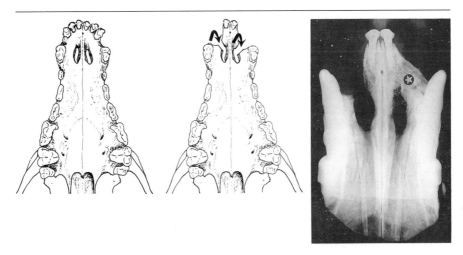

Fig. 6 Left, Maxilla of a dog prior to the clefting procedure. **Center,** The bilateral nasoalveolar clefts (curved arrows). **Right,** Radiographic appearance of the nasoalveolar clefts 2 months postoperatively: right side (*) treated with osteoregenerative composition; left side was untreated.

BMP is pivotal in the cascade of bone healing events,[23–25] and various growth factors are instrumental in proliferation of osteoprogenitor cells.[26] Numerous additional noncollagenous proteins and proteoglycans have key roles in the sequenced, structured scheme of bone formation.[27] A delivery system that contains and releases appropriate substances at optimal times and doses will have to be engineered for use at the selected anatomic site, with attention given to site-specific vascularity, biomechanical properties, and the compendium of cellular, stromal, and humoral components of tissue regeneration.

Delivery Systems

Preliminary Comments

A key attribute of a delivery system is its sequenced removal from the implantation site. Delay in removal will impede new bone formation; removal too quickly will lead to soft-tissue prolapse into the ablation wound. The terminology for removal of a delivery system from the implantation site has evolved into a confusing jumble. However, three basic descriptors define this property: erodible, degradable, and absorbable.[28] In describing polymers, an erodible system involves solubilization of the polymer by chemical reaction (eg, hydrolysis, ionization, protonization). Polymer chain length may decrease. Degradable systems are removed from the host site through decrease in size of the polymeric chain length. Absorbable polymers are removed from the host site by combinations of enzymatic, hydrolytic, and/or phagocytic processes, or by solubilization and metabolic clearing. Ron and Langer[28] note it is permissible to use interchangeable terminology when describing polymers that will be removed from the implantation site by biologic processes; yet, they point out that a particular polymer may have one, two, or all three of these properties. The term biodegradable will be used in this chapter.

Desired Characteristics

A number of characteristics are needed by a biodegradable delivery system.[10] These have been enumerated in the introduction.

Biodegradable Materials: Candidate Delivery Systems for Osteoregenerative Molecules

There are several excellent books and reviews on biodegradable polymers that may have application in medical and dental specialties.[29–32] Broadly, these polymers may be grouped in two categories: natural and synthetic (Outline 1). Because polymers must be biocompatible at insertion and during the biodegradation cycle, the total number of candidate polymer delivery systems is decreased. Moreover, the need for postsynthesis formulation of candidate systems to incorporate a payload and make them suitable for surgical manipulation will eliminate more polymer systems. For example, the solvents and heat required to manufacture a polymer containing BMP may result in solvent inactivation of the protein through conformational change of its secondary or tertiary structure. Heating above 55°C during postsynthesis formulation may inactivate or attenuate the biologic activity of BMP. Therefore, clever strategies must be pursued to package biologically active wound-repair molecules in biodegradable, biocompatible polymer delivery systems.

Outline 1 Biodegradable polymers

Synthetic
  Polyamides
    poly(hydroxylalkyl-co-L-glutamine)
    poly(L-glutamic acid-co-L-glutamate)
  Polyanhydrides
    poly[bis(p-carboxyphenoxy) propane anhydride]
    poly(carboxy phenoxyacetic acid)
  Polyesters (aliphatic)
    poly(α-hydroxy acids)
      poly(lactic acid): isomers D and L, and racemic D,L
      poly(glycolic acid)
      poly(lactic-glycolic)
    poly(β-hydroxybutyrate)
    poly(ε-caprolactone)
    poly(alkene oxalates)
    poly(alkyne diglycolates)
    polydioxanone
  Poly(ortho esters)
  Polyphosphazenes
  Poly(vinyl pyrrolidone)
Natural
  Albumin
  Collagen
  Polysaccharides
    chitosan

The homopolymers poly(lactic acid) (PLA), poly(glycolic acid) (PGA), and their copolymers (PLAGA) and poly(ε-caprolactone) are probably the most extensively investigated biodegradables. Furthermore, their history of safety merits preeminent consideration as delivery systems of choice for molecules such as BMP.[29] Consequently, this class of polymers will be discussed in this chapter. Additional candidate delivery systems have been mentioned.[10]

Poly(α-hydroxy acids)

Researchers and clinicians must be extremely circumspect and cautious when implanting foreign material in human patients. Although the history of poly(α-hydroxy acids) (PLA, PLG, PLAGA) is admirable, a number of reports have surfaced regarding a problem encountered when this polymer is used for rigid fixation.[33–38] Incidences of aseptic draining sinus tracts and swelling (ranging from 5.9% to 22.5% of patients) have been associated with polylactide and polyglycolide homopolymers that were used for long bone and zygoma fixation. A recent report offered circumstantial evidence of efferent lymph involvement from degradation of poly(L-lactic acid).[38] The authors concluded that ". . . the fate and possible role of crystalline degradation products of the polymer may limit the clinical application of poly(L-lactide) and should further remain an item of concern and the subject of further studies."[38] Yet according to Lewis:[39] "When properly prepared under GMP [good manufacturing practices as defined by the U.S. FDA] conditions from purified monomers, the polymers

(. . . of lactic and glycolic acids) exhibit no evidence of inflammatory response or other adverse effects upon implantation.''

The majority of previous reports have focused on biodegradable suture material and not on bulk quantities of polymers fabricated as fixation plates and screws. These devices are resident in the host for substantially longer periods of time than sutures or microparticles. A recent paper described the cellular responses in vivo to PLAGA microspheres.[40] The microsphere size was not identified clearly, and tissue reactions were described in response to the quantity of microspheres injected into the back muscle of rats. Referencing other workers, the authors stated that PLAGA microspheres less than 12 μm in diameter can be phagocytosed by macrophages. In addition, they commented that foreign body giant cells form when implantable materials cannot be phagocytosed by macrophages. Therefore, size and, probably, particle surface profile (smooth, porous, pebbly) appear to be crucial to local cell responses, to biocompatiblity, and, ultimately, to biodegradability. Yamaguchi and Anderson[40] noted that over the 150 days of the in vivo study, PLAGA microspheres were biocompatible.

Clearly, the quantity of foreign material introduced into host tissue must be minimized to promote optimal biologic activity of the osteogenic payload of BMP. Therefore, clever strategies for postsynthesis fabrication of polymer delivery systems must be devised. Furthermore, meticulous attention to synthesis and postsynthesis protocols under GMP conditions must be followed to preclude contaminants and to ensure production of a highly characterized polymer. Possibly, some of the adverse reports on polymer fixation devices were caused by contaminants. Moreover, the analytic properties of homo- or copolymer must be documented when reporting preclinical or clinical applications. Merely noting that a copolymer of lactic and glycolic acids is a 65:35 molar ratio is insufficient detail for other laboratories to repeat studies confirming reported observations.

Examples of Poly(α-hydroxy acid) Systems for Bone Repair In select applications, a strategy to minimize the quantity of polymer inserted in the recipient bed is to prepare a sandwich or tube. The combination of polymer plus osteoregenerative component is referred to as a multiphase system.[41] It consists of two independent compartments: the polymer part and the osteoregenerative part. Kleinschmidt and associates[41] reported on a multiphase system for repairing critical-size defects in the parietal bones of New Zealand rabbits. Disks of PLAGA were placed durally and pericranially with demineralized rabbit bone matrix (rDBM) interposed. The disks prevented soft-tissue prolapse, thereby ensuring marrow interaction with the rDBM. The multiphase system resulted in bone regeneration in the critical-size defects.[41]

Combinations of recombinant human BMP-2 (rhBMP-2) and inactivated demineralized bone matrix have been used to regenerate ostectomized segments of bone.[42–44] However, research was undertaken to determine whether rhBMP-2 would be effective with PLAGA for restoring calvarial critical-size defects in rats and to dispel the notion that collagenous matrix was required for the biologic activity of partially purified BMP (for example, BMP-3, known as osteogenin).[45] Insoluble type I bone collagen has been used successfully to deliver rhBMP-2.[46] However, the potential immunogenicity of collagen has been noted,[47] and a recent case report emphasized the hazard of an animal-derived collagen product.[48] Therefore, it was pleasing to note that results from rhBMP-2 combined with autogenous blood and PLAGA revealed parity to an insoluble collagenous delivery system for rhBMP-2.[49]

The duration of the studies using combinations of rhBMP-2 and biodegradable polymers for regeneration of bone has been substantially less than that of the fixation studies where adverse sequelae were reported. However, at the termination of the rhBMP-2/polymer studies, no remnants of biodegradable polymer were evident histologically.[49]

Conclusion

Investigators are persistently seeking biocompatible, biodegradable polymeric constructs uniquely engineered to deploy tissue-regenerating factors to bone-deficient and cartilage-deficient sites. The pursuit will be fruitful if stringent, objective assessment criteria are accrued from carefully orchestrated, sequenced animal studies of standard-sized, reproducible wounds. Candidate polymeric delivery systems for bone-promoting molecules, such as the BMPs, will be developed and refined by adhering to a rigorous testing protocol that includes meticulous synthesis and postsynthesis management of monomers and polymers, use of appropriately characterized products, and vigorous adherence to the mysterious intricacies governing osseous wound repair.

References

1. Boyne PJ: The restoration of resected mandibles in children without the use of bone grafts. *Head Neck Surg* 1983;6:626–631.
2. Hollinger JO, Kleinschmidt JC: The critical size defect as an experimental model to test bone repair materials. *J Craniofac Surg* 1990;1:60–68.
3. Takagi K, Urist MR: The reaction of the dura to bone morphogenetic protein (BMP) in repair of skull defects. *Ann Surg* 1982;196:100–109.
4. Hollinger JO, Schmitz JP, Yaskovich R, et al: A synthetic polypentapeptide of elastin for initiating calcification. *Calcif Tissue Int* 1988;42:231–236.
5. Frame JW: A convenient animal model for testing bone substitute materials. *J Oral Surg* 1980;38:176–180.
6. Frame JW: A composite of porous calcium sulfate dihydrate and cyanoacrylate as a substitute for autogenous bone. *J Oral Surg* 1980;38:251–256.
7. Chai BF, Tang XM: Ultrastructural investigation of experimental non-union of fractures: A transmission electron microscopic study. *Chin Med J* 1986;99:207–214.
8. Boyne PJ: Special bone grafts in oral and maxillofacial surgery, in Robinson LH, Guernsey LH (eds): *Clinical Transplantation in Dental Specialties.* St Louis, MO, CV Mosby, 1980, pp 232–256.
9. Jowsey J: Studies of Haversian systems in man and some animals. *J Anat* 1966; 100:857–864.
10. Hollinger JO: Factors for osseous repair and delivery: Part 11. *J Craniofac Surg* 1993;4:135–141.
11. Jaworski ZF, Lok E: The rate of osteoclastic bone erosion in haversian remodeling sites of adult dog's rib. *Calcif Tissue Res* 1972;10:103–112.
12. Parfitt AM: The physiologic and clinical significance of bone histomorphometric data, in Recker RR (ed): *Bone Histomorphometry.* Boca Raton, FL, CRC Press, 1983, pp 143–223.
13. Schmitz JP, Hollinger JO: The critical size defect as an experimental model for craniomandibulofacial nonunions. *Clin Orthop* 1986;205:299–308.
14. Marx RE, Miller RI, Ehler WJ, et al: A comparison of particulate allogeneic and particulate autogenous bone grafts into maxillary alveolar clefts in dogs. *J Oral Maxillofac Surg* 1984;42:3–9.
15. Penttinen R: Biochemical studies on fracture healing in the rat, with special reference to the oxygen supply. *Acta Chir Scand* 1972; 432:1–32.

16. McKibbin B: The biology of fracture healing in long bones. *J Bone Joint Surg* 1978; 60B:150–162.

17. Reddi AH, Anderson WA: Collagenous bone matrix-induced endochondral ossification hemopoiesis. *J Cell Biol* 1976;69:557–572.

18. Pan WT, Einhorn TA: The biochemistry of fracture healing. *Current Orthop* 1992; 6:207–213.

19. Marden L, Quigley N, Reddi AH, et al: Temporal changes during bone formation in the calvarium induced by osteogenin. *Calcif Tissue Int*, in press.

20. Burchardt H: The biology of bone graft repair. *Clin Orthop* 1983;174:28–42.

21. Burchardt H: Biology of bone transplantation. *Orthop Clin North Am* 1987;18: 187–196.

22. Goldberg VM, Stevenson S: Natural history of autografts and allografts. *Clin Orthop* 1987;225:7–16.

23. Urist MR: Bone: Formation by autoinduction. *Science* 1965;150:893–899.

24. Urist MR, Silverman BF, Buring K, et al: The bone induction principle. *Clin Orthop* 1967;53:243–283.

25. Reddi AH, Ma SS, Cunningham NS: Induction and maintenance of new bone formation by growth and differentiation factors. *Ann Chir Gynaecol* 1988;77:189–192.

26. Canalis E, McCarthy T, Centrella M: Growth factors and the regulation of bone remodeling. *J Clin Invest* 1988;81:277–281.

27. Hulth A, Johnell O, Lindberg L, et al: Sequential appearance of macromolecules in bone induction in the rat. *J Orthop Res* 1993;11:367–378.

28. Ron E, Langer R: Erodible systems, in Kydonieus A (ed): *Treatise on Controlled Drug Delivery: Fundamentals, Optimization, Applications*. New York, NY, Marcel Dekker, 1992, pp 199–224.

29. Hollinger JO, Battistone GC: Biodegradable bone repair materials: Synthetic polymers and ceramics. *Clin Orthop* 1986;207:290–305.

30. Chasin M, Langer R (eds): *Biodegradable Polymers as Drug Delivery Systems*. New York, NY, Marcel Dekker, 1990.

31. Kydonieus A (ed): *Treatise on Controlled Drug Delivery: Fundamentals, Optimization, Applications*. New York, NY, Marcel Dekker, 1992.

32. Zhang XC, Goosen MFA, Wyss UP, et al: Biodegradable polymers for orthopedic applications. *J Macr S Rm* 1993Ø3:81–102.

33. Bostman OM, Hirvensalo E, Makinen J, et al: Foreign-body reactions to fracture fixation implants of biodegradable synthetic polymers. *J Bone Joint Surg* 1990; 72B:592–596.

34. Bostman OM: Absorbable implants for the fixation of fractures. *J Bone Joint Surg* 1991;73A:148–153.

35. Bostman OM: Intense granulomatous inflammatory lesions associated with absorbable internal fixation devices made of polyglycolide in ankle fractures. *Clin Orthop* 1992;278:193–199.

36. Daniels AU, Taylor MS, Andriano KP, et al: Toxicity of absorbable polymers proposed for fracture fixation devices. *Trans Orthop Res Soc* 1992;17:88.

37. Bergsma EJ, Rozema FR, Bos RRM, et al: Foreign body reactions to resorbable poly(L-lactide) bone plates and screws used for the fixation of unstable zygomatic fractures. *J Oral Maxillofac Surg* 1993;51:666–670.

38. Verheyen CCPM, de Wijn JR, Van Blitterswijk CA, et al: Examination of efferent lymph nodes after 2 years of transcortical implantation of poly(L-lactide) containing plugs: A case report. *J Biomed Mater Res* 1993;27:1115–1118.

39. Lewis D: Controlled release of bioactive agents from lactide/glycolide polymers, in Chaskin M, Langer R (eds): *Biodegradable Polymers as Drug Delivery Systems*. New York, NY, Marcel Dekker, 1990, pp 1–42.

40. Yamaguchi K, Anderson J: In vivo biocompatibility studies of medisorb® 65/35 D,L-lactide/glycolide copolymer microspheres. *J Controlled Rel* 1993;24:81–93.

41. Kleinschmidt JC, Marden LJ, Kent D, et al: A multiphase system bone implant for regenerating the calvaria. *Plast Reconstr Surg* 1993;91:581–588.

42. Toriumi DM, Kotler HS, Luxenberg DP, et al: Mandibular reconstruction with a recombinant bone-inducing factor. Functional, histologic, and biomechanical evaluation. *Arch Otolaryngol Head Neck Surg* 1991;117:1101–1112.

43. Yasko AW, Lane JM, Fellinger EJ, et al: The healing of segmental bone defects, induced by recombinant human bone morphogenetic protein (rhBMP-2): A radiographic, histological, and biomechanical study in rats. *J Bone Joint Surg* 1992;74A:659–670.

44. Kirker-Head CA, Gerhart TN, Hennig G, et al: Long-term healing of large midfemoral segmental defects in sheep using recombinant human bone morphogenetic protein-2. *Clin Orthop*, in press.

45. Ma S, Chen G, Reddi AH: Collaboration between collagenous matrix and osteogenin is required for bone induction. *Ann NY Acad Sci* 1990;580:524–525.

46. Marden LJ, Hollinger JO, Chaudhari A, et al: rhBMP-2/ICBM is superior to DBM in repair of rat craniotomies. *J Biomed Mater Res*, in press.

47. DeLustro F, Dasch J, Keefe J, et al: Immune responses to allogeneic and xenogeneic implants of collagen and collagen derivatives. *Clin Orthop* 1990;260:263–279.

48. Moscona RR, Bergman R, Friedman-Birnbaum R: An unusual late reaction to Zyderm I injections: A challenge for treatment. *Plast Reconstr Surg* 1993;92:331–334.

49. Kenley R, Yim K, Abrams J, et al : Biotechnology and bone graft substitutes. *Pharm Res*, in press.

Chapter 25

Osteoconduction in Hydroxyapatite-Based Materials

Ralph E. Holmes, MD

Biologic Basis for Osteoconduction

Three physiologic functions may be attributed to bone grafts. First, the graft itself may provide a source of bone forming cells. Second, the graft may induce cells to form bone via a process called osteoinduction. And third, the graft may provide a framework for bone deposition via osteoconduction. One century ago Curtis[1] acknowledged the presence of osteoconduction when he wrote that "The Haversian canals, moreover, afford easy avenues for the growth of granulation tissue . . . which probably explain why ossification so soon takes place." Although much has been learned in the ensuing 100 years, much also remains unknown.

A biologic basis for osteoconduction may be found in the general observation that many organs, such as liver, kidney, and bone, have a parenchymal and a stromal component. The parenchyma is the physiologically active part of the organ; the stroma is the framework that supports the organization of the parenchyma. The stroma for kidney and liver is a fibrous tissue framework, whereas that for bone is fibrous tissue that has been mineralized. It has long been appreciated that loss of parenchyma with maintenance of stroma leads to a remarkable degree of regeneration and repair. Loss of hepatic lobules from a viral infection that leaves the stroma intact will permit residual hepatocytes to organize a repair that is capable of near normal function. A bacterial infection, leading to suppuration of parenchyma and stroma alike, heals with scar tissue and no regeneration of hepatic function. This observation is important because it suggests that a bone defect might regenerate more predictably if a stromal substitute were implanted to provide a framework for organization of the osteons. By providing a bone defect with a stromal substitute containing spaces morphologically compatible with osteons and their vascular interconnections, a partnership between biomaterials and skeletal regeneration may be encouraged. This facilitation of bone repair by means of a stromal architecture or framework provided by the biomaterial has been called osteoconduction.

When examined as an organ, cortical bone is noted to have a parenchyma of osteons or haversian systems that are held together by a hard tissue stroma or interstitium (Fig. 1). The parenchymal component is vascularized and populated with cells; the interstitium is devoid of circulation and cells. Interstitial bone accounts for one third of the volume of long bones, such as the femur and tibia, with the remaining two thirds consisting of the parenchymal osteons.[2,3] To design an implant for osteoconduction it would seem logical to mimic the architecture of this interstitial or stromal bone. Because osteons average 190 to 230 µm in diameter and intercommunicate through Volkmann's canals, an idealized bone graft framework might mimic osteon-evacuated cortical bone and have an interconnected porous system of channels having similar dimensions (Fig. 2). These pore dimensions are consistent with the classical studies of Klawitter and Hulbert,[4] which established a minimum pore size of 100 µm for bone ingrowth into ceramic structures. Cancellous bone differs from cortical bone in being open-spaced and trabecular (Fig. 3). The trabeculae represent "unrolled" osteons on both surfaces, which are in apposition to a central framework of interstitial bone. An ideal cancellous bone graft framework would mimic osteon-evacuated cancellous bone and have a thin lattice interconnected by pores of 500 to 600 µm (Fig. 4).

Hydroxyapatite-Based Materials

Sintered Hydroxyapatite

The most widely used process for the fabrication of porous hydroxyapatite (HA) implants utilizes isostatic compaction and sintering of calcium phosphate

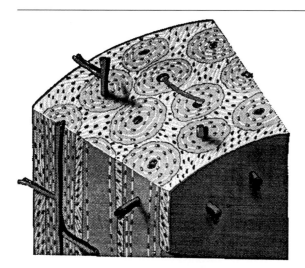

Fig. 1 Microstructure of human cortical bone. The cylindrical osteons or haversian systems represent the parenchymal component of bone. The stroma is represented by the interstitial bone between osteons.

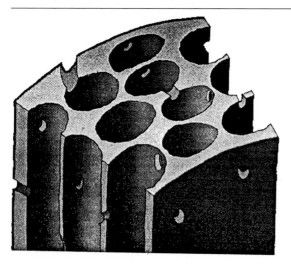

Fig. 2 Idealized microstructure for cortical bone regeneration. After evacuation of the osteons, there remains an osteoconductive structure into which regenerated osteons can naturally fit.

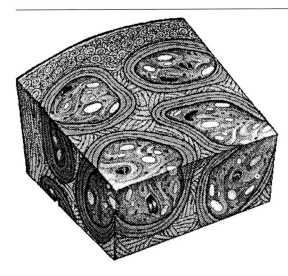

Fig. 3 Microstructure of human cancellous bone. The osteons appear as planar lamellae with interstitial bone filling the spaces in between. The thickness of these planar lamellae, similar to the radius of cylindrical osteons, permits nutrition of osteocytes from blood vessels in the large trabecular spaces.

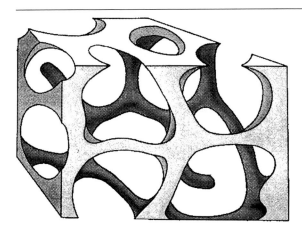

Fig. 4 Idealized microstructure for cancellous bone regeneration. The large interconnected pores can permit ingrowth of fibrovascular tissue, differentiation of osteoblasts, and apposition of new bone against this framework.

powders that contain naphthalene particles.[5] Volatilization of the naphthalene particles leaves a porosity that consists of spherical voids communicating by a narrow-necked aperture wherever the particles were in contact. To permit bone ingrowth of any depth, these apertures must exceed 100 μm or they will represent blind ends and discontinuities in bone. Another sintering process for creating a macroporous structure utilizes pretreatment with hydrogen peroxide.[6]

HA Cement

More recently, water-setting HA cements have been used successfully to create hydroxyapatite materials with various porosities.[7–9] The most completely characterized HA cement in this group[10] is made by reacting tetracalcium phosphate and calcium hydrogen phosphate in an aqueous environment:

$$Ca_4(PO_4)_2 + CaHPO_4 + H_2O \rightarrow Ca_5(PO_4)_3OH + H_2$$

Under in vitro conditions at 37° C, the HA cement sets in approximately 15 min and the isothermal chemical reaction is completed in 4 h. Porosity can be obtained by mixing the cement with sucrose granules before it sets and then removing the granules by dissolution in water.

HA Conversion by Hydrothermal Exchange

During the early 1970s, a process was developed that utilized the skeletal structure of marine invertebrates, especially reef building corals, as a template to make porous structures of other materials.[11] The calcium carbonate skeleton is reacted with diammonium hydrogen phosphate and, by means of a hydrothermal exchange of carbonate and phosphate, is converted to hydroxyapatite:

$$10CaCO_3 + 6(NH_4)_2HPO_4 + 2H_2O \rightarrow$$
$$Ca_{10}(PO_4)_6(OH)_2 + 6(NH_4)_2CO_3 + 4H_2CO_3$$

Under suitable temperature and pressure conditions, the exchange results in a 90% pure hydroxyapatite with residual β-whitlockite and carbonate. The hydroxyapatite structure is an exact replica of the porous marine skeleton, including its interconnected porosity.

Inorganic Bone

Removal of the organic matrix from bone leaves an HA-based material that retains its original architecture and may provide a framework for osteoconduction. One method involves burning the organic matrix and then stabilizing the residual HA matrix with heat fusion.[12] This pyrolysis and sintering is accomplished without destroying the native structural features and is said to result in better developed crystalline structures.

Properties

Porosity

The porosity of sintered and cemented forms of hydroxyapatite frameworks depends on the numbers and dimensions of the volatilized or dissolved particles. The degree of particle compaction and contact helps to determine the interconnectivity of the porosity. As illustrative examples, the sintered HA material studied by Klein and associates[6] had a pore size of 150 to 250 μm. The volume fraction porosity and the pore interconnectivity were not reported. The HA cement material studied by Constantino and associates[10] had a volume fraction porosity of 10% and 20%. The pore dimensions and connectivity were not reported.

Coral-derived forms of hydroxyapatite frameworks depend on the architecture of the original species. To mimic the osteon-evacuated stroma of cortical bone, the coral skeleton from the genus *Porites* was selected. The solid framework and pore network are each a continuous and interconnected domain. The solid components of the implant framework average 75 μm and the interconnections average 95 μm. The pores average 230 μm in diameter and their interconnections average 190 μm in diameter. The void volume fraction is 65%.[13] To mimic the osteon-evacuated stroma of cancellous bone, the genus *Goniopora* was selected. The solid components of its framework average 130 μm with interconnections that average 220 μm in diameter. The pores average 600 μm in diameter and their interconnections average 260 μm in diameter. The void volume fraction is 63%.[13]

For brevity and ease of association with their nominal pore sizes, the hydroxyapatite framework from *Porites* will be called HA200 while that for *Goniopora* will be called HA500. Both of these structures have been compared with human bone. The comparison of the microstructure of HA500 with human cancellous bone is provided in Table 1.[14,15]

Biomechanical Properties

The biomechanical properties of all forms of porous HA depend on the degree of porosity; their strength falls far short of the strength of cortical bone and approximates the strength of cancellous bone. Of greater importance, fatigue properties are low and brittle failure results from inadequate load protection.

Surface Chemistry

The surface chemistry of the porous sintered and cemented HA presumably is no different from that of their dense forms. In coral-derived HA, the crystallite size of the hydroxyapatite is significantly smaller than that within the original coral. Although this reaction has been studied in detail, the explanation for this polycrystalline morphology is not well defined.[16,17] High-power scanning electron photomicrography has demonstrated a high surface area, which may be a factor in osteoconductive behavior.

Osteoconduction

Ingrowth

The tissue response to porous HA implants is inherently different from that to dense HA because of the opportunity for ingrowth. As previously noted, porosity and interconnectivity are key determinants of amount and type of ingrowth. In the osteoconductive channels, fibrovascular tissue ingrowth starts by day 3 or 4. By 28 days, this ingrowth is completed throughout the implant and apposition of bone against the pore walls has begun.[18–20] The spatial apposition of bone then progresses temporally from the implant surface towards the center.[21] A transient appearance of multinucleated giant cells has been reported.[22] The eventual bone-HA bonding within pores is considered to be like

Table 1 Comparison of the microstructure of HA500 and human cancellous bone ($\pm$ SE)

	HA500	Iliac Bone[14]	Iliac Bone[15]
Volume fraction (%)	35.1 ± 1.5	20.5 ± 0.4	20.3 ± 0.4
Surface area (mm²/mm³)	5.3 ± 0.2	3.0 ± 0.1	3.4 ± 0.1
Ratio of surface area to volume fraction	15.3 ± 0.6	14.6 ± 0.6	17.3 ± 0.2
Mean trabecular width (μm)	131.9 ± 4.4	136.6 ± 4.5	120.3 ± 1.6
Mean pore width (μm)	245.0 ± 9.0	529.6 ± 22.9	468.2 ± 27.2

(Reproduced with permission from Holmes RE, Bucholz RW, Mooney V: Porous hydroxyapatite as a bone graft substitute in metaphyseal defects: A histometric study. *J Bone Joint Surg* 1986;68A:904–911.)

that documented for dense HA. Studies in several dog models have found initial bone ingrowth to be nearly complete by 3 months, with maturation to parallel fiber bone occurring by 12 months. Representative of these studies are the data from HA200 in Table 2 and HA500 in Table 3.

In the diaphyseal radius implants of HA200, the intramedullary portion showed a substantial remodeling with removal of the bone ingrowth from the medullary regions.[23] In metaphyseal tibial implants of HA500, the portion of implant within the cancellous interior contained trabecular bone ingrowth, while the portion within the cortical shell contained compact bone ingrowth.[24] These findings suggest that after the completion of osteoconduction, the implant pore architecture plays a secondary role to other signals of bone maintenance.

Incorporation

When bone ingrowth is present throughout the pores of an osteoconductive implant, it is conceptually conceivable that the bone could occupy the pore center without contacting the pore walls, or it could contact the pore walls and thicken into the pore center. Incorporation implies apposition of bone ingrowth against the pore walls and represents another measure of osteoconduction.[25] As exemplified by the data in Table 4, the osteoconduction in porous HA implants can result in a high degree of incorporation.

Table 2 Tissue volume fractions (%) of HA200 implants retrieved from the dog radius ($\pm$ SE)

Months	n	Soft Tissue	Bone	HA Matrix
3	3	12.1 $\pm$ 2.4	49.4 $\pm$ 2.4	38.6 $\pm$ 1.5
6	3	13.7 $\pm$ 1.8	46.1 $\pm$ 2.1	40.2 $\pm$ 3.6
12	3	11.6 $\pm$ 2.3	52.7 $\pm$ 3.1	35.7 $\pm$ 1.2
24	3	7.7 $\pm$ 0.5	54.8 $\pm$ 1.0	37.6 $\pm$ 1.5
48	2	6.2 $\pm$ 1.1	54.3 $\pm$ 4.2	39.6 $\pm$ 3.2

(Reproduced with permission from Holmes RE, Bucholz RW, Mooney V: Porous hydroxyapatite as a bone graft substitute in diaphyseal defects: A histometric study. *J Orthop Res* 1987;5:114–121.)

Table 3 Tissue volume fractions (%) of HA500 implants retrieved from the dog proximal tibial metaphysis ($\pm$ SE)

Months	n	Soft Tissue	Bone	HA Matrix
2	2	57.3 $\pm$ 1.4	10.3 $\pm$ 0.6	32.6 $\pm$ 1.3
4	2	50.1 $\pm$ 1.6	11.6 $\pm$ 0.7	38.3 $\pm$ 1.5
6	2	51.2 $\pm$ 1.6	13.0 $\pm$ 0.7	35.9 $\pm$ 1.4
12	2	49.0 $\pm$ 1.7	17.3 $\pm$ 0.9	33.8 $\pm$ 1.6

(Reproduced with permission from Holmes RE, Bucholz RW, Mooney V: Porous hydroxyapatite as a bone graft substitute in metaphyseal defects: A histometric study. *J Bone Joint Surg* 1986;68A:904–911.)

Effect of Osteoconduction on Strength

In porous HA, the tissue responses result in an implant-bone composite that significantly changes the original biomechanical properties. A high correlation (r = 0.92) was reported between the bending strength of porous HA and the amount of pore space occupied by bone ingrowth.[26] In HA200, compressive strength was found to increase 3.5 to 7.2 fold and anisotropy of the original matrix was neutralized after bone ingrowth (Table 5). In HA500, compressive strength was found to increase 2.7 to 6.8 fold after bone ingrowth.[27]

Biodegradation

Two mechanisms—cell mediated and dissolution—participate in the biodegradation and resorption of HA in the body. The activity of both of these mechanisms is directly related to implant surface area. Because of its low surface area, dense HA has demonstrated very low rates of biodegradation. Osteoconductive HA implants, because of their porosity, can undergo a significant degree of resorption. Coral-derived HA has micropores 1 to 5 μm in diameter in addition to its macropores, resulting in a high surface area, and resorption rates have ranged from 2% to 5% per year. Rather than resorbing along a front, the individual pore walls appear to become thinner by 2% to 5% per year, resulting

Table 4 Porous HA matrix surface areas (mm²/ mm³) and surface fractions (%) covered by bone ingrowth in implant specimens retrieved after 11 to 17 months ($\pm$ SD)

Months	Surface Area	Surface Fraction
11	9.6 $\pm$ 0.8	88.8 $\pm$ 8.8
12	9.3 $\pm$ 0.9	90.2 $\pm$ 6.9
14	9.2 $\pm$ 0.4	89.3 $\pm$ 8.4
15	9.3 $\pm$ 0.4	96.6 $\pm$ 1.8
16	9.0 $\pm$ 0.6	92.2 $\pm$ 5.6
17	9.2 $\pm$ 0.7	90.6 $\pm$ 5.6

(Reproduced with permission from Holmes RE, Roser SM: Porous hydroxyapatite as a bone graft substitute in alveolar ridge augmentation: A histometric study. *Int J Oral Maxillofac Surg* 1987;16:718–728.)

Table 5 Crush strength (psi) in compression of HA200 before and after bone ingrowth

Orientation	Before		After	
	Mean	Range	Mean	Range
Parallel	1343	997–1675	4776	2750–8479
Perpendicular	626	257–963	4529	2475–7562

(Reproduced with permission from Piecuch JF, Goldberg AJ, Shastry CV, et al: Compressive strength of implanted porous replamineform hydroxyapatite. *J Biomed Mater Res* 1984;18:39–45.)

in maintenance of the bulk dimensions of the implant until it is finally "thinned" out of existence.

Clinical Applications

Among the different block forms of porous HA osteoconductive materials, coral-derived HA200 and HA500 have undergone major clinical trials. Clinical applications in maxillofacial and orthopaedic surgery have been and continue to be evaluated. A representative study will be reviewed from each field of application. These studies are small, and a substantially larger database will be required before all the indications and contraindications can be determined.

Maxillofacial Surgery

In 92 consecutive patients undergoing orthognathic surgery, a total of 355 HA200 implants were placed in the maxilla (294), mandible (41), and midface (20).[28] In the 47 patients who had maxillary surgery, 202 implants were positioned directly adjacent to the maxillary sinus. Of these 202, 58 were placed in a maxillary step osteotomy, 99 in the lateral maxillary wall osteotomy, and 45 were placed between the pterygoid plate and maxillary tuberosity. The remaining maxillary implants were placed interdentally (53) and midpalatally (36) after segmentalization and expansion. Of the 41 mandible implants, 28 were positioned in the buccal cortical defect left by a sagittal split osteotomy, 10 were used for chin onlay, and 3 were used for chin interpositional inlay. Of the 20 midface implants, 12 were used for the lateral orbital rim, 7 for infraorbital onlay, and one for nasofrontal interposition.

These procedures, representing a broad spectrum of maxillofacial surgery, were associated with long-term complications in 4 of the 92 patients (4.3%). One patient developed bilateral maxillary sinusitis two months postsurgery, responded well to antibiotics, and had no further problems. Two patients developed intranasal exposure of midpalatal implants, which were removed at 6 and 14 months with no further problems. The fourth patient had persistent drainage from an interdental implant, which was removed 21 months after surgery with no further problems. Cephalometric measurement and analysis of postsurgery facial bone position revealed stability equivalent to that seen after the use of autogenous bone grafts. Biopsies taken from nine patients at 4 to 16 months postsurgery revealed structurally intact implants that were both united and incorporated.[29] The biopsy specimens were composed of 48.5% HA200 matrix (range: 36.5% to 56.7%) and 18% bone (range: 6.7% to 31%); the remainder was soft tissue and vascular space. Up to 9 months, woven bone was still apparent, with longer-term biopsies showing only parallel-fiber lamellar bone. Clinical studies of these applications and longer-term measurement of osteoconduction continue to date.

Orthopaedic Surgery

A series of 46 patients with traumatic defects of their long bones underwent reconstruction with HA500 and stabilization with plate and screw fixation.[30] The mechanism of injury was motor vehicle accidents in 32 patients, falls in 10, and gunshot injuries in 4. There were 25 men and 21 women, with an average age of 34.5 years (range: 17 to 67 years). All operations were performed between 6 hours and 5 days from the time of injury. No supplemental autogenous bone graft was used in any of these 46 cases.

Of the patients, 34 had metaphyseal (end-shaft) defects arising from axial compression injuries to adjacent joint surfaces. The location of the defect was tibial plateau in 23, distal tibia in four, distal radius in three, and distal femur in four. All but three patients had displaced osteochondral fragments impacted into the crushed cancellous bone of the metaphysis. Following reduction and rigid internal fixation of all major components of the fracture, the resultant metaphyseal defects varied in volume from 1 to 120 cm^3 (mean: 9.5 cm^3; median: 2.5 cm^3). A satisfactory press fit of the HA500 block was achieved in all cases.

The remaining 12 patients had diaphyseal (mid-shaft) defects, secondary to high-energy bending forces. The location of the defect was tibia in three, femur in one, humerus in three, radius in three, and ulna in two. The volume of cortical defects implanted with HA500 ranged from 1 to 4 cm^3.

Fracture union was achieved in all patients. As judged by disappearance of all cortical and cancellous fracture lines, fracture union occurred at an average of 28 weeks, identical with that noted in a comparable group of historical autograft controls. Four complications occurred in these 46 patients. These consisted of one early loosening of a humeral plate, one soft-tissue slough, one contiguous septic arthritis, and one loss of reduction followed by a late onset infection. None of these complications were attributable to the porous hydroxyapatite implant.

Biopsy of the HA500 implant was performed in 10 patients at the time of elective hardware removal. Fluoroscopic imaging was used to ensure that the biopsy was taken from the center of the implant. The time from surgery to biopsy averaged 11 months (range: 7 to 18 months). The biopsies were of seven proximal tibial metaphyseal fractures, two distal tibial metaphyseal fractures, and one humeral diaphyseal fracture. Histologic evaluation showed compact bone in the superficial (cortical) portions of the biopsy specimens with regenerated osteons filling the HA pores. The deeper (cancellous) sections demonstrated normal appearing trabeculae in apposition to the HA matrix. Histometric analysis was performed on all biopsies and revealed an average bone volume fraction of 40.7%, HA matrix of 31.8%, and soft tissue and vascular space of 27.5%.

Discussion

The absence of any transplanted cells or inductive factors in the porous HA matrices discussed here suggests that bone ingrowth was a result of an osteoconductive effect. Although I believe osteoconduction to be a real effect, the evidence is still insufficient. To measure the magnitude of an osteoconductive effect would require comparison of the amount of bone ingrowth into a porous implant with the amount of ingrowth into an unimplanted (and unosteoconducted) defect. Unfortunately, the vast majority of unimplanted defect controls do not prevent prolapse of adjacent soft tissues into the defect. In discussing the pathogenesis of the critical size defect, Schmitz and Hollinger[31] stated that the "periosteal sheath, lacking support, may fold inward towards the bony segments and form a fibroblastic barrier."

I believe that a protected or "tissue guided" critical size defect may result in equally rapid and more complete bone regeneration, with the osteoconductive framework representing an unnecessarily complex barrier. To claim an implant framework facilitates bone ingrowth, it must be compared to tissue guided controls and demonstrate a statistically significant increase in quantity.

In addition to demonstrating and measuring their osteoconductive effect, the HA based materials must be composited with collagen or some other polymer to give the implants physical properties more like those of native bone. The surgeon needs to be free to shape, fixate, and load an osteoconductive implant with the confidence that failure will not take place while endogenous and surgically delivered osteoprogenitor cells and growth factors play their part.

References

1. Curtis BF: Cases of bone implantation and transplantation for cyst of tibia; osteo-myelitic cavities, and ununited fracture. *Am J Med Sci* 1893;106:30–37.
2. Currey JD: Some effects of ageing in human Haversian systems. *J Anat* 1964;98: 69–75.
3. Evans FG, Bang S: Physical and histological differences between human fibular and femoral compact bone, in Evans FG (ed): *Studies on the Anatomy and Function of Bone and Joints.* New York, NY, Springer-Verlag, 1966, pp 142–150.
4. Klawitter JJ, Hulbert SF: Application of porous ceramics for the attachment of load bearing orthopedic applications, in Hall CW (ed): *Bioceramics—Engineering in Medicine: Biomedical Materials Research Symposium No 2, Part 1. J Biomed Mater Res* 1971;5:161–229.
5. Hubbard WG: PhD Thesis: Physiological calcium-phosphates as orthopedic bio-materials. Milwaukee, WI, Marquette University, 1974.
6. Klein C, Patka P, den Hollander W: Macroporous calcium phosphate bioceramics in dog femora: A histological study of interface and biodegradation. *Biomaterials* 1989;10:59–62.
7. Brown WE, Chow LC: A new calcium phosphate, water-setting cement, in Brown PW (ed): *Cements Research Progress.* Westerville, OH, American Ceramic Society, 1986, pp 352–379.
8. Capano PJ: PhD Thesis: The chemical synthesis, and biomedical and dental applications of the first truly successful, in vivo replacements for bone, teeth, and similar materials. Austin, TX, University of Texas at Austin, 1987.
9. Constantz B, Young SW, Kienapfel H, et al: Pilot investigations of a calcium phosphate cement in a rabbit femoral canal model and a canine humeral plug model, in *Transactions of the 17th Annual Meeting of the Society for Biomaterials. Scottsdale, AZ, May 1–5, 1991.* Algonquin, IL, Society for Biomaterials, 1991, p 92.
10. Constantino PD, Friedman CD, Jones K, et al: Hydroxyapatite cement: I. Basic chemistry and histologic properties. *Arch Otolaryngol Head Neck Surg* 1991;117: 379–384.
11. Roy DM, Linnehan SK: Hydroxyapatite formed from coral skeletal carbonate by hydrothermal exchange. *Nature* 1974;247:220–222.
12. Katthagen BD: *Bone Regeneration with Bone Substitutes: An Animal Study.* New York, NY, Springer-Verlag, 1987, pp 47–50.
13. Hanusiak WM: PhD Thesis: Polymeric replamineform biomaterials and a new membrane structure. University Park, PA, Pennsylvania State University, 1977.
14. Malluche HH, Meyer W, Sherman D, et al: Quantitative bone histology in 84 normal American subjects: Micromorphometric analysis and evaluation of variance in iliac bone. *Calcif Tissue Int* 1982;34:449–455.
15. Merz WA, Schenk RK: Quantitative structural analysis of human cancellous bone. *Acta Anat* 1970, 75:54–66.
16. Eysel W, Roy DM: Hydrothermal flux growth of hydroxylapatite by temperature oscillation. *J Cryst Growth* 1973;20:245–250.
17. Eysel W, Roy DM: Topotactic reaction of aragonite to hydroxylapatite. *Z Kristallogr* 1975;141:11–24.
18. Finn RA, Bell WH, Brammer JA: Interpositional "grafting" with autogenous bone and coralline hydroxyapatite. *J Maxillofac Surg* 1980;8:217–227.
19. Piecuch JF, Topazian RG, Skoly S, et al: Experimental ridge augmentation with porous hydroxyapatite implants. *J Dent Res* 1983;62:148–151.

20. Butts TE, Peterson LJ, Allen CM: Early soft tissue ingrowth into porous block hydroxyapatite. *J Oral Maxillofac Surg* 1989;47:475–479.
21. Holmes RE: Bone regeneration within a coralline hydroxyapatite implant. *Plast Reconstr Surg* 1979;63:626–633.
22. Itatani C, Marshall GJ: Cellular responses to implanted Replamineform hydroxy-apatite. *Trans Orthop Res Soc* 1984;9:123.
23. Holmes RE, Bucholz RW, Mooney V: Porous hydroxyapatite as a bone graft sub-stitute in diaphyseal defects: A histometric study. *J Orthop Res* 1987;5:114–121.
24. Holmes RE, Bucholz RW, Mooney V: Porous hydroxyapatite as a bone graft sub-stitute in metaphyseal defects: A histometric study. *J Bone Joint Surg* 1986;68A: 904–911.
25. Holmes RE, Hagler HK, Coletta CA: Thick-section histometry of porous hydroxy-apatite implants using backscattered electron imaging. *J Biomed Mater Res* 1987; 21:731–739.
26. Martin RB, Chapman MW, Holmes RE, et al: Effects of bone ingrowth on the strength and non-invasive assessment of a coralline hydroxyapatite material. *Bio-materials* 1989;10:481–488.
27. Holmes R, Mooney V, Bucholz R, et al: A coralline hydroxyapatite bone graft substitute: Preliminary report. *Clin Orthop* 1984;188:252–262.
28. Wolford LM, Wardrop RW, Hartog JM: Coralline porous hydroxylapatite as a bone graft substitute in orthognathic surgery. *J Oral Maxillofac Surg* 1987;45: 1034–1042.
29. Holmes RE, Wardrop RW, Wolford LM: Hydroxylapatite as a bone graft substitute in orthognathic surgery: Histologic and histometric findings. *J Oral Maxillofac Surg* 1988;46:661–671.
30. Bucholz RW, Carlton A, Holmes RE: Hydroxyapatite and tricalcium phosphate bone graft substitutes. *Orthop Clin North Am* 1987;18:323–334.
31. Schmitz JP, Hollinger JOP: The critical size defect as an experimental model for craniomandibulofacial nonunions. *Clin Orthop* 1986;205:299–308.

Chapter 26

The Effects of Cellular Manipulation and TGF-β in a Composite Bone Graft

Meir Liebergall, MD
Randell G. Young, DVM
Naoto Ozawa, MD
James H. Reese, PhD
Dwight T. Davy, PhD
Victor M. Goldberg, MD
Arnold I. Caplan, PhD

Introduction

The clinical demand for bone grafts is a common and problematic issue in orthopaedic surgery. Bone grafts have a unique role in tumor surgery (particularly in limb salvage procedures), fracture repair, and failed total joint surgery, as well as other orthopaedic procedures.[1] There is ongoing research to find a composite bone graft that combines osteogenesis with inductive and conductive properties.[1-3]

Calcium phosphate ceramics are biocompatible and exhibit osteoconductive properties. However, this osteoconduction usually is observed in restricted areas adjacent to the preexisting host bone.[4] The ceramic itself does not appear to be useful for the repair of massive bony defects.[5,6] Ohgushi and associates[3,7] and others[5,6] have reported that syngeneic bone marrow cells initiate osteogenesis in porous calcium phosphate ceramics that have been implanted into subcutaneous, intramuscular, or orthotopic sites. These composite grafts may be improved further by the use of osteoinductive proteins, such as growth factors or other agents.

Many growth factors, including transforming growth factor-beta (TGF-β), are involved in the formation, repair, and remodeling of bone.[8-11] Several investigators have examined the effect of TGF-β on isolated, normal, osteoblast-like cells.[9,10,12,13] Contradictory observations have been made on the effect of low concentrations of TGF-β on these cell types.[13-15] TGF-β was found by one group[13] to be nonmitogenic and to cause a decrease in alkaline phosphatase activity, but was found in another study[12] to be highly mitogenic and have no effect on alkaline phosphatase. TGF-β also was found with periosteal cells to enhance the expression of the chondrocyte phenotype, which suggests that it is important in initiating and promoting cartilage formation in vivo.[16] Data from studies on TGF-β during fracture healing suggest a complex action in the regulation of chondrogenesis, intramembranous ossification, and endochondral ossification.[11] These diverse observations could be a result of the cell type used and/or culture conditions. Indeed, TGF-β may function as an autocrine factor

367

by stimulating the cells that release it,[10] and it can augment other osteoinductive proteins such as the bone morphogenetic proteins (BMPs).[8] Thus, TGF-β may stimulate the proliferation of many responding cells, including cells of the osteogenic lineage. The present study was designed to determine whether ex vivo manipulation of cells and TGF-β pretreatment of bone marrow cells and/or cultured mesenchymal stem cells[17] would affect osteogenesis in orthotopic ceramics in a rat femur defect.

Materials and Methods

Ceramic Implants

The sintered porus ceramic material was from Zimmer, Inc., Warsaw, Indiana, and was composed of 60% hydroxyapatite and 40% β-tricalcium phosphate with a mean pore size of 400 μm. The ceramics were shaped into cylinders approximately 4 to 5 mm in diameter and 8 to 9 mm in length. A 1-mm hole was bored through the center of the entire length of the ceramic with a dental burr or sharp needle. The ceramics were sterilized by autoclave prior to use. In group C, described below, the ceramics were coated with fibronectin by soaking them in a test tube containing a sterile solution of 50 ng/ml fibronectin.[18] After preparation of the different ceramics with cell or serum solutions, all of the suspensions were incubated for 2 hours at 37° C in an incubator with a 5% CO_2, 95% air atmosphere to facilitate cell attachment to the ceramic walls.[18]

Marrow Cell Suspensions

Male Lewis rats weighing 200 to 250 g were anesthetized in an atmospheric chamber of CO_2 and then euthanized by exsanguination. The following procedures were performed under sterile conditions. The blood, collected via cardiac puncture, was centrifuged and the serum drawn off for further use. The femurs and the tibiae were dissected and temporarily stored in saline. The ends of the bones were clipped off, and an 18-gauge needle containing heparinized rat serum was used to hydrostatically force the bone marrow plug from the bone. The marrow cells were dispersed by sequential passage through 16-gauge, 18-gauge, 20-gauge, and 22-gauge needles. During this procedure, the receptacle for the serum was kept in a water bath at 37° C to prevent coagulation or thickening of the cell-serum mixture. The resulting single-cell suspension was then centrifuged at 3,000 rpm for 5 min. Supernatants were discarded, and bone marrow cells were washed twice with cell culture medium, BGJ_b, with 10% fetal bovine serum and antibiotics (Gibco, Inc.). Nucleated cells were counted after adding 4% acetic acid at a 1:1 (v/v) ratio to lyse red blood cells. Serum or medium was added to bring the cell suspension to the desired cell concentration.

Preparation of Cultured Bone Marrow Cells

Lewis rats (200 to 300 g) were sacrificed as above. Bilateral femurs and tibiae were recovered immediately, and the marrow cells were collected and prepared as above. Cells were then seeded onto 100-mm tissue culture dishes and cultured. After 3 days, the nonadherent cells were removed with a complete medium change. The cultured cells were passaged to a new dish 7 to 10 days after the initial seeding before the cells reached confluence. Culture medium used for Group B, described below, was BGJ_b with10% fetal bovine serum and 5%

horse serum. Cultured cells were recovered by treatment with 0.25% trypsin and 1mM ethylene-diaminetetraacetic acid, concentrated by centrifugation, resuspended in serum-free BGJ$_b$ medium, and adjusted to the desired cell concentration.[7] These culture-expanded marrow-derived mesenchymal stem cells are referred to as MSCs.[17]

Surgical Procedure

Lewis male rats weighing 250 to 325 g were anesthetized by intramuscular injection of ketamine (14 mg/kg of body weight) and xylazine (3 mg/kg of body weight). A longitudinal incision was made over the lateral aspect of the right femur. The periosteum with the attached muscle was scraped away from the bone along the diaphysis. A polyethylene plate was attached to the femur with two cerclage wires and four threaded Kirschner wires (Fig. 1). A segment of the femur, 8 mm in length, was then removed from the mid diaphysis; a surgical airtome was used in groups A and B, and a spinal narrow rongeur was used in group C. The implant was placed into the gap and secured with 4–0 silk sutures. The muscles were pulled over the bone and the plate. The muscle layer and skin were separately closed by 4–0 chromic gut sutures. The rats were fed normal laboratory diet.

Study Groups

Three different groups were included in this study. Group A was used to compare the effect of TGF-β on ceramic composite with either serum or fresh marrow cells. Group B was used to compare the effect of TGF-β on ceramic composite with either fresh marrow cells or cultured marrow-derived mesenchymal

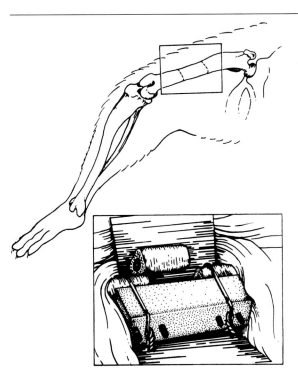

Fig 1. Schematic of the surgical site, illustrating the middiaphysial defect site and the plate fixation with removal of the bone segment.

cells. Group C was used to evaluate the effect of TGF-β on cultured marrow-derived mesenchymal cells in a modified, improved model.

Group A A total of 120 rats were divided into two groups of 60 each for sacrifice at either 4 or 8 weeks after surgery. In each sacrifice group of 60, four sub-groups of 15 animals each received implants treated as follows: (1) ceramic alone; (2) ceramic plus TGF-β (50 ng/ml); (3) ceramic plus whole marrow cells (3×10^6 nucleated cells/ml); and (4) ceramic plus whole marrow cells (3×10^6 nucleated cells/ml) plus TGF-β (50 ng/ml). From each subgroup of 15 animals, ten were used for biomechanical testing in a compression test and the other five were used for histologic testing.

Group B A total of 24 rats were divided into four subgroups of six each for sacrifice at 6 weeks following implantation. The ceramic implants were treated with: (1) fresh whole marrow cells (usually kept overnight in the refrigerator at 4° C); (2) fresh marrow cells plus TGF-β (TGF-β was diluted into a solution of BGJ_b medium containing 10% Lewis rat serum and 1% antibiotic-antimycotic; an aliquot [10 μl] of this solution was added to the marrow cell suspension for a final concentration of 50 ng/ml); (3) cultured MSCs in a final concentration of 5×10^6 cells/ml; and (4) cultured MSCs (5×10^6 cells/ml) plus TGF-β (50 ng/ml added to the culture medium 4 hours before the cells were recovered). All the animals in group B were used for histologic evaluation.

Group C A total of 12 rats underwent the same procedure as those in group B, with two differences. The ceramic implants were coated with fibronectin, and the osteotomy was done with a hand rongeur in an attempt to better preserve the soft tissues and the blood supply at the edges. There were two subgroups: (1) cultured MSCs and (2) MSCs incubated with TGF-β (50 ng/ml) in the presence of the ceramics for 2 hours prior to implantation. Histologic evaluation was done at 4 weeks with the same scoring as in group B.

Biomechanical Testing

This test was performed with the rationale that as the bone content within the ceramics increases, a higher compression force is required before sample failure. The animals were sacrificed in an atmosphere of CO_2, and the operated femurs were dissected. The cerclage wires and the two Kirschner wires were removed at the proximal end of the femur. The proximal end of the femur was sawed off, and the plated femur was mounted on an "Isomet" bone saw fitted with a diamond blade (Bueheler, Inc.). Two cuts were made through the implants to produce a cylindrically shaped, 5.2-mm long segment. A servohydraulic compression tester (Instron Model 1230, Instron, Inc.) was used to apply a compressive force to the cylindrical segments, which were standing on end until the cylindrical material failed. Strength was defined as the force required for failure and is recorded in Newtons (N). As a reference, a 5-mm piece of rat femur cortical bone fails at approximately 980 N.

Histology

The dissected intact plated femurs were fixed with 10% buffered formalin for at least 24 h and then decalcified in a rapid bone decalcifier (RDO, Dupage Kinetic Labs., Inc). After decalcification, the wires and plates were removed, and two different protocols were used for the preparation and evaluation of specimens. In the first (experimental group A), a cylindrical segment was cut from the implant, and then a longitudinal cut was made through the center of the remaining proximal and distal segments of the implant and bone, thereby splitting the bone in the midline. The cylindrical segment of the implant was embedded in paraffin, and sections of 5 μm were cut perpendicular to the long axis to expose the donut-shaped face of the cylinder. The split bones also were embedded in paraffin and were cut longitudinally to focus on the bone-implant interface. The sections were stained with either Mallory-Heidenhain or toluidine blue. In the second preparation (groups B and C), longitudinal sections perpendicular to the plate surface were cut through the complete length, including the ceramic implant. Sections of 5 μm were made and stained with Mallory-Heidenhain.

The evaluation of bone formation in this model was scored by three different parameters related to bony replacement of the defect (Table 1). The first parameter was union between recipient bone and the implant. A full score of 2 was given when the union was made by osseous tissue. This parameter was scored twice in each specimen because there were two interfaces in each sample: proximal and distal. The second parameter is osseous bridging between the proximal and distal components of the recipient femur. When new bone formation was observed outside the implant, the sample was given a score of 1. The third parameter was the incidence in the ceramics of micropores that were filled with bone. This was divided into four categories, depending on the percentage of micropores with bone, and a maximum score of 4 points was given when over 75% of the pores contained osseous tissue. With this scoring system, the maximum score obtainable for a specimen is 9 points.

Statistics

The effects of any treatment in regard to the scores were statistically compared by the Student's t-test and were reported with p values. A difference was considered to be statistically significant when $p < 0.05$.

Results

Group A

This experiment compared the effect of TGF-β on fresh marrow cells with serum-treated ceramics as a control. Compression testing of the middle 5 mm

Table 1 Ceramics score

Situation	Score
Unions at interface (each side)	
Nonunion	0
Osteochondral union	1
Osseous union	2
Bone bridging between the proximal and distal femur	1
Bone formation in ceramic pores	
None	0
<25%	1
25% to 50%	2
50% to 75%	3
>75%	4
Maximum total score $[(2 \times 2) + 1 + 4]$	9

of the ceramic implant was used as a measure of the amount of load-bearing bone that formed in the porous vehicle. The compression force required for failure of the implants of the test groups either 4 or 8 weeks after surgery is presented in Table 2. Not all of the subgroups contain the biomechanical testing results for ten animals. Some animals expired during the course of the experiment because of circumstances unrelated to the experimental conditions. In other cases, the implants were damaged in retrieval, which made them unsuitable for the compression test.

When the average forces (Table 2) required to crush the implants for the subgroups tested after 4 weeks were compared by using the Student's t-test, no differences were found. However, when the subgroups tested after 8 weeks were compared and analyzed statistically, the compression tests showed that the subgroups with implants containing marrow cells had significantly ($p < 0.005$) higher resistance to failure than the subgroups containing no marrow cells. The implants with marrow cells plus TGF-β did significantly ($p < 0.05$) better than both subgroups of ceramics without marrow cells (Table 2). The subgroups with no marrow cells were not statistically different from the subgroup containing marrow cells but no TGF-β. There was no statistically significant difference between the two subgroups of fresh marrow cells with and without

Table 2 (Group A): Compression Test for Strength (Newtons) of Ceramic Implants

Time	Ceramic	Ceramic + TGF-β	Marrow	Marrow + TGF-β
4 Weeks	11.1	50.3	40.1	26.7
	25.8	17.8	42.3	39.2
	15.6	20.0	49.0	UT
	28.9	13.4	21.4	20.0
	13.4	30.3	13.4	25.8
	8.0	21.4	UT	3.6
	UT	35.6	3.6	21.4
		11.1		
		12.5		
		19.1		
Average	17.1	23.1	28.3	22.8
Std Dev	7.6	11.6	16.6	10.6
8 Weeks	45.8	26.7	24.0	31.2
	33.4	26.7	22.3	26.7
	26.7	89.0	16.5	31.2
	13.4	30.3	70.3	128.2
	20.0	46.7	110.4	28.9
	40.1	22.3	207.8	138.0
	24.5	26.7	UT	267.0
	37.8	35.6	356.0	275.9
		42.3	44.5	349.3
			46.7	522.9
Average	30.2	38.5	99.8	179.9
Std Dev	10.3	19.4	106.9	160.7

* UT, not tested.

TGF-β. There is a broad range of actual values for the individual strengths of the implants, especially in the subgroups with marrow cells. This may explain why there was no significant difference between the latter subgroups. However, taken together, these results seem to indicate a positive effect of TGF-β on the marrow cells. There was a statistically significant difference between the 4 and 8 weeks groups; this difference was more significant in the subgroups containing marrow cells ($p < 0.005$ versus $p < 0.01$).

The histology of samples from group A was not quantified in contrast to the histology for groups B and C. However, there was bone formation in the pores of the ceramics at 4 and 8 weeks in both subgroups that received marrow cells. Qualitative evaluations indicated there was much more bone formation at 8 weeks; this correlates with the mechanical properties summarized in Table 2. However, in both specimen groups, the outermost pores did not contain bone, except for those that appeared in contact with substantial bone ingrowth, which appears to originate from a vigorous periosteal reaction. No bone was observed in the serum or serum plus TGF-β subgroups.

Group B

This experiment compared fresh whole marrow cells versus MSCs with and without preexposure to TGF-β. Bone formation within the ceramics in the different composites was evident at 6 weeks. Bone formation in the ceramic pores was more frequently observed in pores located centrally within the ceramic block (Fig. 2). The host bone to ceramic interfaces were either united with

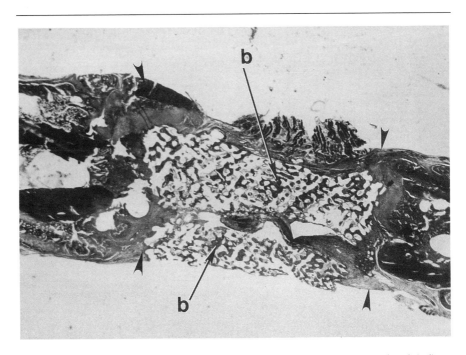

Fig. 2 Ceramics with cultured marrow 6 weeks after surgery. Small black arrowheads indicate the interface between the ceramic and the implant. Most of the ceramics holes were filled with bone (arrows and b); however, there is no bone formation on the surface nor is there bone bridging. (Mallory-Heidenhain stain, × 18)

osseous tissue, fibrous connective tissue, or cartilage. In some cases, the osseous union was observed as new bone formation from the recipient bone into the adjacent ceramic pores. None of the specimens revealed osseous bridging outside the ceramic between the proximal and distal bone margins. Table 3 shows that MSCs treated with TGF-β prior to implantation exhibited the highest histologic score, especially for both the "ceramics" and the "union" scores. The MSC composites had significantly larger numeric scores compared to those containing fresh whole marrow cells ($p < 0.05$). Exposure of MSCs to TGF-β resulted in higher scores than those for MSCs without TGF-β preincubation. These differences, which are significant at $p < 0.05$, were found both in the "ceramic" score and the "total" score.

Group C

This experiment evaluated the effect of TGF-β on MSCs in a modified model. More bone and cartilage formation, especially at the union site, was found at 4 weeks in the TGF-β subgroup (Figs. 3 and 4). Histologic analysis of this experiment revealed that there were significant differences ($p < 0.005$) between the untreated and TGF-β-treated MSCs (Table 4). Of the MSCs preexposed to TGF-β in experimental groups B and C, those in group C exhibited more bone formation at the interface between the host bone and the ceramic, with both periosteal and endosteal bridging (Fig. 4). There was no significant difference in the union scores, but the proximal union score for MSCs preexposed to TGF-β in group C at 4 weeks was higher than that of those in group B at 6 weeks. Because these findings were observed only in the TGF-β-treated ceramic composites of group C, they could not be attributed to the fibronectin used to coat the ceramic prior to cell loading. In addition, the bone formation within the ceramics was significantly greater ($p < 0.005$) in the 6-week group B MSCs than in the 4-week group C MSCs. This result probably reflects increased retention of the MSCs[18] and the contribution of host-derived reparative cells.

Discussion

This study compared whole marrow and cultured MSCs with regard to their osteogenic potential in composite bone grafts in the rat femoral gap nonunion model. In this model, the segmental gap never regenerates or repairs itself, and, therefore, is referred to as a nonunion model. We compared freshly harvested whole marrow cells to cultured MSCs, with or without preincubation with TGF-β, and observed that a cellular composite of either whole marrow or MSCs

Table 3 Histologic Scores of Group B

Treatment*	No. of Specimens	Proximal Union	Distal Union	Pore	Bridge**	Total
FM	4	1	1	0.25	0	2.25
FM + TGF-β	4	1.5	0.5	0	0	2
MSC	5	1.25	0.25	1.75	0	3.25
MSC + TGF-β	5	1.5	1.25	2.5	0	5.25

*FM, fresh dispersed marrow cells; MSC, cultured marrow-derived mesenchymal stem cells. Mean values of the separate specimens.
**Bridging must be completely across to receive a score of 1.

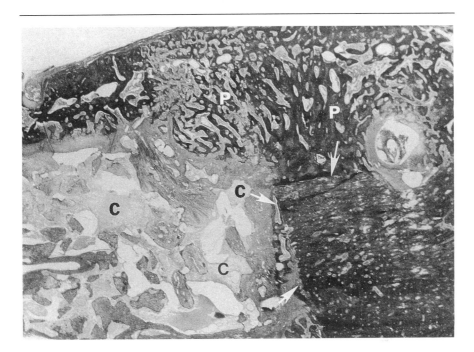

Fig. 3 Ceramics with mesenchymal stem cells treated with TGF-β and the implants harvested 4 weeks after surgery (group C). Note the periosteal bone formation (P) containing cartilage and new bone that bridges the interface between the ceramic (C) and bone edge (white arrows). (Mallory-Heidenhain stain, × 40)

is obligatory for bony repair of the defect. A surgical technique that better preserved the blood supply of the host bone was also shown to be crucial for early and vigorous bony repair. Finally, exposure of the cells to TGF-β enhanced their osteogenic ability. Thus, the donor cells, whether in whole marrow or cultured MSCs, served as a site-specific delivery vehicle for this potent bioactive protein. Whether TGF-β acted directly on the implanted MSCs or stimulated resident host cells or affected systemic events cannot be discerned from these experiments.

Calcium phosphate ceramics have been studied as a bone graft substitute.[1,3] Porous calcium phosphate ceramic functions as a cell anchorage and delivery vehicle; it also spans the gap and protects the site from soft-tissue intrusion, and its porous structure allows vigorous vascularization and osteoconductivity. In addition, the ceramic supports the formation of bone directly on the walls within each of the pores without any histologic evidence of immunoreactivity.[18] The fact that MSCs derived from the marrow seek the walls of the pores and produce bone on these surfaces is a unique and unpredicted feature of this biocompatible delivery vehicle.[2,3,5–7,17] The observations reported here further support the usefulness of porous calcium phosphate ceramics as delivery vehicles for whole marrow or cultured MSCs.

The key to the repair of the bone defect was the presence of marrow-derived MSCs. Careful and precise manipulation of the implanted cells is needed in order to bring enough activated MSCs to the defect. The freshly isolated and dispersed marrow is composed of at least three classes of cells: vascular cells, cells of the hemopoietic lineage, and MSCs. The ability to encourage the latter

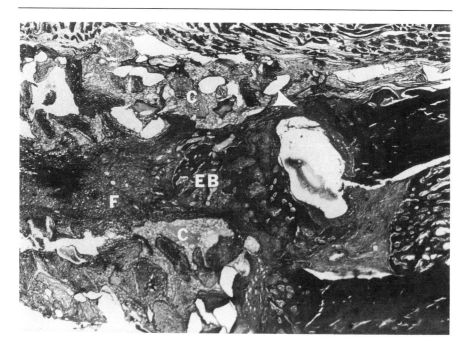

Fig. 4 Bone ceramic interface at 4 weeks (group C). White arrowheads indicate the edges of the host bone. Note the medullary endeosteal bone formation (EB) through the hole in the ceramics (C). The distal end on the hole is filled with fibrous tissue (F). (Mallory-Heidenhain stain, × 40)

Table 4 Histologic Scores of Group B

Treatment*	No. of Specimens	Proximal Union	Distal Union	Pore	Bridge**	Total
MSC	6	0.25	0	0.25	0	0.5
MSC + TGF-β	6	2	1.25	1	0	4.25

*MSC, cultured marrow-derived mesenchymal stem cells.
**Bridging must be completely across to receive a score of 1.

cells to undergo bone formation depends on both the preparation of these cells and the total cell number.[17] As previously reported, with the appropriate treatment, freshly isolated marrow cells will produce bone within the porous ceramic vehicle.[2,6,7,17] The cultured MSCs are a homogeneous cell population[17] and, thus, have a more concentrated osteogenic potential. Increasing the number of these osteogenic progenitors in the implant accelerates osteogenesis in the porous ceramic delivery vehicle.[2] This interpretation provides a rationale for why cultured marrow-derived MSCs were more effective at inducing osteogenesis than fresh marrow cells.

The cellular events involved in bone formation and fracture repair and the analysis of mesenchymal stem cell potential provide evidence of the intimate and direct relationship of osteogenesis to angiogenesis and vasculature.[14] The observation with group C further emphasizes the importance of the surrounding soft tissue and vascularity in bone repair. In this group, the modified surgical technique resulted in an observed increase in the osteogenic potential of the implants. This was achieved by avoiding the use of power instruments that could damage the host bone, and by careful handling of the soft tissues at the osteotomy site. The observed early bone-ceramic union and endosteal bone formation was not seen in the other groups. Because this appears to be a demanding procedure and model, it may also explain the wide range of results in the other groups. The host tissue manipulation seems to be as important as the composition of the implant.

We observed that TGF-β had a positive effect on osteogenesis in this non-union model. TGF-β was incubated with the cells prior to their implantation; thus, the advantage of its use was related to its ex vivo presentation to the marrow cells. This TGF-β effect could be a direct effect on the MSCs or an environmental effect on affected cells adjacent to the surgical site. Again, the most striking effect of TGF-β was in group C and may be related to the vascularity at the surgical site or its effect on other neighboring cells of the host. Although the mechanism of TGF-β action is not clear, this study suggests that the implanted cells served as a delivery vehicle for this drug or for its biologic activity. TGF-β and other bone-inductive proteins play an important role in natural bone remodeling. Their activity depends on concentration as well as on the local environment.[8,10,11,15,16,19-21] It is possible that the TGF-β effect was broad and multifocused, affecting both osteogenesis and angiogenesis.[5,20]

The results of this study indicate the importance of cellular manipulation of both the donor and host components in a composite graft. Isolated and cultured bone marrow-derived MSCs may be used to provide osteogenesis in the porous calcium phosphate vehicle. Moreover, these cells may serve as a delivery vehicle for drugs or other potent biomolecules.[21] These observations encourage the continued exploration of the use of composite grafts, because this approach may be clinically useful.

Acknowledgments

We thank Jack Parr, PhD of Zimmer Corp., Warsaw, Indiana, for the ceramic material. We also thank Debra Fein-Krantz, Jay Bensusan, and Sharon Miller for their technical assistance. This work was supported by grants from the National Institutes of Health and Genentech, Inc.

References

1. Cornell CN, Lane JM, Chapman M, et al: Multicenter trial of collagraft as bone graft substitute. *J Orthop Trauma* 1991;5:1–8.
2. Goshima J, Goldberg VM, Caplan AI: The osteogenic potential of culture-expanded rat marrow mesenchymal cells assayed in vivo in calcium phosphate ceramic blocks. *Clin Orthop* 1991;262:298–311.
3. Ohgushi H, Goldberg VM, Caplan AI: Repair of bone defects with marrow cells and porous ceramic: Experiments in rats. *Acta Orthop Scand* 1989;60:334–339.
4. Cameron HU, Macnab I, Pilliar RM: Evaluation of biodegradable ceramic. *J Biomed Mater Res* 1977;11:179–186.
5. McDavid PT, Boone ME, Kafrawy AH, et al: Effect of autogenous marrow and calcitonin on reactions to a ceramic. *J Dent Res* 1979;58:1478–1483.
6. Nade S, Armstrong L, McCartney E, et al: Osteogenesis after bone and bone marrow transplantation: The ability of ceramic materials to sustain osteogenesis from transplanted bone marrow cells: Preliminary studies. *Clin Orthop* 1983;181:255–263.

7. Ohgushi H, Goldberg VM, Caplan AI: Heterotopic osteogenesis in porous ceramics induced by marrow cells. *J Orthop Res* 1989;7:568–578.

8. Bentz H, Thompson AY, Armstrong R, et al: Transforming growth factor-β$_2$ enhances the osteo-inductive activity of a bovine bone-derived fraction containing bone morphogenetic protein-2 and 3. *Matrix* 1991;11:269–275.

9. Bonewald LF, Mundy GR: Role of transforming growth factor-beta in bone remodeling. *Clin Orthop* 1990;250:261–276.

10. Robey PG, Young MF, Flanders KC, et al: Osteoblasts synthesize and respond to transforming growth factor-type β (TGF-beta) in vitro. *J Cell Biol* 1987;105:457–463.

11. Joyce ME, Terek RM, Jingushi S, et al: Role of transforming growth factor-β in fracture repair. *Ann NY Acad Sci* 1990;593:107–123.

12. Centrella M, McCarthy TL, Canalis E: Transforming growth factor beta is a bifunctional regulator of replication and collagen synthesis in osteoblast-enriched cell cultures from fetal rat bone. *J Biol Chem* 1987;262:2869–2874.

13. Rosen DM, Stempien SA, Thompson AY, et al: Transforming growth factor-beta modulates the expression of osteoblast and chondroblast phenotypes in vitro. *J Cell Physiol* 1988;134:337–346.

14. Caplan AI: Cartilage begets bone versus endochondral myelopoiesis. *Clin Orthop* 1990;261:257–267.

15. Derynck R, Jarrett JA, Chen EY, et al: Human transforming growth factor-β cDNA sequence and expression in normal and transformed cells. *Nature* 1985;316:701.

16. Izumi T, Scully SP, Heydemann A, et al: Transforming growth factor β$_1$ stimulates Type II collagen expression in cultured periosteum-derived cells. *J Bone Miner Res* 1992;7:115–121.

17. Caplan AI: Mesenchymal stem cells. *J Orthop Res* 1991;9:641–650.

18. Dennis JE, Haynesworth SE, Young RG, et al: Osteogenesis in marrow-derived mesenchymal cell porous ceramic composites transplanted subcutaneously: Effect of fibronectin and laminin on cell retention and rate of osteogenic expression. *Cell Transplan* 1992;1:23–32.

19. Roberts AB, Sporn MB, Assoian RK, et al: Transforming growth factor type beta: Rapid induction of fibrosis and angiogenesis in vivo and stimulation of collagen formation in vitro. *Proc Natl Acad Sci USA* 1986;83:4167–4171.

20. Weiss RE, Reddi AH: Role of fibronectin in collagenous matrix-induced mesenchymal cell proliferation and differentiation in vivo. *Exp Cell Res* 1981;133:247–254.

21. Wozney JM, Rosen V, Celeste AJ, et al: Novel regulators of bone formation: Molecular clones and activities. *Science* 1988;242:1528–1534.

Section 4

Future Research Directions

Design and develop a synthetic bone graft using bone growth and morphogenetic factors in an optimal delivery system.

The purification, genetic cloning, and expression of growth factors and bone morphogenetic proteins (BMPs) have set the stage for optimal design of a synthetic bone graft. The availability of recombinant growth and morphogenetic factors will permit combination with a delivery system to determine the optimal synthetic bone graft.

The approach will consist of determining the optimal dose of growth factors and BMPs by examining the osteogenic potency. The recombinant bone and morphogenetic factors should be combined with an appropriate delivery vehicle, and the rate and extent of new bone formation in orthotopic sites should be determined. New bone formation in the experimental nonunion should be evaluated by histomorphometric, biochemical, and biomechanical methods. Further improvements in the delivery system will be made by coating the delivery system matrix with collagens, laminin, and fibronectin to optimize cell attachment and proliferation.

Develop mesenchymal stem cells (MSCs) as a delivery system for introducing novel genes for growth and differentiation factors into synthetic bone grafts.

The emerging knowledge base concerning MSCs provides an opportunity to develop vehicles for gene therapy and gene delivery. The genes for bone growth and morphogenetic factors can be transfected stably into MSCs. This approach may have utility in locally enhancing bone production.

MSCs should be isolated from human marrow. Techniques should be optimized for stable transfection of genes for bone growth and differentiation factors. The secretion of transfected gene products will be determined and optimized. The local and systemic effects of transfected cells in appropriate animal models will be used to assess effects on bone formation. Finally, these cells can be used to test for function in bone grafts.

What are the roles of individual BMPs in bone regeneration?

Multiple families of bioactive factors are available for use in bone regeneration. These include fibroblast growth factors, insulin derived growth factors, platelet derived growth factors, transforming growth factors, and BMPs. Each factor, or type of factor, may have specific effects on cells responsible for bone regeneration, and multiple factors may need to be combined to produce an optimal result.

379

In order to determine the factors necessary/sufficient for bone regeneration, we need to systematically test individual factors in comparable systems to determine their regenerative capabilities alone, in combination with specialized matrices, and as part of bone regenerating devices. These data can then be used to distinguish between bioactive factors and how they can be used in optimal bone regeneration.

Determine physiologic roles for BMPs in skeletal and nonskeletal tissues.

Although BMPs were discovered based on their abilities to induce cartilage and bone formation, evidence now exists that these molecules may be of more fundamental importance during early stages of embryogenesis and also in organogenesis, which occurs later in fetal development.

Using transgenic mice in which loss or overexpression of individual BMPs or BMP-receptors have been engineered, we can begin to assign physiologic roles to individual BMP proteins and determine if specific BMPs are involved in development of one/more organ systems and, once organogenesis is complete, if BMPs play a necessary role in maintenance and repair of differentiated tissues. In addition, our ability to measure relative amounts of BMPs in extracellular matrices and in the circulation may allow us to understand regulation of BMP-responsive cell types in diseased states and aging.

What is the genetic basis for pathologically excessive or deficient bone repair?

Patients often have pathologically excessive or deficient bone. These individuals must be segregated into individual phenotypic groupings, not only to assist in their health-care management but also, and more importantly, to establish the genetic basis for accelerated or suboptimal bone repair. The genes that control such bone repair capacities must then be identified so that potential gene therapies can be established.

Careful clinical criteria must be established to identify different categories of bone repair capacity. In addition, long-term clinical records must be established and maintained for all individuals. Careful screening of such databases will allow for the identification of genes that control bone repair/regeneration.

Are there direct osteoinductive agents? Identify the agents that control individual steps along the osteogenic pathway. Optimize cell delivery vehicles for osteogenic repair.

MSCs can develop along one of several lineage pathways. It is essential to identify the agents that first induce these cells directly into the osteogenic pathway. The current data available do not allow us to conclude that the BMPs do not induce MSCs directly into osteoblasts. Even if BMPs are osteoinductive, it is possible that other osteogenic bioactive agents exist, and these agents should be discovered. Likewise, cells must progress through the osteogenic lineage to become secretory osteoblasts. The bioactive factors that control the osteogenic pathway must be identified in order to understand the molecular control and the dynamics of this pathway. Ultimately, it may be possible to deliver drugs (ie, bioactive factors) or cells treated with drugs to a bone repair site to optimize bone repair/regeneration. The identification of these factors and the appropriate drug/cell delivery vehicles must be the focus of future research.

With the availability of MSCs in culture, assays for osteoinduction can be and have been established. Dexamethasone, for example, has been identified as an osteogenic molecule in vitro. The details of this osteogenesis must be further established including an understanding of the newly synthesized molecules that result from dexamethasone exposure, especially bioactive agents, which may feed back onto the cells themselves to bring them further along the developmental process.

Cell-surface antigens and antibodies to these antigens of osteogenic cells in the osteogenic lineage must be identified as has been done for the chick. With these antibodies, pure populations of cells at specific lineage stages must be obtained. Such intermediate lineage stages can then be subjected to exposure to specific bioactive agents in order to move them further down the lineage. The identity and potency of these agents can then be established. Ultimately, the detailed molecular control of the entire pathway will be established.

With a clear understanding of the molecular control of the pathway of osteogenesis, from MSC to secretory osteoblast, delivery vehicles for MSCs or lineage progressed cells can be designed to facilitate bone repair. Such delivery vehicles must be able to hold cells in the proper orientation to support massive osteogenesis, rapid vascular permeation, and delivery of several bioactive agents to stimulate lineage progression and subsequent osteogenesis.

What is the best osteoinductor to be incorporated into the porous bone graft? What should be the levels and release profiles of these growth factors and of multiple growth factors? Encourage the exploration and development of new biodegradable synthetic bone grafts that might expand the applicability and complement the current polylactic-polyglycolic acids (PLGA) system.

The basic technology of fabricating a bone graft material that is porous with controlled architecture, that has controlled release capability, that has a range of biodegradation rates, and that is reasonably biocompatible can be formulated. Optimal bone graft design can be realized only if the basic information described in the first aim is available. With that information, the graft can be designed to meet the specifications. It is likely that for some applications the graft needs to have characteristics that are beyond the reach of the current PLGA system. We should, therefore, continue to explore and develop other new biodegradable synthetic graft materials that can broaden the range of physicochemical properties. In comparing different graft materials, we might also uncover new information or gain insight into the bone formation process as mediated by osteoinductive factors.

Bone cell biologists and biomaterials scientists should collaborate in tackling the first specific aim. Laboratories working on different matrix materials and growth factors should use a standard animal model so results can be compared in a meaningful way. A systematic study is needed to investigate in vivo release profiles of different growth factors, to determine the biodistribution of these growth factors, and to elucidate the influence of various matrix degradation rates on the bone formation process.

For the second specific aim, efforts should be placed on synthesizing bone graft materials that satisfy four basic requirements. The first is osteoconductivity, which allows construction of porous material with controlled pore size and pore size distribution. The graft should also have initial mechanical stability and an acceptable mechanical degradation profile. The second requirement is the ability to provide controlled release of biologically active molecules that promote bone regeneration. This is a fabrication issue on how to incorporate proteins into a porous structure without damaging their bioactivity. The ability to vary the release rate is more a materials chemistry consideration, as is the next requirement, biodegradability, which means the graft material should have an adjustable degradation rate as specified by the basic studies. The mode of degradation, homogeneous versus heterogeneous, should be clarified. The fourth requirement is biocompatability—compatability with soft and hard tissues as well as nontoxic breakdown products. Clarification/identification of the degradation products is required.

Establish the effects of polymer synthesis method, polymer composition, and polymer postsynthesis modification on cellular response in vitro/in vivo for poly(lactide-co-glycolide) (PLAGA) systems.

PLAGA systems usually are the degradable polymeric materials of choice for use in vitro and in vivo. It has been noted that in vitro growth of cells on polymeric materials based on PLAGA can be highly dependent not only on copolymer composition, but on material crystallinity and monomer sequence. In vivo it has been noted that implants of PLAGA under some conditions exhibit severe reactions during degradation. Mechanisms for these occurrences are unclear. The optimal PLAGA systems obviating these problems have yet to be reproducibly synthesized and fabricated.

The effects of polymer crystalline structure, polymer sequence distribution of monomers, and polymer synthesis modification should be examined systematically with the goal of achieving in vitro systems that allow cell attachment and growth in vivo without adverse histologic events. Once achieved, methods for reproducing this material in significant (large scale) quantities should be found, and methods to provide control during postsynthesis modification should be devised.

Elucidate the basic mechanisms by which cell-matrix interactions take place in vitro/in vivo during tissue regeneration.

In order to successfully design matrix materials that can either support the growth of cells or allow ingrowth of cells from surrounding tissue, a knowledge of the manner in which cells attach, spread, and grow, and possibly undergo changes in phenotype becomes important. For example, how do cells respond to changing shape and chemical environment in erodible systems? What phenotypic changes take place as cells proliferate in matrix systems? What are the characteristics (of the cell substrate) that allow cells to attach and grow?

Cell natural response would be measured in both in vitro (cell culture) and in vivo systems. Cellular expression of matrix attachment proteins should be performed, and the chemical nature of the interface characterized. Changes in the nature of the implant surface, eg, polymer chemical group expression, $CaPO_4$ composition in ceramic systems, should also be determined.

Identify how hydroxyapatite (HA) and osteoconduction facilitate bone regeneration.

Porous HA materials are thought to provide a framework that facilitates the regeneration of bone. Many studies have documented bone ingrowth into gap defects filled with porous HA implants. Woven bone first appears in apposition to the HA surfaces and subsequently remodels into mature bone. When compared to traditional gap defect controls—unprotected against soft-tissue prolapse—these porous implants have demonstrated greater bone regeneration. However, a number of studies have now been reported in which simple protection of gap defects against soft-tissue interposition, eg, guided tissue regeneration, has resulted in bone regeneration equal to or greater than that normally found on porous implants. The existence of an osteoconductive effect is thus now in question. Perhaps it is not the framework architecture, but the adsorption of growth factors, BMP, or cell adhesion molecules to the HA crystal that plays a dominant role in the ingrowth of these porous HA implants. Perhaps the availability of sufficient cells, factors, etc, in young animals makes osteoconduction unnecessary, whereas osteoconduction may play a facilitative role in the elderly or ill. Porous HA implants may play an important role as a delivery material for MSCs, BMPs, etc, and it may contribute to stability of a bone gap. But we should not attribute to these implants an osteoconductive effect without further study.

Defect Models. There is a need to better characterize and understand protected gap defect models. Gap defects of the cranium, mandible, radius, tibia, etc, are available and should be used to measure the amount of bone regeneration when protected against soft-tissue prolapse or interposition. It is suggested that in the presence of intact periosteum, a coarse titanium mesh would suffice. When periosteum is absent, a fine weave mesh may be preferable. The effect of age on protected gap defects should be determined. Because patients have compromising illnesses, animal models with diabetes mellitus or chemotherapeutic treatment should also be used. It should be determined if there is a "window of activation opportunity" after which bone regeneration will no longer take place in these potential gap models.

HA Implant Designs. There is a need to better characterize and understand the effect of different HA implant designs on bone regeneration when placed in the protected gap defect models previously defined. Sintered HA, coralline HA, and HA cement, for example, have different HA crystal sizes that may differ in their adsorption of BMPs, growth factors, other proteins, and in their adherence by cells. The effect of implant pore size on the cell's ability to regenerate cancellous or cortical bone morphology needs to be determined. The pore interconnectivity requirements or thresholds for sufficient vascular invasion to support bone regeneration remain to be determined. Substitutions with carbonate and phosphate should be characterized and their effect on bone regeneration measured in defined protected gap defect models. It has been reported that below a certain size, ie, HA granules rather than HA blocks, a multinucleated cell response is elicited. This size threshold remains to be determined. Finally, the addition of collagen, fibronectin, or laminin to provide cell adhesion should be explored. While the exciting activity in bone regeneration is undoubtedly the result of interactions between cells and their signals, a better understanding of gap defect biology and porous HA implants may increase our ability to clinically utilize these cells and factors.

Investigate the release profiles of bioactive factors (for example, a prototypic molecule such as BMP) from biocompatible, biodegradable delivery systems consistent with the wound healing milieu, eg, to design a delivery system with BMPs that is site-specific for particular needs.

Wound repair at different anatomic sites is affected by different physiologic factors, such as biomechanical function and vascularity. It is supposed, for example, that wounds in the head and neck, appendicular, and axial skeleton will have different requirements for healing gap and fracture wounds.

The goal is to determine if delivery system constructs need to be developed that possess different pharmacokinetic profiles to optimize release of the bioactive factor (or factors) within a certain window of opportunity based on the site of application.

The approach will consist of (1) preparing standardized, reproducible wounds in the appropriate animal model and progressing in a systematic manner to increasingly more physiologically complex species, from rat to nonhuman primate; (2) characterizing the appearance of cells and their products from both untreated and treated defects; (3) designing polymer constructs to release a payload at the appropriate time(s), dose, and duration to ensure bone regeneration as the delivery system biodegrades; and (4) modifying the construct by appropriate synthesis and postsynthesis modifications to fulfill the requirements of the site-specific wound healing milieu. The assessment of bone formation responses will be made by radiohistomorphometry, biochemistry, and histochemistry.

Section 5

Distraction Osteogenesis

Section Editors:
Thomas A. Einhorn, MD
Julie Glowacki, PhD

James Aronson, MD
Jeff Bonadio, MD
Susan V. Brooks, PhD
John A. Faulkner, PhD
André Gächter, MD
Julie Glowacki, PhD
Steven A. Goldstein, PhD
James A. Goulet, MD

Robert Guldberg, MD
Peter C.D. Macpherson, MA
Robert K. Schenk, MD
Laura Senunas, BS
Thomas G. Skoulis, MD
Harald Steen, MD, PhD
Julia Terzis, MD, PhD
Nicholas Waanders, MS

Chapter 27

Histology of Distraction Osteogenesis

Robert K. Schenk, MD
André Gächter, MD

Introduction

Bone tissue exhibits an astonishing regenerative potential and is able to restore its original structure and its mechanical properties almost completely. This capacity, however, has its limits. Factors that endanger or prevent bone repair are, among others, failure of vascularity, mechanical instability, oversized defects, and competing tissues of high proliferative activity. Promotion of callus formation, therefore, plays an important role in the healing of bone defects and in fracture treatment. Bone regeneration can be promoted by such well known principles as osteoinduction and osteoconduction, both of which are responsible for the success of autografts. In recent years, two other methods have been developed and promulgated with quite surprising results: guided bone regeneration and callus distraction. Guided bone regeneration promotes callus formation by using barrier membranes as protection against the invasion of competing, less differentiated tissues. It is discussed in chapter 8. Callus distraction produces even more spectacular results. This method has been systematically developed and perfected by Ilizarov[1-3] and has now gained widespread recognition and application in epiphyseal distraction, bone lengthening, and for bridging of large defects in long bones by segment transport.

Procedure

Numerous modifications of external fixators have been developed and recommended for callus distraction.[4] The fixators must ensure stability and should allow a controlled daily lengthening of 0.5 to 1 mm in small increments or, in case of motorized devices, as a continuous distraction.[5] First, the bone has to be cut in two by corticotomy or osteotomy. The corticotomy has been promulgated by Ilizarov.[1] For this method, the cortex is partially divided with a chisel and then fractured without disrupting the nutrient artery in the marrow cavity. More recent experiments have shown that complete transverse osteotomies function as well, in spite of the temporary interruption of the medullary circulation.[6,7] Distraction is started 5 to 10 days after stable fixation in a neutral position. This time interval allows for the invasion of the osteotomy gap by blood vessels and granulation tissue and the activation of woven bone formation along the cut surface of the host cortices.[2,8]

Radiographic Observations

Bone formation within the gradually widened gap can be monitored by radiographs (Fig. 1). In humans, calcification appears at 2 to 4 weeks, starting from

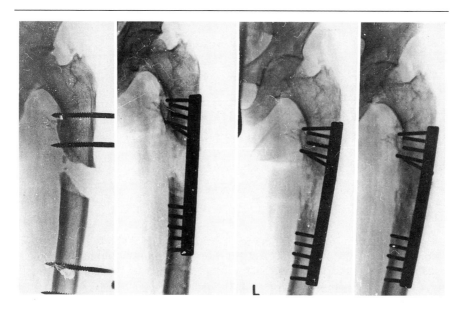

Fig. 1 Radiographs of a patient who underwent bone lengthening of his left femur. **Left,** The femur was transected by a corticotomy and distracted with a modified external fixator at a daily rate of 1 mm for 5 weeks, starting in the second week. **Left center,** Distraction was completed at 5 weeks, when a lengthening of about 30 mm was accomplished. The fixator was replaced by a plate that rigidly fixed the distracted fragment ends. Note the appearance of calcified areas in the distraction space. During this intervention a superficial biopsy was taken. **Right center,** Increased bone density at 3 months. **Right,** Dense bony regenerate at 6 months.

both bone ends and progressing toward a central radiolucent zone. The bony regenerate has a stringy appearance, indicating the formation of parallel columns and plates. They are elongated toward the interzone at a daily rate of up to 500 μm, which is surprisingly high. The radiolucent interzone persists as long as distraction continues, and is full only within weeks after cessation of distraction. On radiographic examination, the initial density of the newly formed bone tissue is low; it takes months for the tissue's compaction and possibly more than a year for the reconstruction of a true diaphysis. Weight-bearing, however, can start much earlier under the protection of the fixation device, and removal of the fixator is recommended before modeling and remodeling of the cortical bone are completed.

Histologic Observations

The light microscopic aspects of callus distraction were originally described by Ilizarov.[1,2] In numerous experiments on dogs, he established the optimal distraction rate; demonstrated the importance of stability; and analyzed the influence of the continuous stretching on angiogenesis, fibrous tissue and bone formation, and adaptive responses in muscles, nerves, vessels, and surrounding soft tissues.[1,2] Most of his observations have been confirmed by different authors in their reports of animal experiments,[6-12] human biopsies,[12-14] and a human amputation specimen.[15]

The radiolucent area represents microscopically a growth zone[9] or fibrous interzone,[11] and it functions as a center for fibroblast proliferation and fibrous tissue formation. The daily distraction aligns the collagen fibrils in parallel bundles that canalize the ingrowing vessels and the accompanying perivascular cells into longitudinal compartments. A microangiographic study shows that the invading vessels arise from both the periosteal envelope and the medullary system at the bone ends, and it confirms the fast revascularization of the bone marrow after osteotomy.[6]

Osteogenesis starts at the level of the cut bone ends. From there, woven bone trabeculae grow into the longitudinal interfibrillar compartments (Fig. 2). The formation of woven bone resembles intramembranous ossification. The osteoblasts are always located close to elongated capillaries, and the vascular net seems to determine the architecture of the growing bony scaffold as much as do the collagen fiber bundles. Whether woven bone trabeculae represent columns or plates is often difficult to decide based on longitudinal sections. Serial transverse sections of a human biopsy, starting in the fibrous interzone and approaching the ossification front, clearly show that the initial trabeculae appear as small columns with a pointed tip (Fig. 3). They measure about 100 μm in diameter; the conical tip is about 200 μm long. The shape is similar to that of a pencil. Each column is covered and lined by a layer of osteoblasts that is continuously supplemented from precursor cells. The cone consists solely of osteoid; mineralization starts in the center of its base. The columnar shape with a conical tip seen in scanning electron micrographs has been described earlier and was compared with stalagmites and stalactites.[10] The preformed and continuously stretched collagen fibers seem to act as a trellis for the advancing trabeculae. The tips of the advancing trabeculae grow preferentially in between the fibers. However, incorporation of collagen fibers also occurs, presumably into the circumferentially enlarging columns and plates.[10]

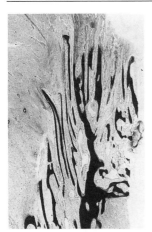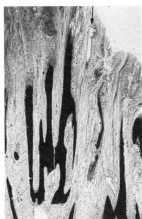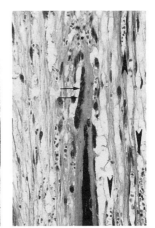

Fig. 2 Longitudinal sections through the distal segment of the distracted callus at 5 weeks (Microtome section, von Kossa stain). **Left,** From the distal fragment end (below), longitudinal bone columns grow out into the fibrous interzone (× 15). **Center,** Proximal ends of bone plates (or columns), growing between longitudinal collagen fiber bundles and blood vessels (arrow) (× 40). **Right,** Proximal tip of a column. Osteoclasts (arrows) line the osteoid surface; longitudinal capillaries are marked by arrowheads (× 250).

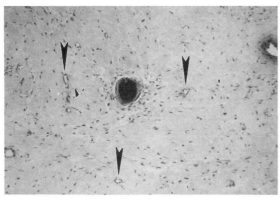

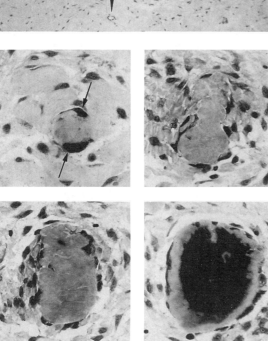

Fig. 3 Serial transverse sections at the borderline of the fibrous interzone 3 (von Kossa-McNeals tetrachrome stain). **Top,** Tip of an isolated column surrounded by fibrous tissue. Arrowheads point to cross sections of small vessels (× 80). **Center left,** Two osteoblasts (arrows) surround the pointed tip of the osteoid cone (× 260). **Center right,** Same column, 60 μm farther distally (× 260). **Bottom left,** Same column, 90 μm farther distally (× 260). **Bottom right,** Same column, 200 μm farther distally; note the mineralized core (× 260).

Toward the parent bone ends, the diameter of the columns increases. Adjacent trabeculae frequently melt into plates and walls that finally surround longitudinal vascular canals (Figs. 4 and 5). At the same time, the structure of the newly formed bone matures from the woven to the parallel-fibered type, and the overall density of the bony scaffold begins to increase.

This level of structural organization is reached after 4 to 6 weeks. The further development leads to a corticalization, ie, a narrowing of the vascular canals and formation of primary osteons by deposition of parallel-fibered and lamellar bone. This process is rather slow and shows a definite gradient from the bone ends toward the former radiolucent interzone. In dogs, formation of compact bone started at 3 months and was not fully achieved at 5 months after the lengthening period.[6] A similar time course was reported for a series of human biopsies.[13] In the radius of sheep, corticalization of the distracted segment was not completed within a follow-up period of up to 28 weeks.[12]

Haversian remodeling represents the last stage of cortical reconstruction. In humans, it begins at 4 months.[13] According to another report (based on an

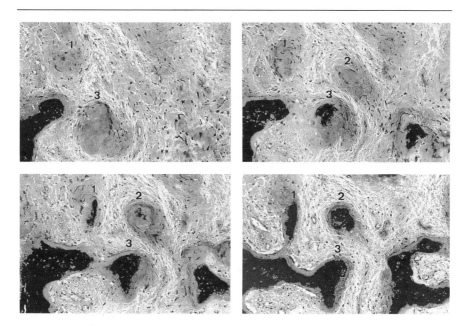

Fig. 4 Serial transverse section at steps of approximately 50 μm, showing the appearance of new columns (identified by numbers 1, 2, and 3), the beginning of their mineralization, and the fusion with neighboring columns that result in plate formation (von Kossa-McNeals tetrachrome, × 100).

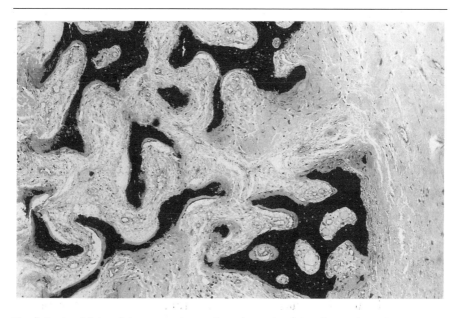

Fig. 5 In the vicinity of the parent bone, the columns have fused into plates that surround vascularized marrow spaces (× 40).

amputation specimen with an excessive segment transport over 15 cm), it has not yet started after 7 months.[15] From the well-known data about the basic metabolizing unit (BMU) dynamics, it is possible to predict that it certainly will take a year or more until a cortical structure comparable to the preexisting one is restored.

Alternative Routes and Complications

Whereas most authors agree with the concept that callus distraction leads to direct or intramembranous bone formation, some studies reveal at least a temporary cartilage or fibrocartilage differentiation and bone formation via the endochondral pathway. This has been documented mainly for rabbits.[7,9] However, cartilaginous nodules or islands and cartilage inclusions into newly formed bone also have been found in dogs[6] and sheep.[12] Ilizarov[1,2] considered cartilage formation an unmistakable indication of unstable fixation, and this may also be the case in some of the other experimental studies.[12] A local disturbance of the blood supply, resulting from ruptured blood vessels caused by extensive distraction, could also account for the appearance of cartilaginous islands, especially in earlier stages of stretching.[13] In later stages, a local ischemia is thought to be responsible for necrotic areas within the bony regenerate.[15]

Microfractures in the bony regenerate are another result of a too rapid distraction. The newly formed bony scaffold is a rather delicate structure and, toward the end of the distraction period, becomes more and more subjected to tensile forces.[13] Fissures and microfractures were a constant and conspicuous finding in a human amputation specimen retrieved at 7 months after a quite successful segment transport over a distance of 15 cm.[15] The microfractures seem to heal readily and without microcallus, and the authors consider this mechanism as a second route for distraction osteogenesis.

Comparative Aspects of Callus Distraction

At present, distraction osteogenesis is certainly the most impressive and, for many experts, unexpected manipulation of (bony) callus formation. The observation that bone formation in the adult organism can match with a daily distraction rate of about 1 mm (500 μm on each side) is indeed surprising, and asks for a comparison with the performance of other, more physiologic growth mechanisms, starting with the growth plate.

In higher mammals, and especially in humans, the growth rate stays far below such values. Rodents, however, come closer. A daily rate of more than 300 μm was measured in the proximal tibia of young rats. Chickens, which were selectively bred for rapid growth, reached values even above 1 mm. Growth cartilage is, indeed, a highly organized tissue. Its contribution to longitudinal growth is based on interstitial growth, ie, on cell proliferation, matrix production, and longitudinal stretching through cell hypertrophy.[16] Finally, a solid framework is elaborated by cartilage mineralization and continuously made available for the ingrowing bone-forming elements as a scaffold for vascular invasion and bone deposition.

The dynamics of bone formation, at this level, must be looked at in two directions. The bone apposition rate, ie, matrix formation and mineralization by osteoblasts, accounts only for the thickening of the primary trabeculae. The axial elongation of the trabeculae, however, depends on the recruitment of new osteoblasts from their precursors, ie, on cell proliferation and differentiation. It is unlikely that osteoblast recruitment is a limiting factor for longitudinal growth. Instead, this restriction is due to the time spent for elaboration of the calcified scaffold in the cartilaginous part of the growth plate. Attempts to speed up interstitial cartilage growth by gentle distraction, without causing an epiphysiolysis, have failed.[17]

Histologically, distraction osteogenesis resembles intramembranous or direct ossification. Intramembranous ossification occurs in three different modes. In early embryonic stages, it starts in the mesenchyme. In defect healing and fracture repair, it takes place in fibrovascular granulation tissues. Bone growth along ligament and tendon insertions and in delayed unions in the fracture gap also belongs to the category of intramembranous ossification. There are, however, quite important differences in the morphology and the dynamics of these modifications. In the mesenchyme and the fibrovascular granulation tissue, woven bone grows quite rapidly and forms a trabecular network or primary spongiosa, often without any incorporation of preexisting collagen fibers. At the site of ligament insertions, collagen fiber bundles are incorporated into the ossification front as Sharpey's fibers; the osteoblasts are pushed apart and become less numerous, resulting in a reduction of the apposition rate. A third modification is seen in tendon insertions; there, the tendon calcifies, and the calcified fibers are substituted by BMU-like elements. The osteoclastic resorption rate of 50 to 70 μm/day limits the daily progress in this type of bony substitution.

Mineralization of fibrous tissue in distraction epiphysiolysis has also been described.[18] In a careful experimental study, Monticelli and associates[19] practiced distraction lengthening in the proximal tibia of growing sheep. Distraction resulted first in an epiphysiolysis and formation of a hematoma. In the following weeks, the hematoma was replaced by fibrous tissue with longitudinally oriented fibers. Ossification started from periosteal elements and from the metaphyseal segment, and it replaced the fibrous tissue with bone. The overall architecture of the stretched collagen fiber bundles and the ingrowing trabeculae is identical to that seen in regular callus distraction. The electron microscope, however, revealed mineral clusters located within the collagen fibers and matrix vesicles possibly detached from degenerating fibroblasts. Subsequently, bone is deposited on a core of mineralized fibrous tissue that is similar to the calcified cartilage cores in the primary spongiosa underneath a growth plate. At present, it is not clear whether this type of ossification, via calcified fibrous tissue, occurs in distraction epiphysiolysis only or also is involved in callus distraction in the adult.

Conclusions

Bony callus formation can be promoted by distraction if stable fixation and a controlled daily distraction of 0.5 to 1 mm is achieved by appropriate external fixators. After corticotomy or osteotomy, the fragments are rigidly fixed in a neutral position for 7 to 10 days, thus allowing the organization of the interfragmentary hematoma and the activation of woven bone formation. Distraction primarily affects angiogenesis and fibrous tissue formation in the continuously widened gap. The tensile forces align the collagen fiber bundles and the outgrowing capillaries longitudinally. Woven bone formation starts in contact with the cut bone surfaces, and it is further canalized by the preformed longitudinal compartment. The columnar trabeculae are elongated at a rate of up to 500 μm/day from both sides toward the fibrous interzone. The fibrous interzone acts as a growth center as long as distraction proceeds. After cessation of distraction, it is replaced by bone. In the following months, the initially formed, rather delicate bony scaffold is reinforced by parallel-fibered and lamellar bone; cortical bone and the marrow cavity are restored; and the bone structure is finally normalized by haversian remodeling. The formation of secondary osteons begins in the fourth to sixth month and continues throughout the following years.

Bone formation in the distracted area follows the pattern of intramembranous ossification. Cartilage formation and endochondral ossification are occasionally reported and are explained by insufficient stability or by local ischemia resulting from vascular damage caused by excessive distraction. Whether fissures and microfractures and their subsequent healing contribute as an alternative route to the bone lengthening has to be clarified.

References

1. Ilizarov GA: The tension-stress effect on the genesis and growth of tissues: Part I. The influence of stability of fixation and soft tissue preservation. *Clin Orthop* 1989; 238:249–281.
2. Ilizarov GA: The tension-stress effect on the genesis and growth of tissues: Part II. The influence of the rate and frequency of distraction. *Clin Orthop* 1989;239:263–285.
3. Ilizarov GA: Clinical application of the tension-stress effect for limb lengthening. *Clin Orthop* 1990;250:8–26.
4. Paterson D: Leg-lengthening procedures. A historical review. *Clin Orthop* 1990; 250:27–33.
5. Korzinek K, Tepic S, Perren SM: Battery driven external fixator for continuous bone lengthening. SICOT 90/XVIII Congres International Montreal, 1990, p 499.
6. Delloye C, Delefortrie G, Coutelier L, et al: Bone regenerate formation in cortical bone during distraction lengthening: An experimental study. *Clin Orthop* 1990; 250:34–42.
7. Kojimoto H, Yasui N, Goto T, et al: Bone lengthening in rabbits by callus distraction: The role of periosteum and endosteum. *J Bone Joint Surg* 1988;70B:543–549.
8. White SH, Kenwright J: The timing of distraction of an osteotomy. *J Bone Joint Surg* 1990;72B:356–361.
9. Alho A, Bang G, Karaharju E, et al: Filling of a bone defect during experimental osteotaxis distraction. *Acta Orthop Scand* 1982;53:29–34.
10. Aronson J, Harrison BH, Stewart CL, et al: The histology of distraction osteogenesis using different external fixators. *Clin Orthop* 1989;241:106–116.
11. Aronson J, Good B, Stewart C, et al: Preliminary studies of mineralization during distraction osteogenesis. *Clin Orthop* 1990;250:43–49.
12. Peltonen JI, Kahri AI, Lindberg LA, et al: Bone formation after distraction osteotomy of the radius in sheep. *Acta Orthop Scand* 1992;63:599–603.
13. Lascombes P, Membre H, Prévot J, et al: Histomorphométrie du régénérat osseux dans les allongements des membres selon la technique d'Ilizarov. (English translation: Histomorphometry of bone regenerate in limb lengthening by the Ilizarov's technique.) *Rev Chir Orthop* 1991;77:141–150.
14. Tajana GF, Morandi M, Zembo MM: The structure and development of osteogenetic repair tissue according to Ilizarov technique in man: Characterization of extracellular matrix. *Orthopedics* 1989;12:515–523.
15. Shearer JR, Roach HI, Parsons SW: Histology of a lengthened human tibia. *J Bone Joint Surg* 1992;74B:39–44.
16. Hunziker EB, Schenk RK, Cruz-Orive LM: Quantitation of chondrocyte performance in growth-plate cartilage during longitudinal bone growth. *J Bone Joint Surg* 1987;69A:162–173.
17. Kenwright J, Spriggins AJ, Cunningham JL: Response of the growth plate to distraction close to skeletal maturity: Is fracture necessary? *Clin Orthop* 1990;250: 61–72.
18. Vauhkonen M, Peltonen J, Karaharju E, et al: Collagen synthesis and mineralization in the early phase of distraction bone healing. *Bone Miner* 1990;10:171–181.
19. Monticelli G, Spinelli R, Bonucci E: Distraction epiphysiolysis as a method of limb lengthening: II. Morphologic investigations. *Clin Orthop* 1981;154:262–273.

Chapter 28
Inflammation and Bone Formation

Julie Glowacki, PhD

Introduction

Tissue Repair

Some features of the healing of bone fractures are similar to those of the process of soft-tissue repair; however, bone has some unique properties that contribute to its remarkable regenerative capacity. Simple forms of life can regenerate complex organs with great fidelity. In higher vertebrates, simple tissues, such as epithelium, connective tissue, and fat, can regenerate; injured organs heal by forming fibrous scar tissue. Although scar tissue does provide for rapid restoration of physical integrity, it does not reestablish the functional properties of the soft tissue it replaces. Currently, principles of wound closure and management are directed at maximal control of the properties of scar tissue. In some situations, fibrosis may be uncontrolled and may lead to serious complications, for example, the formation of abdominal adhesions. On the other hand, insufficient fibrosis may be encountered in chronic and infected dermal wounds. Treatment with growth factors may have potential to ameliorate some of these problems. There is intense research interest in promoting true regeneration of tissues (fascia, tendon) and complex organs (skin, viscera) by exploiting both natural factors and processes that occur in embryogenesis.

Bone tissue undergoes true regeneration rather than simple repair. Although limbs do not regenerate in humans as they do in newts, the characteristic organizational structure, including marrow components, of human osseous tissue can be restored. The skeleton provides a mobilizable reservoir of minerals that can be regulated for mineral homeostasis. The metabolic activity of bone as a tissue sustains its regenerative capacity. The cellular nature of bone gives this tissue properties that allow its successful participation in calcium homeostasis (Fig. 1). The exchange of calcium occurs across lining cells that cover bone surfaces and extend into the canalicular system, thereby linking osteocytes to the vascular supply. In addition, the bone remodeling system contributes to

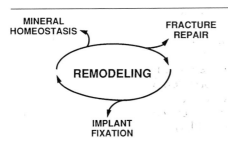

Fig. 1 Central role of bone remodeling in mediating mineral homeostasis, regeneration of bone in fracture repair, and integration with implants.

395

mineral metabolism by the coordinated activity of bone-resorbing osteoclasts and bone-forming osteoblasts.

These vital properties of bone tissue are best appreciated by comparing them with properties of the acellular bone that is found in many teleosts. In these fish, mineral metabolism is regulated primarily by gills, kidney, and skin. Exchange occurs minimally, if at all, in the bones. Bone is produced by the polarized activity of osteoblastic cells, which do not become contained as a network of mature osteocytes. It has been proposed that the acellular, or anosteocytic, quality of such teleost bone is the consequence of diminished reliance on the skeleton as a mineral reserve.

Bone Repair

Just as cellularity confers on bone the capacity to remodel and contribute to mineral homeostasis, it also confers bone with the ability to heal and to incorporate bone grafts and implants. Piscine acellular bone is slower and more limited in healing than fish cellular bone.[1]

Primary fracture repair occurs when the fracture is stable and closely aligned. Treatment with immobilization and anatomic alignment, when possible, can achieve the conditions required for primary union. Cortical repair begins with vigorous osteoclastic resorption of necrotic bone in structures similar to cutting cones. Osteoblasts follow to form new osteons across the gap. These cellular processes are similar to those that contribute to bone remodeling and homeostasis.

Vertebrate bone heals in the face of motion; the rationale for immobilization is to prevent tearing of new vessels and continuous clot formation. The blood supply to cortical bone derives from vessels in the haversian canal. Even a small fracture can form a large hematoma in surrounding tissues. In soft tissue, the clot provides a scaffold for formation of granulation tissue. In fractures, the clot does not appear to be part of callus formation and may, in fact, provide a barrier to repair. The acute inflammatory phase of traumatic repair begins with fibrinous exudate and cellular infiltration. Polymorphonuclear leukocytes are not numerous in the absence of infection. Interruption of vascular integrity across a fracture compromises the nourishment and vitality of proximal bone and marrow cells. Successful healing of fractures depends on the right sequence of cells entering the wound microenvironment, including mast cells, lymphocytes, monocytes, and macrophages.

Inflammation

As with soft tissues, injury of bone usually is followed by some degree of inflammation. In the early stage of secondary repair, disruption of the vascular supply and hematoma formation are accompanied by hypoxia and acidification. Mast cells contribute heparin and vasoactive substances to increase vascular permeability acutely. Proteolysis and kinin release contribute to the synthesis of prostaglandins, primarily PGE_1 and PGE_2, by injured cells. The multiple actions of the prostaglandins include increasing vascular permeability, promoting leukocyte migration by their chemotactic activity, and stimulating the production of extracellular matrix molecules. Subsequent repair of soft-tissue injuries depends on cellular and vascular proliferation, which results in development of granulation tissue. As in other settings, angiogenesis begins with sprouting of endothelial cells from capillaries and small venules.

Fetal soft-tissue wound repair is fundamentally different from that which occurs postnatally.[2-6] Midgestational fetal wounds heal by regeneration rather than by scar formation. There appears to be little or no inflammatory cell infiltrate. It is thus hypothesized that inflammation contributes to scarification in order to provide for rapid restoration of physical integrity at the expense of the more gradual and deliberate interactions needed for morphogenesis and regeneration.

The initial phases of some examples of bone repair also involve aspects of acute inflammatory processes. It is not clear, however, to what extent and in which situations inflammatory cells contribute to, or are necessary for, bone regeneration. Similar acute inflammatory changes accompany necrosis of bone and marrow. The death of these tissues is ischemic in origin and rapid in onset. Capillary sprouts invade the wounded area and expand the vascular network needed to support the proliferation of reactive tissue, which precedes osteogenic activity. The analogy to soft-tissue repair may collapse if inflammation promotes rapid closure and scarification of soft-tissue wounds at the expense of tissue regeneration, which is observed in hard-tissue repair.

Some information is available concerning the effects of anti-inflammatory agents on bone healing. For example, various models show different effects of indomethacin. It has been shown to delay fracture healing as evaluated by histologic and biomechanical parameters.[7,8] Although indomethacin had no effect at early time points, it inhibited bony ingrowth into porous implants after 8 weeks.[9] Indomethacin was reported to inhibit induced osteogenesis in rats if treatment was initiated before implantation of the demineralized bone.[10] It was concluded, therefore, that the early migration and activation of polymorphonuclear leukocytes are essential for the sequence of induced bone formation. It is likely, however, that the early elements of experimentally induced heterotopic osteogenesis differ from skeletal differentiation, fracture healing, and bony ingrowth in response to implants.

The rapidity and fidelity of postnatal bone repair are impressive, especially when compared with soft-tissue repair. Younger bone generally is thought to regenerate more rapidly than the mature skeleton. The fetal lamb model provides an opportunity to understand the biology of immature tissues and to define components that differ in juvenile, adult, and senile phases of life. Although no definitive comparable data were available, a recent study showed that fetal bone healing appeared to be rapid.[11] Moreover, there was no evidence of hematoma, inflammation, or external callus. These observations challenge the presumed importance of inflammation in bone regeneration. If substantiated in postnatal bone, this idea could sharply modify the rationale for therapies to augment bone repair and osteointegration.

The preliminary studies reported here provide information on the effects of frank inflammation on bone repair and on demineralized bone powder (DBP)-induced osteogenesis in rats. These models may be suitable for answering questions about the precise qualitative and quantitative aspects of inflammatory processes that influence bone formation.

Materials and Methods

Rat Tibial Repair Model

Effects of inflammatory materials on osteogenesis were evaluated in a rat tibial defect model. A 2-mm diameter, unicortical defect was constructed 5 mm below the proximal epiphyseal cartilage plates in the tibias of 3-month-old male rats

(CD strain, Charles River Laboratories, MA) that had been anesthetized by methoxyflurane inhalation. A 2-mm drill bit was used to create a standard defect in the flat lateral surface of the bone. A dental amalgam carrier was used to implant particulate materials into the defect. Test materials included ceramic hydroxyapatite (CHA), tricalcium phosphate (β-TCP), synthetic bone-like apatite (Ap), resorbable calcium phosphate (CP), polymethylmethacrylate (PMMA), and polyethylene (PE). The periosteum and soft-tissue envelope were reapproximated with sutures, and the skin was closed with two 9-mm stainless steel clips.

At intervals after implantation, the proximal tibias were harvested and fixed for 2 days in 2% paraformaldehyde in 0.1 M cacodylate buffer, pH 7.4. Some samples were decalcified with 7.5% ethylenediaminetetraacetic acid (EDTA) in the same buffer before being embedded in glycol methacrylate. Three-micrometer cross sections through the defect were stained with toluidine blue and for tartrate-resistant acid phosphatase (TRAP) activity. Sections were assessed histomorphometrically for bridging of the osseous defect and tissue responses to materials.

Osteogenesis Induced by Demineralized Bone Particles

Demineralized bone powder (DBP), 75 to 250 mm, was prepared from long bones of 3- to 4-month-old rats. The DBP was mixed in 3:1 volume ratios with collagen, gelatin, polylactic acid, polysebacic acid, polycarboxyphenoxypropane, or similarly sized β-TCP and PMMA. Materials were deposited into subcutaneous pockets constructed bilaterally in the ventral thoracic region. Reactive tissues were harvested 14 days after implantation and prepared as described above for nondecalcified histology in glycol methacrylate.

Cellular Responses to Particles in Vitro

Balb/c monocyte/macrophage cell line J774A.1 (American Type Culture Collection, Rockville, MD) was maintained in Dulbecco's minimal essential medium (MEM), 10% heat-inactivated fetal bovine serum, 100 U/ml penicillin, and 100 μg/ml streptomycin sulfate. Human dermal fibroblasts were established as outgrowth cultures from foreskin tissue of a 7-year-old child, were maintained in Dulbecco's MEM formulation (10% fetal bovine serum supplemented with 0.292 mg/ml gultamine, 100 U/ml penicillin, and 100 μg/ml streptomycin sulfate), and were used between the third and tenth passages. DBP, 53 to 75 mm, was prepared from rat bone in a manner similar to that described for larger powders.[12] PMMA particles were prepared by polymerization of surgical bone cement in thin strands; the strands were cryofractured, and particles measuring 53 to 75 μm were collected by sieving.

For analysis of attachment, 2×10^5 cells were incubated with 5-mg particles for 2 hours at 37°C. Unattached cells were separated by density centrifugation over Histopaque 1077 (Sigma, St. Louis); the cells were counted, and the percentage of attached cells was calculated relative to the number of cells recovered from controls without particles. Particles were also processed for scanning electron microscopy following fixation, dehydration, mounting on double-faced tape, and sputter-coating with gold.

Results

Tibial Wound Repair

A time-course study of defects that were left empty showed exuberant healing. At 3 days after surgery, the marrow space was filled with organized clot and fine trabeculae of mineralized bone. After 7 days, the marrow space was filled with trabecular bone. By 10 days, the trabecular bone was covered with osteoclasts. After 14 days, the medullary cavity was reduced, osteoclastic activity was still evident, and the cortical gap was completely bridged. After 28 days, the cortex was reorganized into lamellar bone, and the marrow space was repopulated with marrow.

Implantation with CHA did not interfere with osseous repair, and each particle of CHA was incorporated into the reactive bone without evidence of interposing fibrous tissue. If the defects were filled with particulate PMMA, PE, CP, β-TCP, or bone-like apatite, spontaneous regeneration was impaired (Table 1). Only half the animals treated with PMMA demonstrated bony regeneration; each particle of PMMA was surrounded by a fibrous layer interposed between the bone and the particles. A greater inflammatory response was elicited by PE, and there was even less bone formation than with PMMA. Resorbable CPs generated greater inflammatory reactions with less bone formation, and complete inhibition of cortical bridging. In a preliminary study in which 0.65 mg of flurbiprofen was placed in each implant of CP, the defects showed enhanced bone formation (Table 2). These initial results suggest the possibility that local administration of anti-inflammatory agents would inhibit inflammation and permit bone healing.

Table 1 Cortical bone repair 10 days after tibial wounding

Implant*	Bone Fill (% of defect area)**
Empty	96.5 ± 1.6
PMMA	96.3 ± 2.9
CHA	71.6 ± 12.4
β-TCP	64.0 ± 18.1
PE	48.0 ± 16.6
Apatite	48.0 ± 13.5
CP	22.1 ± 20.2

* CHA = ceramic hydroxyapatite; PMMA = polymethylmethacrylate; β-TCP = tricalcium phosphate; PE = polyethylene; and CP = resorbable calcium phosphate.
** Mean ± standard deviation

Table 2 Effect of flurbiprofen on tibial defects

Implant	Medullary Response, Day 10
Empty	Woven bone
Resorbable calcium phosphate	Inflammation, fibrosis
Resorbable calcium phosphate + 0.65 mg flurbiprofen	Woven bone

Ectopic Osteoinduction

Subcutaneous implantation of DBP alone elicited endochondral osteogenesis in rats. Admixtures of DBP with collagen were also osteoinductive. When DBP was mixed with PMMA in a three-to-one ratio, bone induction was totally inhibited, and local inflammation was induced (Outline 1). Large, multinucleated tartrate-resistant acid phosphatase-negative macrophage polykaryons were associated with the PMMA particles throughout the implant. Mixtures of DBP with gelatin, resorbable CP, and other polymers also elicited an inflammatory response with no evidence of bone formation. Thus, in this system, inflammatory responses abolished the osteoinductive potential of demineralized bone. Histologic examination of earlier samples revealed a lack of mesenchymal-cell attachment to the particles of DBP in a polymorphonuclear leukocytic infiltrate. This observation raised the possibility that mesenchymal attachment is an important part of the DBP-induction process.

In one study, the nonsteroidal anti-inflammatory drug (NSAID), flurbiprofen (FL), was added to DBP and to the DBP/PMMA mixtures. The FL had no effect on DBP alone. When FL was combined with the DBP/PMMA mixture, there was no evidence of inflammation, bone formation was vigorous, and the particles of PMMA were incorporated within the induced bone. Some multinucleated cells were present at 3 weeks, but bone formation was no longer blocked by the PMMA-related inflammatory reaction in six of eight samples. This effect was similar to the ameliorating effect of flurbiprofen on impaired osteogenesis in tibial defects.

Specificity of Cellular Attachment in Vitro

Cellular attachment was examined in vitro to characterize the specificity of interactions between cells and osteoinductive DBP or inflammatory PMMA. Dermal fibroblasts and J774A.1 monocytes attached very differently to DBP and PMMA particles. Within 2 hours, > 80% of dermal fibroblasts attached to both DBP and PMMA (Table 3). Less than 15% of the J774A.1 monocytes attached to DBP, and 90% attached to PMMA. Scanning electron microscopy indicated that fibroblasts were well spread on DBP, but were more compact on PMMA (Fig. 2, *top*). Monocytes were adherent to PMMA and appeared activated (Fig. 2, *bottom*). Although some inflammatory cells may be elicited by DBP implants in vivo, the early attachment of mesenchymal cells is a notable feature of the subcutaneous implantation site. The differential attractions of fibroblasts and monocytes to DBP and PMMA in vitro may elucidate the in

Outline 1 Materials that inhibit demineralized bone powder-induced osteogenesis*

Gelatin
Polymethylmethacrylate
Polylactic acid
Polysebacic acid
Polycarboxyphenoxypropane
Resorbable tricalcium phosphate

* Materials were mixed with demineralized bone powder (DBP) in 1:3 composites prior to subcutaneous implantation in rats. Bone induction was assayed histologically 14 days after implantation. Positive control was 1:3 composite of collagen: DBP.

Table 3 Percent attachment of cells to particles after 2 hours

Cells	DBP*	PMMA*
Human dermal fibroblasts	91.6 ± 0.6	79.9 ± 0.6
Mouse monocytes J744A.1	14.3 ± 7.0	90.6 ± 0.3

*DBP = demineralized bone tissue; PMMA = polymethylmethacrylate.

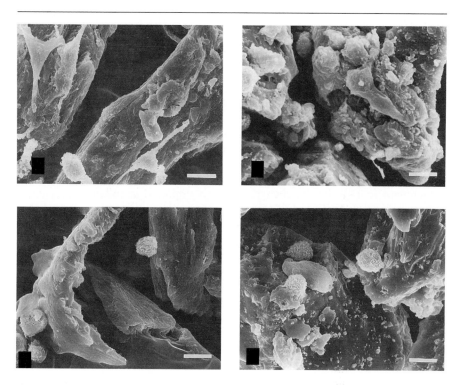

Fig. 2 Scanning electron micrographs of human dermal fibroblasts attached to demineralized bone powder (DBP) **(top left)**, or polymethylmethacrylate (PMMA) **(top right)**, and of murine monocytes J 774A.1 on DBP **(bottom left)** or PMMA **(bottom right)**. Bars represent 10 μm.

vivo results obtained using admixtures of DBP with inflammatory materials. The attachment of target mesenchymal cells to the particles of DBP is likely to be essential for initiating their induction into skeletal cells.

Discussion

Although the role of inflammation in bone repair has been investigated, whether some components of inflammation are necessary for healing and the circumstances under which inflammatory components are inhibitory remain unclear. In my laboratory, models have been developed to examine the influence of various degrees of inflammation of (1) spontaneous bony repair of tibial defects in rats and (2) ectopic osteogenesis induced by DBP. The model of spontaneous bone healing is characterized by distinct stages of medullary and periosteal woven bone formation, bone resorption and remodeling, and repair of the cortical defect and repopulation of marrow. The reproducibility of the model allows the investigation of regulation of these stages and the determination of osteocompatible properties of bone substitute materials. Although an inflammatory phase is part of the normal bone-healing process, excess inflammation provoked by particulate materials impairs bone formation. The model may be useful for screening agents that may modulate local inflammatory and osteogenic processes. The possibility for local pharmacologic management of peri-implant inflammatory responses to wear debris may be supported by these findings.

In these studies no evidence was seen of untoward effects of the NSAID on bone repair, but it would not be unexpected if different doses were inhibitory. It also is possible that different drugs or drug cocktails would be even more effective in inhibiting inflammation and resorption while promoting bone formation. Modulation of the surfaces of implant materials to inhibit attachment and activation of monocytes would also be beneficial. DBP-induced osteogenesis was inhibited by admixture with several inflammatory materials. Osteogenesis was restored when an NSAID was added to the implant. This preliminary study does not show whether higher doses of the drug would block osteogenesis. The attraction of fibroblasts for DBP compared to that of monocytes suggests that attachment may be an important part of the induction phenomenon. Attachment to DBP by mesenchymal cells is impaired in inflammatory composite implants in vivo, and this impairment may be explained by altered chemotaxis or changes in binding sites. An important question remains: could local pharmacologic treatment of inflammation be beneficial in certain osseous defects or around orthopaedic or dental implants? Flurbiprofen has been shown to be beneficial in retarding the inflammatory bone loss associated with periodontal disease.[13]

Some aspects of inflammation or cellular infiltrate are expected to be more important in the initiation of an osteoinductive response to DBP than they are in fracture repair. In a recent report of a study in which DBP was inserted into experimental defects along cranial sutures in fetal rabbits, an osteoinductive response did not occur in utero but was delayed until 2 weeks postpartum.[14] This result is in contrast to accelerated fetal fracture repair during a similar period and could be explained if DBP-induced osteogenesis required a component of the postnatal inflammatory system not required for fracture healing. The precise characterization of this component is not provided by the studies reported herein, but it should be possible.

These studies show that local tissue responses can be modulated to promote osteogenesis. Such a rationale may have applications in managing or preventing focal inflammatory osteolysis, nonunion, or pathologic reactions to implants. These models allow the opportunity to characterize precisely the cellular and molecular components necessary for optimal bone regeneration. Full understanding is needed for rational design of interventional treatments to avoid any risk of untoward consequences.

Acknowledgments

This research was supported in part by NIH grant #AR31330. I would like to thank S. Zelicof, MD, B.P. Perona, MD, S. Marcus, and C. Quinto for their important contributions to these studies.

References

1. Moss ML: Studies of the acellular bone of teleost fist: II. Response to fracture under normal and acalcemic conditions. *Acta Anat* 1962;48:46–60.
2. Adzick NS, Harrison MR, Glick PL, et al: Comparison of fetal, newborn, and adult wound healing by histologic, enzyme-histochemical, and hydroxyproline determinations. *J Pediatr Surg* 1985;20:315–319.
3. Longaker MT, Harrison MR, Crombleholme TM, et al: Studies in fetal wound healing: I. A factor in fetal serum that stimulates deposition of hyaluronic acid. *J Pediatr Surg* 1989;24:789–792.
4. Longaker MT, Harrison MR, Langer JC, et al: Studies in fetal wound healing: II. A fetal environment accelerates fibroblast migration in vitro. *J Pediatr Surg* 1989; 24:793–798.
5. Longaker MT, Whitby DJ, Ferguson MWJ, et al: Studies in fetal wound healing: III. Early deposition of fibronectin distinguishes fetal from adult wound healing. *J Pediatr Surg* 1989;24:799–805.
6. Longaker MT, Chiu ES, Harrison MR, et al: Studies in fetal wound healing: IV. Hyaluronic acid-stimulating activity distinguishes fetal wound fluid from adult wound fluid. *Ann Surg* 1989;210:667–672.
7. Elves MW, Bayley I, Roylance PJ: The effect of indomethacin upon experimental fractures in the rat. *Acta Orthop Scand* 1982;53:35–41.
8. Ro J, Sudmann E, Marton PF: Effect of indomethacin on fracture healing in rats. *Acta Orthop Scand* 1976;47:588–599.
9. Keller JC, Trancik TM, Young FA, et al: Effects of indomethacin on bone ingrowth. *J Orthop Res* 1989;7:28–34.
10. DiCesare PE, Nimi ME, Peng L, et al: Effects of indomethacin on demineralized bone-induced heterotopic ossification in the rat. *J Orthop Res* 1991;9:855–861.
11. Longaker MT, Moelleken BRW, Cheng JC, et al: Fetal fracture healing in a lamb model. *Plast Reconstr Surg* 1992;9:161–171.
12. Glowacki J, Muliken JB: Demineralized bone implants. *Clin Plast Surg* 1985;12: 233–241.
13. Williams RC, Jeffcoat MK, Kaplan ML, et al: Flurbiprofen: A potent inhibitor of alveolar bone resorption in beagles. *Science* 1985;227:640–642.
14. Duncan BW, Adzick NS, Moelleken BRW, et al: An in utero model of craniosynostosis. *J Craniofacial Surg* 1992;3:70–78.

Chapter 29

Stress Morphology Relationships During Distraction Osteogenesis: Linkages Between Mechanical and Architectural Factors in Molecular Regulation

Steven A. Goldstein, PhD
Nicholas Waanders, MS
Robert Guldberg, MS
Harald Steen, MD, PhD
Laura Senunas, BS
James A. Goulet, MD
Jeff Bonadio, MD

Introduction

Throughout the past century, mechanical factors have been considered to have a potent influence on the evolution, formation, and adaptation of bone. Although the principles that relate physical forces to bone response have been used clinically for centuries, it was not until the late 1800s that German anatomists and engineers graphically conceived of the coincidence between trabecular architecture and the presumed principal stress directions that occur during physiologic function.[1,2] This phenomenon, which has become known as Wolff's law, proposes that bone structure is related to the applied loads by mathematical functions. While generally accepted, the law was not based on any formal mathematical quantification, nor was it based on any proposed mechanisms of action. As a result, many investigators have designed both experimental and analytic studies to evaluate the parameters that might relate physical forces to bone adaptation.[2-20]

The incentive for these investigations is the desire to optimize surgical or pharmaceutical intervention for treatment of skeletal trauma or disease, or to predict the onset of skeletal fragility. For example, the treatment of fractures and the response to implants, such as total joint arthroplasties, may depend on specific local responses to mechanical factors. Despite intense investigative efforts dedicated to elucidating the critical parameters associated with mechanically mediated bone formation, the difficulties associated with quantifying or controlling the nature of the mechanical stimulant has slowed progress. Estimating boundary conditions and accounting for the heterogeneous anisotropic material properties of bone have made analytic modeling procedures difficult. Biologic factors have been equally difficult to separate, because bone formation has been documented to occur in the face of very different initiating events. The challenge in continuing and future studies, therefore, is to implement precise control over the mechanical boundary conditions while monitoring the pattern of bone formation temporally. This chapter presents our experience with two models of distraction osteogenesis as means for controlling and perturbing the mechanical environment within a site of active bone formation.

Clinical experience during the past several years has demonstrated that the technique of distraction osteogenesis can reliably use an external fixator to control displacement at an osteotomy site that retains the ability to generate new bone.[21-29] The treatment of fractures, pseudarthroses, osteomyelitis, limb length discrepancies, and deformities has been managed effectively with a variety of devised configurations. Common to many of these procedures is the principle of regulated moderate distraction. Factors that have been shown to contribute to clinical outcome include osteotomy technique, frame mechanics, distraction rate, and limb usage patterns. Although the clinical utility of this technique has been extensively explored, only recently have systematic investigations been designed to isolate and evaluate the relationship between these factors and the course of clinical treatment.

Bone formation in distraction osteogenesis has been reported to be primarily intramembranous. Using a canine model, Aronson and associates[21,22] broadly describe the radiographic and histologic appearance of the regenerated bone in the distraction gap. During the first week of distraction, little bone is observed; whereas at 2 weeks, new bone extends toward the center of the gap from both the proximal and distal osteotomy surfaces. With continual distraction, the new bone continues to extend from the osteotomy surfaces into a central radiolucent interzone. Histologic examination demonstrates that the most active formation occurs at the interface between the newly formed bone and the fibrous interzone. Higher magnification shows thin trabeculae within oriented fibrous tissue with abundant vascular channels. Only sparse evidence of cartilage formation has been documented.[21,22,27]

Based on clinical and experimental work with distraction osteogenesis, we tested the hypothesis that, as an experimental tool, the technique would provide an opportunity to study bone formation under a controlled mechanical environment. Our program of investigation has focused on six specific questions: (1) What are the mechanical characteristics of the external fixator? (2) How does the fixator interact with the bone and the distraction gap tissue? (3) What forces act in vivo to create the mechanical environment in the distraction gap? (4) What is the pattern of bone formation in distraction osteogenesis? (5) What cell types and processes contribute to the bone formation? (6) How can the mechanical environment influence/stimulate/direct the process of bone formation in the distraction gap?

Mechanical Characteristics of the External Fixator

The role of the external fixator is to maintain alignment of the proximal and distal bone segments, to distract the osteotomy site, and (in theory) to provide a mechanical environment that permits osteogenesis. For most clinical applications, the predominate loading mechanism is in the axial direction (muscle contractions, body weight in ambulation, lifting of loads); therefore, we have focused on axial load characteristics of the external fixators.

External fixators (both Ilizarov and conventional monolateral fixators) are made of two major types of hardware. First, there are the components that form the external structure, namely the rings, threaded rods, side bars, distractors, and so forth. This external structure is generally very rigid. The second set of components consists of the wires and pins, which form the interface between the bone and the external structure. These elements are the weak (or low stiffness) link in the system and determine the mechanical properties of the external fixator as a whole. The mechanical properties of isolated tensioned wires have been investigated in previous studies and reported to be nonlinear under large loads.[22] However, under lower loads, the wires demonstrate a relatively linear response. Mechanical testing in our laboratory of a large number of frame configurations has allowed us to generate graphs estimating the contribution of individual wires and half pins to the axial stiffness of the frames, based on the span length of the wire or half pin. Using these graphs (Fig. 1), it is possible to estimate the axial stiffness of any Ilizarov fixator as a summation of the stiffness contributions of each of the wires and half pins.

Interaction of Fixator and Gap Tissue

As load is applied to the bone segments (due to muscle contraction or external loads), force is transferred from the distal segment to the distal wires, through the frame, to the proximal wires and the proximal bone segment. The amount of load transferred to the frame can be thought of as a function of wire deflection, which must relate to the displacement at the distraction site. In essence, this relationship is similar to modeling the external fixator (including wires and half pins) as a spring in parallel with the bone and distraction segment. To investigate the hypothesis that the frame and wires together act as springs in parallel with the bone and distraction gap, we derived a relationship between the percentage of load carried by the frame and the stiffness of the regenerate bone within the distraction gap. This relationship was validated in the laboratory both experimentally and using finite element modeling. The relationship can be written in equation form in terms of the force applied to the limb; the force carried by the frame; and the stiffness of the frame, the native bone, and the osteogenic bone in the gap.

If %LS is used to represent the ratio of the force carried by the frame to the total force applied to the limb, the equation that solves for gap stiffness is:

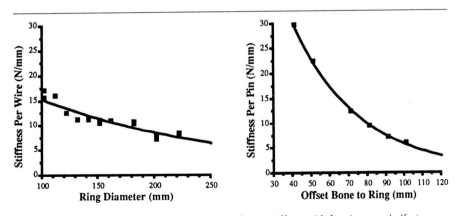

Fig. 1 Left, Average wire contribution to axial frame stiffness. **Right,** Average half pin contribution to axial frame stiffness. (Reproduced with permission from Waanders NA, Lawton JN, Steen H, et al: Clinical estimation of Ilizarov fixator axial stiffness based on wire and half pin contributions. *Bull Hosp Jt Dis*, in press.)

$$\text{Gap Stiffness} = \frac{\text{Bone Stiffness} \times \text{Frame Stiffness} \times (1 - \%\text{LS})}{\text{Bone Stiffness} \times \%\text{LS} - \text{Frame Stiffness} \times (1 - \%\text{LS})}$$

Experimentally, we validated these equations by measuring the forces in frames under applied loads, with a series of springs to simulate various gap stiffnesses. The unit slope of Figure 2 indicates the validity of viewing the frame as a spring in parallel with the bone and distraction gap tissue. The limitation of this approach is the simplification of the nonlinear properties of the bone interface and the distraction gap tissue. However, as a first approximation, a linear estimate for the mechanical properties of the frame/bone composite may be acceptable. We are currently adapting the frame force and applied force measuring system for clinical implementation as a means of noninvasively, mechanically monitoring the maturation of the regenerate bone within the distraction gap.

It is important to recognize the changes in the stiffness of the gap tissue during the phases of the distraction osteogenesis technique. At the time of surgery and during the latency phase, prior to distraction, the bone ends are in contact and the "gap" has a very high stiffness. As distraction creates a gap, filled with unmineralized tissue, the gap stiffness is very low (gap stiffness less than the stiffness of the fixator). After distraction ends and the proximal and distal bone masses unite, the stiffness of the gap tissue increases. As the new bone matures, its stiffness approaches the stiffness of the native bone, becoming much more stiff than the external fixator. The loads and strains acting on the gap tissue in these phases (latency, distraction, maturation) change remarkably. In latency, gap forces are high and strains low. In distraction, gap forces are low, but strains are high. In maturation, gap forces are high and strains are low.

Forces Measured in Distraction Osteogenesis

The forces acting on the fixation frame-bone composite depend on a variety of boundary conditions, including external loads, ground reaction forces, and muscle contractile activity. In general, distraction by the fixator places the gap tissues and associated structures in tension, while the fixator is subjected to compression. Functional activity would tend to compress the gap tissue (reduce or reverse the distraction tension) and to compress the external fixator (increase the compression due to distraction). Clinical and experimental measurements

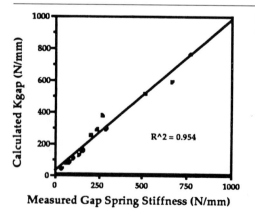

Fig. 2 Calculated gap stiffness versus measured distraction gap stiffness.

of fixator forces[30,31] verify that with distraction of the external fixator, the osteotomy site and the surrounding soft tissues are put into tension. Forces resulting from functional loading of the limb are also a significant part of the mechanical environment. When a patient bears full weight on the limb, the patient's body weight and forces due to muscle contractions must be carried by the frame/bone composite. The net force acting at the distraction site reflects the combination of the distraction tension and the compressive functional loads. We have used a rabbit model to measure fixator forces due to distraction and functional loading during the postdistraction/preconsolidation phase. These forces were then used in an in vitro experiment to estimate the net force and strains that would be acting on the gap tissue in vivo.

A custom-made monolateral fixator (Fig. 3) was used for bilateral middiaphyseal tibial lengthening of 13 male, specific-pathogen-free New Zealand White rabbits. Each fixator was instrumented with strain gages for the measurement of axial loads and applied to the rabbit tibia with four Orthofix M310 tapered stainless steel cortical bone pins (EBI Medical Systems, Inc., Parsippany, NJ) in an anterolateral direction, avoiding interference with normal ambulation. A mid-diaphyseal osteotomy was performed through a medial incision using a fine oscillating saw with elevation and protection of the periosteum. After a 6-day latency period (days 0 to 5), the fixators were distracted 0.25 mm three times per day for 12 days (days 6 to 17). The rabbits were euthanized on day 24.

The force-measuring protocol included 1 minute of monitoring baseline tension with the rabbits suspended in a mesh sling, 9 minutes of monitoring to record the force during distraction and its immediate relaxation with the rabbits still suspended in the sling, and 5 minutes of monitoring functional activity including ambulation. After completion of distraction (days 18 to 23), force monitoring included only the 1-minute baseline while suspended in the sling and the 5 minutes of functional activity. The fixators were recalibrated after

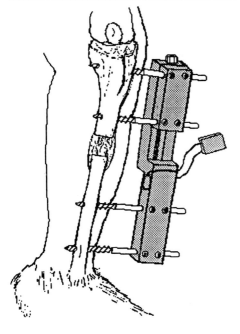

Fig. 3 Custom instrumented fixator for rabbit tibial lengthening.

sacrifice to account for the actual fixator offset at the interface between the bone and pins. To measure the fraction of fixator force carried by the gap tissue as compared to that carried by the surrounding soft tissues, fixator forces in five rabbits were recorded after sacrifice during sequential dissection of the skin, anterior muscles, and posterior muscles. Fixator forces during sequential dissection decreased on average only 7% (less than the 21% reduction reported by Aronson and associates[31] with live dissection of the soft tissues). Following sacrifice, the distraction zone was removed for histologic processing, and the remainder of the tibia was tested to determine in situ stiffness and a corrected fixator-load calibration factor. An example of the force measured in the fixator during distraction can be seen in Figure 4, *left*. Figure 4, *right*, shows the average predistraction fixator force for each day of distraction. The average peak force generated in the fixator during functional loading was 71.2 N (SD 5.1). The average postsacrifice fixator stiffness of 15 fixators was 46.6 N/mm (SD 9.9). Therefore, using spring theory, the associated average deflection and strain of the fixator were calculated to be 1.5 mm and 17%, respectively.

To investigate the net force acting on the distraction gap, a rabbit fixator was mounted on two pieces of acrylic tube with a small spring (stiffness = 4 N/mm) and a load cell in the gap. The fixator was distracted to create a baseline tension of 24 N in the gap spring and five cycles of 0 to 45 N were applied in an MTS testing machine while recording the applied force, the force in the fixator, and the force in the gap spring. The applied force and net gap force are shown in Figure 5. This graph demonstrates that the tension in the gap spring decreased only minimally from 24 to 23 N, as the external load increased from 0 to 45 N.

This combination of in vivo and in vitro measurements taken during distraction (prior to consolidation) suggest that the net force on the gap tissue is predominately tension due to the distraction of the external fixator, with only small superimposed changes due to the functional use of the limb. These small force changes are associated with relatively large (1.5 mm in a 9-mm gap) deflections, resulting in surprisingly high strains (17%) acting on the gap tissue.

We have made similar measurements from frames in the laboratory. Axial testing of these frames with distraction tension did not demonstrate significant changes in axial stiffness. This information indicates that the principle of su-

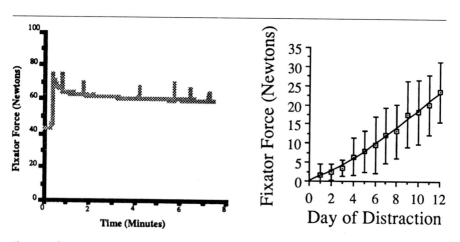

Fig. 4 Left, Fixator force before and after distraction on day 8 of distraction. **Right,** Daily average predistraction fixator force.

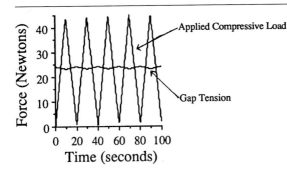

Fig. 5 Measured distraction gap tension with applied compressive loads.

perposition can be applied when analyzing distraction tension and compression loads due to ambulation.

Pattern of Bone Formation in Distraction Osteogenesis

To understand the relationship between the mechanical environment and the process of osteogenesis, it is important to know the macroscopic and microscopic structure of the new bone. A canine model was used in our first in vivo study. A simple two-ring fixator with two wires per ring was applied to the left tibias of 12 large mongrel dogs. After a 5-day latency period, distraction began at a rate of 0.25 mm four times per day until sacrifice or radiographic evidence of 3 mm of lengthening. Radiographs were taken at regular intervals, and the dogs were sacrificed at various times during distraction and during the post-distraction consolidation period, out to 20 weeks.

Several imaging modalities (radiographs, ultrasound, dual-energy x-ray absorptiometry [DEXA], magnetic resonance imaging [MRI], computed tomography [CT] scans) were evaluated for monitoring the progression of bone formation in the distraction gap by comparison with postmortem invasive modalities (microcomputed tomography, microradiography, scanning electron microscopy [SEM], and histology). CT scans were most capable of quantifying the volume, distribution, and density of the new bone, but evaluation with this modality was limited to the macroscopic level. Ultrasound was incapable of penetrating the regenerate bone and was most useful for general monitoring of the interzone between advancing mineralization fronts. DEXA and MRI failed to provide adequate resolution when compared to radiographs and CT scans.

Macroscopically, bone extended into the gap from the periosteal and endosteal surfaces adjacent to proximal and distal osteotomy surfaces, with an interzone of unmineralized tissue existing between the proximal and distal bone masses until after the completion of distraction. On the microscopic level, longitudinal sections demonstrated that the new bone comprised thin trabeculae, highly oriented in the longitudinal direction (up to 83%, much higher than normal metaphyseal trabecular bone). On transverse sections, the thin trabeculae were highly connected with no predominate orientation. The combination of these orientations implies a honeycomb structure uniquely oriented in the direction of distraction (Fig. 6). Evaluation of the thickness of the trabeculae indicated that they grow in length and number, but not in thickness.

Cell Types and Processes of Bone Formation in Distraction Osteogenesis

In our second in vivo experiment, we used a rabbit model shown in Figure 3. After a 6-day latency period (days 0 to 5), fixators were distracted 0.25 mm three times a day for 12 days (days 6 to 17). Rabbits were euthanized on day 24. Within 24 hours of sacrifice, the distraction osteogenic bone segment (still in Bouin's fixative) was scanned in the micro-CT system (Fig. 7) with an approximate resolution of 50 μm per voxel. The stabilizing acrylic plate and nylon

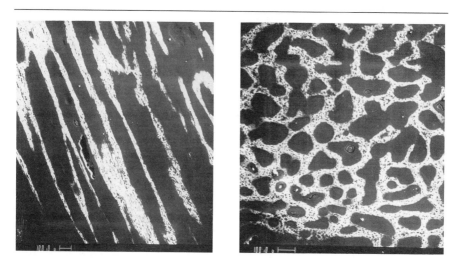

Fig. 6 Scanning electron micrographs of longitudinal (**left**) and transverse (**right**) sections through endosteal new bone.

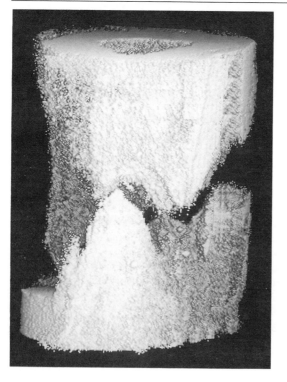

Fig. 7 Three-dimensional micro-computed tomography of rabbit tibia.

bolts did not interfere with the micro-CT scanning. Figure 7 shows a three dimensional (3-D) reconstruction from the micro-CT data set of the new bone in the distraction gap at the time of sacrifice. Immediately after sacrifice, the distraction osteogenic bone segments, stabilized by an acrylic plate, were fixed for 72 hours in Bouin's fixative at 4°C. The specimens were then slowly decalcified in formic acid with citrate buffer. The decalcifying solutions were changed daily until a calcium oxalate precipitate test provided evidence of complete decalcification. The specimens were then processed in the Hypercenter (Shandon Scientific Limited) for dehydration prior to slow paraffin infiltration under vacuum over 10 hours. Specimens were then embedded in paraffin and stored in a 4°C refrigerator until sectioning.

Microscopic review of sections from rabbits confirms that the fixator, the surgery, and the distraction process result in the reliable formation of bone that has a typical histologic pattern. In the postdistraction period, the width of the interzone between the proximal and distal new bone ranged from 2 to 6 mm.

Evaluation of the gap tissue on day 24 revealed heterogeneous tissues. The peripheral margins were fibrous and appeared to extend both proximally and distally along the cortices. Bony tissue was observed proximally and distally in the gap and was longitudinally oriented with many osteoblastic and osteoclastic cells on the surfaces. The interzone tissue was filled with a mixture of cartilage and fibrous and vascular tissues (Fig. 8). In areas identified as cartilaginous, cell morphology varied with the appearance of both proliferative and hypertrophic features. Using immunohistochemical techniques on 8-μm sections, we

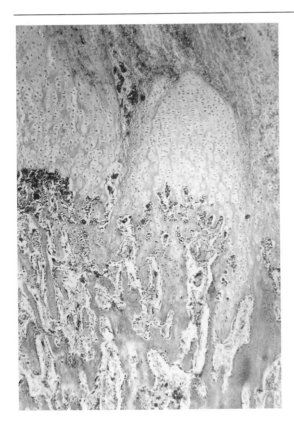

Fig. 8 Low power field of a hematoxylin and eosin stained section at interface of the central nonmineralized zone and new bone.

were able to localize type I procollagen, type II collagen, link protein, and type X collagen. The results demonstrated type I collagen expression by fibroblasts and osteoblasts. Link protein and type II collagen were localized in areas of proliferative chondrocytes, and type X collagen was localized in hypertrophic appearing chondrocytes (Fig. 9).

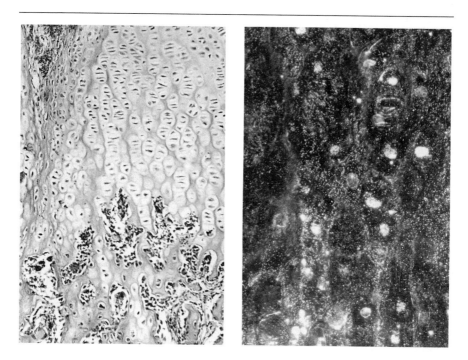

Fig. 9 Left, Detail of the central zone of the new bone interface shown in Figure 8. **Right,** Higher magnification of a region similar to the boxed area on left. Dark field microscopy, immunogold localization of type X collagen in hypertrophic chondrocytes. Bright areas represent immunogold signal.

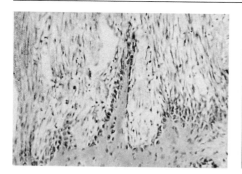
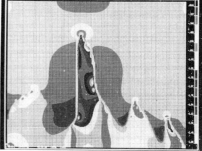

Fig. 10 Left, Histologic section of ossification front used to create the finite element model. **Right,** Finite element model. Contour plot of hydrostatic stress and octahedral stress showing areas of lowest hydrostatic stress and areas of highest octahedral shear correlating with the most active sites of osteoblastic activity.

It should also be noted that the pattern of tissue differentiation was similar in most specimens. This finding further supports the predicted relationship between patterns of local mechanical stresses and bone formation.

Influence of the Mechanical Environment on Bone Formation

In an effort to begin to explore the relationship between local stress conditions and tissue differentiation, two-dimensional (2-D) finite element models were created based on the SEM images from the canine study. It was hoped that the 2-D models would provide the first step in establishing the plausibility of stress/ morphology relationships.

Morphologic measures indicate that the longitudinal walls of the honeycomb structure grow in length but not significantly in width. This measurement suggests that there may be a difference in the mechanical environment along the ossification front such that osteoblastic activity is focused at the tips of the trabeculae. To investigate this possibility, an SEM image was digitized and converted to binary data using a single grayscale threshold to differentiate between bone and fibrous tissue. The image data were used to create a 2-D plane strain finite element model. Bone was assigned properties of 5 GPa and 0.3 Poisson ratio. Fibrous tissue was assigned properties of 500 MPa and 0.3 Poisson ratio. This model was analyzed to produce contour plots of hydrostatic stress and octahedral shear stress. The results of the analysis indicated that the areas of lowest hydrostatic stress coincided with areas of highest octahedral shear (at the tips of the trabeculae). This is at least preliminary evidence that osteoblastic activity is associated with areas of low hydrostatic stress and high octahedral shear (Fig. 10, *left*).

As a second preliminary indication, a histologic section of the ossification front were digitized and converted to binary data delineating bone and fibrous tissue. This image was used to create a new finite element model. Again, the model was analyzed to produce a contour plot of hydrostatic stress and octahedral shear stress. This plot showed that the areas of lowest hydrostatic stress coincided with areas of highest octahedral shear at the tips of the trabeculae. In the histologic slides, the most active areas of bone formation correlated with

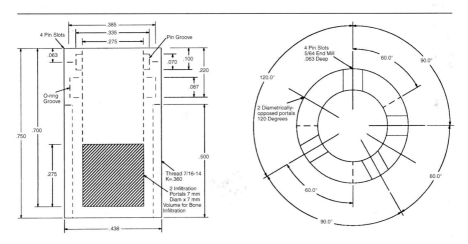

Fig. 11 Bone chamber design.

the analytic model. At the tips of the trabeculae, osteoblasts were cuboidal and several layers deep. Between trabeculae, osteoblasts appeared flat and inactive and in only a single layer. Again, the areas of low hydrostatic stress and high

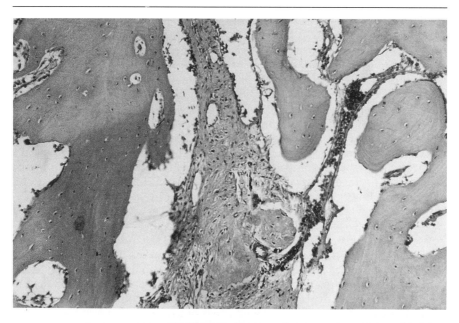

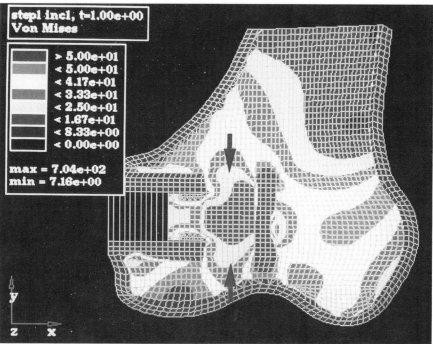

Fig. 12 Top, High power histologic section of bone chamber specimen. **Bottom,** Finite element model.

octahedral shear correlated with the most active sites of osteoblastic activity in the histologic sections (Fig. 10, *right*).

Summary of Distraction Models

The data, to date, provide substantial evidence that the patterns of bone formation during distraction osteogenesis depend strongly on the specific mechanical conditions. Alterations in boundary conditions due to fixator design parameters, external loading conditions, tissue morphology, and material properties eventually may result in significant shifts in formation patterns. Of particular note from these studies was the observation of endochondral bone formation in the rabbit model. This observation, coupled with the estimates of high interzone strains (17%), would suggest that dynamic strain conditions favor an endochondral bone formation process.

Bone Formation Under Low Strain Conditions

In a parallel preliminary study in our laboratories, we have had the opportunity to observe the process of bone formation under conditions of low stress and strain. The experimental model consists of a large volume bone chamber that is placed within metaphyseal regions in large mongrel dogs. The titanium chamber, which has a threaded exterior, incorporates two 120° portals that allow bone tissue infiltration after surgical placement. The internal dimensions of the chamber are 7 mm in diameter by 7 mm in length, which provides a large region for de novo bone formation (Fig. 11).

To date, experience with the bone chamber demonstrates a complete infiltration by cellular fibrous tissue at 4 weeks, significant increase in maturing bone by 8 weeks, and complete filling with trabecular bone and marrow by 16 weeks. Histologic analysis revealed no cartilage at any time during the bone formation process. In contrast to the distraction osteogenesis models, preliminary finite element analysis demonstrates that the bone within the chamber is significantly shielded from mechanical stresses during ambulation of the animal (Fig. 12).

In summary, these data were presented to provide the contrast in what appears to be mechanically modified bone formation processes. Under dynamic loading conditions, as illustrated in our models of distraction osteogenesis, large regions of endochondral bone formation were observed. In contrast, within the stress-shielded bone chamber, the bone formation process was characterized by intramembranous bone formation.

Acknowledgments

This work was supported by funds from the OREF Bristol-Myers Zimmer Research Award, NIH AR-20577, the National Arthritis Foundation, the Frederick J. Fischer Pediatric Endowment, and the University of Michigan Department of Surgery. The authors thank John Germiller, Mark Richards, Mark Stock, and Kathy Sweet for their help with this project.

References

1. Wolff J: *Das Gesetz der Transformation der Knochen*. Berlin, Hirschwald, 1892.
2. Martin RB, Burr DB: *Structure, Function, and Adaptation of Compact Bone*. New York, NY, Raven Press, 1989.

3. Aro HT, Kelly PJ, Lewallen DG, et al: The effects of physiologic dynamic compression on bone healing under external fixation. *Clin Orthop* 1990;256:260–273.

4. Blenman PR, Carter DR, Beaupre GS: Role of mechanical loading in the progressive ossification of a fracture callus. *J Orthop Res* 1989;7:398–407.

5. Burr DB, Schaffler MB, Yang KH, et al: Skeletal change in response to altered strain environments: Is woven bone a response to elevated strain? *Bone* 1989;10:223–233.

6. Carter DR: Mechanical loading history and skeletal biology. *J Biomech* 1987;11–12:1095–1109.

7. Chao EYS, Aro HT, Lewallen DG, et al: The effect of rigidity on fracture healing in external fixation. *Clin Orthop* 1989;241:24–35.

8. Cheal EJ, Mansmann KA, DiGioia AM III, et al: Role of interfragmentary strain in fracture healing: Ovine model of a healing osteotomy. *J Orthop Res* 1991;9:131–142.

9. Cowin SC: Wolff's law of trabecular architecture at remodeling equilibrium. *J Biomech Engr* 1986;108:83–88.

10. Dehne E: The rationale of early functional loading in the healing of fractures: A comprehensive gate control concept of repair. *Clin Orthop* 1980;146:18–27.

11. Frost HM: A determinant of bone architecture: The minimum effective strain. *Clin Orthop* 1983;175:286–292.

12. Fyhrie DP, Carter DR: A unifying principle relating stress to trabecular bone morphology. *J Orthop Res* 1986;4:304–317.

13. Goldstein SA, Matthews LS, Kuhn JL, et al: Trabecular bone remodeling: An experimental model. *J Biomech* 1991;24:135–150.

14. Goodship AE, Lanyon LE, McFie H: Functional adaptation of bone to increased stress: An experimental study. *J Bone Joint Surg* 1979;61A:539–546.

15. Goodship AE, Kenwright J: The influence of induced micromovement upon the healing of experimental tibial fractures. *J Bone Joint Surg* 1985;67B:650–655.

16. Hart RT, Davy DT, Heiple KG: A computational method for stress analysis of adaptive elastic materials with a view toward applications in strain-induced bone remodeling. *Trans ASME* 1984;106:342–350.

17. Huiskes R, Weinans H, Grootenboer HJ, et al: Adaptive bone-remodeling theory applied to prosthetic-design analysis. *J Biomech* 1987;20:1135–1150.

18. Lanyon LE: Experimental support for the trajectorial theory of bone structure. *J Bone Joint Surg* 1974;56B:160–166.

19. Perren SM: Physical and biological aspects of fracture healing with special reference to internal fixation. *Clin Orthop* 1979;138:175–196.

20. Rubin CT, Lanyon LE: Osteoregulatory nature of mechanical stimuli: Function as a determinant for adaptive remodeling in bone. *J Orthop Res* 1987;5:300–310.

21. Aronson J, Harrison BH, Stewart CL, et al: The histology of distraction osteogenesis using different external fixators. *Clin Orthop* 1989;241:106–16.

22. Aronson J, Johnson E, Harp JH: Local bone transportation for treatment of intercalary defects by the Ilizarov technique: Biomechanical and clinical considerations. *Clin Orthop* 1989;243:71–79.

23. De Bastiani G, Aldegheri R, Renzi-Brivio L, et al: Limb lengthening by callus distraction (callotasis). *J Pediatr Orthop* 1987;7:129–134.

24. Delloye C, Delefortrie G, Coutelier L, et al: Bone regenerate formation in cortical bone during distraction lengthening: An experimental study. *Clin Orthop* 1990;250:34–42.

25. Green SA: Osteomyelitis: The Ilizarov perspective. *Orthop Clin North Am* 1991;22:515–21.

26. Ilizarov GA: Clinical application of the tension-stress effect for limb lengthening. *Clin Orthop* 1990;250:8–26.

27. Kojimoto H, Yasui N, Goto T, et al: Bone lengthening in rabbits by callus distraction: The role of periosteum and endosteum. *J Bone Joint Surg* 1988;70B:543–549.

28. Monticelli G, Spinelli R: Distraction epiphysiolysis as a method of limb lengthening: I. Experimental study. *Clin Orthop* 1981;154:254–261.

29. Paley D: Current techniques of limb lengthening. *J Pediatr Orthop* 1988;8:73–92.
30. Wolfson N, Hearn TC, Thomason JJ, et al: Force and stiffness changes during Ilizarov leg lengthening. *Clin Orthop* 1990;250:58–60.
31. Aronson J, Harp JH, Hollis JM: In vivo measurement of mechanical forces generated during distraction osteogenesis. *Trans Orthop Res Soc* 1991;37:440.

Chapter 30

Injury of Nerve Tissue During Stretching

Julia K. Terzis, MD, PhD
Thomas G. Skoulis, MD

Nerve Anatomy

To clarify the mechanism of nerve injury, one has to be acquainted with the microanatomy of the peripheral nerve. The peripheral nerve communicates with the central nervous system via the ventral and dorsal roots; the ventral root is composed of motor fibers whereas the dorsal root receives afferent mechanoreceptive fibers. The motor fibers have their cell body in the ventral horn of the spinal cord and terminate at the neuromuscular junction in the skeletal muscles. The sensory fibers terminate in the skin as free nerve endings or as encapsulated receptors. In addition, proprioceptive fibers reach the musculotendinous organs, and the muscle spindles are involved in constant feedback mechanisms with the higher cortical centers. Nerve fibers may be unmyelinated or myelinated; the unmyelinated fibers contain several axons wrapped by a single Schwann cell, whereas the myelinated nerve fibers involve individual axons, each of which is surrounded by a single Schwann cell.

The nerve fibers are grouped into bundles termed fascicles, enveloped by a distinctive specialized sheath, the perineurium, which is composed of lamellated layers of perineurial cells interspersed with collagen fibers. Individual nerve fibers are surrounded by endoneurial tissue within individual fascicles. The fascicular pattern of a nerve trunk may vary from few fascicles to many fascicles of varying sizes. The connective tissue surrounding each fascicle is called interfascicular epineurium, and the sheath surrounding the entire nerve trunk is termed the extrafascicular epineurium.

The tensile strength and the elasticity of the nerve are derived from the perineurium. The perineurial sheath provides a diffusion barrier and maintains the intrafascicular pressure. The endoneurium has minimal tensile strength. The epineurium forms a protective sheath around the nerve, which allows nutrient blood supply to enter the intraneural contents and provides a medium in which the nerve bundles can glide, especially around the joints.

The peripheral nerves are supplied by a segmental, external blood supply as well as by an intrinsic blood supply.[1] The network of longitudinal nutrient vessels is found in epineurium, perineurium, and the endoneurium with the largest vessels located in the epineurial connective tissue. Studies reveal a very extensive intrinsic blood supply, which allows mobilization of the peripheral nerves over a long distance. The blood supply of the peripheral nerves plays a critical role in its survival and function.[2]

Classification of Peripheral Nerve Injury

Seddon[3] and Sunderland[4] described classification systems for nerve injuries. Seddon's classification is less complicated and easier to use. Nerve injuries are divided into three types. Neurapraxia, the mildest form of nerve injury, refers to a localized conduction block along the nerve. This lesion is not accompanied by axonal degeneration, but involves only focal demyelination. The second type, axonotmesis, refers to a complete disruption of axonal continuity as well as a complete conduction block. Thus, Wallerian degeneration always accompanies an axonotmetic lesion. However, the recovery is good due to continuity of the supportive structures (endoneurium, perineurium, and epineurium). The most severe type of nerve injury is neurotmesis, which refers to a complete anatomic disruption of the peripheral nerve trunk with poor prognosis for normal recovery.[5]

Sunderland's classification, which involves five degrees of nerve injury of increasing severity, allows for a better description of mixed lesions.[4] These are: (1) loss of conduction in axons; (2) loss of continuity of axons without disruption of the endoneurial sheath; (3) loss of continuity of nerve fibers; (4) the involvement of perineurium and individual bundles; and (5) loss of continuity of the nerve trunk.

With a first degree injury, the axonal continuity is preserved with some local thinning and segmental demyelination. Local conduction block occurs, but, because the axons remain intact, the functional loss is brief with eventual restoration of function. There is no Wallerian degeneration. This corresponds to the neurapraxia injury of Seddon.[3] A similar course of conduction block is observed in tourniquet compression injuries, in which mechanical compression produces the block.

In second degree injuries, the axon is severed with preservation of the remaining structures (endoneurium, perineurium, and epineurium). There is Wallerian degeneration (degeneration of the distal axon) but Schwann cells proliferate, providing conduits for nerve regeneration. The axon completely regenerates, replacing the site of injury and allowing for eventual functional recovery. The fiber pattern after recovery is identical to that before the injury because the regenerating axons are confined to their respective endoneurial tubes. Clinically, there is a complete loss of motor, sensory, and sympathetic function in the distribution of the injured nerve until regeneration and functional restoration. The interval before recovery is longer than after first degree injury, and the course of recovery is variable because it depends on the rate of restoration of axonal continuity. The time period for full functional restoration may be months as opposed to the weeks observed in neurapraxia. The second degree injury corresponds to axonotmetic injury. The lesion can be produced by crush or mild traction.

The third degree injury involves axonal disintegration, Wallerian degeneration, and disorganization of the internal structure of the fascicles. The perineurium is affected only minimally, with preservation of the general arrangement of the nerve trunk. The fiber disorganization may be further complicated by intrafascicular hemorrhage, edema, vascular stasis, ischemia, and inflammation leading to fibrosis, which may hinder axon regeneration. Such changes may distort axon elongation, thereby compromising subsequent functional return. The regenerating axons may not be confined to the original endoneurial tubes, resulting in axonal wastage and cross-shunting. Clinically, the involvement of all fascicles results in complete motor, sensory, and sympathetic functional loss in the distribution of the involved nerve. The onset of recovery is delayed for longer periods than after second degree injury because this injury is of greater intensity. Recovery is often incomplete; the patient is left with paresis and/or sensory deficit caused by ineffective regeneration. This injury is commonly caused by traction or crushing forces.

The fourth degree injury involves the entire fascicular structure in which the bundles are so disrupted and disorganized that they are no longer sharply demarcated from the epineurium. The continuity of the nerve trunk is preserved, but the fibrous tissues arrest axonal growth, resulting in neuroma formation. The involvement of all fascicles results in complete loss of function, and spontaneous recovery to a useful degree rarely occurs. This type of injury requires excision of the damaged segment and microsurgical reconstruction.

The fifth degree injury involves a complete loss of continuity of the nerve trunk with loss of function. If untreated, recovery is negligible, even when the ends are in proximity with each other.[5]

Stretch Injury

Background

Stretch injuries are encountered in therapeutic procedures and traumatic accidents. During the second half of the nineteenth century, nerve stretching was transiently popular in treatment of neuralgia.[6] Many war wounds had peripheral nerve damage without loss of anatomic continuity; these may have been due to traction injury. Similar findings are encountered in trauma involving the brachial plexus. Obstetrical trauma, violent accidents associated with fractures and dislocations, and inadvertent retraction during surgery are often complicated by nerve stretch injuries.[5]

Many clinical and experimental studies were performed to study stretch injury of the peripheral nerve.[7] Initial studies showed that the peripheral nerves were highly resistant to stretching. This was further investigated by clarifying the stress-strain properties of peripheral nerves. The structures contributing to the peripheral nerve play an important role in the stress-strain response.[8] The degree of nerve damage appearing at critical points of the stress-strain curve may clarify the extent of nerve injury and its outcome.[9]

Tillaux[10] stretched the median and ulnar nerves of human cadavers until rupture, noting their ability to stretch 34% to 45% of their length with the tensile strength of 20 to 25 kg.

Mitchell[11] reported a case in which the sciatic nerve of a patient was severely elongated, "pushed fully four or five inches out of its path" with intact sense of touch and only resulting pain. His experimental studies with the sciatic nerves of rabbits revealed failure of motor conduction after 25% lengthening.

Takimoto[12] reviewed nerve stretching as a therapeutic procedure in both human and animal experiments. His study revealed that an enormous weight, 32 kg, was required to stretch a human sciatic nerve. He further investigated the histologic changes associated with rapidly elongated rabbit sciatic nerves.

De Rényi[13] claimed that the elasticity of a frog nerve fiber depended on the elasticity of the axon, with stretching of the axon up to 10% resulting in regaining of its original length and structure. Highet and Sanders[14] noted by histologic studies that severe damage to a nerve occurred after elongation by 11%.

Denny-Brown and Doherty[15] felt that the peripheral nerves of cats behaved as a plastic material, allowing 100% stretch with minimal damage. Only slight weakness occurred 24 hours later, with full functional recovery within 14 days. Histologic studies revealed that extreme nerve elongations were associated with severe injuries secondary to tearing of the epineurial vessels, decreased blood flow, and edema. Severe stretch produced a diffuse lesion associated with a variety of changes. Nerves had a benign macroscopic appearance while undergoing irreversible injury. An initial edematous swelling progressed to fibrous scarring with loss of endoneurial structures. Single nerve fibers haphazardly tore within nerve fiber bundles prior to the bundles rupturing, while other surviving bundles withstood the increasing force to preserve their pattern. Examination of the myelin sheaths at these rupture sites revealed globular swelling, fragmentation, and degeneration.

Liu and associates[16] measured the tensile strength of human nerves; they observed the histologic damage at different points of the nerve's stress-strain curve. Their histologic picture revealed that the endoneurium was far less elastic than the perineurium. The tears of endoneurium were seen after stretching to about 20%, and the longitudinal splitting of perineurium at 22%, with herniation of nerve fibers. The elastic properties were retained as long as the perineurium remained intact. Further tension resulted in the whole nerve protruding out of the sheath as it became progressively thinner with a threatened rupture. Patches of edema were found at the earlier stages of stretching secondary to damage to small blood vessels in the epineurium. The perineurial cells prevented the endoneurial fibroblasts from spreading into the neighboring tissue to form a true neuroma.

Schneider[17] studied myelinated nerve fibers from frogs and concluded that nerve fibers are elastic, with the endoneurium acting as the protective layer against stretching. He estimated greater than 50% stretch of the nerve trunk prior to the true stretch of the nerve fibers.

Hoen and Brackett[18] studied peripheral nerve elongation; they achieved increases in length of 2.5 to 9.5 cm. in dogs' sciatic nerves, which normally measured less than 10 cm after exiting the pelvis. Anatomically useful increases of 2.5 to 5 cm were obtained in nerves from six of the nine animals, and these nerves were observed to be normal in structure.

The stress-strain phenomena was further investigated by Sunderland and Bradley,[6] whose results show an initial linear relationship between load and elongation. The elastic properties of the nerve allowed the nerve to stretch and recoil within its soft tissue surrounding. The nerve trunk in its bed, the fasciculi in the epineurium, and the nerve fibers ran an undulating course, which allowed an initial tension-free stretching. As the nerve was further elongated, the straightened nerve was further stretched prior to rupturing. The nerve fibers inside the fasciculi ruptured before the perineurial tissue. The nerve retained its elasticity as long as the perineurium remained intact. The strength of the perineurium was derived from layers of collagen fibers that allowed elongation at the expense of the cross-sectional area. As the cross-sectional area of the nerve was reduced, the intrafascicular pressure was increased, compromising the microcirculation. The even distribution of the microscopic tears throughout the elongated area suggests that the damage was not restricted to the site of visible tear. On rupture of the entire fascicle, the nerve elongated rapidly as would a plastic structure.

Sunderland and Bradley[6] also observed that the greatest elongation (approximately 20%) occurred at the elastic limit, and the maximal elongation (30%) occurred at the point of mechanical failure. The nerve strength and elasticity were greatly influenced by the rate of application of the load. Of the two ways a nerve can suffer a stretch injury—acutely, by an abrupt application of force of considerable load resulting in destructive structural changes and immediate loss of function, or chronically, by slow stretching whereupon considerable deformation occurs before symptoms appear—slow stretch leads to marked increase in length without noticeable disturbance of function. The extent and severity of damage are determined by the magnitude of the load and the rate of deformation.

Studies by Haftek[9] revealed the behavior of rabbit peripheral nerves that were exposed to increasing loads to the point of failure. The stress-strain relationship is illustrated in a curve (Fig. 1), which rises in a straight line to a point where it suddenly declines, with a slower decline later to zero. The initial rise reflects the extension of the epineurium and straightening of the fascicles prior to the nerve stretch, which obeys Hook's law. The elasticity of the peripheral nerve then allows an initial linear relationship between load and elongation until the point of the elastic limit (1, interrupted arrow) at which mechanical failure occurs. At this breaking point, the elasticity no longer holds the load, and the nerve yields. Considerable stretching is required to reach this point prior to the plastic state of the nerve that lies beyond the linear stress-strain curve.

Haftek[9] felt that because the epineurium functions to cushion the fascicles from the stresses applied to the nerve, nerves composed of greater amounts of epineurium should be less vulnerable to stress injury. The sciatic nerve contains a significant amount of epineurial tissue and has a fascicular content as low as 12%. Clinical findings by Platt[19] and Highet and Holmes[20] indicate that the common peroneal division of the sciatic nerve is more susceptible to stress injury than the tibial division. This is explained by the peroneal division containing larger fascicles with less epineurial tissue than the tibial division. Among the peripheral nerves, apart from the brachial plexus, the peroneal nerve is most often exposed to a stretch injury (JK Terzis, personal communication, 1993).

Lundborg and Rydevik[21] observed the effect of stretch on the intraneural microcirculation. Stretching changed the normal intraneural topography, compromising the microvascular structures until there was insufficient blood flow and oxygen supply for proper nerve function. The nutrient vessels had an initial coiled and tortuous appearance that disappeared on stretch. With further elongation, there was a rise in the intrafascicular pressure, which occluded these intraneural vessels. The "lower stretching limit" was observed with 5% to 10% elongation, when venular flow slowed down with normal flow in the arterioles and capillaries. There was evidence of tissue injury seen as microthrombi, emboli, and granulocytosis. The "upper stretching limit" was described as 11% to 18% elongation, when all microcirculation stopped leaving a nonviable nerve.

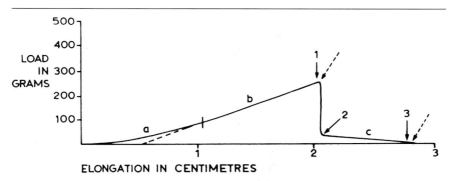

Fig. 1 Typical graph made by the Instron machine during gradual stretching of the nerve to complete rupture. (Reproduced with permission from Haftek J: Stretch injury of peripheral nerve: Acute effects of stretching on rabbit nerve. *J Bone Joint Surg* 1970;52B:354–365.)

Functional Relationship

Previous clinical and experimental studies reveal high peripheral nerve resistance to stretching. The functional changes in a stretched nerve depend on the magnitude of the deforming force and the rate of distraction. The functional changes must be observed along with the morphologic correlates in order to better understand stretch injury and recovery.

In 1917, Takimoto[12] examined the physiologic and histologic changes associated with acute nerve stretching. The rabbit sciatic nerves, stretched by a deforming load of 400 g, had histologic changes that were observed as hyperemia, hemorrhages in the epineurium and perineurium, rupture of connective tissue fibers, and loss of continuity, with degeneration of axons followed by later regeneration. Hemorrhage was not necessarily found in a significantly stretched nerve, and when it occurred, it was found in the epineurium. The immediate changes noted were breaking of the axis cylinders into short segments or thinning to produce beading. On survival to 2 days, the nerve became edematous, with myelin droplets at the nodes of Ranvier. At 3 days, degeneration of the myelin sheath began, with more severe involvement of the periphery of the nerve bundles. These changes correlated with the motor and sensory disturbances and recovery.

Spiegel and associates[22] introduced an in vivo model of stretch injury in the sciatic nerve of the rat. A good degree of functional recovery occurred 2 to 3 weeks after deforming stretch injury when nerves were not stretched beyond the limit of elasticity. The timing of functional return suggested a neurapraxia lesion with rapid and spontaneous recovery rather than the regeneration obtained following Wallerian degeneration. The histologic changes correlated with the level of functional impairment, and the nerves predisposed to failure had degrees of degenerating neurons suggestive of axonotmesis. Many animals, with nerves stretched beyond the limit of elasticity, still recovered a significant degree of function despite gross histologic changes. The signs of nerve recovery appeared in an orderly way with the return of sensory before motor, from proximal to distal areas. Deep sensation and crude touch preceded light touch and pinprick.

By examining the relationship between the degree of nerve stretch and the compound action potential (CAP), it is possible to understand the effect of stretch on nerve function.[23] The CAP is the total potential recorded from a nerve trunk as a result of the excitation of many simultaneously firing nerve fibers, and it is present only if the peripheral nerve is functioning.[24] Studies have shown failure of nerve conduction in crush injuries and entrapment syndromes.[25] CAP is useful in defining the site and extent of the lesion. The shape of the waveform can be examined to identify the extent of injury. In stretch injury, the contour and shape of the CAP would represent the degree of severity of the traction lesion.

Nerve Expansion

Nerve elongation definitely can take place without any negative results in nerve function during such normal conditions as pregnancy, big hernias, and so forth, as well as after surgical intervention, such as the subcutaneous placement of a tissue expander under the skin. In these cases, the slowly elongated intact nerve fibers maintain all the characteristics of normal nerve function.

The placement of a tissue expander under an intact sciatic nerve of a rat, followed by rapid or slow filling of the expander produces nerve elongation, but it has different functional results in each case. Rapid nerve expansion is accompanied by a delay in "onset and peak latency," a decrease in the amplitude of the CAP, and a decrease in the conduction velocity of the axons. After the release of the expansion, all these values eventually return to normal; however, there is an increased threshold to nerve excitability.[26]

On the other hand, gradual, slow nerve expansion over weeks or months produces approximately 30% elongation of the nerve, which is permanent. There is only a transient effect on the behavioral values of the animal during the course of the expansion as measured by the Sciatic Function Index.[27,28] The behavioral as well as the electrophysiologic values return to normal after the end of the expansion period.[29]

Distraction Osteogenesis

Progressive advances in biomechanics and surgical techniques have made limb lengthening possible. It is now possible to achieve a stable elongated limb by external fixation devices along the osteotomy distraction sites. Patients with short stature, achondroplasia, hypochondroplasia, and other skeletal dysplasias can gain greater than 10 cm from a limb, or 8% to 58% more of the original bone length by means of a slow progression of distraction of bone using a unilateral or circular external fixator.[30] The slow rate, 1 mm per day in humans and 0.5 mm per day in rabbits, does not disrupt bone callus, but rather stimulates osteogenesis during lengthening.[31] Distraction begins about 1 week after surgery, whereupon osseous autoregeneration occurs; the fixator is gradually mobilized as the autoregeneration consolidates.

The lengthening procedures have obtained satisfactory results without permanently disabling damage to joints, bone, skin, and muscle. The patients are of the younger age group, with children suffering frequent emotional problems from the initial injury and subsequent lengthy distraction period. Bone complications requiring multiple revision operations and loss of muscle power are rare.

Little is known about the effect of bone elongation on the soft tissue. Although bone receives the direct distractional forces, the soft tissues do undergo a significant indirect local stretching. Upon osteotomy, the bone lengthens only at the osteotomy site, and the soft tissues surrounding the site are exposed to the distraction forces. Often the factors limiting the amount of bone lengthening are related to the soft tissue rather than bone. The most critical soft tissue seems to be the muscle, which has direct attachments to the bone, at the osteotomy site. The muscle is subjected to excessive local tensile stress at its origin and insertion. Other soft tissues of importance are blood vessels, nerves, and skin that attach indirectly to the bone, making them better at adapting to lengthening. Studies reveal that the muscle as a whole elongates, sharing the tensile stress, with possible new muscle tissue formation. Muscle stretch detaches the stable cross bridges between actin and myosin filaments. These cross bridges reform if given enough time between stretches.[32] In one study with rabbit tibias, the periosteum and the muscle fascias were labeled with metal markers prior to a slow progressive distraction. The result was longitudinal migration of the periosteal markers, with the periosteum sliding over the bone cortex and allowing local stretching of the muscle around the osteotomy site. However, the muscle elongation involved not only the osteotomy site, but also the entire muscle substance.[31]

Neurologic injury may be related to the surgical technique or to the rate of distraction. Paley[33] studied 46 patients with 60 limb segments complicated by four sensory and four motor nerve palsies and one reflex sympathetic dystrophy. Of these, three motor and three sensory palsies were due to poor surgical technique. Pin- or wire-related injuries are best avoided by proper insertion techniques, based on knowledge of the anatomy of the peripheral nerve pathways. The osteotome or the oscillating saw may directly injure the nerve. An acute stretch of the nerve may result from rotational osteoclasis maneuver.

Distraction-related nerve injuries were rare in a study by Paley.[33] Such neurologic symptoms were transient, with complete recovery over time. In a study by Faber and associates,[34] 46 leg-lengthening procedures were complicated by seven common peroneal nerve pareses and one common peroneal nerve hyperalgesia. These symptoms disappeared on reducing the speed of lengthening temporarily. Bell and associates[35] treated 32 limb segments with Ilizarov technique, resulting in two transient peroneal nerve palsies during lengthening.

Today, the limb lengthening procedures continue at a slow rate because of the awareness of the dangers of nerve stretching. The amount of tension and the rate of distraction are thought to be the two critical factors in precipitating functional loss. No studies have yet revealed the extent of nerve stretch possible before loss of nerve function. Studies reveal that stretching of normal nerves injures sensory conduction before motor conduction.[36] Peripheral nerves possess an elastic limit of approximately 20% elongation.[6] The individual differences in various peripheral nerves may explain their varying susceptibility to deforming forces.

The distraction rate plays an important role in morphologic changes of the nerve tissue. The nerve fibers from a limb distracted at a rate of 1 mm per day had an uneven diameter of axons and formation of irregular accumulations of cytoplasm. These changes were less pronounced at a distraction rate of 2 mm/day in four steps.[37,38] In addition, limb lengthening of 1 mm/day divided in four steps resulted in minimal change in axons, with newly formed nerve fibers at various stages of differentiation. Schwann cells surrounded the whole group of axons at this slow rate.[37,38]

Despite the favorable response of nerves to distraction, with temporary functional loss and minimal histologic changes, it is important to be aware of possible nerve injury during limb elongation. Frequent neurologic examinations should be made when tension is applied to a limb. Patients with distraction-related injuries have early signs of significant discomfort, pain, and hyperesthesia. With progression, they develop hypoesthesia, decreased muscle strength, and paralysis. Such symptoms should alert a surgeon to thoroughly investigate the duration and nature of onset and the extent of sensory and/or motor loss.

No studies have yet revealed the degree of nerve stretch possible before loss of nerve function in distraction. A better understanding of the reaction of the peripheral nerves to loads increasing to the point of physiologic and mechanical failure is needed to guide the surgeon through clinical nerve elongation procedures. Such data may be obtained through careful study of the pathophysiology of peripheral nerve stretch injuries related to limb elongation.

Acknowledgment

We would like to thank Shinji S. Lee for her assistance in preparation of this manuscript.

References

1. Breidenbach WC, Terzis JK: The blood supply of vascularized nerve grafts. *J Reconstr Microsurg* 1986;3:43–58.

2. Lundborg G: The intrinsic vascularization of human peripheral nerves: Structural and functional aspects. *J Hand Surg* 1979;4:34–41.
3. Seddon HJ: Three types of nerve injury. *Brain* 1943;66:237–288.
4. Sunderland S: A classification of peripheral nerve injuries producing loss of function. *Brain* 1951;74:491–516.
5. Terzis JK, Smith KL: *The Peripheral Nerve: Structure, Function and Reconstruction.* New York, NY, Raven Press, 1990.
6. Sunderland S, Bradley KC: Stress-strain phenomena in human peripheral nerve trunks. *Brain* 1961;84:102–119.
7. Terzis JK, Fabisoff B, Williams B: The nerve gap: Suture under tension versus graft. *Plast Reconstr Surg* 1975;56:166–170.
8. Sunderland S: *Nerves and Nerve Injuries,* ed 2. New York, NY, Churchill Livingstone, 1978, pp 151–157.
9. Haftek J: Stretch injury of peripheral nerve: Acute effects of stretching on rabbit nerve. *J Bone Joint Surg* 1970;52B:354–365.
10. Tillaux P J: *Des affections chirurgicales des nerfs.* Paris, Asselin, 1866.
11. Mitchell SW: *Injuries of Nerves and Their Consequences.* Philadelphia, PA, JB Lippincott, 1872. (American Academy of Neurology, New York, NY, Dover Publications, 1965).
12. Takimoto G: Ueber die Nervendehnung: Experimentelle und klinische untersuchung. *Mitt med Fak Tokyo* 1917;16:73–136.
13. De Rényi GS: Structure of cells in tissues as revealed by microdissection: II. Physical properties of living axis cylinder in the myelinated nerve fiber of frog. *J Comp Neurol* 1929;47:405–425.
14. Highet WB, Sanders FK: Effects of stretching nerves after suture. *Br J Surg* 1943;30:355–369.
15. Denny-Brown D, Doherty MM: Effects of transient stretching of peripheral nerve. *Arch Neurol Psych* 1945;54:116–129.
16. Liu CT, Benda CE, Lewey FH: Tensile strength of human nerves: Experimental physical and histologic study. *Arch Neurol Psych* 1948;59:322–336.
17. Schneider D: Die Dehnbarkeit der markhaltigen Nervenfaser des Frosches in Abhangigkeit von Funktion und Struktur. *Z Naturfo B* 1952;7(b):38–48.
18. Hoen TI, Brackett CE: Peripheral nerve lengthening: Experimental. *J Neurosurg* 1956;13:43–62.
19. Platt H: Traction lesions of external popliteal nerve. *Lancet* 1940;2:612–614.
20. Highet WB, Holmes W: Traction injuries to lateral popliteal nerve and traction injuries to peripheral nerves after suture. *Br J Surg* 1943;30:212–233.
21. Lundborg G, Rydevik B: Effects of stretching the tibial nerve of the rabbit: A preliminary study of the intraneural circulation and the barrier function of the perineurium. *J Bone Joint Surg* 1973;55B:390–401.
22. Spiegel DA, Seaber AV, Chen LE, et al: Recovery following stretch injury to the sciatic nerve of the rat: An in vivo study. *J Reconstr Microsurg* 1993;9:69–74.
23. Terzis JK, Publicover NG: Clinical application of electrophysiologic recordings, in Terzis JK (ed): *Microreconstruction of Nerve Injuries.* Philadelphia, PA, WB Saunders, 1987, pp 203–210.
24. Terzis JK, Dykes RW, Hakstian RW: Electrophysiological recordings in peripheral nerve surgery: A review. *J Hand Surg* 1976;1:52–66.
25. Marinacci AA: The problem of unusual anomalous innervation of hand muscles: The value of electrodiagnosis in its evaluation. *Bull Los Angeles Neurol Soc* 1964;29:133–142.
26. Michelow BJ, Terzis JK, Lovice D, et al: Rapid nerve expansion. *Microsurgery* 1993;14:33.
27. De Medinaceli L, Freed WJ, Wyatt RJ: An index of the functional condi:ion of rat sciatic nerve based on measurements made from walking tracks. *Exp Neuro* 1982;77:634–643.
28. Bain JR, Mackinnon SE, Hunter DA: Functional evaluation of complete sciatic, peroneal, and posterior tibial nerve lesions in the rat. *Plast Reconstr Surg* 1989;83:129–138.

29. Skoulis TG, Terzis JK: Nerve expansion: The answer to the short nerve gap. Presented at the 11th Congress of the International and Microsurgical Society, Rhodes Island, Greece, June 1992.
30. Aldegheri R, Renzi-Brivio L, Agostini S: The callotasis method of limb lengthening. *Clin Orthop* 1989;241:137–145.
31. Yasui N, Kojimoto H, Shimizu H, et al: The effect of distraction upon bone, muscle, and periosteum. *Orthop Clin North Am* 1991;22:563–567.
32. Polus BI, Patak A, Gregory JE, et al: Effect of muscle length on phasic stretch reflexes in humans and cats. *J Neurophysiol* 1991;66:613–622.
33. Paley D: Problems, obstacles, and complications of limb lengthening by the Ilizarov technique. *Clin Orthop* 1990;250:81–104.
34. Faber FW, Keessen W, van Roermund PM: Complications of leg lengthening: 46 procedures in 26 patients. *Acta Orthop Scan* 1991;62:327–332.
35. Bell DF, Boyer MI, Armstrong PF: The use of the Ilizarov technique in the correction of limb deformities associated with skeletal dysplasia. *J Pediatr Orthop* 1992:12:283–290.
36. Rajacich N, Bell DF, Armstrong PF: Pediatric applications of the Ilizarov method. *Clin Orthop* 1992;280:72–80.
37. Ilizarov GA: The tension-stress effect on the genesis and growth of tissues: Part I. The influence of stability of fixation and soft-tissue preservation. *Clin Orthop* 1989;238:249–281.
38. Ilizarov GA: The tension-stress effect on the genesis and growth of tissues: Part II. The influence of the rate and frequency of distraction. *Clin Orthop* 1989;239:263–285.

Chapter 31

Contraction-Induced Injury to Skeletal Muscle: Mechanisms Underlying the Initial and Secondary Injury

John A. Faulkner, PhD
Peter C. D. Macpherson, MA
Susan V. Brooks, PhD

Introduction

Almost 100 years ago, while studying muscle fatigue in the finger flexor muscles of human beings, Hough[1] observed the phenomenon of late onset muscle soreness and concluded that the delayed pain was caused by injury to skeletal muscle fibers. Several research groups have investigated this phenomenon by contrasting injury to muscles in legs involved in stepping down with injury in legs involved in stepping up[2] and by comparing injury to muscles in legs resisting the rotations of the pedals of a bicycle ergometer with injury in legs producing normal forward rotations of the pedals.[3] These studies supported the premise that injury was more likely to occur during physical activities that involved predominantly a lengthening of muscles during contractions rather than during activities that required muscles to shorten. The studies on human beings also indicated that the muscle injury resulted in a significant increase in the plasma concentration of a number of enzymes normally found in skeletal muscles. These enzymes included creatine kinase[2] and lactate dehydrogenase.[4] Light microscopic evidence showed injury to single skeletal muscle fibers,[5] and electron micrographs indicated that the injury was localized within single sarcomeres.[3]

In spite of their insightful designs, studies of human beings performing complex volitional contractions of diverse muscle groups permit neither identification of which fibers are actually contracting nor determination of the velocity of the movement, the magnitude of the displacement relative to fiber length (strain), or the average force normalized for total fiber cross-sectional area (stress). To control simultaneously, or to measure, each of these variables during shortening, isometric, and lengthening contractions (Fig. 1) and during passive lengthening, McCully and Faulkner[6] developed a single in situ extensor digitorum longus (EDL) muscle preparation in the mouse. With use of this single-muscle preparation, only the protocol of repeated lengthening contractions produced an injury comparable to the human experience of late onset muscle soreness associated with physical activities involving predominantly lengthening contractions. Contraction-induced injury may also be studied rigorously by using a single permeabilized fiber model (PCD Macpherson, JA Faulkner, unpublished data). This chapter will report on a series of investigations based on the single-muscle and single-fiber models of contraction-induced

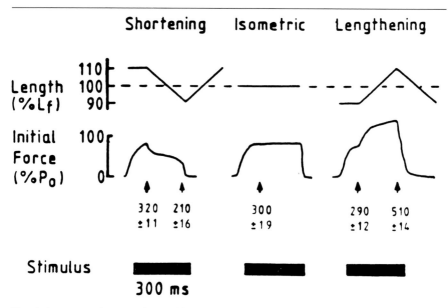

Fig. 1 Representative recordings of length and force for shortening, isometric, and lengthening contractions of extensor digitorum longus muscles of mice. Muscles were stimulated at 150 Hz for 300 ms. Isometric contractions were at the length at which maximum isometric twitch force occurred (L_f). Shortening and lengthening contractions were initiated at 110% and 90% L_f, respectively. After 100 ms of stimulation, the muscle was shortened or lengthened by 20% of L_f at a velocity of 1 L_f/s. Force is expressed as a percentage of the maximum isometric force (P_o). Actual force values (means $\pm$ standard error of the mean expressed in mN) are given below the force traces. (Adapted with permission from McCully KK, Faulkner JA: Injury to skeletal muscle fibers of mice following lengthening contractions. *J Appl Physiol* 1985;59: 119–126.)

injury and will relate the findings to injury to human muscles caused by volitional contractions.

The In Situ EDL Muscle and the Single Fiber Preparations

With the foot at a 90° angle relative to the lower leg, the fibers of the EDL muscle are at the optimum length (L_f) for the development of force. The EDL muscle extends the digits of the foot and dorsiflexes the foot. From L_f, the fibers of the EDL muscle can undergo stretches of approximately 20% strain during full plantarflexion of the foot (E Zerba, JA Faulkner, unpublished data).

To prepare the EDL muscle for contractions in situ, the mouse is anesthetized, and a small incision is made over the tendon of the EDL muscle. The knee is pinned to the baseplate, and the tendon is attached to the lever arm of a servomotor. To obtain single permeabilized fibers, the EDL muscle of the rat is excised and placed in an ice-cold (0°C) skinning solution containing 50% glycerol. Bundles of 50 to 100 fiber segments are immersed in skinning solution and stored for up to 3 weeks at -20°C. The bundles are removed, placed in a low calcium concentration relaxing solution, and single fibers are pulled from the bundles. The single fiber segments are attached to a force transducer and servomotor.

The Lengthening Contraction Protocols

Each lengthening contraction consists of maximally activating (150 Hz stimulation) the EDL muscle or (activating solution with pCa 4.5) the single fiber, allowing the muscle or fiber to develop maximum force, and then stretching the muscle or fiber from L_f to some percentage of L_f at a constant velocity in L_f/s and returning it to L_f. Consequently, throughout this chapter, the magnitudes of all stretches are defined with the assumption that L_f corresponds to zero strain. Two protocols of lengthening contractions are used: a repeated contraction protocol and a single contraction protocol. The repeated contraction protocols consist of 75, 225, or 360 stretches of 20% strain at a velocity of 0.5 L_f/s with one contraction every 4 s. The single contraction protocols for whole muscles consist of single stretches of between 10% and 70% strain at velocities of lengthening ranging from 0.5 to 3 L_f/s. Similarly, the single contraction protocols for single fibers involve single stretches of 5%, 10%, or 20% strain at a velocity of 0.5 L_f/s. The average force during contractions is not controlled. During repeated lengthening contractions, the average force decreases rapidly.

Criteria of Injury

Histologic, histochemical, and electron microscopic techniques provide the only direct measurements of injury. To conclude that a contraction or protocol of contractions has caused injury to skeletal muscle fibers, photomicrographs following the contraction protocol must show evidence of a change in fiber morphology that is consistent with a diagnosis of damage (Figs. 2 and 3). Direct evidence of damage to fibers may include disruption of the thick and thin filament lattice of single sarcomeres, disruption of the structural integrity of whole sarcomeres, damage to the sarcolemma, infiltration of fibers by phago-

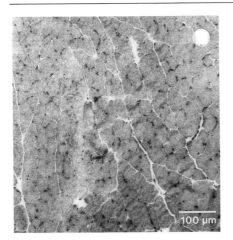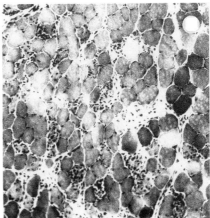

Fig. 2 The two panels show photomicrographs of a portion of the cross section through the belly of a control extensor digitorum longus (EDL) muscle (**left**) and an EDL muscle 3 days after a protocol of 360 lengthening contractions with a contraction occurring every 5 s (**right**). The sections were stained with hematoxylin and eosin. The scale bar applies to both panels. (Reproduced with permission from Faulkner JA, Jones DA, Round JM: Injury to skeletal muscles of mice by forced lengthening during contractions. *Q J Exp Physiol* 1989;74:661–670.)

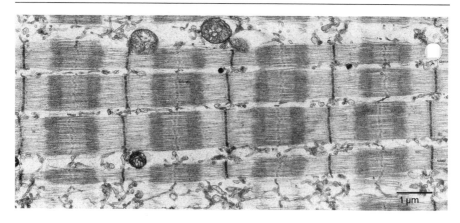

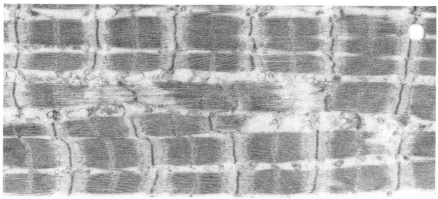

Fig. 3 The two panels show electron micrographs of longitudinal sections of a control single permeable fiber (**top**) and a single permeable fiber immediately after a single maximally activated stretch of 10% strain (**bottom**). The scale bar applies to both panels. Note the damage to single sarcomeres in the bottom panel.

cytes, and, eventually, complete loss of sarcoplasmic elements.[2,3] Although direct morphologic evidence of contraction-induced injury is important, it is not possible to quantify the magnitude of the injury by direct methods. This impossibility results from the highly focal nature of the injury, both in cross sections of the muscle and longitudinally, along the length of individual muscle fibers.[6,7]

Indirect measures of injury to skeletal muscle fibers include enzyme release from muscle fibers,[2,8] increased calcium influx,[8,9] increased ratio of oxidized to reduced glutathione,[10] an increase in the force deficit in the absence of fatigue, and the subjective report of muscle soreness in humans. Most of the indirect measures either vary in magnitude with time or are influenced by intervening variables not directly associated with the injury. Of all the indirect measures, the decrease in the ability of the muscle or fiber to develop maximum isometric force provides the most quantitative measure of the magnitude of the totality of the injury.[6] Because the deficit in maximum force relative to the maximum force developed by the control muscle before injury—[1 − (maximum force after injury/maximum force before injury)] × 100—provides the best prediction of the magnitude of the morphologic damage, this force deficit is the most useful representation of injury. After a protocol of repeated contractions, the force deficit represents both fatigue and injury for some period of time (E Zerba, JA Faulkner, unpublished data).[11] Because fibers recover from fatigue within a matter of hours and certainly by 24 hours,[12] the best estimate of the force deficit attributable to the initial injury is the force deficit at 3 hours (Fig. 4). The estimate of the magnitude of the injury based on the force deficit assumes a recovery from fatigue and that no major change in the magnitude of the contraction-induced injury occurs during the first 3 hours of recovery. In contrast, after a single contraction with no possibility of fatigue present, the force deficit provides a valid estimate of the injury immediately after the initiation of the injury (E Zerba, JA Faulkner, unpublished data).

Time Course of Contraction-Induced Injury

As represented by the force deficit, an initial injury is observed immediately after a protocol of either a single or repeated lengthening contractions. The presence of this initial injury is supported by electron micrographs of damaged fibers (PCD Macpherson, E Zerba, JA Faulkner, unpublished data). The initial injury is followed by a secondary injury that peaks between 1 and 5 days later (Fig. 4). The timing of the secondary injury appears to be a function of the severity of the initial injury.

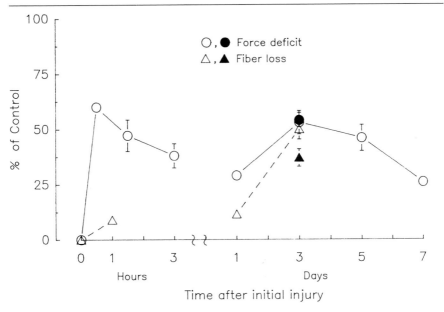

Fig. 4 Data are shown for the force deficit (circles) and fiber loss (triangles) measured prior to and at selected times following a protocol of repeated lengthening contractions administered to the ankle dorsiflexor muscles (open symbols) and the extensor digitorum (EDL) muscles (filled symbols) of mice. The dorsiflexor muscle group was exposed to a protocol of 360 lengthening contractions and the EDL muscle to a protocol of 225 lengthening contractions. All values are expressed as percentages of the control value measured for uninjured muscles and represent means ± standard error of the mean. (Adapted with permission from McCully KK, Faulkner JA: Injury to skeletal muscle fibers of mice following lengthening contractions. *J Appl Physiol* 1985;59:119–126.)

Although slight variations are observed in the timing of the peak values, plasma creatine kinase concentration,[2] subjective assessments of muscle pain,[2] and the number of damaged and missing fibers are in reasonable agreement with the timing of the peak force deficit (Fig. 4). Light microscopy of sections stained with hematoxylin and eosin shows no significant loss of fibers or injury to fibers during the first few hours after a protocol of lengthening contractions. However, electron microscopic evidence of injury to individual sarcomeres is observed within minutes of a single lengthening contraction or of a repeated lengthening contraction protocol.[3] Although the peaks in force deficit and the number of missing or severely damaged fibers peak at about the same time, the magnitude of the deficit in force is usually greater than that based on the number of damaged fibers.[6,13] The discrepancy is attributed to the focal nature of the injury, with some fibers that appear normal in one cross section being injured in another region of the muscle.[6,7]

Mechanisms Underlying the Initial Injury

The mechanism responsible for the initial injury is primarily mechanical in nature. Theoretical support for the mechanical basis of the initial injury is provided by the models of force development during constant velocity lengthening contractions reported by Harry and associates[14] and Morgan.[15] A number of different experimental observations support the mechanical basis of the initial injury to active muscles or muscle fibers.

Following a single lengthening contraction, the force deficit is a function of both the average force developed during the stretch and the magnitude of the displacement. Consequently, the product of average force and displacement, the work done to stretch the muscle, has the highest predictive value. In contrast, during repeated lengthening contractions, the relationship is complicated by the rapid decrease in average force (Fig. 4). Following protocols of repeated lengthening contractions, the variable and eventually negligible values for average force can lead to the erroneous conclusion that displacement (d) or strain (d/L_f) is the determinant of injury.[16] Muscles previously fatigued by a protocol of isometric contractions begin to approach the displacement—average force relationship of a passive muscle. Such fatigued muscles are no longer injured by a protocol of repeated lengthening contractions that initially caused a 55% force deficit at 3 days.[17]

Compared with the stretching of passive muscles, the stretching of maximally activated muscles results in a much greater increase in the heterogeneity in sarcomere lengths.[18] Our hypothesis is that during stretches of active fibers, the heterogeneity in sarcomere length in series along myofibrils arises from intrinsic differences in the relative strengths of different sarcomeres. When fibers with imbalances in sarcomere strength are stretched, the strong sarcomeres are stretched less than the weak sarcomeres.[18,19] Under these circumstances, even with small displacements, weak sarcomeres may be stretched beyond overlap of thick and thin filaments.[20] In support of this conclusion, single stretches of 10% strain of maximally activated single fibers result in the same force deficit as single stretches of 60% strain of passive single fibers.

A stretch of ~55% strain of a passive single fiber extends the average sarcomere to a length beyond the overlap of thick and thin filaments.[21] Repeated stretches of this magnitude result in injury to the thick and thin filament structure of sarcomeres.[21] The injury is quite uniform throughout the sarcomeres of a passively stretched fiber. In contrast, following small stretches of active fibers, the injury to the ultrastructure of sarcomeres is focal, and the injury involves only scattered groups of sarcomeres (PCD Macpherson, E Zerba, JA Faulkner, unpublished data). The exact mechanism responsible for contraction-induced injury is not known. Our hypothesis is that contraction-induced injury results within individual sarcomeres when thick and thin filaments are stretched beyond overlap and do not interdigitate successfully on return to L_f. For stretches of active muscles or fibers, even if sarcomeres are not stretched beyond overlap, injury may be initiated by strain of the cross-bridges, the sarcolemma, or the Z-line.

The observation that repeated lengthening contractions of 20% strain produce an injury of similar magnitude to a single lengthening contraction of 70% strain is consistent with the idea that sarcomere heterogeneity increases during repeated lengthening contractions with small displacements, as has been reported for passive single fibers.[21]

Mechanisms Underlying the Secondary Injury

As evaluated by the force deficit, the secondary injury takes several days to develop, but is usually of greater severity than the initial injury (Fig. 4). This conclusion is supported by the phenomenon of late onset muscle soreness experienced by humans after a variety of different, unusually vigorous, or exhaustive physical activities. The secondary injury gives rise to increased plasma concentration of creatine kinase[2] and lactate dehydrogenase.[4] The increase in the plasma concentrations of enzymes usually found in the sarcoplasm of muscle fibers has led to the conclusion that the muscle membrane integrity is seriously impaired.[2,22] This conclusion is further supported by the increase in the concentration of intracellular calcium,[9] which activates a variety of proteolytic enzymes.[8] The subsequent cascade of events produces an increase in the ratio of oxidized to reduced glutathione[10] and a degradation of sarcoplasmic proteins.[23]

Oxygen free radical damage to muscle fibers that have already suffered mechanical injury was considered a key element in the secondary injury, but the exact role of oxygen free radicals has been difficult to identify. The concentration of oxygen free radicals in skeletal muscles is difficult to measure because of their short half life.[23] As an alternative, the activity of oxygen free radicals can be blocked by increasing the concentration of the oxygen free radical scavenger, superoxide dismutase. Mice were treated with 1,000 U/kg of polyethyleneglycol superoxide dismutase (PEG-SOD) for 3 days before and 3 days after a protocol of lengthening contractions.[13] Without the PEG-SOD treatment, the protocol caused a 50% force deficit at 3 days; whereas, young mice treated with PEG-SOD had a force deficit of 10% (Fig. 5). The conclusion was that oxygen free radical damage was the major factor in the secondary injury.[13] The design did not permit resolution of the cause of the 10% force deficit that remained. This could be due to incomplete recovery from the initial mechanical injury, an incomplete block of oxygen free radical injury, or to a small additional injury from factors other than oxygen free radicals.

Summary

The single in situ whole muscle preparation in the mouse and the single in vitro permeable fiber preparation provide valid models for the study of the mechanisms responsible for contraction-induced injury. The data correlate well in time and magnitude with indirect measures of the secondary injury observed in human beings. In particular, the time and severity of the force deficit are in

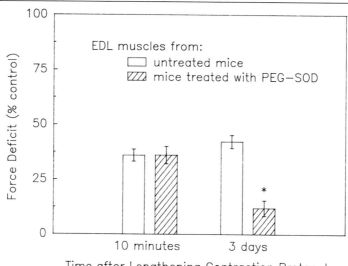

Fig. 5 Force deficits expressed as a percentage of control values at 10 minutes and 3 days following a protocol of 75 lengthening contractions at a rate of 1/4 s. PEG-SOD is polyethyleneglycol superoxide dismutase. Values are means ± standard error of the mean. Asterisk indicates a significant difference (p < 0.05) between muscles from treated and untreated mice.

good agreement with the widely reported phenomena of late onset muscle soreness and elevated plasma creatine kinase.

Acknowledgment

The research work on which this chapter is based was supported by National Institute on Aging grant AG-06157.

References

1. Hough T: Ergographic studies in muscular soreness. *Am J Physiol* 1902;7:76–92.
2. Newham DJ, Jones DA, Edwards RHT: Large delayed plasma creatine kinase changes after stepping exercise. *Muscle Nerve* 1983;6:380–385.
3. Fridén J, Sjöström M, Ekblom B: Myofibrillar damage following intense eccentric exercise in man. *Int J Sports Med* 1983;4:170–176.
4. Schwane JA, Johnson SR, Vandenakker CB, et al: Delayed-onset muscular soreness and plasma CPK and LDH activities after downhill running. *Med Sci Sports Exerc* 1983;15:51–56.
5. Jones DA, Newham DJ, Round JM, et al: Experimental human muscle damage: Morphological changes in relation to other indices of damage. *J Physiol* 1986;375: 435–448.
6. McCully KK, Faulkner JA: Injury to skeletal muscle fibers of mice following lengthening contractions. *J Appl Physiol* 1985;59:119–126.
7. Ogilvie RW, Armstrong RB, Baird KE, et al: Lesions in the rat soleus muscle following eccentrically biased exercise. *Am J Anat* 1988;182:335–346.
8. Jackson MJ, Jones DA, Edwards RHT: Experimental skeletal muscle damage: The nature of the calcium-activated degenerative processes. *Eur J Clin Invest* 1984;14: 369–374.

9. Jones DA, Jackson MJ, McPhail G, et al: Experimental mouse muscle damage: The importance of external calcium. *Clin Sci* 1984;66:317–322.
10. Lew H, Pyke S, Quintanilha A: Changes in the glutathione status of plasma, liver and muscle following exhaustive exercise in rats. *FEBS Lett* 1985;185:262–266.
11. Faulkner JA, Jones DA, Round JM: Injury to skeletal muscles of mice by forced lengthening during contractions. *Q J Exp Physiol* 1989;74:661–670.
12. Faulkner JA, Brooks SV: Fatigability of mouse muscles during constant length, shortening, and lengthening contractions: Interactions between fiber types and duty cycles, in Sargeant AJ, Kernell D (eds): *Neuromuscular Fatigue*. Amsterdam, Royal Netherlands Academy of Arts and Sciences, 1993, pp 116–123.
13. Zerba E, Komorowski TE, Faulkner JA: Free radical injury to skeletal muscles of young, adult, and old mice. *Am J Physiol* 1990;258(3Pt1):C429–C435.
14. Harry JD, Ward AW, NC Heglund, et al: Cross-bridge cycling theories cannot explain high-speed lengthening behavior in frog muscle. *Biophys J* 1990;57:201–208.
15. Morgan DL: New insights into the behavior of muscle during active lengthening. *Biophys J* 1990;57:209–221.
16. Lieber RL, Fridén J: Muscle damage is not a function of muscle force but active muscle strain. *J Appl Physiol* 1993;74:520–526.
17. McCully KK, Faulkner JA: Characteristics of lengthening contractions associated with injury to skeletal muscle fibers. *J Appl Physiol* 1986;61:293–299.
18. Julian FJ, Morgan DL: The effect on tension of non-uniform distribution of length changes applied to frog muscle fibres. *J Physiol* 1979;293:379–392.
19. Julian FJ, Morgan DL: Intersarcomere dynamics during fixed-end tetanic contractions of frog muscle fibres. *J Physiol* 1979;293:365–378.
20. Brown LM, Hill L: Some observations on variations in filament overlap in tetanized muscle fibres and fibres stretched during a tetanus, detected in the electron microscope after rapid fixation. *J Muscle Res Cell Motil* 1991;12:171–182.
21. Higuchi H, Yoshioka T, Maruyama K: Positioning of actin filaments and tension generation in skinned muscle fibres released after stretch beyond overlap of the actin and myosin filaments. *J Muscle Res Cell Motil* 1988;9:491–498.
22. Jones DA, Jackson MJ, Edwards RHT: Release of intracellular enzymes from an isolated mammalian skeletal muscle preparation. *Clin Sci* 1983;65:193–201.
23. Jackson MJ, Edwards RHT: Free radicals, muscle damage and muscular dystrophy, in Quintanilha A (ed): *Reactive Oxygen Species in Chemistry, Biology, and Medicine*. New York, Plenum Press, 1988, pp 197–210.

Chapter 32

Experimental Assessment of Bone Regenerate Quality During Distraction Osteogenesis

James Aronson, MD

Introduction

Ilizarov first introduced the method of distraction osteogenesis both experimentally and clinically during his 40-year career in Siberia.[1,2] Distraction osteogenesis involves the mechanical stretching, using external fixation, of reparative tissue invoked by a low-energy osteotomy. Ilizarov's work implies that this process is regenerative rather than reparative, consequently he referred to the new bone as "regenerate bone."[3,4] His clinical successes, saving the limbs of thousands of patients with conditions that traditionally resulted in amputation, not only have revolutionized the current practice of modern orthopaedic surgery[5,6] but also have complemented the exciting advances being made in stimulation of bone formation by other inductive modes, such as electromagnetic coils, ultrasound, and osteogenic proteins.

Invasive analyses using decalcified and nondecalcified histology, india ink injection with Spalteholz clearing, backscattered scanning electron microscopy (SEM), gravimetric and chemical analysis, and biomechanical testing have all been used in our laboratory to characterize the process of distraction osteogenesis. Relatively noninvasive methods including plain radiography, arteriography, technetium scintigraphy, computed tomography, and strain gauge measurements have been used in order to correlate findings with those of the invasive techniques.

With groups of four adult dogs (the minimum number required for statistical comparison), treatment conditions could be altered to produce significant variations in outcome from those encountered in the normal process. Results obtained using these invasive tests were then compared to data obtained using noninvasive tools in order to develop reliable methods for monitoring patients in the clinical setting.

Canine Tibial Lengthening Model

Ilizarov used the canine tibia to study distraction osteogenesis. By varying the stability of fixation, energy of the osteotomy (ie, degree of vascular damage), and rate and rhythm of distraction, he postulated that all four factors are critical to osteogenesis.[3,4]

I have reproduced Ilizarov's original model of a 28-mm lengthening of the adult canine tibia following a 7-day latency to study the histology, blood supply, and radiology of bone formation during distraction osteogenesis. Most experiments have been run with four animals in each group, using the contralateral, normal tibia as a control. Results summarized here were found to be significant according to a Wilcoxon nonparametric statistical analysis.[7]

Adult (skeletally mature by radiographic closure of physes) mongrel dogs weighing 15 to 25 kg were used in all experiments. Following a timetable outlined by Ilizarov in his early experiments, the operation started at day 0. After a 7-day latency period, distraction was carried out from day 7 to day 35 for a total of 28 days. The distraction rate of 1 mm per day at a rhythm of 4 times per day (0.25 mm every 6 hours) was used for the first few groups of dogs, but a rhythm of two times a day (0.5 mm each) was found to be adequate for normal distraction osteogenesis in the dog model.[8–11] From day 35 to day 77, the frame was left intact for a 42-day consolidation period. At day 77, the dogs were sedated, and the frames were removed. The dogs were finally euthanized 42 days later, on day 119. The dogs were housed in a 4-ft × 8-ft² cage and allowed daily activity. The protocol was consistent with Department of Laboratory Animal Medicine standards. Veterinarians administered anesthesia and postoperative care and observed the animals daily for pain or infection. The dogs were maintained on a normal chow diet.

The surgical procedure was performed on day 0 under sterile conditions. Dogs were premedicated (atropine, ketamine, and innovar) and given general orotracheal anesthesia (metaphase). The external fixator was applied using two pins in both the proximal and distal tibia, 4-mm half-pins for the anteromedial monolateral frames, and 1.6- to 1.8-mm tensioned wires for the two-ring external fixator (Fig. 1). An Ilizarov corticotomy (a low-energy, subperiosteal osteotomy of only the cortex with hammer, chisel, and torsional osteoclasis) was performed for lengthening (Fig. 2). Special care was taken to avoid periosteal damage (subperiosteal retractors) and to preserve the intramedullary blood supply (minimum diastasis ≤ 2 mm). A partial fibulectomy was done to prevent bony tether. Sterile dressings were applied for 2 days postoperatively.

My initial experiments tested the hypothesis that rate and rhythm are critical to distraction osteogenesis. Seven days following external fixation of a corticotomy in the proximal tibia, the entire distraction gap was created under sedation to see whether new bone would bridge between the cut surfaces. In all animals, an atrophic nonunion developed. This experiment reproduced the original method of limb lengthening reported by Codivilla at the turn of the century,[12] which routinely resulted in an empty gap.

In order to further examine the effects of rate and rhythm, the next group underwent the Ilizarov corticotomy with sporadic daily distractions of 1.0 to 1.5 mm, which is similar to the standard and currently accepted technique of limb lengthening developed by Wagner.[13,14] More bone was produced but, again, all trials resulted in nonunion. The Wagner technique is intended to include three stages: to distract, to graft the defect with internal plate fixation, and then, years later, to remove the plate when all of the graft is incorporated and remodeled.

When the corticotomized fragments were distracted at the rate and rhythm recommended by Ilizarov, 0.25 mm every 6 hours, all bones bridged and went on to remodel to normal lengthened bone. Whole bone gravimetrics were used to confirm that new bone was actually produced; the average 12% (26 to 28 mm) lengthening produced an average 27% increase in mass and an average 26% increase in volume, for a minimal change in whole bone density.[15]

Chemical analysis of the newly consolidated bone demonstrated average water (15%), lipid (5%), calcium (25%), phosphorus (12%), and collagen

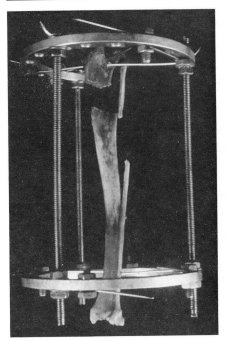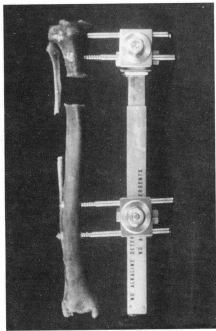

Fig. 1 Canine tibia with metaphyseal separation demonstrating experimental 28-mm gap. **Left,** Two-ring external fixator with tensioned wires, fabricated to specifications of the Ilizarov device. After 1987, similar commercial devices were used (donated by Smith & Nephew Richards, Memphis, TN). Wrenches are necessary to rotate each pair of nuts securing the three connecting rods to one of the rings for bony distraction. **Right,** Wagner monolateral frame with 4-mm half-pins mounted anteromedially (donated by Synthes, Paoli, PA). Distraction is accomplished by manually turning the knob at one end.

(24%) content, as well as calcium:phosphorus (2:1) and calcium:collagen (1:1) ratios similar to those measured in normal bone.[9,16–18]

Rate was further tested by comparing two groups distracted at 1 and 2 mm per day. In both groups, all bones bridged the gap and remodeled to normal-appearing bone; however, noninvasive monitoring techniques—quantitative technetium scintigraphy and quantitative computed tomography (QCT)—detected a trend toward decreased osteoid production and mineralization at weeks 4 and 5 in the more rapid, 2 mm/day group.

Distraction osteogenesis stimulated by the same corticotomy, latency, and rate and rhythm was then tested for fixator specificity by comparing the tensioned-wire ring external fixator modeled after the Ilizarov device used in all previous experiments to the standard half-pin fixator used by Wagner.[10,19–21] The radiographic and histologic appearance of new bone formation was identical, except that the medially placed half-pin device tended toward uncontrolled angulation (valgus) during the distraction process. If any external fixator was destabilized (eg, untensioned wires, loose pins, or flexible frame), the distraction produced bone that either angulated (malunion) or failed to bridge (nonunion).

Histology

Histologic preparations were made using biopsy samples and whole bones sectioned in the coronal and transverse planes.

Low-Energy Corticotomy in adult canine tibia: cortex cracked by osteotome while periosteal tube and spongiosa preserved.

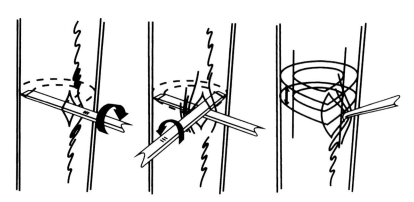

Fig. 2 This drawing depicts the Ilizarov method of producing a low-energy osteotomy by cutting only the cortex (corticotomy), preserving periosteum and endosteal vessels. Torsional osteoclasis completes the corticotomy. (Adapted with permission from Chapman M: The biology of distraction osteogenesis, in *Operative Orthopaedics*, ed 2. Philadelphia, PA, JB Lippincott, 1993, p 877.)

The initial latency period appears to be no different than for routine fracture healing. Fibrin-enclosed hematoma and inflammatory cell infiltration fill the gap at the corticotomy site. At the start of distraction, mesenchymal cells begin to organize a bridge of collagen and immature vascular sinusoids. New bone formation is limited to trabeculae deep within each cut bone segment; cartilage islands are not present.

As distraction begins, the fibrovascular bridge seems to organize itself parallel to the direction of distraction.[9] The collagen network becomes more dense and less vascular, almost resembling tendon, while the vascular channels remain at the edges next to the cut surfaces of the corticotomy segments. During the first week of distraction, this central zone of relatively avascular fibrous tissue bridges the entire 6- to 7-mm gap.[22] I have called it the fibrous interzone (FIZ). Spindle-shaped cells resembling fibroblasts are loosely interspersed between collagen bundles; neither osteoid nor osteoblasts are evident. Bone mineral is distinctly absent by von Kossa staining and backscattered SEM of nondecalcified specimens. Cartilage islands are not seen.

During the second week of distraction, osteoblastic cells appear in clusters adjacent to the vascular sinuses on either side of the FIZ. Collagen bundles become fused with pink-staining matrix resembling osteoid (Fig. 3). The osteoblastic cells initially rest on the surface of these primary bone spicules and eventually become enveloped as the spicules gradually enlarge by circumferential apposition of collagen and osteoid.[5,10] By the end of the second week, the osteoid begins to mineralize (Fig. 4). These early bone spicules, called the primary matrix front (PMF), extend from each corticotomy surface toward the central FIZ, three-dimensionally resembling geologic stalactites and stalagmites.[22] The mineralization within the columns was confirmed by von Kossa staining of the nondecalcified specimens and by backscattered SEM of carbon-coated specimens.[5,23] This osteogenic process uniformly covers the entire cross

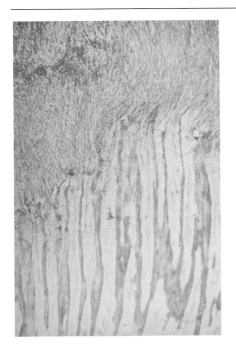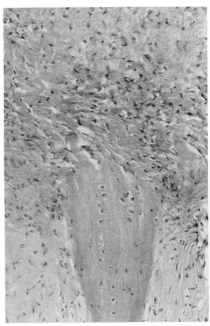

Fig. 3 Decalcified histology of new bone microcolumns, each of which grows parallel to the distraction force from a central collagen bridge. The host bone surfaces are both mechanically and biologically connected by this process. **Left,** Parallel columns of bone (below) arise from central collagen fibers (above) (aniline blue, × 4). **Right,** Collagen fibers incorporate directly into top of new microcolumn of bone (hematoxylin and eosin, × 20).

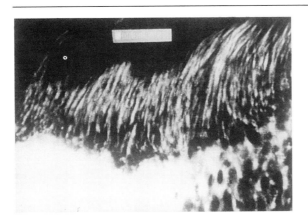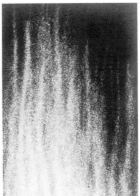

Fig. 4 Microradiographs of nascent microcolumns demonstrating the mineralization patterns within each that produce zonal increases in overall density. **Left,** Newly mineralized microcolumns arise from both cortical and cancellous (endosteal) host surfaces. **Right,** Conical mineralization within each column from the tip at 5 to 10 μm to 200 μm in diameter.

section of the cut bone, including periosteum, cortex, and medullary spongiosa.[5]

From the third week on, this process continues with the FIZ undulating across the center at an average thickness of 6 mm. As the distraction gap increases, the bridge is formed by the elongation of the new bone spicules. These bone spicules are actually bridged by the collagen fibers, as can be seen by routine and polarized light microscopy.[5] The tips of the spicules begin at a diameter of approximately 7 to 10 μm and rapidly expand to diameters of up to 150 μm at each corticotomy surface.[5,10,22] Each microcolumn of new bone is surrounded by large thin-walled sinusoids.[5] The columns have no haversian canals, and no cartilage or osteoclasts are seen. I have called this zone microcolumn formation (MCF).

At the conclusion of distraction, the FIZ ossifies to create one zone of MCF that completely bridges the gap. Cartilage islands may form centrally in areas more than 300 μm from local vessels.[5] This cartilage formation is rarely seen if distraction is carried out at the proper rate and rhythm, and bone fixation remains stable. Cartilage interposition indicates formation of the osseous bridge by very slow endochondral ossification and is seen more often if the tissue has been traumatized by unstable fixation. This phenomenon was noted in cases of local pin osteolysis.

In this experimental model, the frame was removed 6 weeks following the 4-week distraction period. During this 6-week consolidation period, the dogs usually resumed weightbearing.

During the 6 weeks following frame removal, the osteogenic area remodels into cortex and medullary canal. The bony columns take on the staining characteristics of mature lamellar bone, with cement lines and smaller osteocytes resting in lacunae. The fibrovascular tissue that filled the spaces around bone columns is replaced by normal-appearing marrow elements. Normal osteoclastic remodeling is present.

Some clinicians using the Ilizarov method have referred to this area of bone regeneration as a growth plate, and in the sense of new bone formation it is. However, histologically, distraction osteogenesis involves intramembranous and not endochondral ossification. This direct appositional bone growth of distraction osteogenesis with osteoblasts laying down osteoid, which is then mineralized, is seen in normal bone remodeling. It is also seen with periosteal new bone formation. In fact, the only part of a growth plate that resembles distraction osteogenesis is at the zone of Ranvier, where periosteum is stretched across the physis.[24]

Cartilage and an endochondral sequence have been noted in some of my specimens when the local blood supply has been disrupted or when bone-fixator instability occurred. The endochondral sequence of ossification seems to occur much more slowly, and residual islands may persist indefinitely. In all of my experimental canine tibial lengthenings, as well as those reported by others,[25] and in two biopsies on my patients, intramembranous ossification has been the predominant finding.

Blood Supply

Physiologically, the regional and local blood supply is probably the most absolute requirement for new bone formation. Based on a combination of angiography, histology, india ink injections, and quantitative technetium scintigraphy, my findings substantiate this assertion and provide some additional insights.

Histologically, each column of new bone is completely surrounded by large vascular sinusoids (Fig. 5). Clusters of osteoblasts at the tip of each column are in close proximity to these sinusoids.[5] India ink injection studies with Spalteholz clearing technique demonstrate that these vessels parallel the bone columns and

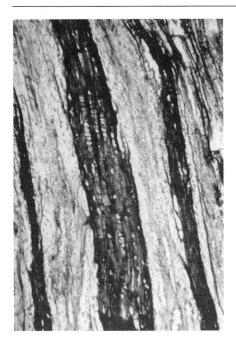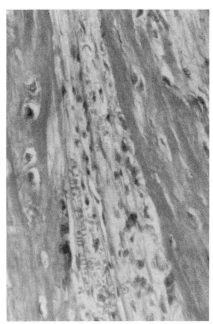

Fig. 5 The blood supply is intimately arranged with the new microcolumns of bone. **Left,** Fibrovascular tissues separate and surround each microcolumn (aniline blue, × 10). **Right,** Polymorphic mesenchymal cells lie in the loose matrix with these vessels (aniline blue, × 40).

the distraction force; however, very few vessels actually cross the FIZ, which remains relatively avascular.[5]

Technetium scintigraphy of the osteogenic area is intensely hot, with a central cool area corresponding to the FIZ. We developed a method of quantitative technetium scintigraphy to automatically outline the hottest 40% of the distracted tibia and measure the average number of counts per pixel in this region of interest.[26] The computer program then creates a mirror image region of interest on the contralateral control tibia, providing the average counts per pixel for comparison.

The initial or flow phase of the quantitative technetium scan (QTS) correlates best with blood flow.[27] During the 4 weeks of distraction, flow in the experimental side peaks at seven times the normal (baseline preoperative intact bones) side and then decreases to three times normal for at least the next 3 months. The curve pattern of these measurements resembles that for simple fracture healing in a similar study, although the actual values during distraction osteogenesis are twice those of the fracture model.[28]

Pathophysiology

Conditions, documented from experimental animals and patients, that reliably lead to poor osteogenesis are excessive rate of distraction, sporadic rhythm, initial diastasis, frame or bone-fixator instability, inadequate consolidation period, poor regional or local blood supply, and an excessively traumatic corticotomy. The massive increase in regional blood flow (measured experimentally) must circulate uniformly throughout the tissue at the microscopic level. The orderly zones of bone formation seen in normal distraction osteogenesis involve collagen deposition, osteoid formation, and mineralization. It is easy to speculate that an initial diastasis between the cut bone surfaces would inhibit the formation of a primary fibrovascular bridge, which seems essential to transmit distraction force to the tissue level. External fixation frame instability results in macromotion, especially shear forces, which could disrupt the delicate bone and vascular channels (Fig. 6).

Regulation of rate and rhythm is important for rate-limited steps, such as protein synthesis and mitosis, in the biosynthetic pathways on the cellular level, especially those steps involved in angiogenesis. If the host bone suffers from inadequate vascularity initially, the regional hyperemic response to the corticotomy may be insufficient to drive the local biology. Systemic factors such as diabetes, smoking, or peripheral vascular disease may limit vascularity, or a traumatic corticotomy could severely disturb the local flow. In my clinical practice, distraction osteogenesis of patients with these conditions has been more likely to result in nonunion. Biopsies from such sites of failed osteogenesis reveal ischemic, atrophic fibrous tissue with the host bone surface devoid of osteocytes in lacunae and red blood cells absent from vascular spaces.

If the bone ends are initially separated by more than a centimeter or are distracted too quickly, islands of cartilage proliferate in the gap. Gaps and motion[29] have traditionally been implicated in the formation of nonunions and pseudarthroses. Even after successful osteogenesis, remodeling to lamellar bone and normal macrostructure is necessary for normal weightbearing. Experimental premature destabilization of the frame has led to late breakdown of the microcolumns and subsequent replacement with a fibrocartilaginous nonunion.[11]

Noninvasive Monitoring

During the process of distraction osteogenesis, it is clinically helpful to assess the progress of bone formation. Early on, the surgeon might adjust the length

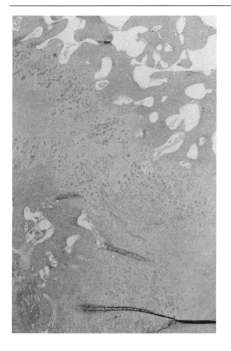

Fig. 6 Fibrocartilage interposition within the distraction gap replaces the intramembranous bone columns when the external fixator is unstable (hematoxylin and eosin, × 4).

of latency to enhance the osteogenic potential. During distraction, rate or rhythm adjustments may be necessary to optimize osteogenesis. During consolidation it is important to know when the osteogenic area is strong enough to remove the fixator.

Standard radiography provides a good weekly or biweekly check on the progress of the distraction gap (length and alignment). Usually, by the third week of distraction, new bone mineral appears as fuzzy, radiodense columns extending from both cut surfaces toward the center.[9,11,30] As distraction proceeds, the central FIZ remains as an undulating radiolucent zone, between 4 and 8 mm wide, while more and more new bone is added from each end.[22] The new bone should span the entire cross-sectional area of the host bone surfaces on both orthogonal views. If the new bone appears to be bulging and the FIZ is narrowing, osteogenesis is proceeding too rapidly, risking premature consolidation, and the distraction rate should be accelerated. If the new bone forms an hourglass appearance and the FIZ is widening, osteogenesis is proceeding too slowly, risking nonunion, and the distraction rate should be decelerated.

The absence of new radiodensity by the third week of distraction is cause for concern (Fig. 7). Sensitivity of ultrasonic examination to mineral depositions within cartilage prior to their appearance on plain radiographs was confirmed by my extensive clinical experience with the neonatal hip. Unfortunately, my experience with ultrasound during distraction osteogenesis was not as reliable. Vascular channels are also echogenic and may mimic the new microcolumns of bone. The high resolution probe may not fit easily between rings, even with silicone spacers. Circumferential examinations are usually obscured by the rings, rods, and anatomy. Occasionally, the distraction gap appears empty by ultrasound, indicating a cystic cavity. In this rare instance, distraction should cease and the gap should be gradually closed until the corticotomy surfaces engage for a repeat latency prior to redistraction.

QCT is a technique [31–34] that I have found extremely useful. The histologic zones of distraction osteogenesis create a predictable pattern of mineralization that can be detected and measured with QCT. The average number of Housfield units (HU) per pixel in a freehand region of interest drawn around the perimeter of the osteogenic area is computer generated at each level in a series of transverse cuts spanning the distraction gap. These values are reproducible with minimal interference by the connecting rods or aluminum telescopic rods.[35] (Heavy metal, such as rings, wire fixation bolts, or the steel head of the clicker units will cause significant interference, so measurements in these areas should be avoided.) When compared to a similar anatomic region on the contralateral, normal side, the average QCT density is converted to a percentage of normal. The FIZ usually is about 25% to 35% of normal, the PMF usually rises to about 40% to 55% of normal, and the MCF remains at about 60% to 75% of normal during distraction.[22] These values are roughly supported by a similar increase in the calcium to collagen ratios measured experimentally from the different zones. The chemical analysis of specimens taken from the different radiologic-histologic zones reflects the QCT density in the corresponding zones. Calcium was measured from dried, defatted bone (µg of calcium per mg of bone) and expressed as a percentage of the normal contralateral bone: FIZ, 30%; PMF, 40% to 50%; and the MCF, 60% to 70%.[22] If this uniform sequence is present by QCT, then distraction can continue despite radiolucency on plain films.

When new bone mineral cannot be demonstrated by plain radiography or QCT, I have found the triphase technetium bone scan to be quite useful. Based on experimental evidence, the distraction gap should be very hot in all three

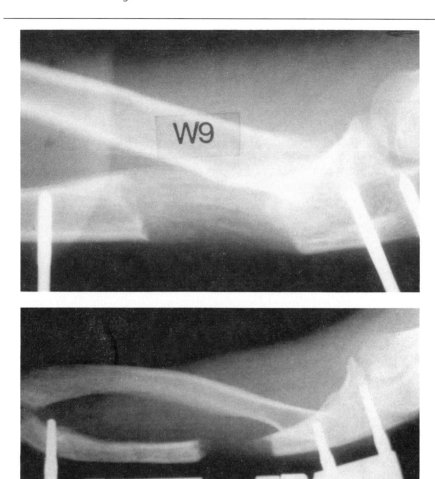

Fig. 7 Two patients with identical diagnosis of multiple hereditary exostoses, short ulna, and monolateral distraction devices. The only difference between them was the initial diastasis of the corticotomy at surgery. **Top,** Excellent distraction osteogenesis bridges the distracted bone surfaces with a central radiolucent fibrous interzone. The corticotomy was held in contact for a latency of 5 days prior to distraction. **Bottom,** No radiographic signs of new bone after the same amount and time of distraction in the patient with an initial corticotomy diastasis of 10 mm despite the same latency and 1 mm per day distraction rate. The gap failed to form bone and required subsequent bone grafting. The tissue within the gap revealed ischemic fibrous tissue with a few small islands of bone formation.

phases.[5,26] It is important to discern that technetium uptake is increased on both sides of the osteogenic gap. In cases of poor vascularity or traumatic corticotomy, a triphase bone scan can also be performed after the predicted latency to confirm that both sides of the corticotomy have adequate flow (Fig. 8). If the scan is cold, distraction must be discontinued and the local problem carefully assessed. Arteriography, which is rarely indicated in these circumstances, can be helpful preoperatively if congenital or posttraumatic variation in the major

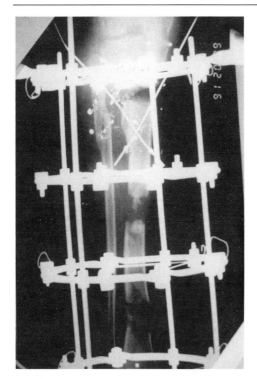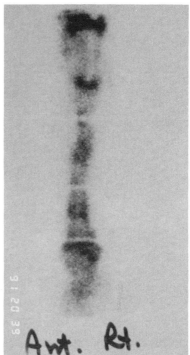

Fig. 8 This patient had a posttraumatic vascular insufficiency with only one major artery left to supply the lower leg. She underwent two corticotomies to regenerate the 50-mm proximal tibial defect (following resection of chronic osteomyelitis) by retrograde, serial bone transportation.[6] Technetium scintigraphy was used to confirm both vascularity and early osteoid production from both sides of each corticotomy following a 10-day latency prior to initiation of distraction. Subsequent bone formation was successful. **Left,** Radiograph of the tibia during transportation demonstrating proximal defect, two corticotomies in the mid and distal tibia, and the four-ring external fixator. **Right,** The technetium scan demonstrated increased blood flow to each of the corticotomy surfaces, with the hot sites separated by linear cold areas representing the four steel rings.

arteries is suspected. In these cases, special care can be taken to avoid injury to the dependent vessels.

During consolidation, plain radiography can be obtained on a monthly basis until the osteogenic area has cortex and a medullary canal on orthogonal views. Despite the appearance of these radiographic findings, the overall bone density may be severely reduced. QCT is helpful in demonstrating quantitatively that the new bone is strong enough by mineral density and cross-sectional distribution.[36]

Recent Experimental Work

Quantitative Technetium Scintigraphy for Assessment of Distraction Osteogenesis[26]

Ten dogs were randomized into three groups, based on rate and duration of distraction. The normal rate of distraction and twice the normal rate were selected to test the effect, if any, of rate of stretching on the blood flow. The third group was subjected to twice the distraction time and length (at the normal rate) in order to see whether the peak flow period could be extended by temporarily prolonging the distraction. Eight dogs underwent a 28-mm distraction (15% lengthening), four at a rate of 1 mm/day × 28 days (group I) and four at 2 mm/day × 14 days (group II). The two other dogs underwent a 56-mm distraction (30% lengthening) at a rate of 1 mm/day × 56 days (group III). Baseline QTS values for the preoperative tibiae compared to the experimental and opposite (unoperated) sides were used as controls.

The eight dogs in groups I and II each underwent eight scans: preoperative baseline; weeks 1, 2, 3, 4, and 5 postoperatively (through the entire distraction period), and during the consolidation period, at weeks 11 (fixator removal) and 17 (presacrifice). The two dogs in group III each underwent scans on weeks 3 and 7 postoperatively during the prolonged distraction period.

All scans were performed with the dogs under sedation (ketamine, rompun) in a standardized position, using a wooden dog-holding cradle that secured the hindlimbs in extension (Fig. 9). At the time of each scan, orthogonal radiographs were also taken. Because all dogs were closely matched for weight and skeletal maturity, standard dosages of 10 mCi of Tc 99m MDP were administered intravenously via the forepaw. The Technicare 550 (Cleveland, OH) gamma camera was placed directly over the tibial crests held parallel to the surface of the collimator. Dynamic data were accumulated at the rate of one image per 3 s for the first 3 min postinjection to calculate flow (60 s) and pool (3 min) images. Two hours later, static bone images of 500,000 counts were accumulated. All data were saved on hard-copy bone scan film and on Polaroid color prints of color-enhanced computer images (Informatek 64 × 64 matrix) with the calculated region of interest (ROI) and then stored on magnetic disks for backup.

Using the left leg (experimental side), a computer color-enhanced isocontour map was used to outline an ROI that corresponded to the 40% region of highest uptake, quantitated as the average number of counts per pixel in each ROI.[5]

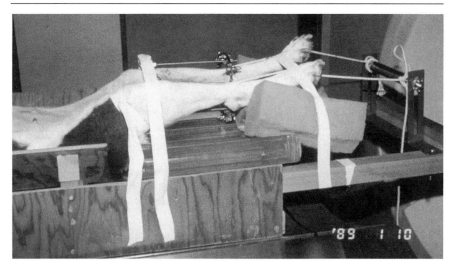

Fig. 9 A sedated dog lies in the standardized cradle for both technetium and computed tomography scanning.

The mirror image of this ROI was then transferred to the control side in order to measure the average number of counts per pixel in the exact same anatomic position and area. A third ROI, a fixed rectangular area, was placed over the lateral soft tissues adjacent to the tibial diaphysis on the control right side for the average counts per pixel in the soft tissues. After correcting for decay and actual body weight and subtracting the soft-tissue uptake, the experimental side was divided by the opposite to determine the ratio or increase over normal. The control side was compared to baseline (preoperative) measurements and between dogs to confirm its use as a common denominator for the experimental side. Data from the three groups were compared over time and to previously published data on injury models.[28]

The geographic distribution of the isotope along the entire lengths of the tibiae was measured from proximal to distal as ratio of the opposite side using MacIntosh IIcx (Image 1.49, NIH, Bethesda, MD) from digitized video images (Mediagrabber, Rasterops 24STV, Santa Clara, CA) of the flow scan hard copy. Identical rectangular ROI were selected from the proximal half and distal half of each tibia, the lengthened and opposite control, and of the background between the two legs. The profile of the gray shades was plotted on a 0 to 255 scale, and then the area under each curve was calculated to make quantitative comparisons. After subtracting the background, the value for the experimental lengthened side was divided by the value from the identical anatomic area on the opposite side to express a ratio of normal.

The preoperative baselines demonstrated left-right equality within 25% variation, while the postoperative increases always exceeded 100% of baseline. The opposite leg was noted to decrease its uptake from the preoperative baseline in all future scans during the experiment, a so-called "steal effect" in which the massive increase in flow to the experimental limb sequestered enough of the isotope to decrease the scan uptake in the normal unoperated limb (Fig. 10). This steal effect was quite consistent in all animals throughout the experiment; therefore, the data were thought to be consistent and normalized by a left:right ratio.

In group I, the average flow phase within the distraction area increased by 8.5 times that of the opposite leg, peaking at week 1 of distraction and then decreasing to six times that of the opposite leg (week 2), 3.5 to four times the opposite leg (weeks 3 and 4), and reaching a plateau at twice that of the opposite leg until sacrifice at week 17. In group II, the average flow phase within the distraction area increased by 9.5 times that of the opposite leg, peaking at week 2 and then decreasing to four to 5.5 times that of the opposite leg from week 3 through week 11 and finally falling to twice that of the opposite leg by week 17. In group III, the data were normalized to group I at week 3; at week 7 of prolonged distraction, the blood flow measured by this technique was almost three times that of the opposite leg but fell within the same range of the other two groups. By a Wilcoxon two-sample test, all values during distraction were significantly greater than the control ($p = 0.05$). None of the increases measured between groups I, II, and III were significantly different at any one point in time.

When both the distracted left tibiae and control right tibiae were divided into proximal and distal halves for comparison of relative blood flow, the flow in the proximal halves was always greater than that in the distal halves at each time point from preoperative baseline until week 17. The proximal to distal ratios ranged from 1.6 to five, with an average of three, even in the unoperated leg.

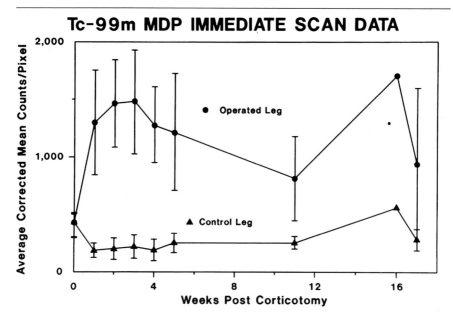

Fig. 10 Graphic display of average technetium uptake per pixel in all animals during flow phase as measured with the osteogenic area (region of interest) compared to the same anatomic area on the control limb. Peak flow occurs at 2 to 4 weeks of distraction. The steal effect on the opposite side (control) is minimal and consistent.

The blood flow measured in the distal half of the left tibiae (distant from the distraction osteogenesis zone in the proximal metaphysis) was always increased when compared to that in the right opposite controls. The mean ratios were calculated for dogs from groups I and II. The peak flow of seven to eight times control occurred at weeks 2 and 3, reaching a plateau at two to three times control from weeks 4 through 17.

One dog from each of groups I and II had nonunion. The dog from group I demonstrated the normal pattern of increased blood flow; the dog from group II had only a moderate increase in blood flow that was consistently below the average for the group and for all dogs tested. The difference was not significant, however.

QCT Based Finite Element Analysis Model[36]

An animal bone model producing a wide range of apparent densities was required to test the accuracy of the QCT based finite element analysis (FEA) model. The canine tibia was lengthened by distraction osteogenesis to supply an isolated segment of bone with a wide range in apparent density, which was confirmed by prior studies using gravimetrics, calcium analysis, and QCT scanning.[9,22] The contralateral side served as the source of anatomically equivalent normal bone. Forty-two days after the fixator was removed (day 119 of the experimental model), the dog was sedated and in vivo QCT scans were made of the newly formed bone zone and the corresponding zone on the contralateral leg, using a dipotassium hydrogen phosphate solution phantom.

The dog was then euthanized and the tibiae were harvested, mechanically macerated, and frozen. Before mechanical testing, the tibiae were thawed and placed in steel mounts consisting of a 65-mm square tube welded to a 10-mm plate with a central 12-mm stud. An alignment jig was used to hold the steel mounts so the mechanical load axis would fall along the axis of the tibia. The tibiae were fixed to the mount by 5-mm diameter threaded full pins and potted with Wood's Metal. The assemblies were mounted in an MTS Bionix™ Test system. A clip-on strain gauge that had been modified for a 25-mm gauge length was attached to each tibia, and the assembly was loaded axially to two times body weight (400 N) in both tension and compression. A total of six strain gauge readings were obtained from each tibia along the anterior, medial and lateral aspects of the tibiae and spanning the zones 65 to 91 mm and 91 to 117 mm from the tibial plateau.

Numerical matrices of the QCT images were obtained and processed to determine the cortical geometry and material properties. The endosteal and periosteal surfaces were delineated by using 500 HU as the threshold value for cortical bone. Each QCT slice was modeled as a ring of eight three-dimensional (3-D) plate elements using an FEA program preprocessor (MTab, Structural Analysis, Inc., Austin, TX). The plate element height was the QCT slice thickness, and plate thickness was the average cortical thickness of each segment. The coordinates of each element corner were derived by interpolating between the cortical midpoint coordinates. Each model had 210 nodes and 216 plate elements; 25 boundary elements were used to restrain the lower steel plate and to form the applied load.

The four highest QCT numbers in each segment were averaged; this was thought to decrease volume averaging effects at the edge of the dense cortical areas without discounting the high stiffness of denser regions in the cortex. The QCT values were adjusted for differences in phantom readings. The distracted tibia mean QCT number was 1,174 HU; the control tibia mean was 1,476 HU. The average QCT number was then used to calculate the apparent density of each segment.[37]

A finite element model[38,39] was constructed for both distracted and control tibiae by calculating the modulus of elasticity from the segment apparent density (Fig. 11). Separate finite element models of each tibia were constructed; the Carter and Hayes[40] equation was used for one model (model I), and the Schaffler and Burr[41] relationship for the other (model II).

FINITE ELEMENT MODEL OF QCT SLICE

SUBJECT 1004, SERIES V, SCAN II, L, TIBIA

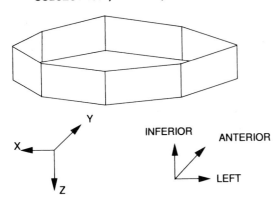

Fig. 11 Finite element model of experimental tibia generated from the numerical display of serial transverse computed tomography scans that were geometrically converted to apparent density and then modulus of elasticity.

An axial loading of 400 N in compression was applied to the actual bone and simulated in the FEA. Displacements were interpolated from the computer analysis at points that were 65, 91, and 117 mm from the tibial plateau and on the anterior, medial, and lateral periosteal surface, which matched the strain gauge locations during mechanical testing.

The predicted axial displacements in compression from the finite element models were compared with the measured displacements in compression using a simple regression. Both models (I and II) of the control and distracted tibiae had significant correlations when the displacements from both tibiae were pooled together (n = 12). The Carter and Hayes[40] formulation had a higher correlation coefficient (R^2 = 0.671) than the models based on Schaffler and Burr[41] (R^2 = 0.423). When the displacements were correlated by tibia (n = 6), the Carter and Hayes formula (model I) predicted the displacements better in the distracted tibia (R^2 = 0.914) versus model II (R^2 = 0.654); the Schaffler and Burr formula (model II) predicted displacements better in the control tibia (R^2 = 0.820) compared to model I (R^2 = 0.652). Based on this experiment, a larger series of metaphyseal versus diaphyseal tibial lengthenings was further evaluated by QCT.

Metaphyseal Versus Diaphyseal Corticotomy Sites[11]

As a test of the effect of the osteotomy site on the osteogenic potential,[14] 32 dogs underwent left tibial corticotomy for a 28-mm lengthening and were randomized into two groups by corticotomy location: 16 in the proximal metaphysis and 16 in the mid-diaphysis. Because different latency periods are advocated for optimal osteogenesis,[1,42,43] each major group was then divided into four subgroups of four dogs each on the basis of 0, 7-, 14-, and 21-day latency periods. On day 0, with the dog under general orotracheal anesthesia, a subperiosteal corticotomy was performed at either the inferior third of the tibial tuberosity for metaphyseal lengthening or at the mid-diaphysis for diaphyseal lengthening. The operated tibiae were stabilized by a ring external fixator with two percutaneous 1.8-mm transosseous wires above and two below the corticotomy. The wires were bolted under tension to standard fixation points on the two rings that were then interconnected with three threaded rods, also positioned in standardized locations. The distraction protocol followed day 0 (surgery) according to the four different latency periods. The standard distraction rate of 1 mm/day (at a rhythm of 0.5 mm twice a day) for 4 weeks led to a 28-mm elongation. All animals had the fixator and wires removed on day 77, for postdistraction consolidation phases of 49, 42, 35, and 28 days, which corresponded to the 0, 7-, 14-, and 21-day latency groups, respectively. The dogs exercised daily and most bore full weight by day 77.

Standardized anteroposterior and lateral projection radiographs were taken weekly from before surgery to the end of distraction and biweekly until sacrifice at day 119. The criteria used for evaluation of the radiographs were: (1) the initial appearance of faint radiodense new bone formation in the lengthening zone; (2) the first radiodense callus connecting the bone ends; (3) the first increase in peripheral radiodensity such that the bone ends were connected by a cortex equal to the adjacent cortices in thickness; and (4) the appearance of the initial medullary canal in the lengthening zone, surrounded by cortices on all surfaces. If a transverse radiolucency persisted within the osteogenic zone by day 77, a nonunion was presumed. If the wires became bowed toward the center of the fixator, and the radiographs showed no gap of the bone ends and early bridging callus after distraction, a premature consolidation was diagnosed. At day 77, the final distraction gap between proximal and distal bone ends was measured on the radiograph using a dial caliper (Mitutoyo #505–635–50, Tokyo, Japan). The bone healing index or treatment time per centimeter of new bone[42] was used to compare bone production between the groups and subgroups.

The serial, in vivo density measurements of the new bone mineralization, by QCT (Siemens DR3), were standardized with graduated dibasic potassium phosphate phantoms immediately beneath the foam rubber leg holder. Under ketamine hydrochloride (7 mg/kg) sedation, each dog underwent a total of five CT scans: preoperation, start of distraction, end of distraction, day 77 (fixator removal), and day 119 (presacrifice) (Fig. 12). The mean density per pixel, in HU, represented the average radiodensity of each outlined region of interest from contiguous 4-mm CT slices of the new bone. In this way, density changes were monitored from proximal to distal across the osteogenic area and compared with the equivalent levels on the control side. The three minimum QCT readings taken from contiguous cuts were averaged for each dog at each time point. The density ratio of the experimental to the control side was calculated to compare average bone density between groups and subgroups.

All 32 dogs survived the experiment. Of these, 23 had successful lengthening to the predetermined length (72%) and nine fused prematurely (28%). Of the 32 lengthenings, four resulted in nonunion (12.5%). Among 16 metaphyseal lengthenings, there were six premature consolidations (37.5%), four with a 21-day latency and two with a 14-day latency, and one nonunion (6.2%).

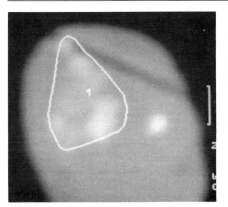

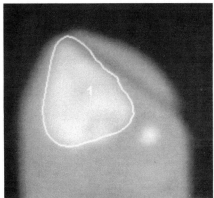

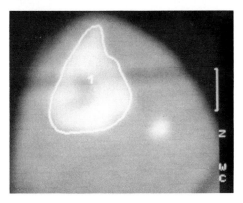

Fig. 12 Serial bone formation, consolidation, and remodeling of metaphyseal distraction osteogenesis in computed tomography scans, which can predict stiffness. **Top left,** Week 4 of distraction demonstrates early bridging of new bone growth within the central osteogenic area. **Top right,** Week 6 of consolidation shows early cortex formation. **Center,** Week 12 of consolidation confirms nearly normal macrostructure and density with remodeling of the medullary canal.

Among the 16 diaphyseal lengthenings, three fused prematurely (18.7%), two fused with a 21-day latency, one had an incomplete corticotomy with a 7-day latency, and three resulted in nonunion (18.7%). All corticotomies, both metaphyseal and diaphyseal, successfully bridged the distraction gap after a 0-day latency. The average length gained, excluding premature consolidation, was 23.9 (SD = 3.7) mm in metaphyseal and 23.8 (SD = 2.0) mm in diaphyseal lengthening.

Evaluation of radiographs showed that in metaphyseal sites, the first new bone was seen 7 days earlier; the first bone bridge, 10 days earlier; the first cortex, 5 days earlier; and the first canal formation, 6 days earlier than in the diaphyseal sites.

Although the bone-healing index averaged 6 days earlier in metaphyseal than in diaphyseal sites, no significant difference was found by t-test. Comparison of the latency groups showed that new bone consolidation occurred soonest, at a 0-day latency in both metaphyseal and diaphyseal lengthenings, with a significant difference between 0-day and 7-day latency groups ($p = 0.01$).

The minimum QCT density ratio of the experimental to the contralateral side, excluding the nine premature consolidations, decreased during distraction, reached a minimum at the end of distraction, and then increased gradually during the consolidation period. Among the subgroups, no significant difference was found preoperatively or at the start of distraction. When the metaphyseal (n = 10) and diaphyseal (n = 13) lengthenings were compared, significant differences in the minimum QCT were found at the end of distraction ($p = 0.001$), at fixator removal ($p = 0.001$), and at sacrifice ($p = 0.04$).

Load Measurements During Distraction[44]

A subgroup of these 32 dogs was used to measure load readings during distraction in order to predict outcome. This group consisted of 21 dogs with either metaphyseal or diaphyseal corticotomies and varying latency periods (0, 7, 14, or 21 days) between surgery and the start of distraction.

At 1-week intervals during the 4-week distraction phase, the dogs were sedated and positioned supine on a holding frame. The external fixator was suspended so the tibia was horizontal to eliminate gravity loads. The dial caliper was used to measure the baseline ring separation at the three distraction rod locations. Load cell assemblies were installed (Fig. 13), and the load was transferred from the distraction rods to the load cell assembly by loosening the nuts on the distraction rods, which were left loosely in place to provide translational control between the rings. Load measurements were recorded[45] for 1 minute before distracting each rod 0.5 mm. Loads were then measured for an additional 9 minutes. After the monitoring period, the load cell assemblies were removed and the rings reset to the proper position.

Each dog had a CT scan prior to surgery and at the end of distraction. The baseline tibia length was measured from the scout view. The cross-sectional area of the osteogenic zone at the end of distraction was computed at the scanner console by outlining a freehand ROI around the new bone. The axial images were later processed to obtain the area of soft tissue at the osteogenic zone using a video image processing computer program (Image Analyst, Automatix, Billerica, MA) running on a Macintosh IIx system.

The clinical outcome of the lengthening procedure was determined from examination of the last radiograph prior to sacrifice. Observer bias was prevented by having the radiographs analyzed by an investigator who was unaware of the load measurement results. An outcome was judged to be a nonunion if

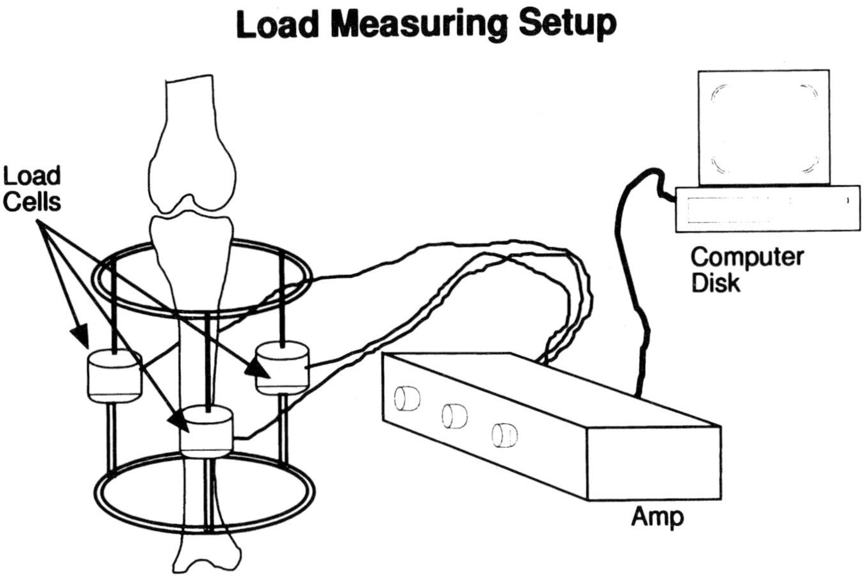

Load Measuring Setup

Fig. 13 Load cell set-up with in-line strain gauges connected to an amplifier and then into computer for load measurements predicts healthy or pathologic biomechanical bridging of the osteogenic area at as early as 2 to 3 weeks of distraction.

there was a continuous radiolucency in the osteogenic area. An outcome of malunion was assigned if angular deformity ($> 5°$) existed without signs of a nonunion.

The variables for each subject were baseline tibia length, osteogenic zone area, soft-tissue area at the osteogenic zone, latency from surgery to start of distraction, and distraction loads at weekly intervals. These data were grouped by both osteotomy site and outcome and then analyzed using the BMDP statistics package (BMDP Statistical Software, Inc., Los Angeles, CA). The BMDP programs used were 3D (T-Tests), 1R (Linear Regression by Groups), and 5V (Unbalanced Repeated Measures Models with Structured Covariance Matrices).

Six dogs had premature fusions early during the distraction phase. These were easily discerned on the plain radiographs. Loads were measured in these subjects within the safety limits of the load cells so as not to overload the gauges and endanger the instrumentation system.

Fifteen dogs were included in the distraction load measurement phase of the study. Diaphyseal ($n = 40$) and metaphyseal ($n = 20$) observations from 15 subjects were divided evenly over the four observation periods. One animal died of lymphosarcoma (unrelated to the experimental protocol) prior to scheduled sacrifice. Fourteen dogs completed the entire protocol to final bone healing for outcome assessment. The clinical outcomes of these 14 dogs were assessed radiographically prior to sacrifice at day 119 after surgery. There were 11 unions and three nonunions at the completion of the study. Two of the unions developed angular deformity that was felt to be secondary to premature removal of the fixator.

No significant difference (t-test) was found in the baseline tibia length when data were grouped by corticotomy site, metaphyseal versus diaphyseal ($p =$

0.6424). There was a significant difference between osteogenic cross-sectional areas ($p = 0.0138$) as calculated by CT scans; the means were 3.31 cm² (SD = 0.57) for the metaphyseal sites and 2.34 cm² (SD = 0.43) for the diaphyseal sites.

The mean weekly load measurements were grouped by corticotomy site. Diaphyseal (n = 40) and metaphyseal (n = 20) observations from 15 subjects were divided evenly over the four observation periods. The mean load at the end of distraction was 155 N for metaphyseal (n = 5) and 111 N for diaphyseal (n = 10) sites. That the load increased steadily over time from surgery was highly significant ($p < 0.0001$). The effect of corticotomy site on load was also significant ($p = 0.0207$). A linear regression for all dogs tested based on the distraction loads versus time was significant, $R^2 = 0.55$ ($p < 0.0001$). An analysis of variance of regression coefficients over groups was highly significant ($p = 0.00161$), indicating that the slopes of the regression lines between metaphyseal and diaphyseal sites are statistically different for measured loads over time.

The individual distraction loads were then divided by the respective cross-sectional area of the osteogenic zone in each subject. The resulting quantity was called the osteogenic zone stress. The regression analysis on these data increased significantly with time, $R^2 = 0.50$ ($p < 0.0001$). An analysis of variance of regression coefficients between metaphyseal and diaphyseal groups was not significant ($p = 0.87$), which indicates there was no statistical difference in the slopes of the regression lines for calculated stress.

There was a significant difference in the ultimate tibial length ($p = 0.0292$) when grouped by outcome. The mean lengths and standard deviations were 175 mm (sd = 5.24) and 185 mm (sd = 9.70) for the unions and nonunions, respectively. The three nonunions had osteotomies at the diaphyseal site. There were no significant differences in latency, osteogenic zone area, or soft-tissue area. A linear regression of the load readings demonstrated a significant difference in the slopes ($p < 0.0023$) between unions and nonunions. When compared by t-test, there was a significant difference in loads between unions and nonunions at the end of the third week ($p = 0.044$). There was even a suggestive change as early as the end of the second week ($p = 0.056$).

This study statistically supports earlier case reports that suggest distraction loads increase with time[46,47] and vary with corticotomy site.[43,48] I hypothesized that this load is directly related to distraction of the collagenous bridge central to the osteogenic interzone. The measured loads were therefore converted to stress by dividing the osteogenic zone area into the load. When metaphyseal stresses were compared to diaphyseal stresses by linear regression, there was no longer a statistically significant difference between groups, and the regression lines for the two groups were essentially parallel and colinear. This does not prove, however, that the distraction rod load results primarily from deformation of the osteogenic zone tissue, because another parameter, such as muscle mass, also varies with corticotomy location and may be a contributing factor.

Differential Stress During Distraction Osteogenesis[49]

Four dogs underwent a 30% (56 mm) left tibial lengthening (twice the standard experimental model) in order to measure loads during distraction of larger magnitude and to differentiate the effects of soft-tissue resistance from that in the osteogenic zone.

Weekly radiographs and load measurements were made as described previously. Following a 7-day latency, distraction at 0.5 mm twice a day was carried out for 56 days. On the last day of distraction, each dog was placed under general anesthesia. Using sterile and hemostatic surgical technique, with strain gauges in place for ongoing load measurements, the lengthened leg was differentially dissected in order to observe the changes in resistance to the distraction load as each layer of soft tissue was released. In sequence the skin, fascia, individual muscle groups, and finally the periosteum were circumferentially released until only the tibia itself remained with the external fixator and in-line strain gauges.

The loads continued to rise over time throughout the 56-day experiment. The major resistance to distraction was determined to be in the distraction zone itself. Each of the soft-tissue layers accounted for 3% to 5% of the load; the bone itself still contained 75% to 80% of the baseline load.

These findings are consistent with the previous assumption that the fibrous interzone carries the primary distraction load and, therefore, the cross-sectional area of this zone is directly proportional to the load. It is postulated that the width or thickness of this zone (length of unmineralized collagen) is indirectly proportional to the load. As distraction proceeds, the collagen matrix becomes progressively more mineralized and, therefore, stiffer. More of the resistance is thus concentrated on shorter lengths of collagen, giving rise to higher loads over time. The load increment seems to decrease with time as the fibrous interzone reaches a stable length. A proper range of osteogenic zone stress is probably critical for perpetuation of the distraction osteogenesis process. The data suggest that by week 3 of distraction, an osteogenic zone stress in the range of 47 N/cm^2 is consistent with healthy distraction osteogenesis, and an osteogenic stress below 27 N/cm^2 will lead to nonunion, secondary to an abnormal biologic bridge.

Acknowledgments

This work was done with the support of UAMS Institutional Biomedical Research Support Grant RR 05350–22; Whitbeck Research Award, UAMS Foundation Fund; Orthopaedic Research and Education Foundation Grant 88–469; UAMS Department of Orthopaedics Musculoskeletal Research Institute; Arkansas Children's Hospital; Smith and Nephew Richards, Memphis TN; and Synthes, Paoli, PA.

References

1. Ilizarov GA: Clinical application of the tension-stress effect for limb lengthening. *Clin Orthop* 1990;250:8–26.
2. Ilizarov GA, Lediaev VI, Shitin VP: The course of compact bone reparative regeneration in distraction osteosynthesis under different conditions of bone fragment fixation: Experimental study. *Eksp Khirurgiia Anesteziol* 1969;14:3–12.
3. Ilizarov GA: The tension-stress effect on the genesis and growth of tissues: Part I. The influence of stability of fixation and soft tissue preservation. *Clin Orthop* 1989; 238:249–281.
4. Ilizarov GA: The tension-stress effect on the genesis and growth of tissues: Part II. The influence of the rate and frequency of distraction. *Clin Orthop* 1989;239:263–285.
5. Aronson J: Biology of distraction osteogenesis, in Bianchi-Maiocchi A, Aronson J (eds): *Operative Principles of Ilizarov: Fracture Treatment, Nonunion, Osteomyelitis, Lengthening, Deformity Correction*. Baltimore, MD, Williams & Wilkins, 1991, pp 42–52.

6. Aronson J, Johnson E, Harp JH: Local bone transportation for treatment of intercalary defects by the Ilizarov technique: Biomechanical and clinical considerations. *Clin Orthop* 1989;243:71–79.

7. Sokal RR, Rohlf FJ (eds): *Biometry: The Principles and Practice of Statistics in Biological Research*, ed 2. San Francisco, CA, WH Freeman, 1981, pp 400–453.

8. Aronson J, Harrison B, Boyd CM, et al: Mechanical induction of osteogenesis: The importance of pin rigidity. *J Pediatr Orthop* 1988;8:396–401.

9. Aronson J, Harrison B, Boyd CM, et al: Mechanical induction of osteogenesis: Preliminary studies. *Ann Clin Lab Sci* 1988;18:195–203.

10. Aronson J, Harrison BH, Stewart CL, et al: The histology of distraction osteogenesis using different external fixators. *Clin Orthop* 1989;241:106–116.

11. Aronson J, Shen X: Experimental healing of distraction osteogenesis comparing metaphyseal to diaphyseal sites. *Clin Orthop* 1994;301:25–30.

12. Codivilla A: On the means of lengthening in the lower limbs, the muscles and tissues which are shortened through deformity. *Am J Orthop Surg* 1904;2:353–369.

13. Wagner H: Operative beinverlangerung. *Chirug* 1971;42:260–266.

14. Wagner H: Operative lengthening of the femur. *Clin Orthop* 1978;136:125–142.

15. Robinson RA, Elliot SR: The water content of bone: I. The mass of water, inorganic crystals, organic matrix, and "CO_2 space" components in a unit volume of dog bone. *J Bone Joint Surg* 1957;39A:167–188.

16. Glimcher MJ: Recent studies of the mineral phase in bone and its possible linkage to the organic matrix by protein bound phosphate bonds. *Philos Trans R Soc Lond Biol* 1984;304:479–508.

17. Herring GM: The organic matrix of bone, in Bourne GH (ed): *The Biochemistry and Physiology of Bone*, ed 2. New York, NY, Academic Press, 1972, vol 1, pp 127–189.

18. Lane JM, Boskey AL, Li WKP, et al: A temporal study of collagen, proteoglycan, lipid and mineral constituents in a model of endochondral osseous repair. *Metab Bone Dis Rel Res* 1979;1:319–324.

19. Aronson J: Proper wire tensioning for Ilizarov external fixation. *Tech Orthop* 1990;5:27–32.

20. Aronson J, Harp JH Jr: Factors influencing the choice of external fixation for distraction osteogenesis, in Greene WB (ed): *Instructional Course Lectures, Volume XXXIX*. Park Ridge, IL, American Academy of Orthopaedic Surgeons, 1990, pp 175–183.

21. Aronson J, Harp JH Jr: Mechanical considerations in using tensioned wires in a transosseous external fixation system. *Clin Orthop* 1992;280:23–29.

22. Aronson J, Good B, Steward C, et al: Preliminary studies of mineralization during distraction osteogenesis. *Clin Orthop* 1990;250:43–49.

23. Boyde A, Jones SJ: Back-scattered electron imaging of skeletal tissues. *Metab Bone Dis Rel Res* 1983;5:145–150.

24. Lacroix P: The internal remodelling of bones, in Bourne GH (ed): *The Biochemistry and Physiology of Bone*, ed 2. New York, NY, Academic Press, 1971, vol III, pp 119–144.

25. Delloye C, Delefortrie G, Coutelier L, et al: Bone regenerate formation in cortical bone during distraction lengthening: An experimental study. *Clin Orthop* 1990;250:34–42.

26. Aronson J: Temporal and spatial increases in blood flow during distraction osteogenesis. *Clin Orthop* 1994;301;124–131.

27. Nutton RW, Fitzgerald RH Jr, Brown ML, et al: Dynamic radioisotope bone imaging as a noninvasive indicator of canine tibial blood flow. *J Orthop Res* 1984;2:67–74.

28. Williams EA, Rand JA, An KN, et al: The early healing of tibial osteotomies stabilized by one-plane or two-plane external fixation. *J Bone Joint Surg* 1987;69A:355–365.

29. Urist MR, Mazet R Jr, Mclean FC: The pathogenesis and treatment of delayed union and non-union: A survey of eighty-five ununited fractures of the shaft of the

tibia and one-hundred control cases with similar injuries. *J Bone Joint Surg* 1954; 36A:931–968,980.

30. Walker CW, Aronson J, Kaplan PA, et al: Radiologic evaluation of limb lengthening procedures. *Am J Roentgenol* 1991;156:353–358.

31. Genant HK, Block JE, Steiger P, et al: Quantitative computed tomography in assessment of osteoporosis. *Semin Nucl Med* 1987;17:316–333.

32. Kuhn JL, Goldstein SA, Feldkamp LA, et al: Evaluation of a microcomputed tomography system to study trabecular bone structure. *J Orthop Res* 1990;8:833–842.

33. Markel MD, Morin RL, Kuo RF, et al: Noninvasive determination of the local and structural properties of intact bone and delayed union with quantitative CT. *Trans Orthop Res Soc* 1991;16:437.

34. Snyder SM, Schneider E: Estimation of mechanical properties of cortical bone by computed tomography. *J Orthop Res* 1991;9:422–431.

35. Aronson J, Boyd C, Amerson D, et al: Reliable sampling techniques using quantitative computed tomography for density of long bones. *Trans Orthop Res Soc* 1988;13:533.

36. Harp J, Aronson J, Hollis JM: Noninvasive determination of bone stiffness for distraction osteogenesis by quantitative computed tomography. *Clin Orthop* 1994; 301:42–48.

37. Brooks RA, Mitchell LG, O'Connor CM, et al: On the relationship between computed tomography numbers and specific gravity. *Phys Med Biol* 1981;26:141–147.

38. Keyak JH, Meagher JM, Skinner HB, et al: Automated three-dimensional finite element modeling of bone: A new method. *J Biomed Eng* 1990;12:389–397.

39. Marom SA, Linden MJ: Computer aided stress analysis of long bones utilizing computed tomography. *J Biomech* 1990;23:399–404.

40. Carter DR, Hayes WC: The compressive behavior of bone as a two-phase porous structure. *J Bone Joint Surg* 1977;59A:954–962.

41. Schaffler MB, Burr DB: Stiffness of compact bone: Effects of porosity and density. *J Biomech* 1988;21:13–16.

42. De Bastiani G, Aldegheri R, Renzi-Brivio L, et al: Limb lengthening by callus distraction (callotasis). *J Pediatr Orthop* 1987;7:129–134.

43. White SH, Kenwright J: The timing of distraction of an osteotomy. *J Bone Joint Surg* 1990;72B:356–361.

44. Aronson J, Harp J: Mechanical forces as predictors of healing during tibial lengthening by distraction osteogenesis. *Clin Orthop* 1994;301:73–79.

45. Halter MA: *Data Acquisition System for Automatically Monitoring the Forces Applied During Bone Distraction in Canines.* Little Rock, AR, University of Arkansas, 1989. Master's Thesis.

46. Leong JC, Ma RY, Clark JA, et al: Viscoelastic behavior of tissue in leg lengthening by distraction. *Clin Orthop* 1979;139:102–109.

47. Wolfson N, Hearn TC, Thomason JJ, et al: Force and stiffness changes during Ilizarov leg lengthening. *Clin Orthop* 1990;250:58–60.

48. Steen H, Fjeld TO, Miller JA, et al: Biomechanical factors in the metaphyseal- and diaphyseal-lengthening osteotomy: An experimental and theoretic analysis in the ovine tibia. *Clin Orthop* 1990;259:282–294.

49. Hollis JM, Aronson J, Hofmann OE: Differential loads in tissues during limb lengthening. *Trans Orthop Res Soc* 1992;17:14.

Section 5
Future Research Directions

The production of a controlled, low-energy fracture of bone followed by its gradual distraction, termed distraction osteogenesis, has led to the observation that the osteogenic regenerative capacities of the human body are enormous. For over 40 years, Russian surgeons (and more recently, Western surgeons) have exploited this phenomenon for the purposes of lengthening bones, transporting bone segments to fill gaps, correcting skeletal deformities, and treating other skeletal conditions, such as osteomyelitis and nonunions. Clinical experience shows that the application of the principles of distraction osteogenesis to orthopaedic surgery is accompanied by a variety of complications. These include inadequate bone formation, pain, inflammation and infection at pin sites, joint contracture, joint dislocation/subluxation, articular cartilage damage/adhesion, malunion, and others. Clinical questions such as the optimum length of treatment and the time to frame removal remain unanswered. Concerns regarding the effects of metabolic state, drug usage, cigarette smoking, and chronic disease have to be addressed. However, it is perhaps most important that clinicians and scientists recognize the uniqueness of this phenomenon to the entire spectrum of bone formation and regeneration. The charge to investigators will be to elucidate the individual components of the process, understand the conditions that govern them, and gain further knowledge in order to develop new approaches to osteogenesis research and treatment.

What roles do periosteum, cortical bone, bone marrow, and blood supply play in distraction osteogenesis?

When an osteotomy or corticotomy is produced, responses will occur in periosteum, cortical bone, bone marrow, muscle, nerve, and blood supply. The contributions of each of the tissues to the overall process will dictate the healing response. Determining how each of these tissue responses affects the potential for and rate of healing will require significant research efforts.

The periosteal contribution can be studied in several ways. The source of osteoprogenitor cells, roles of attached tendons (Sharpey's fibers) and ligaments, and the possible "barrier function" (ie, how the periosteal lining blocks contributions by the external soft tissues) should be investigated. In addition, because the size and thickness of the periosteum may change between the diaphyseal and metaphyseal regions, the role of the periosteum in this process should be studied at several anatomic sites.

Bone marrow is another potentially important tissue contributor to this process. Experiments must be designed to identify the osteoprogenitor cells within the marrow compartment that participate in this phenomenon and to determine how they are involved from both a time-specific and site-specific perspective. The importance of bone marrow blood supply must also be investigated. Experiments should be designed to determine, for example, the importance and mechanistic contribution of a latency period before distraction, the length of the latency period, and, most importantly, the scientific basis for this latency period.

Although it does not seem that bone cells in the cortical bone ends would contribute to the formation of new bone to the same degree as cells in the periosteum or endosteum, that hypothesis will have to be tested. Further experiments in which these different tissue pools are inhibited from participating in the response can help to answer this question.

Finally, the way by which the rate of the regeneration process can be altered should be investigated. Experiments should be planned to test the ability to accelerate lengthening, change the rate of regeneration during the lengthening period, and assess the effects of continuous versus intermittent lengthening.

During distraction osteogenesis, in what ways do skeletal muscles serve as a rate limiting factor?

The traditional rate of distraction osteogenesis (1 mm/day) produces a contracture in skeletal muscles and, consequently, appears to be beyond the capability of skeletal muscle fibers to adapt, both acutely and chronically, to the magnitude of the stretch. For single skeletal muscle fibers, passive stretch beyond the overlap of thick and thin filaments of the average sarcomere, which occurs at approximately 55% strain, will damage the morphology of the sarcomeres. For fully activated single skeletal muscle fibers, each stretch beyond a 10% strain will result in focal injury to some sarcomeres. Compared with the values for single fibers, the thresholds for injury of passive and activated whole skeletal muscles are increased approximately 20%. The increase in thresholds is due to the series compliance introduced by the tendons of the whole muscles. Skeletal muscle fibers are able to adapt to chronic stretch by adding sarcomeres at the myotendinous junction, but such an adaptation requires time; therefore, addition of sarcomeres during distraction osteogenesis may not be possible.

During distraction osteogenesis, in what way do nerves serve as a limiting factor?

Based on the existing data, nerves appear to tolerate stretches of the magnitude induced by distraction osteogenesis without irreversible injury as long as the stretching occurs over a prolonged period. Consequently, the stretching of peripheral nerves does not appear to constitute a limiting factor. The pain experienced by patients may reflect activation of stretch receptors in skeletal muscle rather than a direct effect on nerves. Pain is the major clinical complication of this technique. Nerve dysfunction due to direct stretch, although less frequent, may be directly related to ischemia, toxic metabolites, or structural damage.

Peripheral nerve injury mechanisms are well studied and documented but not in relation to controlled displacement during distraction osteogenesis. Because pain is involved, clinical studies would be required to determine the source of the pain.

How can we define the cellular components in the regenerating bone and the mechanism of bone formation in distraction osteogenesis?

Histologically, the mechanism of bone formation in distraction osteogenesis appears similar to the mechanism of bone formation in other types of systems, such as fracture healing and bone remodeling. However, because of potential variables in technique, hardware, and the animal species being studied, it is not known to what extent maintenance of vascularity, injury to periosteum, and inflammation influence osteogenesis. Further, the origins of cells in regenerating bone are unknown. Some tools are available to determine the origin of these cells.

The relative contributions of periosteal and cortical bone and marrow pools of osteoblasts and preosteoblasts need to be determined. It is possible that the latency period introduces or modulates environmental factors that regulate bone cell or precursor mitogenesis, differentiation, or function. Once stimulated in this initial period, the osteoblasts appear to organize around matrix elements, including vessels or collagen fibers.

In many studies, bone formation appears to be of the intramembranous type, without substantial chondrogenesis. Mechanisms of matrix production include deposition of new bone on calcified or uncalcified collagen fibers in the distraction site. There are other studies that demonstrate endochondral osteogenesis in distraction, but it is not known whether this component influences outcome, nor whether different local mediators stimulate chondrogenesis from the same population of progenitor cells that develop into osteoblasts. Propagation of bone formation may also involve recruitment of osteoblasts from pools distinct from those recruited in the latency or initiation phases.

Understanding the nature of matrix formation in response to different mechanical, surgical, or technical treatment parameters should provide sound scientific bases for improving clinical outcomes. Further, from a different perspective, experimental models of distraction osteogenesis could provide new and fundamental information on bone cell biology and matrix formation that could have significance for and applications in other bone formation situations.

Markers of osteoblastic and chondroblastic phenotypes are not abundant for dogs and rabbits, species commonly used for studies in distraction osteogenesis. Efforts are needed to develop cellular and molecular probes to establish the origin of the regenerate cells. Development and validation of models in other species such as rats, chickens, and mice may provide additional opportunities to use markers to definitively identify the origin(s) of the osteoblasts and chondroblasts. Markers for endothelial cells, perivascular cells with skeletogenic potential, and potential accessory cells of the connective tissue, marrow, immune, and inflammatory tissues are also needed for full understanding of the mechanism of distraction osteogenesis. Quantitative assays for these different cell types need to be developed.

Relative contributions of periosteum, cortex, marrow, vasculature, and soft tissue to cell differentiation and function can be evaluated experimentally by ablation of specific compartments by surgical manipulation, use of barriers, specific pharmacological treatments, use of bioactive factors, mutants, or gene-knockout models.

What are the factors and signals involved in distraction osteogenesis?

The osteotomy and the controlled displacement that initiate and propagate bone formation during distraction osteogenesis produce well-organized functional bone of normal anatomic appearance. Histologically, this process may follow a sequence of events that resemble either intramembranous or endochondral bone osteogenesis, dependent on undefined circumstances. It is important from the clinical perspective, and it would be fundamentally instructive to identify the factors/signals that govern/modulate the various steps in this process and the pathways of signal transduction. Specifically, are there growth factors such as bone morphogenic proteins, transforming growth factor-betas, insulin-derived growth factors, protein-derived growth factors, and so forth that are locally produced or activated? Are they necessary or permissive? Are they stage specific? Are "inflammatory" mediators involved, such as interleukins, prostanoids, and others? What are the magnitude and distribution of mechanical strain and electrical potentials in the tissue? Is there a correlation between the local mechanical changes and biochemical mediators? What are the mechanisms of signal transduction, both for the mechanical perturbations and the other factors involved?

The greatest merit of distraction osteogenesis in the context of factors and signals is the combination of controlled mechanical stimulation with all other factors that affect osteogenesis.

Factors initiated by the distraction osteogenesis-inducing perturbations can be identified by applying immunochemistry, in situ hybridization, Northern hybridization analyses, and tissue extraction of factors/activities. The importance of specific factors can be tested by adding antibodies during the procedure or inhibitors such as nonsteroidal anti-inflammatory drugs (NSAIDs). It also is possible to change the hormonal milieu of the organism by ablation of endocrine glands (surgical or chemical hypophysectomy, thyroidectomy, gonadectomy, etc.) or by inducing pathologic states such as diabetes. Genetic mutations could be used, especially if methods are developed to produce distraction osteogenesis in mice. Transgenic animals, gene deletions, and natural genetic defects could serve as valuable models.

The obvious drawback of these approaches is the need to conduct experiments in vivo, where results reflect multiple influences and the resolution of single variables is difficult.

What are the effects of local mechanical or electric conditions on the cellularly based processes of bone formation during distraction osteogenesis? What are the contributions of intrinsic or extrinsic factors to the generation of these local mechanical/electric conditions, ie, frame construct design, tissue properties, functional loading? What are the temporal effects of the distraction procedure on the relationships between biophysical influences and bone formation?

It is clear that biophysical factors significantly influence the initiation, propagation, and maturation of bone formation. Exploring the biologic processes that are engendered during distraction osteogenesis may provide a unique opportunity to advance our understanding of the mechanisms associated with biophysically-mediated bone formation. However, critical to this advancement is the need to precisely measure and/or model the three-dimensional state of biophysical conditions acting locally at sites of active or reactive bone formation. It will then be possible to begin to correlate the contribution of biophysical parameters to specific cell functions.

The approach to addressing these issues must likely involve the following issues. In vivo models of distraction osteogenesis must be developed that precisely control the extrinsic biophysical factors. Techniques must be developed to quantify the contribution of both intrinsic and extrinsic factors to the pattern of local biophysical conditions and correlate these to patterns of cell function and activity. Through the use of normal, transgenic, or diseased animal models, we must attempt to isolate the role of specific cellular factors in responding to biophysical influence.

Section 6

Fracture, Etiology, Biomechanics, and Outcome

Section Editors:
Wilson C. Hayes, PhD
Joseph M. Lane, MD

Charles N. Cornell, MD
John L. Esterhai, Jr, MD
Wilson C. Hayes, PhD

Joseph M. Lane, MD
Paul P. Weitzel, BA

Chapter 33

Osteoporosis: Cause of Geriatric Fractures

Joseph M. Lane, MD

Although the loss of bone substance occurs naturally with aging in all individuals, in some older adults, this process is expedited and leads to profound fragility of the skeleton.[1] Osteoporosis affects 20% to 30% of women older than 65 years and accounts for at least 70% of the fractures of both the appendicular and axial skeleton in the elderly. Osteoporosis is eight times more common in women than in men; more women are more likely to develop this condition because the maintenance of bone mass in women is related to the female hormone estrogen.[2–8] This hormone is produced in much smaller quantities after menopause and is almost absent in 20% of women.

Consequences of Osteoporosis

When the amounts of bone mass decrease as a result of osteoporosis, bones are weakened and may fracture.[1,5,9,10] In the spine, vertebrae can be compressed and lead to kyphotic circumstances. The secondary effects of this process include prominence of the ribs against the pelvic rim, foreshortening of the height of the abdomen, and protuberance of the abdominal contents. In addition to spinal problems, osteoporosis leads to vulnerability of the appendicular skeleton to fractures, particularly of the hip, wrist, and humerus. In North America, in those individuals living to 85 years of age, 17% of men and 32% of women will also sustain a hip fracture.[2,5] Of these individuals 20% will have an increased mortality rate during the first year and only one third will return to a lifestyle approximating their previous circumstance.

Although all individuals lose bone with age, certain individuals have higher risks.[1,2,10] Significant factors are gender (female), poor diet, and lack of exercise. Malnutrition represents a critical element for osteoporosis. Anorexia nervosa patients lose the ability to produce matrix and also sustain long periods of amenorrhea. Even after correction of anorexia nervosa, the bone growth lost to the syndrome is never replaced. Other factors associated with osteoporosis include premature menopause and abnormal menstrual cycle, particularly before the age of 25; Caucasian or Oriental background; fair complexion; petite thin body build; family history; smoking; alcohol; and scoliosis.

Scoliosis appears to be a primary risk factor for osteoporosis.[11,12] Scoliosis has been suggested to be related to underlying genetic disease in collagen synthesis and maturation. Patients in all age groups who have scoliosis, when compared to controls, have significantly less bone mass. At The Hospital for Special Surgery, more than 75% of patients past the age of 65 with a 10° curve were noted to have at least one compression fracture. Thus, it has been concluded that scoliosis represents a high risk for osteoporosis and, therefore, preventive measures should be established early.

Bone is formed during childhood and reaches its peak mass by the age of 25.[13,14] Thereafter, bone mass is lost at a rate of 0.5% per year in women up to the point of menopause, at which time there is an expedited loss of bone at 2% per year for approximately 10 years.[1,2,10,15] Following this, bone loss resumes at 0.5% per year. Trabecular bone, which has a high surface and low volume, is lost more rapidly than cortical bone. Men lose bone at the rate of 0.5% per year and mirror women's rate of loss after the age of 65.

Bone strength is related to bone structure as well as density.[16] Bone structure and architectural connectivity account for over 50% of the variants in strength, whereas apparent density by itself accounts for 80% of the strength and 80% of the attributable risk of fracture. Both density and connectivity account for over 100% of the strength variables because these two properties closely correlate. As the percentage of trabecular bone decreases with age, it plays a smaller role in providing inherent strength to the bone. In the young individual, 50% of vertebral strength is related to trabecular bone, but this decreases to 30% in the elderly. Even less of the strength of the femoral bone is related to trabecular bone, which thus carries only 30% of the weight load. The connectivity of the various components of the trabecular bone also plays a critical role.[17]

In the elderly, compact bone contributes twice as much to vertebral strength as trabecular bone.[18] In addition, compact bone surrounding trabecular bone can significantly increase trabecular bone strength. Biomechanical and anthropologic studies have suggested that the strength of the bone is related to the percentage of trabecular and compact bone, to the architectural relationship of these various bones, and to structural characteristics, such as connectivity.[19] Noninvasive methodologies, such as dual x-ray densitometry and quantitative computed tomography (QCT) scanning, give rise to figures of apparent density and can approximate only 80% of the integral strength of bone, at best.[20,21]

Controversy arises over the relative role of bone mass and hip fracture risk. Many factors other than bone density contribute to hip fractures; these include balance, frequency of falls,[22] falling to the side,[23] padding of the hip areas, and the structure of the femur itself. Cross-sectional studies have demonstrated a significantly enhanced risk associated with femoral bone mineral density; relative risk is three to four times greater for each one standard deviation change in the femoral bone density. Cummings and associates[24] have confirmed that bone density measurements at the femoral site are superior to those at other sites for predicting future hip fracture.

Thus, hip fractures are related to falls in osteoporotic individuals, and the figures that have been generated indicate that somewhere between 65% and 95% of the hip fractures are related to the falls with the rest related to the underlying osteoporotic condition.[5] Further discussion can be found in chapter 35. Clearly, the purported role of underlying metabolic bone disease in hip fracture has not been definitely identified. The correlation between bone density and spine fractures is much stronger. Spine fractures are related to underlying metabolic bone disease in the face of normal activity levels rather than to specific trauma to the spine.

The distinction between vertebral fracture and vertebral deformation is ill defined. The implications of this controversy are great in that as the fracture definition is expanded to include more minor changes, the efficacy of drug interventions becomes clouded. Thus the definition of the fracture is critical to the entrance and endpoint criteria used in trials of osteoporosis treatments. Consensus meetings have noted that radiographic deformation, even with height loss of 20% to 30%, is not always due to a vertebral fracture. Kleerekoper and Nelson[25] have indicated the problematic nature of deformation. Only 25% of significant radiographic deformations of the spine were associated with clinical symptoms and increased nucleotide uptake. Association with a true clinical fracture occurred only when vertebral deformations crossed a 30% loss of height. Thus, it is unclear whether deformations up to 30% are indicative of osteoporosis and represent risk of fractures. Storm and associates[26] and Watts and associates[27] in their articles on determination of the efficacy of etidronate defined fractures as a 20% to 25% reduction in anterior, middle, or posterior height accompanied by reduction of an area of approximately 10% to 20%. Riggs and associates,[28] on the other hand, accepted a 15% change within the vertebral body as evidence of a fracture.

Bone density measurements that look at correlations between density and fracture risk have a much higher correlation at 20% to 25% deformation and a very weak correlation between 15% and 25%, which places drug trials using the latter criterion in question. In addition, with the 15% definition lack of precision between multiple readings makes it very difficult to identify these minor changes with consistency. Thus, the issues of deformation and fracture, entrance criteria for studies, and changes that would demonstrate efficacy of treatment have not yet been agreed to by either the investigators or the U.S. government.

Bone Turnover

Riggs and Melton[10] postulated two types of osteoporosis: type I (early perimenopausal and early postmenopausal phases) in which there is a high turnover osteoporosis with increased resorption, excellent response to estrogen, and loss of trabecular bone; and type II (late onset), which is more related to a failure of bone formation and a relative lack of response to estrogen occurring in individuals who are in their 70s. Recent studies have raised issues about rates of turnover, the percentages of patients undergoing high and low turnover, and the continuity of a single form of bone loss in individuals. Nordin[29] and others have suggested that there is, in fact, a high temporal variability in the rate at which bone loss occurs. Most women go through a period of rapid bone loss at the onset of menopause. This is followed by a relative stability with occasional short-term episodes of high loss.

Recent studies by Browne and associates[30] have suggested that rapid bone loss is episodic, not continuous, and that only 30% of osteoporotic women at any age are in high turnover states. Thus, there is histologic heterogeneity in osteoporosis at any time point (Fig. 1). In an effort to gain a better understanding of bone metabolism at the time of analysis, a number of biochemical markers have been developed, including osteocalcin, bone specific alkaline phosphatase, and pyridinoline peptide cross-link analysis. At this time, the high imprecision of the biochemical markers and the temporal variability of the bone turnover have made their clinical use questionable. Several investigators, most notably Christiansen and associates,[31] suggested that individuals with high rates of bone loss at menopause run a higher risk for a fracture. High rates of resorption and osteoclast formation lead to loss of connectivity and porosity within the cortical bone. These structural aberrations also may contribute to the risk for fracture.

Accepted Therapies

In the treatment of osteoporosis the goals must be clear.[32] Hip fractures have the greatest impact on morbidity, mortality, and cost.[5] Of elderly patients with

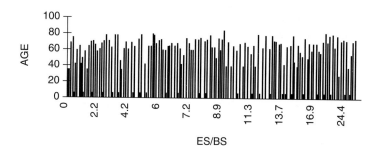

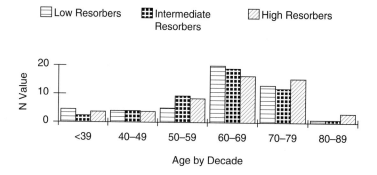

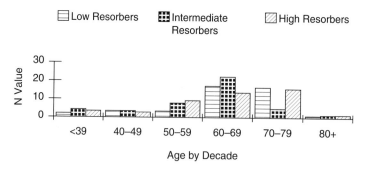

Fig. 1 These graphs address the resorption profile in osteoporotic women with vertebral fractures. **Top,** The eroded surface is plotted against the age of the biopsied patients. **Center,** Lowest, middle, and upper third of resorption types as measured by eroded surface/total bone surface are broken down for all osteoporotic women. **Bottom,** Lowest, middle, and upper third of resorption types as measured by osteoclast surface/total bone surface are broken down.

femoral fractures, 25% die within a year; another 50% never recover and often require long-term care. Only 25% return to full function. In contrast, vertebral fractures, which may be associated with back pain and invariably cause loss of height, rarely result in major morbidity and mortality. Therefore, the primary goal is to prevent hip fractures.

In theory, there are two basic thrusts to treatment of osteoporosis: prevention of bone loss and promotion of bone formation (Table 1). Currently accepted therapies such as estrogen, calcitonin, and calcium generally seek to prevent bone loss. Several experimental therapies are aimed at increasing bone mass.

Calcium

Calcium is critically important to bodily functions aside from those of the skeleton.[2,33–35] Ninety-eight percent of calcium is found within the skeleton, and bone plays a pivotal role in calcium turnover and maintenance to the body. During the growing years, the body uses calcium to build strong bones and to store reserves for later life. After menopause, estrogen levels decline, and calcium is released from the bone. This calcium is used to meet the demands of the body. Dietary calcium requirements are related to the age of the individual (Table 2). Most modern individuals fall far short of these requirements, particularly at age 12. This shortfall leads to a continual tendency toward negative calcium balance, which leads to ultimate loss of bone throughout life. The role of vitamin D is one of maturation of the intestinal lining and enhancement of calcium absorption across the gut. Vitamin D also plays a role in mobilizing calcium from the bone when dietary intake is inadequate. In Northern climates with inadequate sunlight, vitamin D levels may be quite sparse, particularly in certain areas of Europe.

Calcium is one of the most widely used agents in the management of osteoporosis. It has been demonstrated to be effective for postmenopausal women

Table 1 Therapies for treatment of osteoporosis

Antiresorptive	Formative
Calcium (Vitamin D)	Sodium fluoride
Estrogen	Parathyroid hormone*
Calcitonin	
Bisphosphonates*	
Thiazides*	
Anabolic steroids*	

*Experimental

Table 2 Calcium requirements

Age/Condition	Dosage (mg elemental Calcium)
Child (< 11)	400 to 750
Adolescent→young adult (11 to 15)	1,300
Premenopausal	700
Postmenopausal	1,500
Major fracture	1,000 to 1,500

with dietary intakes of less than 400 mg per day.[36] Studies have demonstrated that although calcium intake is quite effective in enhancing bone mass in children,[37] it has little influence in preventing the initial bone loss that occurs in the first 5 years after menopause. However, supplements given to older patients significantly prevented loss of femoral bone mass and lowered vertebral fracture rates.[38] More importantly, Chapuy and Meunier[39] demonstrated in France that low doses of vitamin D and calcium not only prevented loss of femoral bone mass, but also significantly decreased the rate of hip fractures in elderly persons. Thus, there is a role for calcium supplementation, particularly in individuals with low calcium diets. It is important in growing children and in the older individuals,[37] and it appears to have a significant role in maintaining hip bone mass and preventing hip fractures.

Estrogen

Estrogen is the cornerstone of support for the skeletal system.[4,6,40,41] Estrogen has a profound effect in preventing bone resorption and, in fact, favors bone formation. The benefits of estrogen have been demonstrated in menopause, during which it can actually lead to augmentation of up to 2% per year of skeletal bone mass rather than loss of 2% per year. Recent data indicate that estrogen benefits individuals long past early menopause.[6] Although bone mass may no longer increase in the elderly, estrogen can enhance the quality of bone, and there is strong evidence that it decreases hip fractures. Case control and cohort studies have shown that estrogen therapy protects against postmenopausal fractures.[32,41–44] Combined data from the various studies show the incidence of osteoporotic fractures of the spine and hip to be decreased by 50% and 10%, respectively, with estrogen use as compared to controls. There are a number of problems with these studies, which include inability to exclude selection bias among the women who received estrogen, the control of dose, and the duration of therapy. New studies confirm that estrogen dramatically decreases the risk of fracture although bone density is only maintained or slightly increased.[45]

There is a small enhancement of breast cancer in the population on estrogen supplementation with or without progesterone.[46–48] In patients who have had breast cancer, the increased risk rises.[48] Counterbalancing the breast cancer risk is the observation that estrogen will decrease cholesterol and prevent heart disease.[49–51] The sum result of these two conflicting points leads to an increased longevity of up to 4 years in individuals who are taking estrogen.[52] Preliminary data indicate that tamoxifen, an oncologic antiestrogen with some estrogen-like properties, is used for treatment of breast cancer but also has an estrogen-like effect on bone. Tamoxifen could be a promising drug because it could protect against death, disfigurement, and disability in elderly women,[53] but at an increased risk of endometrial cancer.[54] It stops bone loss in the spine[55] and perhaps in the femur.[56] In light of these studies, new analogs of estrogen are under investigation.

Calcitonin

Salmon calcitonin is the only drug other than estrogen approved by the FDA for osteoporosis. Short-term prospective studies have shown that calcitonin, when injected subcutaneously, can prevent bone loss and even increase bone mass.[32,57–61] Gruber and associates[62] found that the protective effects on bone persisted for 18 months. By 24 months, the rate of bone loss was similar to that of the controls. A 2-year prospective randomized study in 70 postmeno-pausal women[63] indicated that calcitonin was as effective as, but not better than, estrogen. Combination therapy had no additive effect.

When given for periods of 12 to 18 months, calcitonin has been shown to be effective in turning off bone resorption and stabilizing a modestly increased bone mass measured as total body calcium.[32] This effective period has led to a transient uncoupling of bone remodeling, so that bone formation is allowed to continue while remodeling spaces from prior resorption are repaired.

New studies have demonstrated that calcitonin is effective in reducing frac-ture rates although it has a modest influence on spinal bone mass and almost no influence on peripheral bone mass.[32,60] In spite of modest skeletal changes in terms of bone mass, the spinal deformation rates have been reported to be decreased to one fourth that of calcium controls.[64] In general, calcitonin appears to be most successful in high-turnover disease.

Calcitonin has little effect on compact bone.[65] It does not alter the biome-chanics of long bones or the histology of trabecular bone. It is uncertain how calcitonin might act on hip fractures. A recent study by Kanis and Passmore[33,34] demonstrated a 25% reduction in hip fracture risk with calcitonin treatment.

Exercise

Exercise is often prescribed as part of the treatment regimen for osteoporosis. Prospective studies have been undertaken to test a variety of exercise regimens that differ in duration, intensity, and measurement of end point. Several early nonrandomized studies have suggested that exercise was effective in increasing bone mass in osteoporotic women.[66–69] Efforts included weightbearing exer-cises, jogging, walking, and stair climbing. A program that used walking alone did not prevent bone loss.[70–72] Exercise has been demonstrated to be a remedy for bone loss from weightlessness and immobilization, but there has been con-cern about excessive exercise, and numerous studies have demonstrated loss of bone in amenorrheic women who are runners and athletes. This loss is asso-ciated with lower circulating levels of gonadal hormones.[73] Although exercise is not a substitute for medical and hormonal management, many studies have demonstrated that bone loss can be partially inhibited in older men and women who are routinely physically active.[32]

Experimental Therapies

Bisphosphonates

Bisphosphonates represent a class of drugs that now has come to the fore.[26,27,74–77] They were previously called diphosphonates, compounds char-acterized by a phosphorus carbon phosphorus (PCP) structure. They are ana-logs of naturally occurring pyrophosphates, which have a phosphorus oxygen phosphorus structure. The essential functional difference is that the PCP bonds in bisphosphonates are resistant to enzymatic hydrolysis by pyrophosphatases. There are many analogs available, which differ primarily in the side chains off the central carbon atom.[78] Their primary effect is to inhibit bone resorption, but at higher doses they can inhibit bone formation. Etidronate was the first agent used effectively in a cyclic program to prevent osteoporosis.[26,27] Newer agents currently available and under trial throughout Europe show greater promise, particularly in the ability to enhance resorption with less compromise of formation. Clinical trials indicate that bisphosphonates increase spinal bone mineral density in older women and osteoporotic patients, but have little effect on peripheral bone density.[26,27] Fracture rates appear to be reduced in the spine by bisphosphonate treatment, but there is concern over the consequences of long-term depression of bone turnover, which may result in accumulation of microfractures. The newer generation of bisphosphonates appears to have no negative effect on structurally important compact bone and to lead to mild increases in vertebral strength. Long-term studies of fracture risk are being performed to demonstrate protective value for the spine fracture and to answer the question about the potential risk for hip fracture.

Fluoride

Fluoride has a long career in the treatment of osteoporosis. Unlike other therapeutic agents fluoride may significantly increase bone mass instead of just stopping further loss.[2,28] The mechanism of fluoride action in bone is not fully understood. In addition to a physicochemical effect on stabilizing the hydroxyapatite crystal, there appears to be a direct bone stimulatory effect. Fluoride has been shown to increase osteoblastic proliferation and enhance enzymatic activities.[79–82]

Studies at the Mayo Clinic have demonstrated a rate of spinal deformation with high dose sodium fluoride over 4 years similar to that of calcium-treated controls in spite of an increase of 10% per year in the bone density of fluoride-treated patients.[28] Questions raised by these studies were whether fluoride induced an adverse effect on trabecular structure and decreased strength of the compact bone. Riggs and associates[28] suggested an increased hip fracture rate in patients receiving 70 mg/day of sodium fluoride. Studies performed by Aaron and associates[83] and by Vesterbey and associates[84] have demonstrated histologically that fluoride therapy thickens trabecular bone without adversely affecting bone structures. Similarly, compact bone does not show increased porosity when a slow-release form of sodium fluoride is used. In fact, Einhorn and associates[85] have demonstrated that the bone is stronger. Recent information from Farley and associates[86] shows that spinal fracture rates were decreased as a function of time when patients were treated with sodium fluoride, and the results were related to the initial spinal bone density. Patients on fluoride who had fractures were not responsive to the fluoride in terms of bone density enhancement, were older individuals, had more fractures prior to initiation of therapy, and had lower initial bone densities.

Recent information has suggested that fluoride induces a secondary hyperparathyroidism from an associated calcium defect. Of fluoride-treated osteoporotics, 70% have a serum calcium deficiency because of large mineral increases induced in trabecular bone. This deficiency can lead to a decrease in bone density of the peripheral bones, including the femur, coupled with elevated parathyroid hormone.[87] This calcium deficit can be corrected by treating with vitamin D (calcitriol, 0.5 µg/day). Current investigators now use a lower dose of sodium fluoride (50 mg/day), but administer it in a cyclic fashion and with an antiresorptive agent.[5] The concerns about the adverse effects on compact bone are that it may increase hip fractures. These data are somewhat in question. Epidemiologic studies performed by Jacobsen and associates[88] suggest areas of the United States with water fluoridation have a higher rate of hip fractures. However, a longitudinal study performed by Jacobsen and associates[89] in Rochester, Minnesota, demonstrated that hip fracture rates actually decreased slightly in the 10 years after water fluoridation began in that location.

Thiazides

Thiazide diuretics decrease urinary excretion of calcium and increase serum calcium.[90] Two large retrospective studies have shown that long-term thiazide use is associated with increased bone mineral content in both men and women.[91,92] Prospective studies of postmenopausal osteoporotics have failed to demonstrate effectiveness of thiazides in protecting against bone loss[93,94] with the exception of individuals with absorptive hypercalciuria. A large study from the Framingham group has shown that pure thiazide users among women experienced significant protection against fractures, whereas combination drug users experienced no protection.[95]

Anabolic Steroids

Derivatives and analogs of testosterone have profound anabolic effects on a number of tissues. Methyltestosterone, stanozolol, and nandrolone decanoate[96–100] have all been reported to increase bone mass but also to cause liver abnormalities and have virilizing effects and adverse effects on serum lipoproteins. The use of anabolic steroids in women must be considered experimental, and future use will depend on the synthesis of less androgenic compounds.

Summary

Osteoporosis weakens both the axial and appendicular skeleton. Strength of the bone appears to be related to the bone density, its microarchitecture, and the ratios of compact to trabecular bone. Antiresorptive and bone stimulative agents are currently under investigation as means of overcoming this problem. Questions abound as to the ability of intervention to restore bone or whether most therapies at this time merely prevent further skeletal erosion. There appears to be a clear difference in steps needed to prevent vertebral body fractures and those associated with prevention of hip fractures. This difference is related to the difference in bone composition and anatomic structure. Calcium preparations, anabolic steroids, vitamin D compounds, calcitonin, and estrogen in a recent review by Kanis and associates[101] and in the study by Chapuy and associates[38] have been suggested to have a protective role in the prevention of hip fractures. Sodium fluoride is the sole agent that has been associated with a higher hip fracture rate, but that may, in part, be related to the high dose, the immediate fluoride-release mechanism, and the absence of adequate calcium and vitamin D supplementation, which has been recently popularized.

Although osteoporosis clearly increases the risk for fracture, all studies indicate that anywhere from 65% to 95% of the time appendicular fractures are related to falls. There is a combination of trauma and bone stock that accounts for the specific fractures in which the relationship of trauma to fractures of the spine is lower and the relationship to fractures of the appendicular skeleton is much greater. Although falls are the final cumulative event leading to appendicular fractures, there is very strong epidemiologic evidence that osteoporosis places an individual at risk for the fracture following the fall. Consequently, therapies should be directed not only at preventing falls but also at enhancing the quantity, quality, and architectural alignment of the axial and appendicular skeleton.

References

1. Riggs BL, Melton LJ III: The prevention and treatment of osteoporosis. *N Engl J Med* 1992;327:620–627.
2. Barth RW, Lane JM: Osteoporosis. *Orthop Clin North Am* 1988;19:845–858.
3. Gallagher JC, Goldgar D, Moy A: Total bone calcium in normal women: Effect of age and menopause status. *J Bone Miner Res* 1987;2:491–496.
4. Genant HK, Cann CE, Ettinger B, et al: Quantitative computed tomography of vertebral spongiosa: A sensitive method for detecting early bone loss after oophorectomy. *Ann Intern Med* 1982;97:699–705.
5. Lane JM, Healey JH (eds): *Diagnosis and Management of Pathologic Fractures.* New York, NY, Raven Press, 1993.
6. Lindsay R, Hart DM, Aitken JM, et al: Long-term prevention of postmenopausal osteoporosis by oestrogen: Evidence for an increased bone mass after delayed onset of oestrogen treatment. *Lancet* 1976;1:1038–1041.
7. Nordin BEC, Need AG, Bridges A, et al: Relative contributions of years since menopause, age, and weight to vertebral density in postmenopausal women. *J Clin Endocrinol Metab* 1992;74:20–23.
8. Quigley ME, Martin PL, Burnier AM, et al: Estrogen therapy arrests bone loss in elderly women. *Am J Obstet Gynecol* 1987;156:1516–1523.
9. Cummings SR, Rubin SM, Black D: The future of hip fractures in the United States: Numbers, costs, and potential effects of postmenopausal estrogen. *Clin Orthop* 1990;252:163–166.
10. Riggs BL, Melton LJ III: Involutional osteoporosis. *N Engl J Med* 1986;314:1676–1686.
11. Healey JH, Lane JM: Structural scoliosis in osteoporotic women. *Clin Orthop* 1985;195:216–223.
12. Healey JH, Vigorita VJ, Lane JM: The coexistence and characteristics of osteoarthritis and osteoporosis. *J Bone Joint Surg* 1985;67A:586–592.
13. Matkovic V, Fontana D, Tominac C, et al: Factors that influence peak bone mass formation: A study of calcium balance and the inheritance of bone mass in adolescent females. *Am J Clin Nutr* 1990;52:878–888.
14. Slemenda C, Hui SL, Johnston CC: Patterns of bone loss and physiologic growing: Prospects for prevention of osteoporosis by attainment of greater peak bone mass, in Christiansen C, Overgaard K (eds): *Osteoporosis 1990: Proceedings of the Third International Symposium on Osteoporosis, Copenhagen, Denmark, October 14–20, 1990.* Copenhagen, Denmark, Osteopress ApS, 1990, vol 2, pp 948–953.
15. Parfitt AM: Bone remodeling: Relationship to the amount and structure of bone, and the pathogenesis and prevention of fractures, in Riggs BL, Melton LJ III (eds): *Osteoporosis: Etiology, Diagnosis, and Management.* New York, NY, Raven Press, 1988, pp 45–93.
16. Einhorn TA: Bone strength: The bottom line. *Calcif Tissue Int* 1992;51:333–339.
17. Brinckmann P, Biggemann M, Hilweg D: Prediction of the compressive strength of human lumbar vertebrae. *Spine* 1989;14:606–610.
18. Faulkner KG, Cann CE, Hasegawa BH: Effect of bone distribution on vertebral strength: Assessment with patient-specific nonlinear finite element analysis. *Radiology* 1991;179:669–674.
19. Mazess RB: Fracture risk: A role for compact bone. *Calcif Tissue Int* 1990;47:191–193.
20. Sandor T, Felsenberg D, Kalender WA, et al: Regional analysis of the loss of bone mineral density from spinal cortical bone. *Radiology* 1992;185(suppl):266.
21. Squillante RG, Williams JL: Videodensitometry of osteons in females with femoral neck fractures. *Calcif Tissue Int* 1993;52:273–277.
22. Nevitt MC, Cummings SR, Hudes ES: Risk factors for injurious falls: A prospective study. *J Gerontol Med Sci* 1991;46:M164-M170.

23. Hayes WC, Myers ER, Morris JN, et al: Impact near the hip dominates fracture risk in elderly nursing home residents who fall. *Calcif Tissue Int* 1993;52:192–198.

24. Cummings SR, Black DM, Nevitt MC, et al: Bone density at various sites for prediction of hip fractures: The study of Osteoporotic Fractures Research Group. *Lancet* 1993;341:72–75.

25. Kleerekoper M, Nelson DA: Vertebral fracture or vertebral deformity. *Calcif Tissue Int* 1992;50:5–6.

26. Storm T, Thamsborg G, Steiniche T, et al: Effect of intermittent cyclical etidronate therapy on bone mass and fracture rate in women with postmenopausal osteoporosis. *N Engl J Med* 1990;322:1265–1271.

27. Watts NB, Harris ST, Genant HK, et al: Intermittent cyclical etidronate treatment of postmenopausal osteoporosis. *N Engl J Med* 1990;323:73–79.

28. Riggs BL, Hodgson SF, O'Fallon WM, et al: Effect of fluoride treatment on the fracture rate in postmenopausal women with osteoporosis. *N Engl J Med* 1990;322:802–809.

29. Nordin BEC: Bone mass, bone loss, bone density and fractures. *Osteoporos Int* 1993;3(suppl 1):1–7.

30. Browne MG, Bansal M, DiCarlo E, et al: Resorption parameters in the classification of osteoporosis. *Bone* 1992;13:A6.

31. Christiansen C, Riis BJ, Rodbro P: Prediction of rapid bone loss in postmenopausal women. *Lancet* 1987;1:1105–1108.

32. Weinerman SA, Bockman RS: Medical therapy of osteoporosis. *Orthop Clin North Am* 1990;21:109–124.

33. Kanis JA, Passmore R: Calcium supplementation of the diet: I. Not justified by present evidence. *BMJ* 1989;298:137–140.

34. Kanis JA, Passmore R: Calcium supplementation of the diet: II. Not justified by present evidence. *BMJ* 1989;298:205–208.

35. Nordin BEC, Heaney RP: Calcium supplementation of the diet: Justified by present evidence. *BMJ* 1990;300:1056–1060.

36. Dawson-Hughes B, Dallal GE, Krall EA, et al: Effect of vitamin D supplementation on wintertime and overall bone loss in healthy postmenopausal women. *Ann Intern Med* 1991;115:505–512.

37. Johnston CC Jr, Miller JZ, Slemenda CW, et al: Calcium supplementation and increases in bone mineral density in children. *N Engl J Med* 1992;327:82–87.

38. Chapuy MC, Arlot ME, Duboeuf F, et al: Vitamin D3 and calcium to prevent hip fractures in elderly women. *N Engl J Med* 1992;327:1637–1642.

39. Chapuy MC, Meunier PJ: Calcium et vitamine D3, une prévention des fractures du col du fémur chez les femmes âgés. *Presse Med* 1993;22:615–616.

40. Ettinger B, Genant HK, Cann CE: Long-term estrogen replacement therapy prevents bone loss and fractures. *Ann Intern Med* 1985;102:319–324.

41. Weiss NS, Ure CL, Ballard JH, et al: Decreased risk of fractures of the hip and lower forearm with postmenopausal use of estrogen. *N Engl J Med* 1980;303:1195–1198.

42. Hutchinson TA, Polansky SM, Feinstein AR: Postmenopausal oestrogens protect against fractures of hip and distal radius: A case-control study. *Lancet* 1979;2:705–709.

43. Kiel DP, Felson DT, Anderson JJ, et al: Hip fracture and the use of estrogens in postmenopausal women: The Framingham study. *N Engl J Med* 1987;317:1169–1174.

44. Paganini-Hill A, Ross RK, Gerkins VR, et al: Menopausal estrogen therapy and hip fractures. *Ann Intern Med* 1981;95:28–31.

45. Spector TD, Brennan P, Harris PA, et al: Do current regimes of hormone replacement therapy protect against subsequent fractures? *Osteoporos Int* 1992;2:219–224.

46. Hulka BS: Hormone-replacement therapy and the risk of breast cancer. *CA Cancer J Clin* 1990;40:289–296.

47. Key TJA, Pike MC: The role of oestrogens and progestagens in the epidemiology and prevention of breast cancer. *Eur J Cancer* 1988;24:29–43.

48. Steinberg KK, Thacker SB, Smith SJ, et al: A meta-analysis of the effect of estrogen replacement therapy on the risk of breast cancer. *JAMA* 1991;265:1985–1990.

49. Barrett-Connor E, Bush TL: Estrogen and coronary heart disease in women. *JAMA* 1991;265:1861–1867.

50. Lobo RA: Cardiovascular implications of estrogen replacement therapy. *Obstet Gynecol* 1990;75(suppl):18S–25S.

51. Stampfer MJ, Colditz GA, Willett WC, et al: Postmenopausal estrogen therapy and cardiovascular disease: Ten year follow-up from the nurses' health study. *N Engl J Med* 1991;325:756–762.

52. Hillner BE, Hollenberg JP, Pauker SG: Postmenopausal estrogens in prevention of osteoporosis: Benefit virtually without risk if cardiovascular effects are considered. *Am J Med* 1986;80:1115–1127.

53. Powles TJ: The case for clinical trials of tamoxifen for prevention of breast cancer. *Lancet* 1992;340:1145–1147.

54. Lahti E, Blanco G, Kauppila A, et al: Endometrial changes in postmenopausal breast cancer patients receiving tamoxifen. *Obstet Gynecol* 1993;81:660–664.

55. Love RR, Mazess RB, Barden HS, et al: Effects of tamoxifen on bone mineral density in postmenopausal women with breast cancer. *N Engl J Med* 1992;326:852–856.

56. Maclean JP, Leslie WD: Estrogen and bone density: A comparison of tamoxifen and hypoestrogenemia. *J Nucl Med* 1993;34:165P.

57. Aloia JF, Vaswani A, Kapoor A, et al: Treatment of osteoporosis with calcitonin, with and without growth hormone. *Metabolism* 1985;34:124–129.

58. Civitelli R, Gonnelli S, Zacchei F, et al: Bone turnover in postmenopausal osteoporosis: Effect of calcitonin treatment. *J Clin Invest* 1988;82:1268–1274.

59. Gennari C, Chierichetti SM, Bigazzi S, et al: Comparative effects on bone mineral content of calcium and calcium plus salmon calcitonin given in two different regimens in postmenopausal osteoporosis. *Curr Therapy Res* 1985;38:455–464.

60. Mazzuoli GF, Passeri M, Gennari C, et al: Effects of salmon calcitonin in postmenopausal osteoporosis: A controlled double-blind clinical study. *Calcif Tissue Int* 1986;38:3–8.

61. Wallach S, Cohn SH, Atkins HL, et al: Effect of salmon calcitonin on skeletal mass in osteoporosis. *Curr Ther Res* 1977;22:556–572.

62. Gruber HE, Ivey JL, Baylink DJ, et al: Long-term calcitonin therapy in postmenopausal osteoporosis. *Metabolism* 1984;33:295–303.

63. MacIntyre I, Stevenson JC, Whitehead MI, et al: Calcitonin for prevention of postmenopausal bone loss. *Lancet* 1988;1:900–902.

64. Rico H, Hernandez ER, Revilla M, et al: Salmon calcitonin reduces vertebral fracture rate in postmenopausal crush fracture syndrome. *Bone Miner* 1992;16:131–138.

65. Whitehead MI, Ellerington MC, Marsch MS, et al: Intranasal calcitonin for prevention of postmenopausal osteoporosis. Presented at the Fourth International Symposium on Osteoporosis, Hong Kong, 1993.

66. Aloia JF, Cohn SH, Ostuni JA, et al: Prevention of involutional bone loss by exercise. *Ann Intern Med* 1978;89:356–358.

67. Krolner B, Toft B, Nielsen SP, et al: Physical exercise as prophylaxis against involutional vertebral bone loss: A controlled trial. *Clin Sci* 1983;64:541–546.

68. Smith EL Jr, Reddan W, Smith PE: Physical activity and calcium modalities for bone mineral increase in aged women. *Med Sci Sports Exerc* 1981;13:60–64.

69. Smith EL Jr, Smith PE, Ensign CJ, et al: Bone involution decrease in exercising middle-aged women. *Calcif Tissue Int* 1984;36:S129–S138.

70. Cavanaugh DJ, Cann CE: Brisk walking does not stop bone loss in postmenopausal women. *Bone* 1988;9:201–204.

71. Sandler RB, Cauley JA, Hom DL, et al: The effects of walking on the cross-sectional dimensions of the radius in postmenopausal women. *Calcif Tissue Int* 1987;41:65–69.

72. White MK, Martin RB, Yeater RA, et al: The effects of exercise on the bones of postmenopausal women. *Int Orthop* 1984;7:209–214.
73. Snead DB, Weltman A, Weltman JY, et al: Reproductive hormones and bone mineral density in women runners. *J Appl Physiol* 1992;72:2149–2156.
74. Reginster JY, Lecart MP, Deroisy R, et al: Prevention of postmenopausal bone loss by tiludronate. *Lancet* 1989;2:1469–1471.
75. Reid IR, King AR, Alexander CT, et al: Prevention of steroid-induced osteoporosis with (3-amino-1-hydroxypropylidene)-1, 1-bisphosphonate (APD). *Lancet* 1988; 1:143–146.
76. Sato M, Grasser W, Endo N, et al: Bisphosphonate action: Alendronate localization in rat bone and effects on osteoclast ultrastructure. *J Clin Invest* 1991;88: 2095–2105.
77. Valkema R, Papapoulis SE, Fismans F-J, et al: A four year continuous gain in bone mass in APD-treated osteoporosis, in Christiansen C, Johnsen JS, Riis BJ (eds): *Osteoporosis 1987: Proceedings of the International Symposium on Osteoporosis, Denmark, September 27—October 2, 1987.* Copenhagen, Denmark, Osteopress ApS, 1987, vol 2, pp 836–839.
78. Shinoda H, Adamek G, Felix R, et al: Structure-activity relationships of various bisphosphonates. *Calcif Tissue Int* 1983;35:87–99.
79. Farley JR, Tarbaux N, Hall S, et al: Evidence that fluoride-stimulated 3[H]-thymidine incorporation in embryonic chick calvarial cell cultures is dependent on the presence of a bone cell mitogen, sensitive to changes in the phosphate concentration, and modulated by systemic skeletal effectors. *Metabolism* 1988;37:988–995.
80. Farley JR, Wergedal JE, Baylink DJ: Fluoride directly stimulates proliferation and alkaline phosphatase activity of bone-forming cells. *Science* 1983;222:330–332.
81. Hauschildt S, Hirt W, Bessler W: Modulation of protein kinase C activity by NaF in bone marrow derived macrophages. *FEBS Lett* 1988;230:121–124.
82. Wergedal JE, Lau KHW, Baylink DJ: Fluoride and bovine bone extract influence cell proliferation and phosphatase activities in human bone cell cultures. *Clin Orthop* 1988;233:274–282.
83. Aaron JE, Vernejoul MC, Kanis JA: Bone hypertrophy and trabecular generation in Paget's disease and in fluoride-treated osteoporosis. *Bone Miner* 1992;17:399–413.
84. Vesterby A, Gundersen HJG, Melsen F, et al: Marrow space star volume in the iliac crest decreases in osteoporotic patients after continuous treatment with fluoride, calcium and vitamin D2 for five years. *Bone* 1991;12:33–37.
85. Einhorn TA, Wakley GK, Linkhart S, et al: Incorporation of sodium fluoride into cortical bone does not impair the mechanical properties of the appendicular skeleton in rats. *Calcif Tissue Int* 1992;51:127–131.
86. Farley SM, Wergedal JE, Farley JR, et al: Spinal fractures during fluoride therapy for osteoporosis: Relationship to spinal bone density. *Osteoporos Int* 1992;2: 213–218.
87. Dure-Smith BA, Farley SM, Linkhart SG, et al: Increased spinal bone density in response to fluoride is associated with calcium deficiency, secondary hyperparathyroidism and appendicular bone loss. *Trans Orthop Res Soc* 1993;18;561.
88. Jacobsen SJ, Goldberg J, Cooper C, et al: The association between water fluoridation and hip fracture among white women and men aged 65 years and older: A national ecologic study. *Ann Epidemiol* 1992;2:617–626.
89. Jacobsen SJ, O'Fallon WM, Melton LJ III: Hip fracture incidence before and after the fluoridation of the public water supply in Rochester, Minnesota. *Am J Public Health* 1993;83:743–745.
90. Yendt ER, Cohanim M: Prevention of calcium stones with thiazides. *Kidney Int* 1978;13:397–409.
91. Wasnich RD, Benfante RJ, Yano K, et al: Thiazide effect on the mineral content of bone. *N Engl J Med* 1983;309:344–347.

92. Wasnich RD, Ross PD, Heilbrun LK, et al: Differential effects of thiazide and estrogen upon bone mineral content and fracture prevalence. *Obstet Gynecol* 1986;67:457–462.

93. Christiansen C, Christensen MS, McNair P, et al: Prevention of early postmenopausal bone loss: Controlled 2-year study in 315 normal females. *Eur J Clin Invest* 1980;10:273–279.

94. Transbol I, Christensen MS, Jensen GF, et al: Thiazide for the postponement of postmenopausal bone loss. *Metabolism* 1982;31:383–386.

95. Felson DT, Sloutskis D, Anderson JJ, et al: Thiazide diuretics and the risk of hip fracture: Results from the Framingham study. *JAMA* 1991;265:370–373.

96. Aloia JF, Kapoor A, Vaswani A, et al: Changes in body composition following therapy of osteoporosis with methandrostenolone. *Metabolism* 1981;30:1076–1079.

97. Chestnut CH III, Ivey JL, Gruber HE, et al: Stanozolol in postmenopausal osteoporosis: Therapeutic efficacy and possible mechanisms of action. *Metabolism* 1983;32:571–580.

98. Chestnut CH III, Nelp WB, Baylink DJ, et al: Effect of methandrostenolone on postmenopausal bone wasting as assessed by changes in total bone mineral mass. *Metabolism* 1977;26:267–277.

99. Dequeker J, Geusens P: Anabolic steroids and osteoporosis. *Acta Endocrinol* 1985;271(suppl):45–52.

100. Need AG, Morris HA, Hartley TF, et al: Effects of nandrolone decanoate on forearm mineral density and calcium metabolism in osteoporotic postmenopausal women. *Calcif Tissue Int* 1987;41:7-10.

101. Kanis JA, Johnell O, Gullberg B, et al: Evidence for efficacy of drugs affecting bone metabolism in preventing hip fracture. *BMJ* 1992;305:1124–1128.

Chapter 34

Age-Related Hip Fractures: Biomechanics of Fracture Risk

Wilson C. Hayes, PhD

Introduction

Hip fractures are a public health problem of crisis proportions. In the United States, more than 280,000 such fractures occur each year, with the numbers continuing to increase along with the average age of the population. A recent AAOS Position Statement projected an expected incidence of 350,000 fractures annually by the year 2000, and 650,000 by 2050.[1] Current annual costs of hip fractures are close to $10 billion, and are increasing at an alarming rate. Patients with hip fractures routinely are hospitalized for surgical treatment and, in many hospitals, they occupy roughly 50% of orthopaedic beds. If the prevalence of hip fracture continues to rise at current rates, it may well be that in the next few decades, orthopaedists will do little else but treat this problem.

The design and implementation of intervention efforts aimed at reducing the number of hip fractures are complicated by: (1) uncertainty as to the relative importance of reduced bone strength and increased incidence of falling in the etiology of hip fractures; (2) the complex multifactorial nature of falls; and (3) the nearly complete lack of understanding about what distinguishes injurious from noninjurious falls.[2-4] The steep rise with age in hip fracture incidence, coupled with demonstrated age-dependent reductions in bone density and strength[5-8] have led to the predominant view that age-related bone loss, or osteoporosis, is the most important determinant of hip fracture incidence.[9] However, a number of authors have suggested that it is the increased tendency of the elderly to fall and to experience falls of increased severity that dominate hip fracture risk.[10-13] Indeed, most densitometric indicators of femoral osteopenia have failed to discriminate between hip fracture patients and age- and gender-matched controls.[8,14,15] On the other hand, bone mineral density at the hip is known to decline with age, reaching lower levels in women than in men.[6-8,16] In-vitro biomechanical studies of cadaveric hips have shown that these reductions in density are associated with reduced bone strength.[17-24] There is also growing clinical evidence that the frequency of hip fracture increases as femoral bone mineral density declines.[7,16,25] More recent studies have shown statistically significant differences in densitometric measures at the hip between hip fracture patients and controls.[26-32]

Faced with this conflicting evidence, Melton and associates[7,33] and Cummings and Nevitt[34] have suggested that reduced skeletal resistance to trauma and an increased propensity for falling together determine hip fracture risk. Over 90% of hip fractures are the result of a fall.[35-41] Yet, for reasons that are not well understood, fewer than 2% of all falls result in hip fracture.[42-44] In

485

addition, as with interventions directed toward bone density, fall prevention programs have met with only limited success in preventing hip fractures.[45,46] It thus appears that some unexplained, confounding factor is limiting both the ability to discriminate hip fracture patients from controls and the attempts to reduce hip fracture incidence. Moreover, the relative risks associated with bone loss and the trauma associated with falling have not until recently been estimated from clinical surveillance studies.[47,48]

The group at the Beth Israel Orthopaedic Biomechanics Laboratory has taken the position that fall severity is a potentially dominant factor in the etiology of hip fracture. Defining a high-risk fall and placing in context the relative importance of fall biomechanics and bone fragility have been central thrusts of our research efforts. This chapter summarizes some of those efforts, beginning with evidence from fall surveillance studies, which help define a high-risk fall and provide first-order estimates of the relative importance of fall severity and bone fragility. It then introduces a new paradigm, called the factor of risk, for the examination of fracture risk. This parameter, the inverse of the factor of safety, reflects the standard engineering practice that the risk of fracture is expressed as a ratio of the loads applied to a structure divided by the loads necessary to cause failure of that structure. Based on that paradigm, recent studies from the Laboratory are reviewed to estimate the numerator and the denominator of the factor of risk. From these estimates, it is concluded, as it was by Melton and Riggs,[33] that hip fractures are both a disease and an injury, and beyond that, that it is possible to estimate the relative importance of these two components of fracture risk.

Hip Fracture: Disease or Injury?

A fall has four distinct phases: (1) an instability phase that results in a loss of balance; (2) a descent phase; (3) an impact phase; and (4) a postimpact phase during which the subject comes to rest. Previous research on falling in the elderly has focused almost entirely on those factors that result in a loss of balance, ie, the instability phase. The work has emphasized the importance of gait disturbances, dementia, visual impairment, neurologic and musculoskeletal disabilities, postural hypotension, medications, and environmental hazards.[36,38,43,44,49-54] By contrast, little is known about the mechanics of the fall itself; thus, it might be said that a great deal is known about why people fall but very little about how they fall. There are also no verified definitions of fall severity or what constitutes a high-risk fall. Cummings and Nevitt[34] hypothesized that three conditions must be met for a fall to cause a hip fracture: (1) impact near the hip; (2) failure of active protective mechanisms such as using the outstretched arm to break the fall; and (3) insufficient passive energy absorption by local soft tissues. They suggested that, under these conditions, sufficient force can be transmitted to the proximal femur to exceed its fracture load. Others have suggested that much more energy is available in a typical fall than is required to fracture the elderly hip.[3,55] However, until recently, data have not been available that allow these hypotheses to be tested.

In an attempt to characterize fall severity and to determine which aspects of the descent and impact phases of a fall are associated with a high risk of hip fracture, a fall surveillance study of nursing home residents was undertaken. To address these issues, elderly fallers or reliable witnesses were asked several open-ended questions about falls. The study design was a case-control observational study. Case subjects sustained a hip fracture after a fall and control subjects did not fracture the hip after a fall. The source of the study subjects was the Hebrew Rehabilitation Center for the Aged (HRCA), a life-care environment for approximately 720 residents. The average resident age at the HRCA is 87 years, and the women to men ratio is three to one. Falls were surveyed consecutively from December 1986 to July 1990, a period during which approximately 1174 residents were under observation for falls. All ambulatory residents of age 65 years and older were eligible. A subject was entered if an examination of the HRCA computerized reports and daily logs revealed that the subject had fallen. Multiple fallers were entered only once. A total of 395 subjects who fell during the study were included; 82 of these fell and fractured a hip and 313 fell and did not sustain a fracture. Characteristics of the fall were determined by personal interview with the faller and with any witnesses. When possible, the interviews were conducted within 24 hours of the event by a research assistant at the HRCA. The following variables were assessed: date and time of the fall, height of the fall, fall direction, impact location on the body, and activity and location of the subject at the time of the fall. The continuous and dichotomous variables assessed in this study are described in detail by Hayes and associates.[56]

The average age ($\pm$ standard deviation) of the nursing home residents at the time of the first recorded fall was 88 ($\pm$ 6) years. The falls that resulted in hip fracture occurred in subjects who were taller, lighter, and had a reduced body mass index than those whose falls did not result in fracture (Table 1). Potential energies (estimated as mgh) were 442 ($\pm$ 143) Joules (J) for those falls that resulted in hip fracture and 424 ($\pm$ 143) J for those falls that did not; the energies were not significantly different ($p = 0.38$). From a univariate analysis, walking at the time of the fall, mental impairment, falling to the side, and impacting the body in the region of the hip were all associated with hip fracture from a fall (Table 2). In particular, impacting the side or side of the leg was associated with an odds ratio of 21. Independent variables associated with the occurrence of a hip fracture by a multiple logistic regression model included impact location on the hip, body mass index (kg/m^2), and potential energy content of the fall. From the logistic regression, the odds ratio for having a hip fracture, given that impact was on the hip or side of the leg, was 21.7. Low body mass index and high energy content of the fall were also found to be independent predictors of hip fracture. The univariate associations of hip fracture with mental impairment, falling to the side, and walking at the time of the fall (Table 2) did not result in significant associations in the multiple logistic regression.

This study was undertaken to characterize fall severity and to determine which aspects of fall mechanics are associated with a high risk of hip fracture. The risk of hip fracture from falls among these elderly nursing home residents was found to be associated independently with impact site, body mass index,

Table 1 Mean values and standard deviations of characteristics of patients with hip fracture and controls without hip fracture

Property*	Fracture cases	Fall controls	Significance (t test)
Age (years)	88.9 (6.2)	87.8 (5.9)	0.13
Weight (kg)	53.3 (10.7)	56.9 (11.1)	0.01
Height (m)	1.57 (0.08)	1.52 (0.08)	< 0.001
BMI (kg/m^2)	21.5 (3.5)	24.7 (4.4)	< 0.001

* BMI is body mass index.

Table 2 Frequency distributions of subject and fall characteristics for subjects with hip fracture and control subjects without fracture.

Characteristic	Fracture cases (%)	Fall controls (%)	Odds ratio	95% CI*	Significance (χ-square)
Female	77	77	1.0	0.6–1.8	0.98
Fall from standing height or higher	81	73	2.5	0.8–2.9	0.21
Walking	59	35	3.6	2.6–4.4	< 0.001
Mental impairment	74	43	4.6	3.2–6.2	< 0.001
Fall to side	60	23	5.9	3.5–10	< 0.001
Impact hip or side of leg	59	6	32.0	9.2–48	< 0.001

* CI is confidence interval.

and potential energy content of the fall. Fracture of the hip was not associated with gender or age in this sample of elderly nursing home residents. Impact on the hip or side of the leg was the strongest determinant of hip fracture compared with the other variables measured, raising the risk of fracture by about 20-fold. The value of the odds ratio for impacting the hip was a function of two effects, the increased odds of hip fracture when the subject impacted the hip and the decreased odds for impacting the hip for subjects without fracture.

Comparison of the potential energies available in these falls with the energies required to fracture the elderly cadaveric femur in vitro indicates that much less energy is needed to fracture the proximal femur than is available in simple falls from sitting or standing height. Fracture energies required to break elderly cadaveric hips loaded on the lateral greater trochanter range from 5 to 51 J.[21] By contrast, the potential energies associated with falls among elderly nursing home subjects were on average more than 400 J, or an order of magnitude greater. There are two important implications of this finding. First, a fall from standing height should no longer be viewed as representing "minimal trauma" and used as an operational definition of an osteoporotic hip fracture. Data indicate that a fall from standing height, especially if impact occurs near the hip and energy-absorbing mechanisms are inadequate, provides more than sufficient energy to fracture the hip in elderly fallers. Second, for falls from standing height that involve impact near the hip but do not result in hip fracture, significant energy-absorbing mechanisms must reduce the force actually delivered to the femur. In probable order of importance, these energy-absorbing mechanisms are likely to include eccentric contraction of the muscles of the lower extremities, the use of the outstretched arm or hand to break the fall, and the absorption of energy by soft tissues at the site of impact. The combined effects of these energy-absorbing mechanisms and the relatively low probability of impact near the hip probably account for the fact that fewer than 2% of all falls result in hip fracture.[42–44]

Furthermore, the potentially dominant confounding role of fall severity is a likely explanation for the failure of most densitometric studies to distinguish clearly between patients with hip fractures and age- and gender-matched controls, especially in the population over age 70 in whom over 90% of hip fractures occur.[57] The importance of fall severity may also help to explain the generally disappointing results of intervention efforts directed toward the maintenance of bone strength in this population.[58]

More precise determinations of the relative risks associated with fall mechanics, body habitus, and bone fragility require simultaneous characterization of fall severity, body habitus, and bone fragility at the hip. Such data are just beginning to emerge. Nevitt and Cummings[47] recently reported measurements of bone density and some determinants of fall severity in a large prospective cohort of nonblack women aged 65 and older living in the community. Those who subsequently suffered hip fractures as a result of a fall (n = 130) and a consecutive sample of those who fell without a fracture (n = 467) were interviewed. In multivariate analyses, women who suffered hip fractures were more likely to have fallen sideways or straight down (odds ratio 3.3) and to have landed on or near the hip (odds ratio 32.5) than women who fell without a fracture. Among women who fell on their hips, the risk of fracturing that site more than doubled for each standard deviation decrease in bone density at the hip.

In a prospective case-control study designed to determine the relative importance of fall characteristics, body habitus, and femoral bone mineral density in predicting hip fracture among community-dwelling elderly, Greenspan and associates[48] enrolled 149 people (126 women, 23 men). Enrollees were age 65 and above, and included 72 who fell and sustained a hip fracture and 77 who fell with no hip fracture. Direction of the fall (odds ratio 6.0), a decrease of one standard deviation in femoral neck bone mineral density (odds ratio 2.8), an increase of one standard deviation in the potential energy of the fall (odds ratio 3.0), and a decrease of one standard deviation in the body mass index (odds ratio 2.1) were all significant and independent risk factors for hip fracture in both sexes. Greenspan and associates[48] concluded that among elderly persons who fall, in most of whom hip bone mineral density is already well below the fracture threshold, fall characteristics and body habitus are important risk factors for hip fracture and touch on a domain entirely missed by knowledge of bone mineral density.

Although these data clearly suggest that hip fracture risk is multifactorial, and that both fall severity and bone fragility play important etiologic roles, such data exhibit the typical limitations of clinical research, including recall bias and reliability of the outcome variables. Another perspective on the relative risks associated with the severity of trauma and bone fragility can be obtained from a standard engineering approach for the assessment of fracture risk in engineering structures.

Factor of Risk: A New Paradigm

In order to predict the risk of fracture of any structure, it is necessary to have information on: (1) the geometry of the structure; (2) the materials from which the structure is made; and (3) the loads to which the structure is subjected (Fig. 1). Based on this information, engineering analyses can be used to predict, under the given loading conditions, how close the structure is to failure. Alternatively, if experimental data are available on the ultimate load-carrying capacity of the structure, knowledge of the imposed loads leads directly to an estimate of fracture risk. Consider a simple example. If a structural beam supporting a roof is known to withstand 10,000 N before failure and the beam is subjected to only 1,000 N, it is possible to be relatively certain that the beam will not fail and the roof will not collapse. However, if, because of wind or snow loads, the beam is subjected to close to or greater than 10,000 N, there is at least a strong likelihood that the beam will fail. This approach to fracture risk prediction can be formalized by defining a factor of risk F as the ratio of

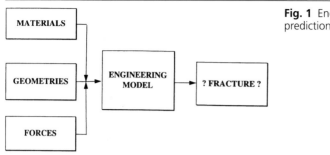

Fig. 1 Engineering fracture risk prediction.

the applied loads divided by the loads necessary to cause fracture. This can be written

$$\Phi = \text{Applied Load/Fracture Load} \qquad \text{(Eq. 1)}$$

in which Φ is known as the factor of risk. Equation 1 simply states that for a factor of risk much less than 1, fracture is unlikely. For a factor of risk close to or exceeding 1, fracture is considered likely.

For a skeletal structure such as the proximal femur, estimates of the factor of risk require information both on the forces to which the proximal femur is subjected and on the forces necessary to cause fracture of the proximal femur. The forces in both the numerator and denominator of equation 1 should be for the same loading conditions. That is, to determine the risk of fracture during normal gait, information is needed on the maximum forces to which the hip is subjected during gait and on the forces necessary to cause fracture under those same loading conditions. To determine the factor of risk for impact loading from a fall, data must be available on the maximum forces applied to the hip during a fall and on the forces required to cause fracture under the same loading conditions. It would be inappropriate and inaccurate to compute a factor of risk by calculating the ratio of the forces applied during gait to the forces that cause fracture of the proximal femur under fall loading conditions.

Although the assessment of the factor of risk requires information both on the ultimate load-carrying capacity of the femur and on the forces to which the femur is subjected, these latter forces have been largely neglected in the literature on age-related fractures and osteoporosis. Reflecting the dominant view that age-related fractures are primarily the consequence of bone loss and increased bone fragility, researchers have focused on densitometric estimates of the denominator of Equation 1, neglecting the intuitively obvious but largely ignored notion that the applied forces can easily dominate the fracture process. For example, if a person falls from a great height and lands on the hip, it makes very little difference whether the femoral bone mineral density is one standard deviation below or above age- and gender-matched norms. The hip will fracture simply because the forces are well in excess of those necessary to fracture the hip of even a young, vigorous adult. The question that is then immediately raised by this approach is whether a fall from standing height represents minimal trauma, as most have suggested, or represents trauma of sufficient magnitude to fracture the hip every time such a fall occurs. The first step in addressing this question is to examine the process of falling in an attempt to estimate the forces that can be expected in simple falls from standing height.

Fall Impact Forces: The Numerator of Φ

To provide estimates of the hip impact force from a fall from standing height, Robinovitch and associates[59] developed a simple experiment that they call the pelvis-release experiment. In addition to providing estimates of the hip impact force and rate of loading, these pelvis-release experiments examined how fall impact forces are influenced when the body contacts the ground in a state of muscle relaxation as opposed to muscle contraction. Robinovitch and associates[59] tested human volunteers of varying height and weight and examined the differences in impact response arising when subjects were encouraged to contract the trunk muscles.

Seven men and seven women ranging in age from 20 to 35 years and in body weight from 489 to 916 N participated. Each subject lay with the lateral aspect of the greater trochanter contacting a high-fidelity force plate, the lower leg and shoulder resting on rigid support, and the pelvis cradled in a canvas sling (Fig. 2). Before the test, the pelvis was raised slightly and then released. The resulting oscillatory force versus time record was fit with a mass-spring-damper model used to determine the effective mass of the body at impact, the spring stiffness k, and the damping factor b of the soft tissues overlying the greater trochanter. Just prior to the experiment, the subject was instructed either to completely relax the body (muscle-relaxed) or to contract the trunk and back muscles in an attempt to raise the head and shoulder off their supports (muscle-active). Muscle activity was monitored in all trials through electromyographic surface electrodes placed on the spinalis portion of the erector spinae muscles at the level of the tenth rib, the posterior superior portion of the external oblique, and the gluteus medius 5 cm superior to the greater trochanter.

In order to estimate the typical force applied to the proximal femur for falls in both muscle-relaxed and muscle-active states, average values of the effective mass m and the values of the trochanteric soft tissues' stiffness and damping were incorporated into equations describing the dynamics of impact, with velocity given by a free-fall of the effective mass from an initial height of 0.7 m. For men, the effective mass averaged 39 kg in the muscle-relaxed state and 49 kg in the muscle-active state; these values represented 50% and 63% of the average whole body mass, respectively. In women, the effective mass averaged 31 kg in the muscle-relaxed state and 38 kg in the muscle-active state; values represented 50% and 60% of average whole body mass, respectively. The pre-

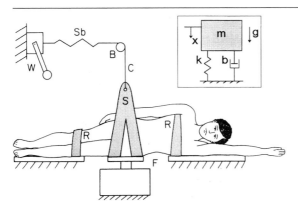

Fig. 2 Apparatus for pelvis release experiments. F, high fidelity force platform; S, pelvis holding sling; R, shoulder and knee restraints; C, steel chain; B, electromagnetic brake; Sb, bias spring; W, winch. The mass-spring-damper model used to simulate the impact response of the body in pelvis release experiments is shown in the inset. (Reproduced with permission from Robinovitch SN, Hayes WC, McMahon TA: Prediction of femoral impact forces in falls on the hip. *J Biomech Eng* 1991; 113:366–374.)

dicted peak forces as a function of fall height demonstrated dramatic increase in peak force for the muscle-active state in men, but not in women (Fig. 3). At a fall height of 0.7 m (a reasonable average value for a fall from standing height), the peak force in men was 6,100 N in the muscle-relaxed state and 12,100 N in the muscle-active state. Corresponding values for women were 5,050 N in the muscle-relaxed state and 6,370 N in the muscle-active state.

These results suggest that the state of muscle activity at impact is an important determinant of fall fracture risk, at least in men. For example, muscle activation in men caused a 100% increase in predicted average peak force. These changes reflect two phenomena caused by contraction of the trunk muscles at impact: (1) an increase in the effective mass as more of the trunk and lower extremities participate in the impact and (2) an increase in the rigidity of the muscular connection between the trunk, pelvis, and lower limbs. Therefore, although neuromuscular control in the descent phase of the fall may reduce the velocity of impact and allow the faller to adjust the body into a safe landing configuration, striking the ground in a stiff state actually increases the impact force. These findings also confirm the well-established notion that falling while relaxed reduces the injury potential of a fall.

Strength of the Proximal Femur: The Denominator of Φ

To estimate the factor of risk Φ, the estimated impact force must be divided by the estimated strength of the proximal femur. Such estimates of fracture force can be provided by in vitro studies of cadaveric femora tested in a loading configuration that would simulate a fall with impact on the greater trochanter. Such data were provided by Lotz and Hayes[21] from a study in which fracture load under quasistatic conditions in a fall loading configuration were related to a densitometric variable determined by quantitative computed tomography (QCT). The average fracture forces were about 2,100 N and average fracture energies were about 26.5 J. Moreover, a QCT variable based on density and cross-sectional area of bone was strongly correlated ($r^2 = 0.93$) to the measured fracture load. More recently, Courtney and associates[60,61] conducted similar experiments in which paired specimens of elderly cadaveric femora were tested in a fall-loading configuration under quasistatic conditions or under high loading rates equivalent to those that would occur in a fall. In addition, the measured fracture loads at both loading rates were correlated with densitometric

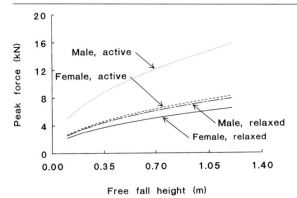

Fig. 3 Effect of drop height, gender, and muscle activity on predicted peak impact force. (Reproduced with permission from Robinovitch SN, Hayes WC, McMahon TA: Prediction of femoral impact forces in falls on the hip. *J Biomech Eng* 1991;113:366–374.)

measures of the femoral neck determined by dual-energy x-ray absorptiometry (DXA).

Increasing the loading rate from quasistatic values (2 mm/s) to realistic impact values (100 mm/s) increased the fracture load from 3,440 ($\pm$ 1,330) N to 4,170 ($\pm$ 1,590) N, an increase of 21% ($p < 0.05$) (Fig. 4). However, due to a 92% increase in stiffness at the higher loading rate, the energy-absorption capacities did not increase significantly at the higher rate (55 ($\pm$ 30) J [2 mm/s] versus 67 ($\pm$ 59) J [100 mm/s]) (Fig. 4). As with the earlier QCT study, densitometric variables measured by DXA were correlated with fracture load (Fig. 5). At both loading rates, fracture load correlated with bone mineral density of the femoral neck ($r^2 = 0.85$ [2 mm/s] and $r^2 = 0.72$ [100 mm/s]). Because the slopes and intercepts of the two linear regressions were not significantly different, the data were pooled, again resulting in a strong linear correlation between femoral fracture load and femoral neck bone mineral density ($r^2 = 0.68$) (Fig. 5).

These results may be compared with those of Weber and associates,[62] who reported increases in fracture load of 19.5% and 104% for femurs loaded at displacement rates of 14 mm/s and 4,000 mm/s, respectively, compared to femurs loaded at 0.7 mm/s. They also reported coefficients of determination (r^2) between bone mineral density of the femoral neck and fracture load of 0.89

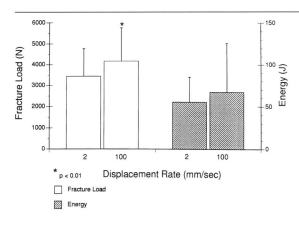

Fig. 4 Effect of increasing the displacement rate on fracture load and energy absorption capacity.

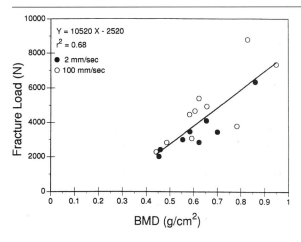

Fig. 5 Correlation of fracture load with bone mineral density (BMD) of the femoral neck at quasistatic and fall impact loading rates.

and 0.60 for the lowest and highest displacement rates, respectively. However, it should be noted that the high displacement rates of 4,000 mm/s used by these researchers probably exceed the impact velocity from a fall from standing height by about 25% and, moreover, do not account for rate reductions from the compliance of the pelvis and the soft tissue over the greater trochanter. Robinovitch and associates[59] established their high displacement rate by matching the time to peak load and a simulated fall on the hip, which was estimated from pelvis released experiments to be about 30 ms. Weber and associates[62] suggested the different fracture patterns and the increased comminution observed at the highest displacement rate might help explain the weaker correlations with fracture load at high rates. These factors might also help explain the observed increases in energy absorption capacity at the highest displacement rate. In their experiments, Robinovitch and associates[59] observed no significant increase in energy absorption capacity even for a 50-fold increase in displacement rate, nor did they observe different fracture patterns or increased comminution at the higher displacement rate.

Hip Fracture: Disease and Injury

Clinical data from fall surveillance studies in which estimates of fall severity and measures of bone mineral density at the hip were available suggest that both fall severity and bone fragility are important determinants of hip fracture risk. Nevitt and Cummings,[47] for instance, suggested an increased risk of fracture of over 30-fold for a fall involving impact on or near the hip and a twofold increase in risk for each standard deviation decrease in bone density at the hip. Similarly, Greenspan and associates[48] indicated that simply falling to the side raised the risk of fracture sixfold, that increasing the potential energy of the fall by one standard deviation raised the risk threefold, and that a decrease in one standard deviation in the body mass index decreased the risk of fracture about twofold. In comparison to these indices of fall severity, a decrease in one standard deviation in bone mineral density at the hip raised the risk of fracture from a fall by nearly threefold.

Although these odds ratios begin to give a picture of the relative importance of fall severity and bone fragility, a different perspective is provided by estimating the factor of risk for simple falls from standing height. Based on the pelvis-release experiments of Robinovitch and associates,[59] lumping the muscle-relaxed fall impact force estimates for both men and women results in a predicted fall impact force of about 5,600 N. Using the high loading rate data of Courtney and associates[61] results in an in vitro average fracture load for an elderly specimen population of mixed gender of 4,170 N. Based on the definition of the factor of risk (Eq 1), under these conditions $\Phi = 1.35$, ie, the estimated femoral impact forces are about 35% higher than the mean fracture load of the elderly femur. Due to the higher rate of loading, this difference is smaller than the 50% difference reported in previous low-rate experiments.[60] However, either value suggests that a fall with impact directly on the hip is associated with a high risk of hip fracture in the elderly. Given these findings, it is surprising that even in the elderly, only 1% of all falls result in hip fracture.[43] This lower than expected fracture rate is explained in part by experimental and epidemiologic evidence, which shows that both fall characteristics and bone fragility are important determinants of hip fracture risk.

In real falls, some of the energy available can be absorbed by the leg muscles during the descent phase[63] or by use of the outstretched hand to break the fall.[47,49,57,64,65] At impact, the skin and fat over the greater trochanter can absorb energy,[59,66] thereby further reducing the load applied to the hip. Favorable combinations of these factors could, therefore, reduce the load applied to the femur to below the fracture load and, thus, explain the much lower incidence of hip fracture from falls than would be expected by simply calculating a factor risk, Φ.

These results thus confirm previous findings that the average fracture load of the elderly femur is well below the loads that can be expected in a relaxed fall from standing height. Moreover, the relationship between bone mineral density and fracture load indicates that an increase of more than 20% in femoral neck bone mineral density would be required to raise the mean fracture load to the level of the impact loads from a fall on the hip. However, controlled trials of pharmacologic interventions have at best demonstrated increases of only a few percent in femoral neck bone mineral density,[67] especially in the older elderly who are at greatest risk of fracture.[68] For instance, Felson and associates[68] recently showed that in women over the age of 75 who had taken estrogen, bone density was only 3.2% higher than in women who had never taken estrogen. Results from my laboratory therefore emphasize the continuing need for intervention strategies that focus on fall prevention and reductions in fall severity, if major reductions are to be made in hip fracture incidence.

These findings on the etiology of hip fracture also have implications for the design and implementation of fracture-prevention efforts. Because fall impact forces appeared to exceed the strength of the elderly femur by at least 35%, it is unlikely that sufficient protection can be afforded by the use of osteodynamic agents, especially in this elderly population in whom bone density is already well below clinically recommended fracture thresholds. Moreover, because fall-prevention efforts have proven disappointing,[48,58] it seems likely that more productive intervention strategies would involve attempts to reduce the severity of those falls that do occur. Such reductions in fall severity can be accomplished either through passive energy absorption strategies, through the use of trochanteric padding or energy-absorbing floors,[69] or through exercise programs directed toward increasing lower extremity strength and maintaining neuromuscular response mechanisms.[70] Indeed, preliminary results with trochanteric padding systems[71-74] suggest these to be a productive strategy to pursue. Moreover, data from my laboratory indicate that such trochanteric padding systems can be designed so that impact forces are reduced to levels below the fracture threshold for elderly cadaveric femora.[48,75] Based on such approaches and the improving understanding of the complex interplay between fall biomechanics and bone fragility in the etiology of hip fracture, there is hope that the rising epidemic of hip fractures among the elderly can be substantially abated.

References

1. American Academy of Orthopaedic Surgeons: A position statement: Prevention of hip fractures. Rosemont, IL, American Academy of Orthopaedic Surgeons, 1993.
2. Melton LJ III, Riggs BL: Risk factors for injury after a fall. *Clin Geriatr Med* 1985; 1:525–539.
3. Muckle DS, Bentley G, Deane G, et al: Basic science of the hip, in Muckle DS (ed): *Femoral Neck Fractures and Hip Joint Injuries.* New York, NY, John Wiley and Sons, 1978.
4. Tinetti ME: Factors associated with serious injury during falls by ambulatory nursing home residents. *J Am Geriatr Soc* 1987;35:644–648.
5. Hayes WC, Gerhart TN: Biomechanics of bone: Applications for assessment of bone strength, in Peck WA (ed): *Bone and Mineral Research: 3.* Amsterdam, Elsevier Science Publishers, 1985, pp 259–294.

6. Mazess RB: On aging bone loss. *Clin Orthop* 1982;165:239–252.

7. Melton LJ III, Wahner HW, Richelson LS, et al: Osteoporosis and the risk of hip fracture. *Am J Epidemiol* 1986;124:254–261.

8. Riggs BL, Wahner HW, Seeman E, et al: Changes in bone mineral density of the proximal femur and spine with aging: Differences between the postmenopausal and senile osteoporosis syndromes. *J Clin Invest* 1982;70:716–723.

9. Consensus Conference: Osteoporosis. *JAMA* 1984;252:799–802.

10. Aitken JM: Relevance of osteoporosis in women with fracture of the femoral neck. *Br Med J* 1984;288:597–601.

11. Cummings SR: Are patients with hip fractures more osteoporotic? Review of the evidence. *Am J Med* 1985;78:487–494.

12. Evans RA, Ashwell JR, Dunstan CR: Lack of metabolic bone disease in patients with fracture of the femoral neck. *Aust N Z J Med* 1981;11:158–161.

13. Wicks M, Garrett R, Vernon-Roberts B, et al: Absence of metabolic bone disease in the proximal femur in patients with fracture of the femoral neck. *J Bone Joint Surg* 1982;64B:319–322.

14. Bohr H, Schaadt O: Bone mineral content of femoral bone and the lumbar spine measured in women with fracture of the femoral neck by dual photon absorptiometry. *Clin Orthop* 1983;179:240–245.

15. Eriksson SAV, Widhe TL: Bone mass in women with hip fracture. *Acta Orthop Scand* 1988;59:19–23.

16. Riggs BL, Melton LJ III: Involutional osteoporosis. *N Engl J Med* 1986;314:1676–1686.

17. Alho A, Husby T, Hoiseth A: Bone mineral content and mechanical strength: An ex-vivo study of human femora at autopsy. *Clin Orthop* 1988;227:292–297.

18. Dalen N, Hellstrom LG, Jacobson B: Bone mineral content and mechanical strength of the femoral neck. *Acta Orthop Scand* 1976;47:503–508.

19. Esses SI, Lotz JC, Hayes WC: Biomechanical properties of the proximal femur determined in-vitro by single-energy quantitative computed tomography. *J Bone Miner Res* 1989;4:715–722.

20. Leichter I, Margulies JY, Weinreb A, et al: The relationship between bone density, mineral content, and mechanical strength in the femoral neck. *Clin Orthop* 1982;163:272–281.

21. Lotz JC, Hayes WC: The use of quantitative computed tomography to estimate risk of fracture of the hip from falls. *J Bone Joint Surg* 1990;72A:689–700.

22. Phillips JR, Williams JF, Melick RA: Prediction of the strength of the neck of femur from its radiological appearance. *Biomed Eng* 1975;5:367–372.

23. Sartoris DJ, Sommer FG, Marcus R, et al: Bone mineral density in the femoral neck: Quantitative assessment using dual-energy projection radiography. *Am J Roentgenol* 1985;144:605–611.

24. Vose GP, Mack PB: Roentgenologic assessment of femoral neck density as related to fracturing. *Am J Roentgenol* 1963;89:1296–1301.

25. Melton LJ III, Kan SH, Wahner HW, et al: Lifetime fracture risk: An approach to hip fracture risk assessment based on bone mineral density and age. *J Clin Epidemiol* 1988;41:985–994.

26. Mazess RB, Barden H, Ettinger B, et al: Bone density of the radius, spine and proximal femur in osteoporosis. *J Bone Miner Res* 1988;3:13–18.

27. Aloia JF, McGowan D, Erens E, et al: Hip fracture patients have generalized osteopenia with a preferential deficit in the femur. *Osteoporos Int* 1992;2:88–93.

28. Chevalley T, Rizzoli R, Nydegger V, et al: Preferential low bone mineral density of the femoral neck in patients with a recent fracture of the proximal femur. *Osteoporos Int* 1991;1:147–154.

29. Duboeuf F, Braillon P, Chapuy MC, et al: Bone mineral density of the hip measured with dual-energy x-ray absorptiometry in normal elderly women and in patients with hip fracture. *Osteoporos Int* 1991;1:242–249.

30. Libanati CR, Schulz EE, Shook JE, et al: Hip mineral density in females with a recent hip fracture. *J Clin Endocrinol Metab* 1992;74:351–356.

31. Perloff JJ, McDermott MT, Perloff KG, et al: Reduced bone-mineral content is a risk factor for hip fractures. *Orthop Rev* 1991;20:690–698.

32. Vega E, Mautalen C, Gomez H, et al: Bone mineral density in patients with cervical and trochanteric fractures of the proximal femur. *Osteoporos Int* 1991;1:81–86.

33. Melton LJ III, Riggs BL: Hip fracture: A disease and an accident, in Uhthoff HK, Stahl E (eds): *Current Concepts of Bone Fragility*. Berlin, Springer-Verlag, 1986, pp. 385–389.

34. Cummings SR, Nevitt MC: A hypothesis: The causes of hip fracture. *J Gerontol* 1989;44:M107-M111.

35. Alffram PA: An epidemiologic study of cervical and trochanteric fractures of the femur in an urban population: Analysis of 1,664 cases with special reference to etiologic factors. *Acta Orthop Scand Suppl* 1964;65:1–109.

36. Waller JA: Falls among the elderly: Human and environmental factors. *Accid Anal Prev* 1978;10:21–33.

37. Melton LJ III, Chao EYS, Lane J: Biomechanical aspects of fracture, in Riggs BL, Melton LJ (eds): *Osteoporosis: Etiology, Diagnosis and Management*. New York, NY, Raven Press, 1988, pp 111–131.

38. Grisso JA, Kelsey JL, Strom BL, et al: Risk factors for falls as a cause of hip fracture in women: The Northeast Hip Fracture Study Group. *N Engl J Med* 1991;324: 1326–1331.

39. Hedlund R, Lindgren U: Trauma type, age and gender as determinants of hip fracture. *J Orthop Res* 1987;5:242–246.

40. Cummings SR, Rubin SM, Black D: The future of hip fractures in the United States: Numbers, costs, and potential effects of postmenopausal estrogen. *Clin Orthop* 1990;252:163–166.

41. Cummings SR, Black DM, Nevitt MC, et al: Appendicular bone density and age predict hip fracture in women: The Study of Osteoporotic Fractures Research Group. *JAMA* 1990;263:665–668.

42. Gryfe CI, Amies A, Ashley MJ: A longitudinal study of falls in an elderly population: I. Incidence and morbidity. *Age Ageing* 1977;6:201–210.

43. Nevitt MC, Cummings SR, Kidd S, et al: Risk factors for recurrent nonsyncopal falls: A prospective study. *JAMA* 1989;261:2663–2668.

44. Tinetti ME, Speechley M, Ginter SF: Risk factors for falls among elderly persons living in the community. *N Engl J Med* 1988;319:1701–1707.

45. Hindmarsh JJ, Estes EH Jr: Falls in older persons: Causes and interventions. *Arch Intern Med* 1989;149:2217–2222.

46. Hornbrook MC, Wingfield DJ, Stevens VJ, et al: Prevention of falls among the noninstitutionalized elderly: Strategy for assessing outcomes of a randomized trial. Presented at the Annual Meeting of the American Public Health Association, New Orleans, LA, October 1987.

47. Nevitt MC, Cummings SR: Type of fall and risk of hip and wrist fractures: The study of osteoporotic fractures. The study of Osteoporotic Fractures Research Group. *J Am Geriatr Soc* 1993;41:1226–1234.

48. Greenspan SL, Myers ER, Maitland LA, et al: Fall severity and bone mineral density as risk factors for hip fracture in ambulatory elderly. *JAMA* 1994;271:128–133.

49. Campbell AJ, Borrie MJ, Spears GF: Risk factors for falls in a community-based prospective study of people 70 years and older. *J Gerontol* 1989;44:112–117.

50. DeVito CA, Lambert DA, Sattin RW, et al: Fall injuries among the elderly: Community-based surveillance. *J Am Geriatr Soc* 1988;36:1029–1035.

51. Lipsitz LA, Jonsson PV, Kelly MM, et al: Causes and correlates of recurrent falls in ambulatory frail elderly. *J Gerontol* 1991;46:M114-M122.

52. Prudham D, Evans JG: Factors associated with falls in the elderly: A community study. *Age Ageing* 1981;10:141–146.

53. Ray WA, Griffin MR, Schaffner W, et al: Psychotropic drug use and the risk of hip fracture. *N Engl J Med* 1987;316:363–369.

54. Robbins AS, Rubenstein LZ, Josephson KR, et al: Predictors of falls among elderly people: Results of two population-based studies. *Arch Intern Med* 1989;149:1628–1633.

55. Frankel VH, Burstein AH: *Orthopaedic Biomechanics: The Application of Engineering to the Musculoskeletal System.* Philadelphia, PA, Lea & Febiger, 1970.

56. Hayes WC, Myers ER, Morris JN, et al: Impact near the hip dominates fracture risk in elderly nursing home residents who fall. *Calcif Tissue Int* 1993;52:192–198.

57. Cummings SR, Kelsey JL, Nevitt MC, et al: Epidemiology of osteoporosis and osteoporotic fractures. *Epidemiol Rev* 1985;7:178–208.

58. Resnick NM, Greenspan SL: "Senile" osteoporosis reconsidered. *JAMA* 1989;261: 1025–1029.

59. Robinovitch SN, Hayes WC, McMahon TA: Prediction of femoral impact forces in falls on the hip. *J Biomech Eng* 1991;113:366–374.

60. Courtney AC, Wachtel EF, Myers ER, et al: Age-related reductions in the strength of the femur tested in a fall loading configuration. *J Bone Joint Surg,* in press.

61. Courtney AC, Wachtel EF, Myers ER, et al: Effects of loading rate on strength of the proximal femur. *Calcif Tissue Int,* in press.

62. Weber TG, Yang KH, Woo R, et al: Proximal femur strength: Correlation of the rate of loading and bone mineral density, in *Advances in Bioengineering.* New York, NY, The American Society of Mechanical Engineers, 1992, pp 111–114.

63. Van den Kroonenberg A, Munih P, Weigent-Hayes M, et al: Hip impact velocities and body configurations for experimental falls from standing height. *Trans Orthop Res Soc* 1993;18:24.

64. Myers ER, Hecker AT, Rooks DS, et al: Geometric variables from DXA of the radius predict forearm fracture load in vitro. *Calcif Tissue Int* 1993;52:199–204.

65. Myers ER, Sebeny EA, Hecker AT, et al: Correlations between photon absorption properties and failure load of the distal radius in vitro. *Calcif Tissue Int* 1991;49: 292–297.

66. Maitland LA, Myers ER, Hipp JA, et al: Read my hips: Measuring trochanteric soft tissue thickness. *Calcif Tissue Int* 1993;52:85–89.

67. Riggs BL, Melton LJ III: The prevention and treatment of osteoporosis. *N Engl J Med* 1992;327:620–627.

68. Felson DT, Zhang Y, Hannan MT, et al: The effect of postmenopausal estrogen therapy on bone density in elderly women. *N Engl J Med* 1993;329:1141–1146.

69. Streit DA, Casalena J, Cavanagh PR: Preliminary design of a dual-stiffness floor for injury prevention due to falls, in *Proceedings of the 2nd World Conference on Injury Control.* Atlanta, GA, Centers for Disease Control, 1993, p 184.

70. Wolf SL: Exploring novel interventions to reduce falls in older individuals, in Apple DF Jr, Hayes WC (eds): *Prevention of Falls and Hip Fractures in the Elderly.* Rosemont, IL, American Academy of Orthopaedic Surgeons, 1994, pp 119–126.

71. Lauritzen JB, Petersen MM, Lund B: Effect of external hip protectors on hip fractures. *Lancet* 1993;341:11–13.

72. Wallace RB, Ross JE, Huston JC, et al: Iowa FICSIT trial: The feasibility of elderly wearing a hip joint protective garment to reduce hip fracture. *J Am Geriatr Soc* 1993;41:338–340.

73. Sellberg MS, Huston JC, Kruger DH: The development of a passive protective device for the elderly to prevent hip fracture from accidental falls. *Adv Bioeng* 1992; 22:505–508.

74. Huston JC, Sellberg MS, Kundel C, et al: A passive protective device to prevent hip fracture from falls in the elderly, in Apple DF Jr, Hayes WC (eds): *Prevention of Falls and Hip Fractures in the Elderly.* Rosemont, IL, American Academy of Orthopaedic Surgeons, 1994, pp 127–141.

75. Hayes WC, Robinovitch SN, McMahon TA: Energy-shunting hip padding system reduces femoral impact force from a simulated fall to below fracture threshold, in Yang K (ed): *Proceeding of the Third CDC Symposium on Injury Prevention Through Biomechanics.* Detroit, MI, Wayne State University, 1993.

Chapter 35

Current Assessment of Fracture Healing

Charles N. Cornell, MD

The current goals of fracture management are solid skeletal union and complete rehabilitation of the soft tissues and joints of the injured limb. These simultaneous goals are somewhat conflicting because early physical therapy and use of the limb may jeopardize fracture healing, especially in unstable fractures treated by internal fixation. The fracture surgeon needs a method to judge the stage of healing and, thereby, the stiffness and strength of the fracture callus. Armed with this information, the surgeon can effectively advance the stage of physical rehabilitation to maximize outcome. Without such methods, premature, excessive loading of the fracture can lead to failure of healing or unnecessarily prolonged immobilization can lead to severe muscle atrophy and joint stiffness.

This chapter is intended to review the current experimental and clinical methods that are available to assess the extent of fracture healing. These current methods will be contrasted with traditional methods that have assisted simple clinical judgment in the past as well as with more objective technologies that are being developed for future use.

Assessment of Experimental Fracture Healing

In the past decade much has been learned of the biochemistry of fracture healing. As a result, there has been an explosion in the number of studies in which there has been an attempt to manipulate fracture healing by influencing the biochemistry and biophysics of the fracture callus. To prove definitively that such manipulations influence the quality, rate, or extent of healing, very objective and quantitative methods of assessment are needed. Many of the existing classifications of the stages of fracture healing are based on biochemical observations, histologic appearance, roentgenographic criteria, clinical judgment, or some combination thereof.[1,2] These methods have remained qualitative and cannot be used to quantify moderate differences in the rate and extent of fracture healing.[2,3] White and associates[2] have pointed out the importance of biomechanical testing in evaluating fracture healing. This is the crux of the matter. Skeletal tissues must have stiffness and strength to perform their structural function. Although a specific histologic and radiographic appearance may imply a certain stage of healing, no studies to date have conclusively correlated these variables with biomechanical tests of strength or stiffness, the true measure of skeletal healing.[2-5]

The reasons that histologic and radiographic studies of the callus are not definitive monitors of the biomechanical changes in the callus have been suggested by Whiteside and associates.[3] They point out that the final stage of fracture healing, the stage of remodeling of the callus, is the stage in which the greatest biomechanical gain in strength occurs. However, because this healing occurs by internal remodeling of the callus, no detectable biomechanical or radiographic density changes are noted in this stage. Work by Tiedeman and associates[6] has confirmed this. In their studies, quantitative radiographic methods correlate with gains in strength and stiffness only until 50% of the strength and stiffness in the intact bone is reached. These data confirm the principle that all studies involving manipulations of fracture callus must use biomechanical tests of strength and stiffness to assess the effect of such manipulations.

Experimental fractures can be mechanically evaluated by tests of four-point bending and by torsion testing using the methods described by Hayes[7] and by Burstein and Frankel.[8] These tests are easily performed, reproducible, and closely correlated to the stages of fracture healing.[1,2,9] Using the method of Burstein and Frankel[8] allows measurement of several mechanical parameters of the callus including ultimate strength, stiffness, and energy absorption to failure (Fig. 1). These parameters can be quantified and examined as a ratio of a normal contralateral limb permitting valid comparisons between animals. These biomechanical tests have become the standard for evaluating experimental fracture models.[1,2,6,9]

Recently, several authors have begun to quantify more accurately the relationship between noninvasive and biomechanical tests of fracture healing. These methods rely on the relationship between mineral density, which can be measured by photon absorptiometry or radiographic density measures, and developing stiffness at the fracture site. Tiedeman and associates[6] have found a very high correlation between bending rigidity of fractures and radiographic density. These authors point out that the method loses predictive value after the experimental fracture reaches 50% of the rigidity of the contralateral intact

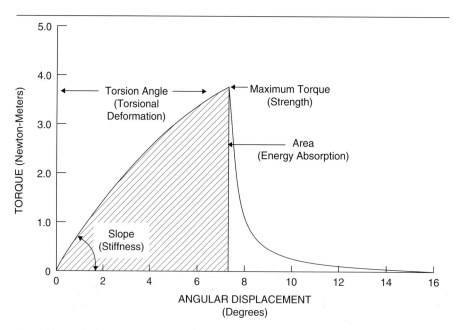

Fig. 1 The typical torque versus angular displacement curve when bone is torsionally tested to failure. Stiffness of the bone is calculated from the slope of the linear portion of the curve. Maximum torque represents strength. The area under the curve represents the energy absorption to failure or fracture toughness.

bone. Furthermore, a gap-healing model is required. Oblique fractures or fractures with internal fixation make assessment more difficult. Aro and associates[10] have found similar results using micro-bone densitometry. In this study, high resolution single photon absorptiometry correlated linearly with ash weight of the fracture callus as well as nonlinearly with fracture hardness. As with the study of Tiedeman and associates,[6] the authors[10] cite the difficulties of using this technique in the clinical setting. Finally, computed tomography (CT) scanning has been explored. Braunstein and associates[11] found it superior to plain radiography in evaluating experimental plated osteotomies in sheep. Although this technique may have considerable promise in the clinical setting, the relationship between the CT scan appearance of a fracture and its biomechanical properties has not been studied. In spite of these advances, the basic test for assessing experimental manipulation of the callus must remain biomechanical testing.

Assessment of Fracture Healing in the Clinical Setting

In the management of fractures of long bones, the physician must decide when the injured limb may assume normal function unsupported by an external support or ambulatory aids. This decision traditionally has been based on criteria such as time elapsed since injury, resolution of pain and tenderness at the fracture site, restoration of local muscle function, radiographic appearance, and the perception of stability at the fracture site during manual testing. The correlation of patient symptoms and limb function with completeness of fracture healing is very poorly understood. Matthews and associates[12] have studied an orthopaedist's ability to sense motion at a fracture site. They have found that experienced surgeons can detect[11,13] degrees of angular deformation with consistency and can use this skill to predict completeness of healing with some accuracy.[4–6,14]

The usefulness of plain radiographics has been evaluated carefully. Most fracture surgeons rely heavily on the radiographic appearance of a fracture without any knowledge of how the appearance and healing correlate. In actuality, routine radiographs probably are the only method available to the clinician if a cast or internal fixation device is in place. Nonetheless, Panjabi and associates[4,5] have shown that plain radiographs are a very poor predictor of healing (Fig. 2). The most important radiographic finding that is predictive of healing is restoration of cortical continuity. Callus area, fracture displacement, and callus thickness do not correlate with strength of healing.[4,5] Luckily, in spite of the fact that radiographs are not predictive, most clinicians underestimate the degree of healing from these studies. CT scanning with multiplanar reconstruction improves the predictive value of radiographs,[15] but would add considerably to the expense of routine fracture care. In the clinical setting, direct measurement of the properties of the healing fracture is possible when external fixators are used. Burny and associates[16] developed considerable experience with these methods and found this technology to be highly predictive of the condition of the callus. In fact, a classification scheme describing eight conditions of healing has been developed from strain gauge data.[16] Clearly, these techniques will become useful if the technology can be made available and affordable on a routine basis.

In the absence of an external fixator, a noninvasive method that could combine physical examination and radiographic testing is mandatory in the clinical setting. Although the traditional methods have served the clinician well, as fracture management becomes more complex, with newer devices for internal

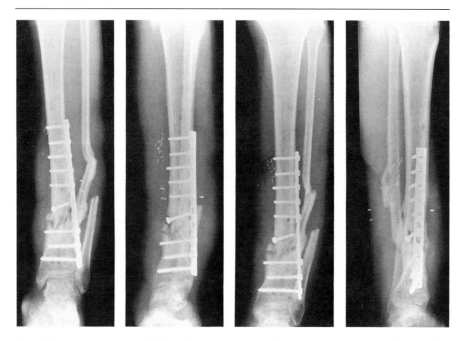

Fig. 2 Plain anteroposterior (**left**), oblique (**center**), and lateral (**right**) views of a slow-healing tibial fracture. Cortical continuity appears established on some views, but not others.

fixation or with callus distraction, more objective methods for assessment of healing will be extremely useful.

Recently, considerable progress has been made in the understanding of vibrational transmission of waves through bone and across fracture sites.[17] This has lead to the development of vibrational analysis and acoustic emission measurements of fracture healing. The principles of acoustic or other wave propagation across fracture sites are complex. Such wave propagation is a material property; defects or fractures alter the transmission of waves in a measurable way. Therefore, a stress wave in bone can be used to measure the progress of healing.

This technology is clearly in its developmental stages, but several investigators have begun to study its usefulness in the clinical setting.[13,17] Benirschke and associates[13] have found that resonant frequency of healing tibial fractures correlates well to flexural rigidity. In this study, the authors[13] used an electronic hammer to provide a "tap" and measured wave propagation across the fracture with an accelerometer (Fig. 3). The measurement of the injured limb could be compared to that of the intact contralateral limb for a prediction of solid healing. Unfortunately, the use of plates, pins, rods, and fixators alters the transmission of waves across the fracture in far more complex ways.[17] Considerable further development of this technology is needed before it becomes practical in the clinical setting.

Summary

Objective assessment of fracture healing needs further development. Traditional methods of assessment, such as manual manipulation and radiographs

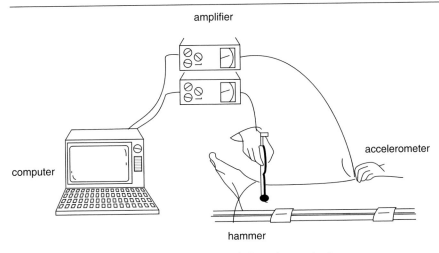

amplifier

computer

accelerometer

hammer

Fig. 3 Schematic diagram of the vibrational analysis testing method.

of the limb, are useful, but as complexity of internal fixation increases or the use of callus distraction methods is introduced, these traditional methods lose accuracy. Use of strain gauges is helpful but requires that pins be implanted into the bone above and below the fracture. Acoustic emission testing and other means of measuring wave propagation across the fracture site is a technology in development that, perhaps, holds the greatest promise for the future.

References

1. Lane JM, Sandhu HS: Current approaches to experimental bone grafting. *Orthop Clin North Am* 1987;18:213–225.
2. White AA III, Panjabi MM, Southwick WO: The four biomechanical stages of fracture repair. *J Bone Joint Surg* 1977;59A:188–192.
3. Whiteside LA, Lesker PA, Sweeney RE: The relationship between the biochemical and mechanical characteristics of callus during radiographically determined stages of fracture healing. *Trans Orthop Res Soc* 1978;3:36.
4. Panjabi MM, Lindsey RW, Walter SD, et al: The clinician's ability to evaluate the strength of healing fractures from plain radiographics. *J Orthop Trauma* 1989;3:29–32.
5. Panjabi MM, Walter SD, Karuda M, et al: Correlations of radiographic analysis of healing fractures with strength: A statistical analysis of experimental osteotomies. *J Orthop Res* 1985;3:212–218.
6. Tiedeman JJ, Lippiello L, Connolly JF, et al: Quantitative roentgenographic densitometry for assessing fracture healing. *Clin Orthop* 1990;253:279–286.
7. Hayes WC: Biomechanics of fracture treatment, in Heppenstall RB (ed): *Fracture Treatment and Healing*. Philadelphia, PA, WB Saunders, 1980, pp 124–172.
8. Burstein AH, Frankel VH: A standard test for laboratory animal bone. *J Biomech* 1971;4:155–158.
9. Einhorn TA, Lane JM, Burstein AH, et al: The healing of segmental bone defects induced by demineralized bone matrix: A radiographic and biomechanical study. *J Bone Joint Surg* 1984;66A:274–279.
10. Aro HT, Wipperman BW, Hodgson SF, et al: Prediction of properties of fracture callus by measurement of mineral density using micro-bone densitometry. *J Bone Joint Surg* 1989;71A:1020–1030.

11. Braunstein EM, Goldstein SA, Ku J, et al: Computed tomography and plain radiography in experimental fracture healing. *Skeletal Radiol* 1986;15:27–31.
12. Matthews LS, Kaufer H, Sonstegard DA: Manual sensing of fracture stability: A biomechanical study. *Acta Orthop Scand* 1974;45:373–381.
13. Benirschke SK, Mirels H, Jones D, et al: The use of resonant frequency measurements for the noninvasive assessment of mechanical stiffness of the healing tibia. *J Orthop Trauma* 1993;7:64–71.
14. Ebraheim NA, Savolaine ER, Patel A, et al: Assessment of tibial fracture union by 35–45° internal oblique radiographs. *J Orthop Trauma* 1991;5:349–350.
15. Kuhlman JE, Fishman EK, Magid D, et al: Fracture nonunion: CT assessment with multiplanar reconstruction. *Radiology* 1988;167:483–488.
16. Burny F, Donkerwalcke M, Baurgois R, et al: Twenty years experience in fracture healing measurement with strain gauges. *Orthopedics* 1984;7:1823–1826.
17. VanderPere G: Non-invasive monitoring of fracture healing. Presented at the 3rd Conference of the International Society for Fracture Repairs. Brussels, September 24–26, 1992.

Chapter 36

Delayed Union, Nonunion, and Synovial Pseudarthrosis

Paul P. Weitzel, BA
John L. Esterhai, Jr, MD

Introduction

Many problems in orthopaedic surgery now have definitive solutions and represent the success that can be achieved with combined basic and clinical research. Such is not the case with delayed unions, nonunions, and synovial pseudarthroses—failures of initial management. The lost wages, psychological, and medical care costs associated with treating patients with nonunions are exorbitant. Despite the improvements in the understanding of fracture repair and treatment techniques as presented in the preceding chapters of this text, delayed unions and nonunions occur all too frequently in our violent society. These occur partly because, in many cases, the precise reason a given patient's fracture did not heal is unknown. This chapter will elucidate a number of the underlying etiologies as well as current and possible future methods available to treat nonunion. Special emphasis is placed on the cellular principles, where known, because it is only through a detailed and improved understanding of events at the cellular and molecular levels that future clinical advances can be made.

Definitions

Delayed union is defined as the failure of a fractured bone to heal in the usual period (2 to 6 months, depending on the bone involved, vasculature, and microenvironment) while maintaining the clinical and radiographic evidence of further potential healing if given additional time.[1-4] Delayed union is a clinical diagnosis. Tenderness and minimal motion are characteristic on physical examination. Bone callus formation and a persistent radiolucency at the fracture site are noted on radiography.

Various definitions exist for nonunion.[1,4-6] We define nonunion as clinical and or radiographic evidence of incomplete healing at least 6 months after injury combined with radiographic evidence that healing will not occur. Radiographic signs include persistent fracture lines accompanied by fracture bone end sclerosis, progressive radiolucency around osteosynthetic biomaterials, hypertrophic callus formation, or atrophic bone resorption (Fig. 1).[1,5,6] The incidence of nonunion varies with the quality of the bone, the bone involved, and the mechanism and energy of the injury. When nonunion sites are stratified by bone, the tibia accounts for 45%; femur 16%; humerus 9%; ulna 7%; radius, carponavicular, and clavicle 5% each.

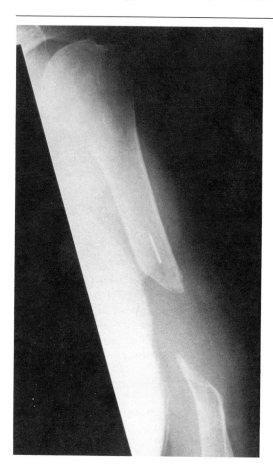

Fig. 1 Radiograph of atrophic non-union of the left humerus of a post-menopausal woman. Note the large nonunion gap, diffuse osteopenia, and atrophic bone ends.

Synovial pseudarthrosis is defined as a nonunion in which a fluid-filled, membrane-lined cavity is present at the site of the fracture (Fig. 2, *left*).[7] Radiographic examination classically reveals a mortar and pestle bone configuration (Fig. 2, *right*). Incidence again varies, with as many as 50% of the nonunions of the humerus complicated by synovial pseudarthrosis.

Classification Systems

Weber and Cech[8] categorized nonunions into hypertrophic/hypervascular and atrophic/avascular by radiographic and histologic appearance. Hypertrophic nonunions show excessive vascularity and callus formation, with the classic horseshoe or elephant foot configurations of the fracture site. Hypertrophic nonunions maintain osteogenic capability but excessive motion at the fracture site inhibits endochondral ossification. Stabilization is the foundation of treatment.

Atrophic nonunions radiographically show little callus formation about the fibrous tissue-filled fracture gap. It is believed that atrophic nonunions are devoid of osteogenic material. Therapy focuses on providing osteoconductive and osteoinductive stimuli as well as stabilization.

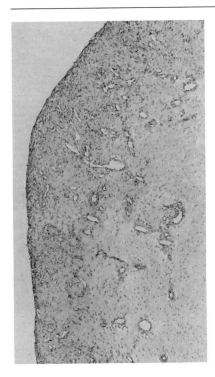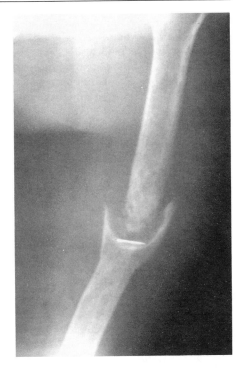

Fig. 2 Left, Photomicrograph of synovial pseudarthrosis (hematoxylin and eosin, × 40). **Right,** Radiograph of synovial pseudarthrosis of the humerus. Note mortar and pestle bone configuration.

Paley and associates[9] classified nonunions on the basis of bone loss, fracture laxity, deformity, and shortening, and used these parameters as a guide for treatment with the Ilizarov device.[9] A type A pseudarthrosis has less than 1 cm of bone loss. Subdivisions include A-1, lax; A-2, stiff; A-2-1, stiff without deformity; and A-2-2, stiff with fixed deformity. Type B nonunions have more than 1 cm of bone loss. Subtypes include B-1, a bony defect; B-2, shortening without a bony defect; B-3, shortening with a bony defect.

Infected nonunions are categorized on the basis of the extent of infection and bony stability. Cierny and associates[10] classified osteomyelitis into four groups based on the local extent of the disease: type I, medullary osteomyelitis due to an endosteal nidus; type II, superficial osteomyelitis most often due to a defect in the soft-tissue envelope; type III, localized osteomyelitis with a well demarcated sequestrum; and type IV, diffuse infection possibly involving an entire bone segment. Types I to IV are further subdivided based on the host's ability to withstand the infection and on morbidity associated with treatment: A, hosts are normal physiologically; B, hosts have either local or systemic compromise to wound and fracture healing; and C, hosts are sufficiently fragile that the risk of treatment outweighs the benefits of cure.[10]

May and associates[11] reviewed and classified posttraumatic osteomyelitis of the tibia, with types III, IV, and V involving nonunions. This classification was based on the size of the tibial bony defect and the condition of the fibula. Patients with a type III tibia have a bony defect of 6 cm or less and an intact fibula. Patients with type IV have a tibial bone defect greater than 6 cm and an intact fibula. Patients with type V have a bone defect of more than 6 cm with no usable, intact fibula. This classification system was designed to guide treatment choices and help predict the duration needed for healing.[11]

Although the classification systems described above all provide therapeutic guidelines for treatment of nonunions of long bones, they fail to define the underlying defect, be it cellular or structural, which has caused the nonunion. In order to prevent delayed union, nonunion, and synovial pseudarthrosis and to improve the success of treatment, with minimal morbidity, these underlying etiologies must be elucidated and addressed.

Etiology

Impaired blood supply constitutes the major injury-related etiology of delayed union, nonunion, and synovial pseudarthrosis. Rhinelander[12] described three vascular supplies integral to fracture repair: the dominant medullary arterial supply, the periosteal arterioles, and the extraosseous blood supply derived from vessels disrupted by the fracture. Immediately after fracture, a newly formed extraosseous vessel network supplies the hematoma and areas of bone stripped of periosteum by the energy of the fracture. The plexus plays a critical role in the inflammatory and reparative phase of healing until the periosteal and medullary arterioles restore the normal centrifugal flow supplying the cortex and newly formed external callus.[13] Delays in restoration of medullary flow due to nutrient artery laceration, segmental or comminuted fractures, destruction by canal reaming, large fracture gaps, excessive motion, and systemic factors can all result in nonunion.

Fractures of the middle and distal thirds of the tibia have an increased incidence of nonunion caused, in part, by the proximal third insertion of the nutrient artery in the tibia.[14] Displaced femoral neck, talar neck, and scaphoid fractures may interrupt the intraosseous supply, leading to subsequent segmental avascular necrosis, and increase the risk of nonunion.[4,14] High-energy, comminuted fracture fragments lose soft-tissue attachments and, thus, blood supply. Canal reaming destroys the intramedullary contents resulting in decreased perfusion to the long bone and fracture site. Vascular ingrowth through the fracture bed occurs only in an environment with minimal shear. Excessive shear may stimulate perifracture angiogenesis, but the vessels will be unable to bridge the gap, creating a hypertrophic/hypervascular nonunion.

Another injury-related factor is the fracture level. Fractures through the diaphysis of long bones take longer to heal, in part, because cortical bone has a smaller surface area and fewer cells per unit area than metaphyseal bone. Conversely, metaphyseal fractures are closer to joints and often are more difficult to immobilize adequately. Both of these anatomic considerations must be assessed by the surgeon to limit the potential for a delayed union or nonunion.

Alignment, reduction, and immobilization are the three factors, which reduce the risk of nonunion, over which the surgeon has the most control (Fig. 3). Bone healing tolerates a wide variety of reductions; however, widely displaced or distracted fractures, or those with interfragmentary soft tissue have a higher incidence of delayed union and nonunion.[4]

Rigid immobilization (ie, a well-placed dynamic compression plate) creates an environment suitable for internal callus formation (direct bone healing) and vascular bridging of the fracture gap, but inhibits external callus formation (indirect bone healing). The time for the fractured bone to return to prefracture strength can be slow because only the fracture ends themselves undergo remodeling to repair the fracture. By comparison, external callus leads to a more

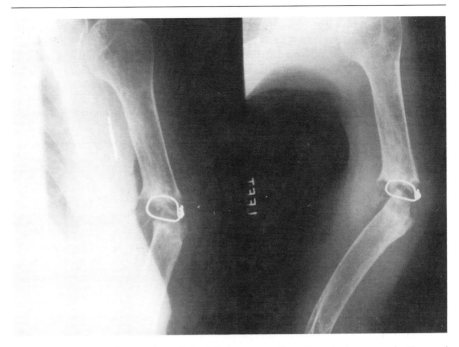

Fig. 3 Radiographs of nonunion of the left humerus after attempted open reduction and internal fixation with inadequate, cerclage wire fixation.

rapid return to normal bone strength because the torsional strength of the bone increases with the cube of the radius.

Orthopaedists continue to debate the optimal rigidity for fracture immobilization. At present, the consensus suggests rigid immobilization with return to physiologic loading and adjacent joint motion as early as possible. Animal models[15] and tissue models[16] have shown that compression (axial micromotion) stimulates osteoblast formation of the external callus of closely apposed bones. The timing of initiation of mechanical stimulation is important. Goodship and associates[17] documented in the ovine model that beginning small displacement, low load, and high rate movement during the first week after osteotomy led to a significant increase in the rate of healing when compared to starting the loading at 6 weeks. Shear and lateral motion do not induce bone formation; instead they stimulate production of disorganized fibrocartilage, which cannot mineralize and ossify due to lack of vascular ingrowth.

Open fractures, high-energy destructive fractures, degloving injuries to the soft tissues, and excessive surgical damage to the periosteum and the soft tissues increase the risk of delayed unions and nonunions.[18] Richards and associates[19] demonstrated in the devascularized canine tibia model that many of the osteogenic cells responsible for fracture repair arose from the periosteum and surrounding soft tissue. Bone union is promoted when dog model osteotomy sites are covered with vascularized muscle instead of skin alone.[20] All efforts in the treatment of fractures of this nature should try to reduce further soft-tissue damage and surround the fracture with as much native vital tissue as possible.

Systemic factors influencing fracture healing include patient age, nutritional status, systemic diseases (diabetes, lupus, and profound anemia), corticosteroid therapy, metabolic bone diseases, tumors, and antineoplastic drugs. In chapter

26, Caplan addresses the decreased number of mesenchymal stem cells present in the bone marrow as a person ages, and in chapter 20, Friedlaender discusses the adverse consequences of therapeutic drugs on fracture healing. To date, no one has evaluated the effects of these phenomena on the polymorphic mesenchymal cells, transformed endothelial cells, and reticular cells described by Brighton and Hunt[21] as possible osteoblast progenitor cells. An additional local factor not already addressed would be local radiation therapy.[22] Every effort to minimize the impact of these factors should be undertaken when treating a fracture.[23]

Infection causes tissue necrosis and inhibits vascular and cellular invasion of the fracture bed which can delay or prevent union (Fig. 4).[24] Evidence points to direct bone degradation by inflammatory cell enzymes. As a response to toxins and bacterial antigens, polymorphonuclear leukocytes and macrophages produce interleukin-1 and prostaglandin E_2, and osteoclastic bone resorption occurs.[25] Proper treatment of the osteomyelitis includes debridement of all necrotic and devitalized tissue; removal of loose, infected hardware; and appropriate antibiotic therapy. Unless the infection is adequately drained, suppressed, or eradicated, efforts to heal the nonunion are wasted.

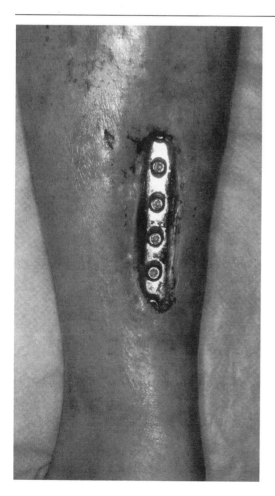

Fig. 4 Photograph of wound dehiscence status after anterolateral dynamic compression plating of distal tibial fracture.

The etiology of a given patient's nonunion is often unclear, especially when there appears to have been adequate fixation. The surgeon must investigate all the possible etiologies and then minimize the influence of each in an effort to stimulate union. From a basic science viewpoint, a nonunion can be approached as a signal failure or a failure of cellular proliferation, differentiation, maturation, migration, mineral deposition, or remodeling. Fortunately for the clinician and his patient, the vast majority of nonunions respond to the present treatment modalities.

Histology

At the light microscopic level, delayed unions appear only slightly different from normally healing fractures. Prominent or even abundant callus formation and interfragmentary fibrous tissue or fibrocartilage that is undergoing slow bony substitution are seen. In nonunions, the interfragmentary cartilage has spread out within the fracture gap, and there is arrest of endochondral ossification. In the adult dog model of Markel and Chao,[26] trabecular bone volume, osteoid surface, and osteoid volume plateaued between 8 and 12 weeks, and osteoblast number increased for 8 weeks and then declined. In hypertrophic nonunions, a vast vascular plexus is seen invading the external callus but not bridging the fracture gap. Atrophic nonunions have disorganized fibrous tissue within the fracture gap.[12] The critical event in nonunion is the cessation of fibrocartilage mineralization, which in turn leads to an inability for vascular invasion across the fracture gap. A synovial pseudarthrosis has cleft-like spaces filled with synovial fluid and lined by papillary projection of cuboidal epithelium at the fracture.[7]

Natural History and Long-Term Course

Without treatment, nonunions will not heal because the underlying etiology has not been addressed. Depending on the level of activity desired by the patient and the bone involved, a person can be reasonably asymptomatic (eg, nonunion of the anterior colliculus of the medial malleolus) or have his or her life devastated by the injury (eg, femoral or tibial nonunion). Given sufficient time and fracture fragment motion, all biomaterials will fail and a synovial pseudarthrosis will form.

Diagnostic Evaluation

A detailed history should include assessment of nutritional status; systemic disease; and fracture history including mechanism, type and duration of treatment, degree of physiologic loading, subsequent motion, and potential presence of infection.

During the physical examination, the patient should be evaluated for signs of infection (fever, chills, diaphoresis, erythema, warmth, swelling, exudate, drainage), instability at the fracture site (motion, crepitus), pain, tenderness, and degree of functional loss (range of joint motion, strength, and weightbearing status).

Serum albumin, total lymphocyte count, and electrolyte values should be checked for indications of nutritional deficiencies. A complete blood cell count with differential is indicated. Some clinicians feel that an erythrocyte sedimentation rate has value.

Radiographs including anteroposterior, lateral, and two oblique views are standard for the evaluation of most long bone nonunions (Fig. 5). Given that some authors define nonunion as radiographic evidence of motion, fluoroscopy and stress views are commonly used in assessing patients whose clinical examination is equivocal.

Detection of acute and chronic infection as well as the presence of a synovial pseudarthrosis affects management, and nuclear medicine provides the best tools to evaluate these areas. Technetium scans have been shown to detect synovial pseudarthrosis with a high sensitivity. The scan will demonstrate a high uptake of the radionuclide at the nonunion site with a "cold" cleft between (Fig. 6).[7] Neither triple phase technetium nor gallium scans have proven useful in differentiating osteomyelitis from soft-tissue infection in the context of nonunion.

Indium 111 white blood cell scans detect acute osteomyelitis with sensitivity reported at 83% to 100%, although they have a somewhat diminished sensitivity for chronic osteomyelitis complicating nonunion.[27] Results of studies using polyclonal IgG suggest similar accuracy with less technical difficulty.

Recent studies have suggested that magnetic resonance imaging (MRI) may be valuable in the evaluation of nonunion because of its ability to accurately assess medullary osteomyelitis and the vascular supply of bones. The most promising study for osteomyelitis detection reports a 100% sensitivity and a 63% specificity.[28] Knowledge of the bone vascularity provides a preoperative indication of bone viability, which affects treatment decisions. One study investigating scaphoid vasculature showed MRI accurately predicted viability in all ten nonunions studied.[29]

Tomography and computed tomography (CT) scans clearly demonstrate fracture lines in situations in which plain radiographs are unable to visualize individual bones (eg, carpus, pelvis) or determine if a gap persists within the abundant callus formation seen with hypertrophic nonunions.

Osteomedullography demonstrates the continuity of the intramedullary veins across the healing fracture site. Radiopaque contrast material is injected into the distal medullary canal and visualized fluoroscopically as it traverses the nonunion. A nonunion is likely if the venous pattern is not reestablished.[30]

Percutaneous or open bone biopsy is indicated in situations of questionable infection, tumor, or systemic disease. Multiple samples should be sent for microbiology and pathology analysis (Fig. 7).

Prevention

Appropriate initial treatment of a fracture, which invokes the principles of restoration of the soft-tissue envelope, reduction, immobilization, and resumption of physiologic loading, provides the best strategy for preventing delayed union and nonunion. In situations of extensive soft-tissue destruction, coverage of the fracture with vascularized muscle must be considered. Furthermore, taking all appropriate measures to minimize the risk of infection will further decrease the potential for nonunion. Opening a closed fracture site surgically increases the infection risk approximately 1% to 2%. Given that traumatic wounds cannot be uniformly and completely sterilized and that adequate reduction, immobilization, and loading are not always possible, nonunions will continue to occur with some degree of regularity.

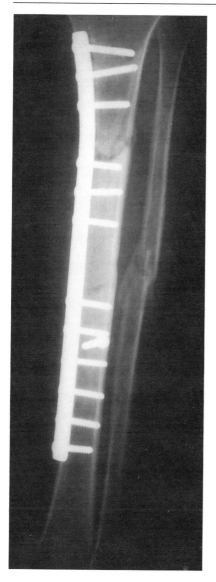

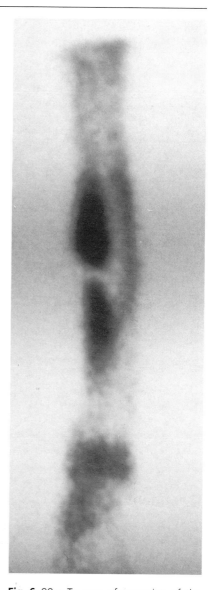

Fig. 5 Radiograph of left tibia 5 months after dynamic compression plating of a segmental fracture. The midshaft fracture has healed. The proximal fracture has not healed, there is no significant bone formation, and there is bone resorption about the most proximal screw. An open bone biopsy after obtaining a positive ^{111}In-labeled leukocyte scan revealed *Staphylococcus aureus* and *Pseudomonas aeruginosa*. (Reproduced with permission from Infection, in Poss R (ed): *Orthopaedic Knowledge Update 3*. Park Ridge, IL, American Academy of Orthopaedic Surgeons, 1990, pp 145–156.)

Fig. 6 99m Tc scan of nonunion of the tibia. Photon deficient (cold) cleft at the synovial pseudarthrosis site.

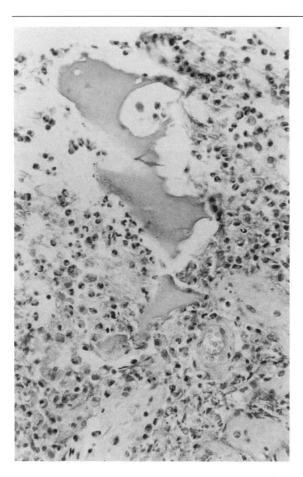

Fig. 7 Photomicrograph of bone biopsy specimen from infected nonunion with necrotic bone and acute inflammatory cell exudate.

Treatment Options

Bone regeneration incorporates three basic mechanisms: osteogenesis, osteoinduction, and osteoconduction. Osteogenesis is the production of bone and cartilage by cells differentiated into osteoblasts and chondrocytes.[31] Osteoinduction is the process of recruitment of mesenchymal-type cells to form cartilage and bone under the influence of a stimulus.[32] Osteoconduction provides a framework that facilitates the migration of cells used for angiogenesis, chondrogenesis, and osteogenesis. Therefore, treatment modalities must function at the cellular level to stimulate osteogenesis through osteoinductive and osteoconductive measures. At the present time, various forms of treatment exist, which overall have excellent union rates with variable morbidity.

Benign Neglect

Depending on the age and functional/physiologic requirements of the patient, some nonunions, such as those involving fractures of the medial malleolus, clavicle, or ulnar styloid, may be left untreated if the patient is asymptomatic. These fractures will not heal with time, but minimal functional loss will be noted by the patient. Other nonunions, such as those of the humerus or greater trochanter, may cause significant limitations, which a patient may choose to tolerate rather than undergo additional surgery (Fig. 8).

Physiologic Loading

Nonunions due to lack of physiologic loading can result from patient noncompliance or the form of fixation creating and maintaining too great a fracture gap. For example, long-bone fractures treated with plates or statically locked intramedullary (IM) rods can have an iatrogenically maintained fracture gap. Mathematical algorithms for simulating bone remodeling in response to mechanical loading have been developed.[33] The deleterious effects of disuse associated with spinal cord injury and bed rest on bone mass[34–36] and the potential to increase bone mass in response to exercise[37–40] have been well described. Treatment would involve dynamization and resumption of physiologic loading.

Stabilization

Persistent motion at the fracture site defines nonunion. Bone healing requires a significant degree of fracture stabilization. Therefore, appropriate stabilization of nonunions must be the foundation of treatment on which other mo-

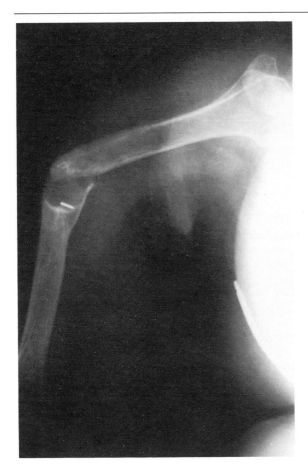

Fig. 8 Radiograph of the right (nondominant) humerus of a woman with a persistent synovial pseudarthrosis after several surgeries, including percutaneous insertion of constant direct current electrodes for electrical stimulation of osteogenesis. The radiograph was obtained during active humerus abduction. The patient opted for continued conservative care with limitation of function rather than accept additional intervention.

dalities can be added. Various forms of stabilization exist: casts, braces, and internal and external fixation.

Casting and bracing are excellent options for initial management of most uncomplicated fractures, but most patients with nonunions have already undergone and failed a trial of casting and bracing. Patients who have not had trials of appropriate stabilization and patients in whom surgery is contraindicated may benefit from casting and bracing. However, most patients with nonunions need more definitive forms of stabilization to promote union.

Internal Fixation

Open reduction, internal fixation (ORIF) presently is the mainstay of treatment for nonunions with and without bone grafting. Some nonunions are perfectly suited for intramedullary nailing, while others can only be treated with a compression plate. This chapter does not provide guidelines for the use of different forms of internal fixation, but rather elucidates the objective of the treatment and the cellular response.

IM Rods IM rods are used effectively in treating humeral, femoral, and, most commonly, tibial nonunions that have failed plating or external immobilization. Debate exists among orthopaedic surgeons on their utility in the presence of infection. Most feel IM rods should be avoided if possible with infected fractures. IM nailing allows immediate partial weightbearing while bringing the fracture ends into closer apposition. To obtain a stable nail configuration in nonunions, canal reaming is recommended. Although this reaming transiently destroys the endosteal blood supply, Rhinelander[12] has shown that blood flow is partially restored in 4 weeks and fully restored in 12 weeks. In the interim period, the periosteal vessels supply the outer third of the cortex. If the medullary canals are sclerosed closed or if an inadequate amount of motion exists at the site of nonunion to allow the surgeon to align the fragments and insert the rod, the fracture site must be opened to guarantee proper alignment and reduction. Osteotomies to provide better alignment and bone-to-bone contact can be indicated. Overall, union after treatment with IM rods has been reported in 94% to 100% of cases.[5,41,42] It must be noted that many of these cases had adjuvant bone grafting.

Plating Plating provides only the environment for bone healing; therefore, many surgeons use bone grafts with plating because of the osteogenic stimulus the bone grafts provide. Overall, treatment of nonunion with plating with or without grafting has been extremely successful, with reported union rates of 92% to 99%.[43]

Dynamic compression plates (DCP) were designed to provide stability while stimulating osteogenic proliferation by axial loading. A DCP allows self-compression axially while maintaining its congruent fit between screw and plate.[44] Union rates have shown to be excellent and comparable to those for compression plating.

Problems with conventional plates include areas of osteoporosis beneath the plate due to stress shielding, compromised periosteal blood flow,[12] infection, lack of axial compression if an iatrogenic gap is maintained by rigid fixation, metal fatigue with resultant plate failure, and screw loosening permitting excessive motion.[44]

Presently investigators are researching the use of flexible resin plates. These plates permit micromotion, which stimulates external callus formation, while maintaining enough rigidity to allow vascular ingrowth through the fracture bed.[45] The resins biomechanically are less prone to fatigue failure than metal, but like metal cause periplate osteoporosis, which some researchers have described as more significant than that seen with metal.[44] The resins are expensive and have limited malleability, which limits their use at this time. Currently, the benefits derived in the treatment of nonunions are not great enough to warrant regular use, but with further research and knowledge these plates could prove beneficial.

Limited contact-dynamic compression plates (LC-DCP) are the latest design available. The plate design incorporates the benefits of dynamic compression plating while affecting periosteal flow less than do regular plates.[44] Given that blood flow is crucial for nonunion healing, this plate might prove a valuable tool when enough clinical experience has been gained. Presently, the plate remains in the clinical investigative stages.

External Fixation

Currently, stabilization with external fixation is the mainstay of treatment for most grade III open fractures, infected fractures, and infected nonunions. External fixation rigidly immobilizes the bony fragments without implanted hardware, minimally disrupts blood flow, and allows access to the soft tissues. Disadvantages include minimal axial loading, pin-tract infection, and the limitation of use to bones in which adequate bone purchase can be obtained.

In the past decade, use of the Ilizarov external fixator has gained popularity in the West. The device has all the characteristics of the traditional external fixator with the added capacity to correct angular deformities and fill in bony defects without the need for bone grafting. The Ilizarov method presently is used for leg lengthening, filling in large segmental bone gaps, correcting angular deformities, and treating uninfected and infected nonunions of long bones.[1] The underlying concept of the Ilizarov method in treatment of nonunions is distraction-compression osteogenesis. If bone lengthening is required, a precisely made subperiosteal corticotomy in the metaphyseal region of the bone is performed, with the surgeon taking care to avoid unnecessary damage to the periosteum, medullary contents, or nutrient artery. This guarantees that the transport segment of bone maintains its periosteal and medullary/nutrient blood supply. The involved bone is divided into three segments by the nonunion and the corticotomy. The bone segments are stabilized and controlled via bicortical cross wires that are attached under tension to external rings. Threaded rods connect the rings and are used to move individual rings with attached bone towards other rings in a longitudinal manner.

A 5- to 7-day latency period after corticotomy allows preliminary callus formation before bone transportation commences. The bone segment is then transported at a rate of 1 mm per day towards the nonunion, reducing the gap. Bone forms at the lengthening corticotomy site by direct membranous ossification. When the transported bone segment reaches the other bone fragment, compression is applied via the device thereby stimulating union.

For hypertrophic nonunions, union occurs secondary to stabilization induced enchondral ossification. Atrophic nonunions often unite because the corticotomy increases regional blood flow by more then 200%.[9] Additional, optional technical stimuli include percutaneous decortication of the nonunion by drilling or opening the medullary canal and modifying the fracture fragments to provide an improved degree of internal stability.[9]

For infected nonunions, wide debridement of infected dead bone, infected soft tissue, and sinus tracts are prerequisites for further treatment of the nonunion. After debridement and resection, the infected nonunion can be treated as a nonunion with a segmental bone gap.

The Ilizarov device provides the surgeon with a proven method for lengthening bone without the morbidity of cancellous or cortical bone harvest. In infected nonunions in which bone grafts are ill-advised because of the potential for recurrent infection, the Ilizarov device allows the surgeon to more radically debride the infected bone, anticipating that the limb length can be restored.[46] Union rates of 74% to 100%[9,10] have been reported, which prove that the efficacy of the device is comparable to internal and external fixation. Side effects associated with use of the device include pin infection, lengthy treatment, iatrogenic neuropathies, soft-tissue contractures, cutaneous scarring, and pain.

Bone Grafting: Osteoconduction, Osteogenesis, and Osteoinduction

It has been known for more than a century that transplanted bone segments could survive, grow, and even stimulate additional bone formation. The biologic principles for these characteristics are being clearly defined as presented in the earlier chapters of this book. Biologic bone graft placed at the site of a nonunion can function via three separate mechanisms: osteogenesis, osteoconduction, and osteoinduction. Currently, only two sources of biologic bone graft are widely used: autograft and allograft. Xenograft bone is no longer used because it elicits a hypersensitive immunologic response. The various forms of bone graft available today are fresh or frozen autograft and frozen, freeze-dried, demineralized, or AAA (autolyzed, antigen-extracted, allogeneic) allograft. These grafts can be cancellous or cortical bone.

Only fresh autografts contribute viable cells for graft-derived osteogenesis. The vast majority of fresh autograft cells perish, but a portion survive by receiving flow via microanastomoses. These surviving cells join the local host cells in bone formation. A higher proportion of cells survive in cancellous bone autograft than in cortical bone due to increased surface area. Recipient fracture fragment osteogenesis probably occurs with all grafts that have osteoconductive and osteoinductive properties.

All grafts, biologic and nonbiologic, function as osteoconductive materials. The three-dimensional composition of mineralized collagen matrix provides an infrastructure on which the local host's capillaries, osteogenic cells, and supporting tissue can grow. These materials are discussed in the section of this chapter on the bone morphogenetic protein (BMP) delivery system.

The primary benefit of bone grafting is osteoinduction. The osteoinductive ability of bone was first noted more than a century ago when Senn[47] reported rapid ossification in bone cavities filled with hydrochloric acid treated decalcified bone. Yet it was not until 1965, when Urist[48] demonstrated bone formation induced by demineralized matrices in rabbits, mice, rats, and guinea pigs, that the osteoinductive capacity of demineralized matrix was proven. In 1979 Urist and associates[49] isolated a hydrophobic, low-molecular-weight protein from rabbit bone matrix, which induced bone formation in rabbit and rat muscle, and called it BMP. The cells targeted by BMP are believed to be the undifferentiated perivascular mesenchymal-type cells in the host bone bed.[50] These cells, under the influence of BMP, will differentiate and form bone and cartilage, thereby healing the fracture.

Cancellous and cortical bone grafts differ in their mechanical properties and incorporation into the host bone bed. Cancellous bone has little inherent strength and serves primarily as an inductor and conductor of bone formation. Cortical bone has tensile and compression strength and is useful where bone stability is desired.

In terms of incorporation, cortical and cancellous bone act identically in the first 2 weeks postimplant. Initially, a hematoma surrounds the implant, with vascular buds soon invading the graft. By the second week, osteoclastic activity, formation of granulation tissue, and donor osteocyte autolysis predominate. Small-volume cancellous bone grafts become revascularized. Creeping substitution and repair by differentiated mesenchymal cells begin. Osteoblasts begin to deposit osteoid onto the devitalized trabecular scaffolding. In the next several months, the newly formed bone will slowly gain strength and begin to be remodeled.

Cortical bone grafts, which initially were structurally strong, undergo osteoclastic resorption, which weakens them to 50% of initial strength by 6 months, depending on the size of the implant.[32] After approximately 6 months, appositional bone growth begins to predominate and returns the bone slowly to its initial strength. Patients treated with cortical bone grafts typically are at risk for fatigue fractures because of the mechanism of incorporation.

Cancellous bone grafting in conjunction with internal and external fixation has been the standard form of treatment of nonunions, with excellent union rates of 90% to 95%. Cortical bone grafts are used with segmental bone defects and in other situations in which the surgeon desires a stability component within the graft material. Bone grafts, however, are limited by a number of factors. First, bone grafting is relatively contraindicated in infected nonunions because the devitalized donor bone can serve as a nidus for recurrent infection. Second, in patients who have already undergone several bone grafting procedures, more autogenous cancellous bone may not be available. Third, there can be significant morbidity at the cancellous bone donor site. In a retrospective review of 243 bone graft procedures in 239 patients, Younger and Chapman[51] revealed that major complications occurred in 8.6% of the procedures and minor complications developed in 20.6%. It is for these reasons that one of the major areas of research in orthopaedics today is the development of a bone grafting material with the characteristics of fresh autogenous cancellous/cortical bone, but without the morbidity of a harvesting procedure.

In contradistinction to cancellous autografts, cortical bone allografts can provide significant initial structural strength, appropriate shape and size to match the host defect, and the potential for being osteoinductive. Antibody- and cell-mediated rejection phenomena develop, but the precise target for this remains unclear. Incorporation depends on the host response, immunogenicity of the graft, adequacy of internal fixation, and the mechanical stressing of the graft.[52]

Bone-Marrow Injection

Bone marrow injection incorporates the osteoinductive properties of bone grafting with a lower harvest site morbidity. Bone marrow is obtained via percutaneous iliac crest aspiration. The sample is immediately injected percutaneously into the fracture site with radiographic guidance. This method has been successfully studied in canine nonunion models[53] and in ten patients with delayed union.[54] Union was reported with nine patients. The potential for this method is great, given the low morbidity. Larger studies are warranted to determine the utility of bone marrow injections in nonunion.

BMP

Since the potential use of BMP in fracture healing was first discovered by Urist and associates,[49] two separate but closely related avenues of research have been followed: (1) biochemical investigation into the characteristics, mechanisms of action, and effects of BMP on various cells and tissues; and (2) clinical investigation of BMP incorporated into a delivery system and its ability to induce bone formation. The substance that originally was termed BMP in 1979 has now been shown to consist of at least seven glycoproteins ranging in molecular weight from 17,000 to 20,000 d, with four having been shown to induce bone formation. Those that have been isolated, purified, and synthesized appear to share a characteristic 15,000-d dimer protein chain. Furthermore, it is now believed that BMP is a member of the transforming growth factor-beta (TGF-β) superfamily.

BMP has been isolated from human and animal bone, dentin, and osteosarcoma tissue.[55] It takes nearly 1 kg of wet bone to synthesize 1 mg of BMP[56] and tens to hundreds of milligrams are required to treat bony defects and nonunions.[57] With the genome for BMP characterized and recombinant synthesis a reality, the issue of quantity of product will no longer be a problem. Its effect at the cellular level has been clearly demonstrated. Bioassays of BMP have shown cartilage differentiation at day 7, woven bone at day 14, and lamellar bone and marrow at 21 days.[58] The biologic effects can be summarized as the ability to recruit, differentiate, mature, and proliferate preosteogenetic cells. Biomechanically, the strength, energy absorption, and angular displacement of BMP-induced bone are comparable to that of normal developing bone.[31,59] These induction characteristics make BMP a superb tool for use in the treatment of nonunions because the host cells at the site of a nonunion maintain their osteogenetic abilities and begin to mineralize fibrocartilage as soon as the environment and osteoinduction signals are appropriate.[1]

BMP Delivery System

BMP implanted alone will disperse from the field and induce minimal local bone formation. An ideal delivery system should (1) deliver a localized sustained release of BMP over time; (2) have a composition and structure similar to that of bone; (3) be adequately porous to permit bonding with the host bone bed; (4) be osteoconductive; (5) lack immunogenicity; and (6) be biodegradable as bone forms and remodeling occurs.[60,61] Delivery systems under investigation are osteoconductive compounds and include AAA (autolyzed, antigen-free, allogenic) alloimplants, true bone ceramic (TBC), hydroxyapatite (HA), B-tricalcium phosphate (B-TCP), collagen, fibrin, and polylactic and polyglycolic acid based materials. It is important to note that BMP and a delivery system alone cannot treat a delayed union or nonunion, but require immobilization in the form of internal or external fixation.

BMP-AAA alloimplants have been shown in human and baboon trials to promote bony union;[50,62] these alloimplants provide structural stability until union, by means of incorporation into the host tissue, has been accomplished without inducing a foreign body reaction. In 1992, Johnson and associates[50] reported 24 of 25 patients with resistant nonunions healed when treated with BMP-AAA and internal or external fixation. Seven patients received additional cancellous bone grafting. Radiographs at 8 weeks showed an augmented host bone bed response indicating an additive effect of BMP with internal fixation. Johnson and associates[50] noted that the precise influence of BMP-AAA was difficult to assess because so many patients do well with fixation alone.

TBC, HA, and B-TCP are all porous ceramic matrices that provide an osteoconductive framework to the host bone bed. Experimentally it has been shown that the optimal pore diameter for incorporation of implanted materials is 100 to 400 μm.[63,64] All these materials have pore diameters within this range.

TBC is formed by delipidized, deproteinated cancellous bone sintered at 1100° and formed into a cylindrical matrix. Only animal studies have been undertaken with BMP-TBC. The implant is an osteoconductive, biodegradable, nonimmunogenic, noncytotoxic compound with a framework similar to that of cancellous bone with varying pore sizes.[60] Katoh and associates[60] recently reported on a rabbit model used to compare BMP-TBC and TBC implanted in iatrogenic bony defects in femoral condyles. The results revealed greater and faster bone growth with BMP-TBC than with TBC alone. The authors suggest that BMP-TBC provides a more favorable environment for bone formation than BMP-HA and BMP-TCP in promoting adhesion, proliferation, and differentiation of osteoprogenitor cells.[60] Future areas of investigation include determining whether the nonimmunogenetic and noncytotoxic characteristics apply to humans and whether a BMP-TBC compound has properties that make it useful for treatment of nonunions.

HA and B-TCP are nonimmunogenic, osteoconductive, synthetic bioceramics. HA is nonbiodegradable, whereas B-TCP is biodegradable and replaced by new bone over time. Structurally, these materials can be synthesized with pore sizes from 50 to 600 μm. Mechanically, HA and B-TCP are brittle and have low impact resistance and low tensile strength,[31,64] which limit their usefulness if structural strength is required. BMP-HA and BMP-TCP have been evaluated in various animals models[63,65,66] with favorable results. Limitations are posed by surrounding tissue affinity, mechanical characteristics, and delayed resorption of material. Areas of investigation, as with TBC, need to focus on biocompatability of BMP-HA/TCP in humans and applicability to orthopaedic problems and nonunions in particular.

Because collagen constitutes the majority of demineralized bone matrix, efforts to use collagen as a BMP delivery system are logical. Initial animal studies revealed an immunogenic response to the implants and inconsistent amounts of bone formation. Recent studies in which antigen-depleted collagen was used in an attempt to eliminate the immunologic reaction have shown initial success,[61] but further investigation is required.

Human fibrin is a biodegradable organic compound derived from human plasma; it has relatively little antigenicity and hemostatic and osteoconductive characteristics.[67] Initial studies in mice suggest that fibrin functions not only as a delivery system but also as a hemostatic with immunochemical properties as well. Presently, fibrin preparations are difficult to produce, but further investigation is warranted to determine if fibrin could be used to function as a carrier for BMP. This is the only implant being investigated today that has characteristics other than osteoconduction, which are beneficial to the patient.

Polylactic and polyglycolic acid polymers (PLA/PGA) are osteoconductive, biodegradable synthetic homopolymers that have been studied in human patients[68] and animal models.[69] BMP-PLA/PGA implants have been shown to induce bone formation without eliciting foreign body reactions if the polymer has a low molecular weight. Miyamoto and associates[69] showed in the mouse model that only PLA650 had no foreign body reaction and induced bone formation. Higher molecular weight compounds caused no bone formation, but caused foreign body reactions, chronic inflammation, or tissue necrosis, which was attributed to the high molecular weight materials being slowly biodegraded. Further investigation is warranted into the low molecular weight polymers as BMP carriers. The perfect delivery system for BMP remains to be determined, and it is hoped that further investigation into the compounds discussed will provide the clinician with a valuable tool for treating delayed unions, nonunions, and segmental bone defects. A double-blind study of fixation with a BMP delivery system versus fixation with bone graft and fixation alone must be undertaken to prove the efficacy of BMP, for which there currently is only strong circumstantial evidence. Until this type of study is undertaken, the precise benefits of BMP cannot be accurately analyzed.

Other Forms of Osteoinduction

The complex process of bone formation is regulated by hormones and local growth factors. Many investigators are examining whether exposing delayed unions and nonunions to these substances could stimulate union. Systemic growth factors including platelet-derived growth factor, insulin-like growth factor (somatomedins), and local growth factors, including bone-derived growth factor, cartilage-derived growth factor, and angiogenic factors have all been shown to increase DNA, collagen matrix synthesis, and cell replication in vitro. Efforts to use these factors clinically remain in the investigative phase.

Prostaglandins, specifically PGE_2, stimulate DNA and collagen synthesis in vitro and in vivo[70] at low concentrations. At high concentrations, PGE_2, like other prostaglandins, has been shown to have an inhibitory effect on collagen and bone formation.[70] This remains an area of intensive examination and only time will tell if injection of prostaglandins will enter the clinical arena.

Vascularized Grafts

With the rapid improvement in microvascular techniques in recent years, more surgeons are looking at vascularized bone grafts as methods of treating infected nonunions and nonunions with segmental bone defects. Vascularized grafts maintain their viability, strength, and osteogenic capacity when transplanted to the recipient site.

Han and associates[71] evaluated 160 patients treated with vascularized fibular or iliac grafts. Of the 60 patients with infected nonunions, 48% had initial union with an overall union rate of 77% after another procedure. Twenty-five patients with segmental bone defects had initial union rates of 76%, with an overall union rate of 92% after a second procedure. Zaidemberg and associates[72] reported that, of ten patients with scaphoid nonunion treated with a vascularized distal radius transplant, nine had union (average, 7 weeks) and seven had complete resolution of symptoms. The complications of vascularized bone grafts include stress fractures, recurrent infection, neuropathies, soft-tissue adhesions, malunion, and the morbidity of harvesting. The benefits are great but the surgery is tedious, and there can be a high degree of donor-site morbidity.

Electrical Stimulation

Electrical stimulation (ES) has been available to the orthopaedic surgeon for treatment of delayed unions and nonunions since the early 1970s. Various authors have reported union rates with ES of 75%, which is comparable to cancellous bone grafting alone, but less than the 90% reported with IM rodding.[73,74] Yet in 1993, fewer than one in five nonunions is treated with electrical stimulation.[74] Perhaps, a lack of understanding of the biologic principles of ES and the success of surgical methods have kept surgeons from using ES.

Currently, three forms of ES are available for treatment of nonunion: inductive coupling (IC), direct current (DC), and capacitive coupling (CC). The biologic principle of ES is based on the observation that mechanically stressed bone cells elicit a measurable electrical field, which is believed to mediate bone cell proliferation. Exogenous ES strives to stimulate bone proliferation by mimicking the electrical stimulus of mechanical stress. The mechanism of action at the cell membrane level remains unknown. One theory suggests that calcium channels are opened.[75] Evaluation of the various forms of ES, therefore, focuses on the cellular and tissue-level effects of ES. Cellular parameters include alkaline phosphatase levels to measure bone proliferation, radiolabeled isotope uptake to evaluate DNA and RNA synthesis, and bone cell proliferation. At the tissue level, histologic examination, fracture biomechanical characteristics, and radiographic appearance are studied.

Current research has two predominate foci: trying to ascertain in animal models and in vitro the dose-response parameters for bone cell stimulation,[76,77] and determining the clinical indications for ES. ES alone is not indicated in the clinical setting of angular deformities, synovial pseudarthrosis, and segmental bone defects. It is used as adjuvant therapy for synovial pseudarthroses, osteoporosis-complicated nonunions, and recalcitrant nonunions treated with ORIF, with or without bone grafting. Two of the most important factors in the use of ES are patient compliance and initiation of therapy before complications develop.[75] The efficacy of treatment with ES decreases once complications such as infection, osteoporosis, and excessive motion at the fracture site become apparent.

The benefits of ES include low cost, reduced morbidity, no need for hospitalization, and encouragement of functional weightbearing during therapy.[78] The devices can be placed and monitored in the physician's office. Although nonweightbearing ambulation had been required when direct current electrodes were inserted into lower extremity nonunions, patients receiving CC or IC are encouraged to load their limbs. The limitations of electrical stimulation are long treatment periods (3 to 6 months), long periods of immobilization, and a reduced union rate as compared with ORIF. The benefits are significant and in select patients outweigh the limitations.

Low Intensity Ultrasound

The effects of nonthermal pulsed ultrasound on fresh fracture and nonunion repair have been reported. It is believed that ultrasound can affect ionic permeability and second messenger activity. In the animal model, healing with stimulation at 17 days equalled controls at 28 days. Treated fractures healed approximately twice as fast as controls.[79] Low intensity pulsed ultrasound may be useful for healing nonunion fractures.

Psychological Impact of Nonunions

Multiple surgeries, long periods of immobilization, and repeated hospitalizations may be necessary to treat the nonunion but, traditionally, little attention has been directed to treating the patient's psyche.[80] Patients experience depression, narcotic addiction, maladaptive behavior, and altered sexuality as a result of orthopaedic problems that require prolonged care.[81] It is imperative that the orthopaedic surgeon treat the patient as a whole person and not focus only on fracture management. The surgeon must be prepared to discuss treatment options with the patient and involve the patient in decision making. A multidisciplinary team, including specialists in infectious diseases, nursing, orthopaedics, pharmacology, psychology, and rehabilitation, is required to achieve the optimal result.

Conclusion

Delayed union and nonunion fractures remain a challenge for the orthopaedic surgeon and the patient. The surgeon must accurately determine what cellular mechanisms are inhibited and take appropriate therapeutic measures to create an environment in which the bone can heal. The patient must be integrally involved in the treatment process.

References

1. Browner BD, Jupiter JB, Levine AM, et al (eds): *Skeletal Trauma: Fractures, Dislocations, and Ligamentous Injuries.* Philadelphia, PA, WB Saunders, 1992.
2. Rosen H: Fracture healing and pseudarthrosis, in Taveras JM (ed): *Radiology: Diagnosis-Imaging-Intervention.* Philadelphia, PA, JB Lippincott, 1986, vol 5.
3. Rosen H: Treatment of nonunions: General principles, in Chapman MW (ed): *Operative Orthopaedics.* Philadelphia, PA, JB Lippincott, 1988, vol 1, pp 489–507.
4. Cohen J, Bonfiglio M, Campbell CJ: *Orthopaedic Pathophysiology in Diagnosis and Treatment.* New York, NY, Churchill Livingston, 1990, pp 160–178.
5. Johnson KD: Management of malunion and nonunion of the tibia. *Orthop Clin North Am* 1987;18:157–171.
6. Connolly JF: Selection, evaluation and indications for electrical stimulation of ununited fractures. *Clin Orthop* 1981;161:39–53.
7. Esterhai JL Jr, Brighton CT, Heppenstall RB, et al: Detection of synovial pseudarthrosis by 99mTc scintigraphy: Application to treatment of traumatic nonunion with constant direct current. *Clin Orthop* 1981;161:15–23.
8. Weber BG, Cech O (eds): *Pseudarthrosis: Pathophysiology, Biomechanics, Therapy, Results.* Berne, Switzerland, Hans Huber Medical Publisher, 1976.
9. Paley D, Catagni MA, Argnani F, et al: Ilizarov treament of tibial nonunions with bone loss. *Clin Orthop* 1989;241:146–165.
10. Cierny G, Mader JT, Penninck JJ: A clinical staging system for adult osteomyelitis. *Contemp Orthop* 1985;10(5):17–37.
11. May JW Jr, Jupiter JB, Weiland AJ, et al: Clinical classification of post-traumatic tibial osteomyelitis. *J Bone Joint Surg* 1989;71A:1422–1428.
12. Rhinelander FW: Tibial blood supply in relation to fracture healing. *Clin Orthop* 1974;105:34–81.
13. Rhinelander FW: The normal microcirculation of diaphyseal cortex and its response to fracture. *J Bone Joint Surg* 1968;50A:785–800.
14. Nagel A: The clinical significance of the nutrient artery. *Orthop Rev* 1993;22:557–561.
15. Goodship AE, Kenwright J: The influence of induced micromovement upon the healing of experimental tibial fractures. *J Bone Joint Surg* 1985;67B:650–655.
16. Brighton CT, Strafford B, Gross S, et al: The proliferative and synthetic response of isolated calvarial bone cells of rats to cyclical biaxial mechanical strain. *J Bone Joint Surg* 1991;73A:320–331.
17. Goodship AE, Adams MA, Kenwright J: The influence of mechanical stimulation on different stages of fracture healing. *Trans Orthop Res Soc* 1989;14:592.
18. Hulth A: Current concepts of fracture healing. *Clin Orthop* 1989;249:265–284.

19. Richards RR, Orsini EC, Mahoney JL, et al: The influence of muscle flap coverage on the repair of devascularized tibial cortex: An experimental investigation in the dog. *Plast Reconstr Surg* 1987;79:946–958.

20. Richards RR, McKee MD, Paitich CB, et al: A comparison of the effects of skin coverage and muscle flap coverage on the early strength of union at the site of osteotomy after devascularization of a segment of canine tibia. *J Bone Joint Surg* 1991;73A:1323–1330.

21. Brighton CT, Hunt RM: Early histologic and ultrastructural changes in medullary fracture callus. *J Bone Joint Surg* 1991;73A:832–847.

22. Widmann RF, Pelker RR, Friedlaender GE, et al: Effects of prefracture irradiation on the biomechanical parameters of fracture healing. *J Orthop Res* 1993;11:422–428.

23. Frost HM: The biology of fracture healing: An overview for clinicians. Part I. *Clin Orthop* 1989;248:283–293.

24. Webb LX: Biomaterial implant based infection. *Complic Orthop* 1993;8:55–60.

25. Gillespie WJ, Allardyce RA: Mechanisms of bone degradation in infection: A review of current hypotheses. *Orthopedics* 1990;13:407–410.

26. Markel MD, Chao EYS: Gap histomorphometic, material and structural changes in a canine delayed fracture healing model. *Trans Orthop Res Soc* 1991;16:115.

27. Schauwecker DS, Park HM, Mock BH, et al: Evaluation of complicating osteomyelitis with Tc-99m MDP, In-111 granulocytes, and GA-67 citrate. *J Nucl Med* 1984;25:849–853.

28. Mason MD, Zlatkin MB, Esterhai JL Jr, et al: Chronic complicated osteomyelitis of the lower extremity: Evaluation with MR imaging. *Radiology* 1989;173:355–359.

29. Perlik PC, Guilford WB: Magnetic resonance imaging to assess vascularity of scaphoid nonunions. *J Hand Surg* 1991;16A:479–484.

30. Puranen J, Punto L: Osteomedulloangiography: A method of estimating the consolidation prognosis of tibial shaft fractures. *Clin Orthop* 1981;161:8–14.

31. Lane JM, Sandhu HS: Current approaches to experimental bone grafting. *Orthop Clin North Am* 1987;18:213–225.

32. Prolo DJ, Rodrigo JJ: Contemporary bone grafting physiology and surgery. *Clin Orthop* 1985;200:322–342.

33. Nauenberg T, Bouxsein ML, Mikic B, et al: Using clinical data to improve computational bone remodeling theory. *Trans Orthop Res Soc* 1993;18:123.

34. Biering-Sorensen F, Bohr HH, Schaadt OP: Longitudinal study of bone mineral content in the lumbar spine, the forearm and the lower extremities after spinal cord injury. *Eur J Clin Invest* 1990;20:330–335.

35. Krolner B, Toft B: Vertebral bone loss: An unheeded side effect of therapeutic bed rest. *Clin Sci* 1983;64:537–540.

36. Donaldson CL, Hulley SB, Vogel JM, et al: Effect of prolonged bed rest on bone mineral. *Metabolism* 1970;19:1071–1084.

37. Margulies JY, Simkin A, Leichter I, et al: Effect of intense physical activity on the bone-mineral content in the lower limbs of young adults. *J Bone Joint Surg* 1986;68A:1090–1093.

38. Leichter I, Simkin A, Margulies JY, et al: Gain in mass density of bone following strenuous physical activity. *J Orthop Res* 1989;7:86–90.

39. Dalsky GP, Stocke KS, Ehsani AA, et al: Weight-bearing exercise training and lumbar bone mineral content in postmenopausal women. *Ann Intern Med* 1988;108:824–828.

40. Snow-Harter C, Bouxsein ML, Lewis BT, et al: Effects of resistance and endurance exercise on bone mineral status of young women: A randomized exercise intervention trial. *J Bone Miner Res* 1992;7:761–769.

41. Bone LB, Johnson KD: Treatment of tibial fractures by reaming and intramedullary nailing. *J Bone Joint Surg* 1986;68A:877–887.

42. Zickel RE : Nonunions of fractures of the proximal and distal thirds of the shaft of the femur, in Bassett FH III (ed): *Instructional Course Lectures XXXVII*. Park Ridge, IL American Academy of Orthopaedic Surgeons, 1988, pp 173–179.

43. Wiss DA, Johnson DL, Miao M: Compression plating for nonunion after failed external fixation of open tibial fractures. *J Bone Joint Surg* 1992;74A:1279–1285.

44. Perren SM: The concept of biological plating using the limited contact-dynamic compression plate (LC-DCP): Scientific background, design, and application. *Injury* 1991;22(suppl 1):1–41.

45. Pemberton DJ, McKibbin B, Savage R, et al: Carbon-fibre reinforced plates for problem fractures. *J Bone Joint Surg* 1992;74B:88–92.

46. Ehrnberg A, DePablos J, Martinez-Lotti G, et al: Comparison of demineralized allogeneic bone matrix grafting (the Urist procedure) and the Ilizarov procedure in large diaphyseal defects in sheep. *J Orthop Res* 1993;11:438–447.

47. Senn N: On the healing of aseptic bone cavities by implantation of antiseptic decalcified bone. *Am J Med Sci* 1889;98:219–243.

48. Urist MR: Bone formation by autoinduction. *Science* 1965;150:893–899.

49. Urist MR, Mikulski A, Lietze A: Solubilized and insolubilized bone morphogenetic protein. *Proc Natl Acad Sci USA* 1979;76:1828–1832.

50. Johnson EE, Urist MR, Finerman GAM: Resistant nonunions and partial or complete segmental defects of long bones: Treatment with implants of a composite human bone morphogenetic protein (BMP) and autolyzed, antigen-extracted, allogeneic (AAA) bone. *Clin Orthop* 1992;277:229–237.

51. Younger EM, Chapman MW: Morbidity at bone graft donor sites. *J Orthop Trauma* 1989;3:192–195.

52. Stevenson S, Horowitz M: The response to bone allografts. *J Bone Joint Surg* 1992;74A:939–950.

53. Tiedeman JJ, Connolly JF, Strates BS, et al: Treatment of nonunion by percutaneous injection of bone marrow and demineralized bone matrix: An experimental study in dogs. *Clin Orthop* 1991;268:294–302.

54. Connolly JF, Guse R, Tiedeman J, et al: Autologous marrow injection for delayed unions of the tibia: A preliminary report. *J Orthop Trauma* 1989;3:276–282.

55. Nogami H, Ono Y, Oohira A: Bioassay of chondrocyte differentiation by bone morphogenetic protein. *Clin Orthop* 1990;258:295–299.

56. Urist MR, Kovacs S, Yates KA: Regeneration of an enchondroma defect under the influence of an implant of human bone morphogenetic protein. *J Hand Surg* 1986;11A:417–419.

57. Sato K, Urist MR: Induced regeneration of calvaria by bone morphogenetic protein (BMP) in dogs. *Clin Orthop* 1985;197:301–311.

58. Urist MR: New bone formation induced in post fetal life by bone morphogenetic protein, in Becker RO (ed): *Mechanisms of Growth Control.* Springfield, Il, Charles C Thomas, 1981, pp 406–434.

59. Einhorn TA, Lane JM, Burstein AH, et al: The healing of segmental bone defects induced by demineralized bone matrix: A radiographic and biomechanical study. *J Bone Joint Surg* 1984;66A:274–279.

60. Katoh T, Sato K, Kawamura M, et al: Osteogenesis in sintered bone combined with bovine bone morphogenetic protein. *Clin Orthop* 1993;287:266–275.

61. Takaoka K, Koezuka H, Nakahara H: Telopeptide-depleted bovine skin collagen as a carrier for bone morphogenetic protein. *J Orthop Res* 1991;9:902–907.

62. Ripamonti U: Calvarial regeneration in primates with autolyzed antigen-extracted allogenic bone. *Clin Orthop* 1992;282:293–303.

63. Kawamura M, Iwata H, Sato K, et al: Chondroosteogenetic response to crude bone matrix proteins bound to hydroxyapatite. *Clin Orthop* 1987;218:281–292.

64. Jarcho M: Calcium phosphate ceramics as hard tissue prosthetics. *Clin Orthop* 1981;157:259–278.

65. Ono I, Ohura T, Murata M, et al: A study on bone induction in hydroxyapatite combined with bone morphogenetic protein. *Plast Reconstr Surg* 1992;90:870–879.

66. Urist MR, Nilsson O, Rasmussen J, et al: Bone regeneration under the influence of a bone morphogenetic protein (BMP) beta tricalcium phosphate (TCP) composite in skull trephine defects in dogs. *Clin Orthop* 1987;214:295–304.

67. Kawamura M, Urist MR: Human fibrin is a physiologic delivery system for bone morphogenetic protein. *Clin Orthop* 1988;235:302–310.
68. Johnson EE, Urist MR, Finerman GAM: Distal metaphyseal tibial nonunion: Deformity and bone loss treated by open reduction, internal fixation, and human bone morphogenetic protein (hBMP). *Clin Orthop* 1990;250:234–240.
69. Miyamoto S, Takaoka K, Okada T, et al: Evaluation of polylactic acid homopolymers as carriers for bone morphogenetic protein. *Clin Orthop* 1992;278:274–285.
70. Flanagan AM, Chambers TJ: Stimulation of bone nodule formation in vitro by prostaglandins E1 and E2. *Endocrinology* 1992;130:443–448.
71. Han CS, Wood MB, Bishop AT, et al: Vascularized bone transfer. *J Bone Joint Surg* 1992;74A:1441–1449.
72. Zaidemberg C, Siebert JW, Angrigriani C: A new vascularized bone graft for scaphoid nonunion. *J Hand Surg* 1991;16A:474–478.
73. Paterson D : The use of electricity in the treatment of nonunion, in Bassett FH III (ed): *Instructional Course Lectures XXXVII*. Park Ridge, IL, American Academy of Orthopaedic Surgeons, 1988, pp 155–156.
74. Clancey GJ, Winquist RA, Hansen ST Jr: Non-union of the tibia treated with Kuntscher intramedullary nailing. *Clin Orthop* 1982;167:191–196.
75. Gershuni DH, Aaron RK, Brighton CT, et al: Symposium: Recent advances in electrical stimulation. *Contemp Orthop* 1993;26:609–636.
76. Pienkowski D, Pollack SR, Brighton CT, et al: Comparision of asymmetrical and symmetrical pulse waveforms in electromagnetic stimulation. *J Orthop Res* 1992;10:247–255.
77. Brighton CT, Okereke E, Pollack SR, et al: In vitro bone-cell response to a capacitively coupled electrical field: The role of field strength, pulse pattern, and duty cycle. *Clin Orthop* 1992;285:255–262.
78. Gossling HR, Bernstein RA, Abbott J: Treatment of ununited tibial fractures: A comparison of surgery and pulsed electromagnetic fields. *Orthopedics* 1992;15:711–719.
79. Pilla AA, Khan S, Nasser P, et al: Low intensity pulsed ultrasound accelerates fracture repair in a rabbit model. *Trans Orthop Res Soc* 1989;14:591.
80. Lerner RK, Esterhai JL Jr, Polomano RC, et al: Quality of life assessment of patients with posttraumatic fracture nonunion, chronic refractory osteomyelitis, and lower-extremity amputation. *Clin Orthop* 1993;295:28–36.
81. Cheatle MD: The effect of chronic orthopaedic infection on quality of life. *Orthop Clin North Am* 1991;22:539–547.

Section 6
Future Research Directions

What is the definition of a fracture?

Fractures that do not involve displacement can be hard to define. Newer technology, including magnetic resonance imaging (MRI) and bone scanning, can be used to identify many nondisplaced fractures. However, spinal fractures are more controversial. The anterior end plate may have some inclination from development or disease and not represent a true fracture. A vertebral fracture has been classified as a 10% inclination, but densitometry studies have indicated that there is no correlation of bone mass with the presence of this minor change. Newer drug trials have used a 20% inclination, which does correlate with bone mass. Thus, there is a need for a clear definition of fracture.

A mechanical study and better densitometry correlations are needed to define fractures. Newer noninvasive methodology needs to be developed.

What are the noninvasive parameters that define bone strength?

Bone strength is currently inferred by radiology, quantitative computed tomography (CT) scan, and dual energy x-ray absorptiometry. These methods identify apparent bone density and do not fully correlate with bone strength. Some studies have suggested that the microstructure is a second important component for bone strength. Noninvasive and minimally invasive methods need to be established that can be used to recognize the relative contributions of density and structure and provide a better measurement of true bone strength.

Newer methodology has to be developed to characterize the micro architecture of bone. CT methods and acoustic methods offer possible avenues of advancement.

Does exercise affect bone strength?

Bone strength is reported to be affected by exercise. There is inadequate knowledge about the mechanism by which loads affect bone, the type of load, the rate and duration of load, and the signal mechanism. Individuals and bones that are immobilized have decreased bone mass and increased susceptibility for fracture. Women who overexercise not only can develop osteoporosis with concomitant amenorrhea but also can develop stress fractures. Both men and women who are marathon runners have less bone mass than their peers. The optimum exercise profile is not known.

Better epidemiologic studies are needed to evaluate the role of exercise in multiple populations. Appropriate animal studies may help define the relative role of type and forms of exercise in establishing the best bone mass and strength. The micromechanical, local, and systemic signals need investigation.

How does metabolic bone disease affect bone strength?

Two populations of postmenopausal women with osteoporosis have been defined. Type 1 was described as high turnover osteoporosis that occurred in recently menopausal women, whereas type 2, low turnover osteoporosis, occurred in older postmenopausal women. It has recently been demonstrated that one third of postmenopausal women at all ages have high turnover osteoporosis and one third have quiescent osteoporosis. There are no data as to which of the turnover groups has more fragile bone nor is there any means of identifying which of the two groups is at higher risk for fracture. The fact that metabolic bone disease fractures do not correlate totally with bone mass implies that there are different types of metabolic bone disease fractures.

Better noninvasive biochemical indices are needed to identify the state of turnover. The degradative products of collagen currently offer the best potential to recognize high turnover states.

Does treatment of osteoporosis prevent fractures?

Estrogen and recently calcitonin, calcium, and etidronate have been shown to diminish spinal fractures. Although sodium fluoride has increased bone mass, there is no diminution of spinal fractures and there is an increase in hip fractures. No agent has markedly decreased hip fractures although calcium, estrogen, and thiazide in the elderly have minimally decreased the rate. What are the opportunities for therapeutic intervention, and is there a subset of osteoporosis patients who would respond to drug intervention?

Clarification of osteoporosis type might lead to selective drug trials in terms of fracture prevention. High turnover osteoporosis patients might be targeted for antiresorptive therapy trials.

Can nonradiographic methods be developed to assess the progression of fracture repair in clinical practice?

Fracture healing is difficult to define and establish. Radiographic analysis of fracture repair fails to give an exact determination of when a healing injury has developed adequate mechanical properties to allow increased function. There are few studies correlating biomechanical strength and radiographic state. Orthopaedic intervention with instrumentation further obscures recognition of healing. To avoid the risks of refracture associated with a premature return to function, orthopaedists take a conservative approach in evaluating fracture repair and in returning patients to full activity or to work. This may result in overtreatment, increased medical costs, and lost wages. In addition, frequent radiographic evaluation of fractures during healing may be associated with a small increase in the risk of cancer and other complications. There is a need for establishing a true mechanical definition of healing. A nonradiographic assessment of fracture repair that was highly correlated with the return of mechanical properties in the fracture would be more accurate and provide a more rational basis for treatment.

Studies should establish a clear definition of healing through mechanical testing and correlation with minimally invasive methodology. Gait parameters and patient feedback should be correlated. Develop methodology to define the progress of fracture repair for both animal models and human fractures.

What are the morbidity, mortality, and nonunion rates associated with fracture repair in elderly and young patient populations? What change in patient function, ability to conduct activities of daily living, and health care costs are associated with fractures?

Newer methods of fracture treatment and changes in the patient population at risk may impact on morbidity, mortality, and nonunion rates seen after fracture. Studies from other countries suggest that fracture-related mortality may be seen in the hospital and in the postinjury period after the patient has left the hospital. Newer developments in devices used for fracture treatment may significantly decrease the rate of nonunion, although an older population may have an increased rate of nonunion. These factors should be assessed to determine the efficacy of treatment and the total costs associated with these injuries.

Current epidemiologic techniques should be applied to this problem.

What are the mechanisms by which infection alters bone fracture repair?

Acute and chronic osteomyelitis, whether hematogenous, associated with an open fracture, or related to the open reduction and internal fixation of a closed fracture has a profound adverse effect on patient outcome. Although prevention remains the primary goal, not all acute infections will be eliminated in the near future.

In vivo and in vitro studies are needed to define the specific actions by which infection perturbs fracture healing. Molecular biologic and biochemical methods are needed to elucidate the underlying mechanisms. It remains to be seen whether the primary problem is one of infection per se or simply the inflammation that accompanies infection. These studies would include the effects of infection and inflammation on cell proliferation, synthesis of matrix, and ossification.

Is there an optimal rate at which physiologic loading can be resumed during the healing of a fracture? Is any form of loading beneficial to the healing of an upper extremity fracture?

Orthopaedists agree that one of the goals of fracture management is the early resumption of weightbearing ambulation for fractures involving the tibia and femur. However, if that loading is started prematurely, the patient is placed at risk of refracture, hardware failure, and increased rate of nonunion.

Develop an in vivo model to define optimal time of initiation, character, and rate of loading of the fractured extremity.

Is there an optimal time for physician intervention in fracture healing to provide stimulation of bone formation?

In the recent past, the orthopaedic community has waited for 6 months or more before intervening with bone graft, modification of open reduction and internal fixation, or electrical stimulation of osteogenesis. More recent trauma center studies have suggested the advantages of bone grafting severely damaged limbs as soon as the soft tissue envelope has stabilized.

Develop an adequate patient data base to allow for randomized patient trials in which the time of intervention is varied, time to healing is measured, acute and long term complications are tracked, and adequacy of return to function is determined.

Can we identify the major epidemiologic and environmental factors that lead to fractures across the age spectrum? How can we work to prevent them?

The cost of health care in the United States continues to rise. A large proportion of the expenditure in orthopaedics is devoted to trauma care. Each physician who cares for patients realizes that violence in our society and physical risk-taking contribute significantly. Fractures are anecdotally associated with multiple factors that either alone or in combination cause falls or injury. These factors include, but are not limited to, alcohol abuse, motor vehicle accidents, blindness, and the consequences of patient frailty, including impaired balance, neural control, or motor function. The specific contribution of these factors to the incidence of fractures is not known. If we could define the percentage of orthopaedic care costs that could be attributed to one or a combination of adverse choices (alcohol or drug consumption, high-speed driving, inner-city personal violence), health-care cost managers would have the powerful information they need to more aggressively develop health care and social welfare policy.

This represents an epidemiologic study requiring collaboration between inner city, suburban, and rural hospitals within a health-care system tracking ICD 9 and CPT 4 codes; costs of prehospital, hospital, and posthospital care; and loss of work time.

What is the role of nerve supply in fracture healing?

There is renewed interest in neurotransmitter peptides as the controlling agents for maintaining bone mass and as particpants in the repair process. Preliminary work with bone morphogenic protein (BMP) probes has documented high concentrations of BMP on nerve fibers. Are the factors present in nerve tissue significant for fracture healing?

Investigations should identify the neuropeptides and other transmitters that are present in the osseous environment. Current immunohistology methods need to be supplemented by methods to quantitate the presence of these agents and to determine their biologic role.

Can we identify mechanical and metabolic risk factors that contribute to delayed union and nonunion? What are the specific risk factors?

Controversy continues as to those factors that complicate fracture healing in patients. Initial injury to the soft-tissue envelope, energy absorbed by the limb at the time of the fracture, adequacy of reduction, motion permitted at the fracture site, local host phenomena, and systemic factors have yet to be defined. These factors mainly are related to the mechanical and physiologic fracture configuration.

Develop in vivo and in vitro models to determine the local effect on the osteocyte at the time of fracture. Just as with normal bone formation, protocols are needed that allow meticulous analysis of the histologic and biochemical response to carefully applied variables.

The study of clinical animal cases may also be helpful. These evaluations should include study of the relationship between fracture configuration and methods of fixation.

Index

Page numbers in italics refer to figures or figure legends.